Biotechnology to Combat COVID-19

Edited by Megha Agrawal and Shyamasri Biswas

Published in London, United Kingdom

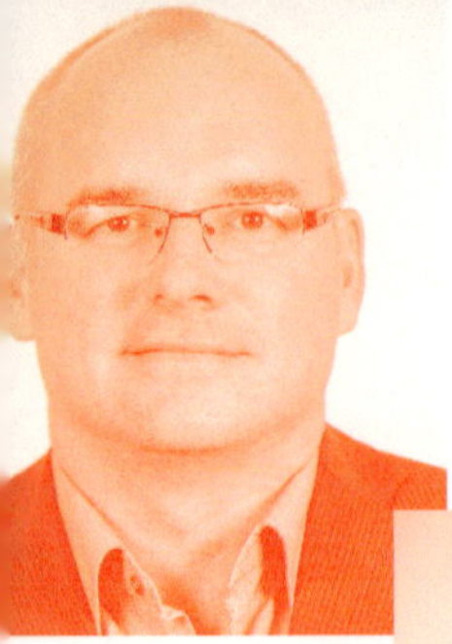
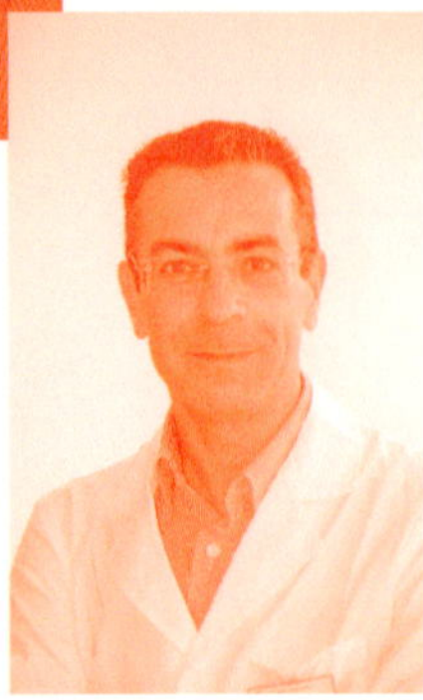
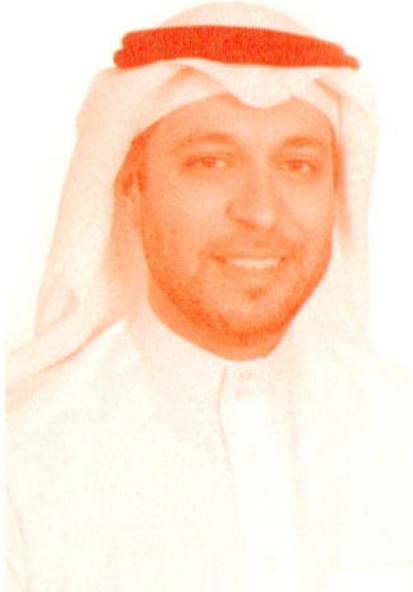
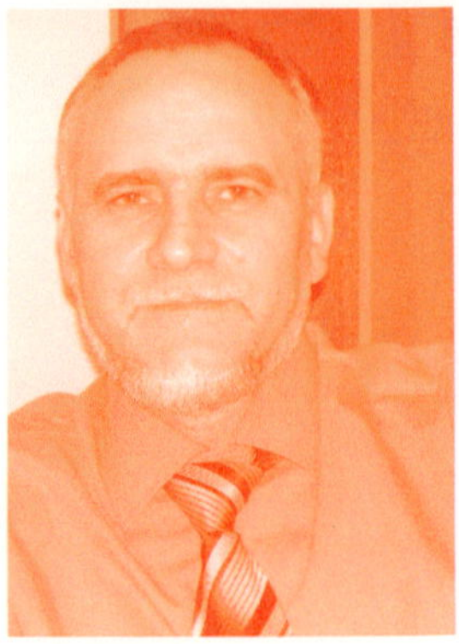
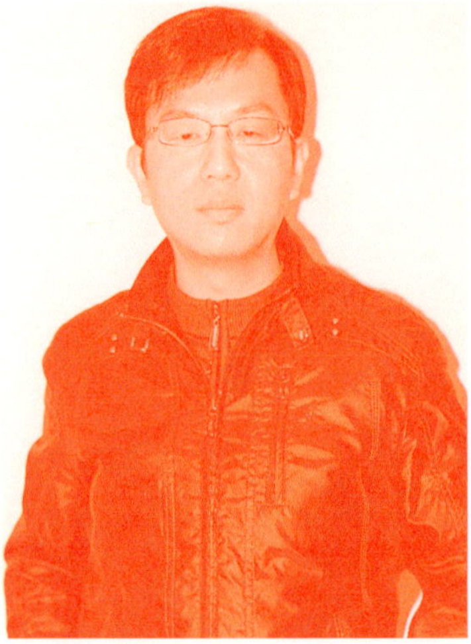
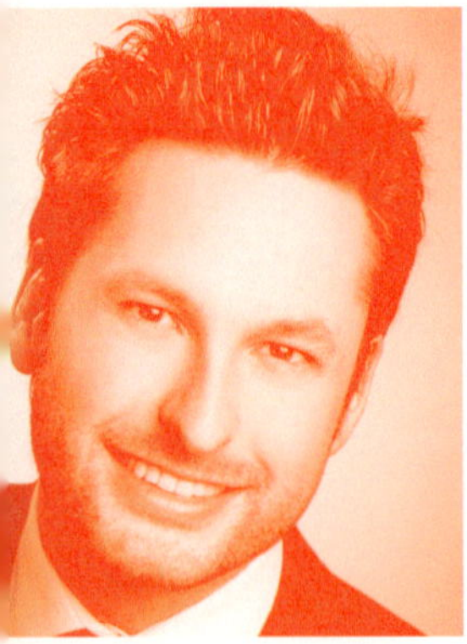
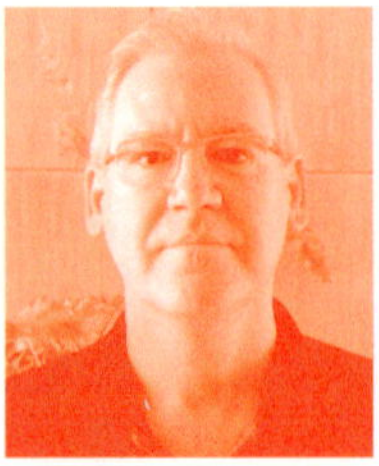

IntechOpen

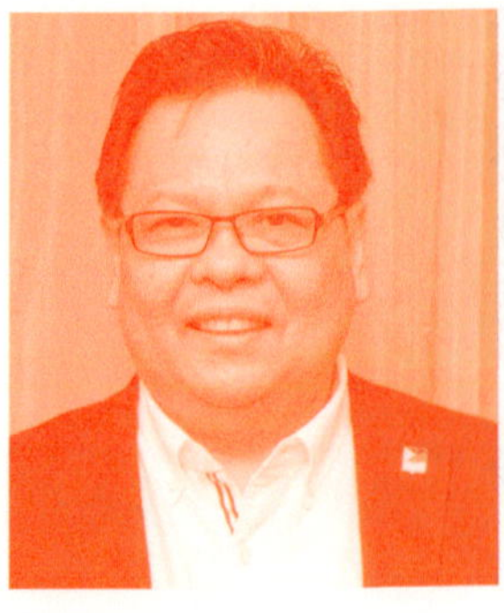
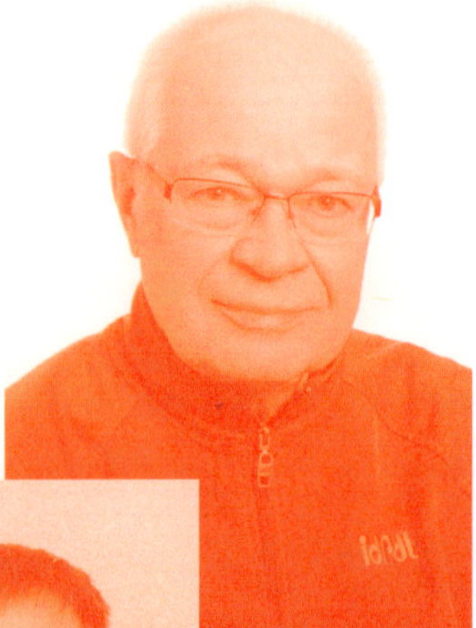
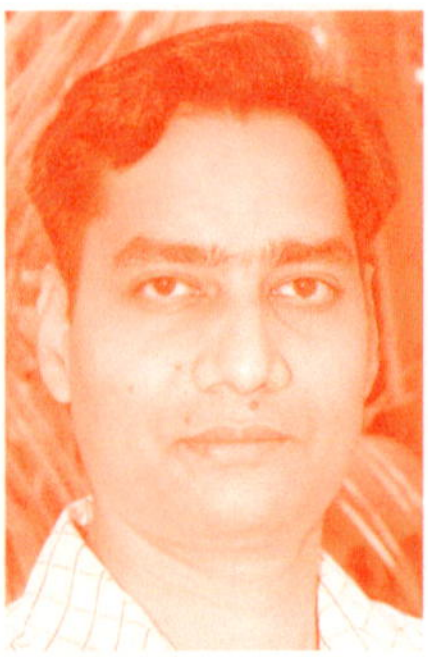
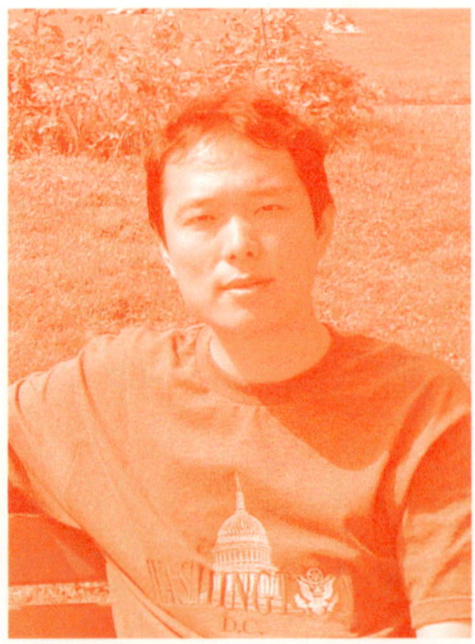
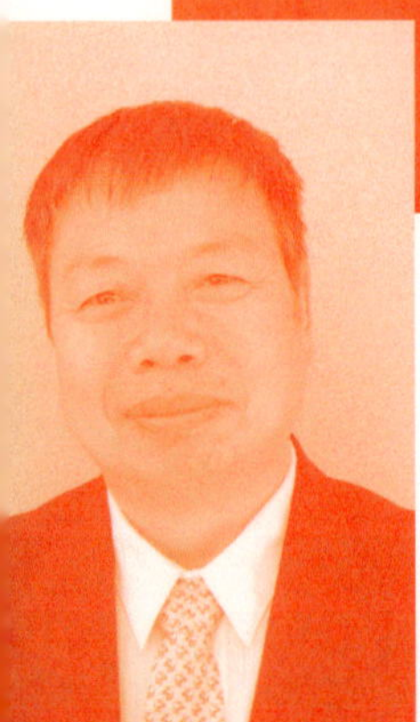
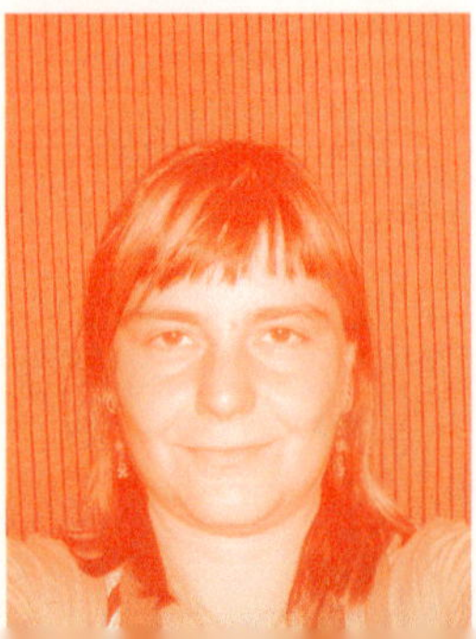

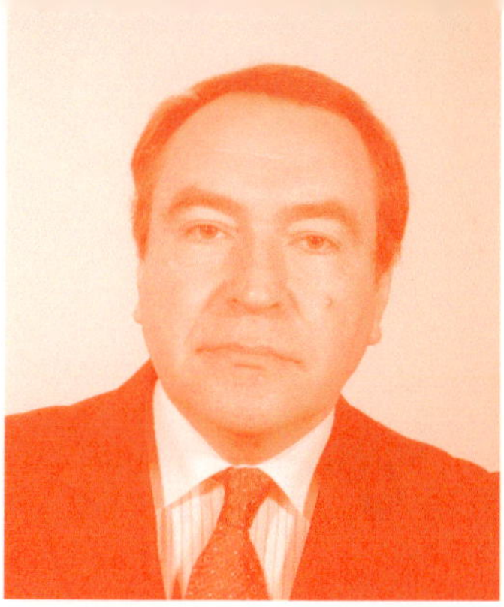
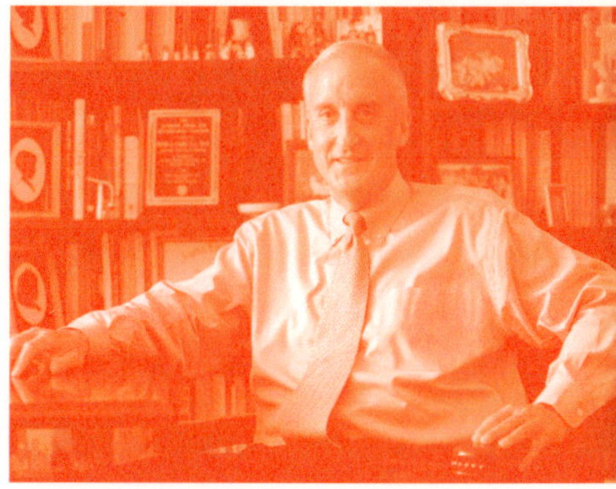
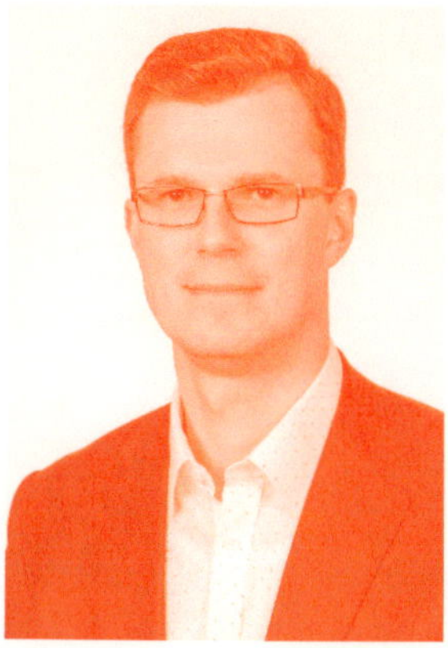
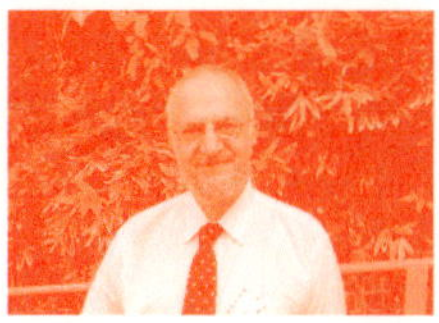
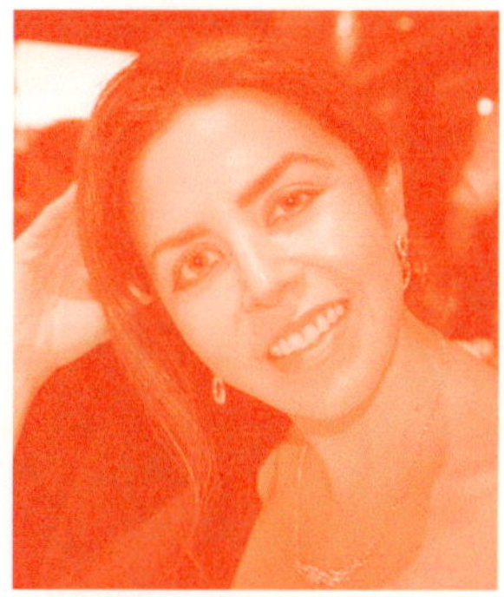

Supporting open minds since 2005

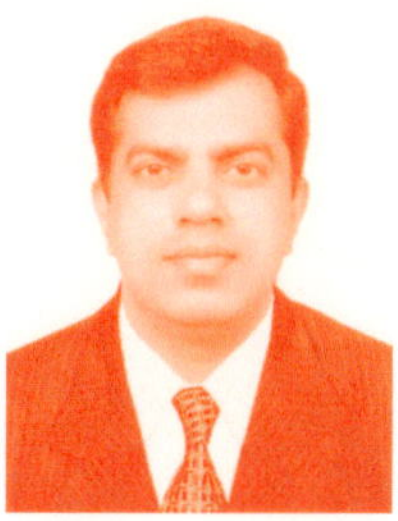
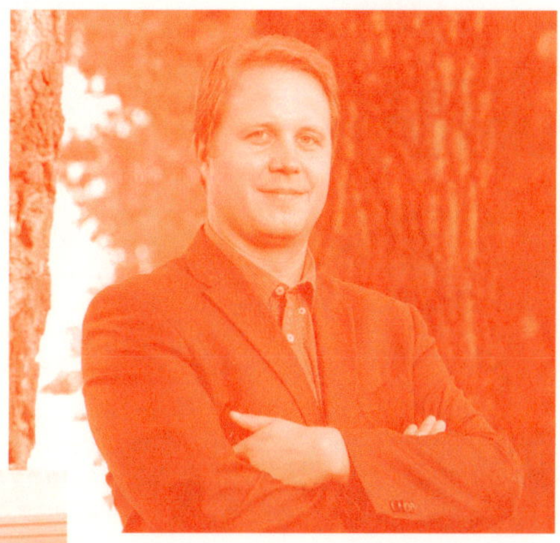
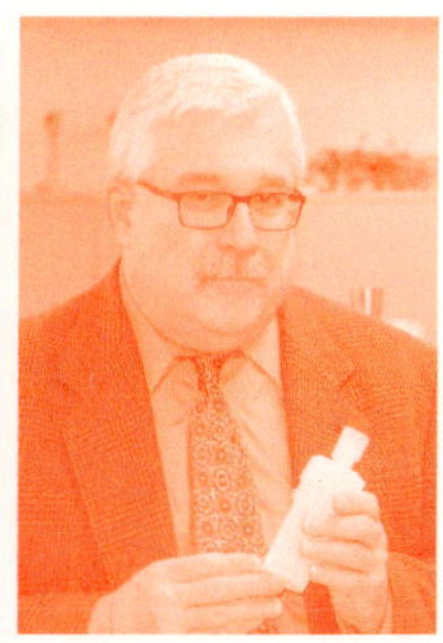
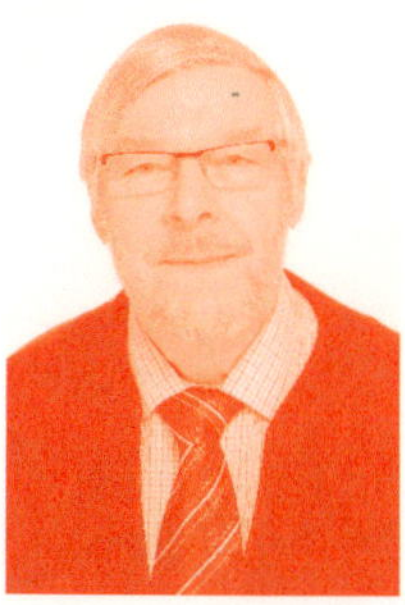
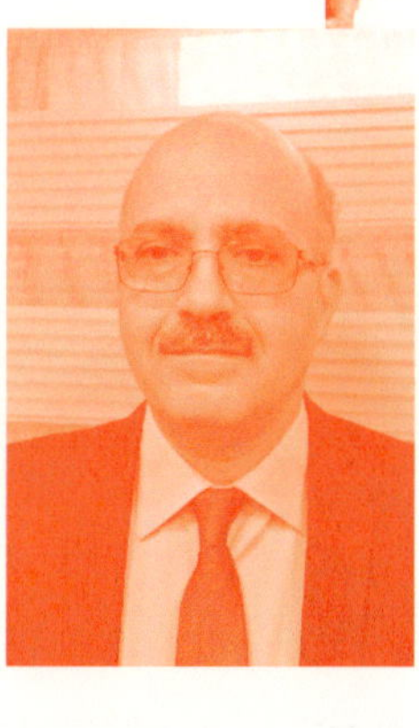
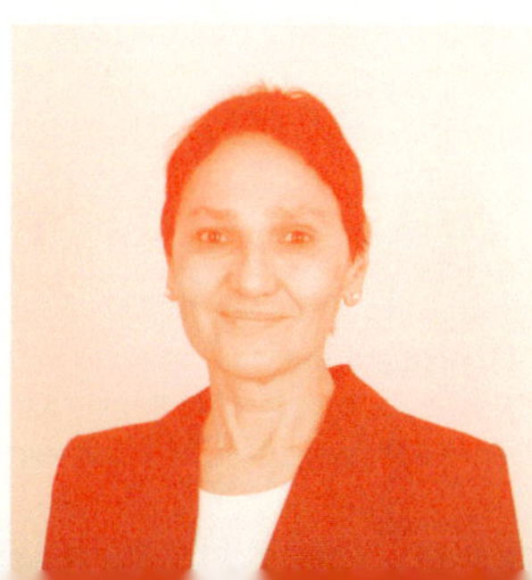
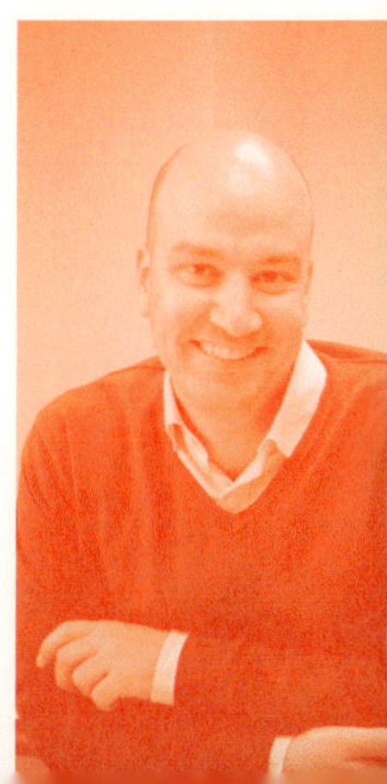

Biotechnology to Combat COVID-19
http://dx.doi.org/10.5772/intechopen.93713
Edited by Megha Agrawal and Shyamasri Biswas

Contributors
Rajeev Gupta, Vamsi Krishna Kudapa, Ajay Mittal, Tejendra Kumar Gupta, Ishita Agrawal, Humphrey Simukoko, Adonis Sfera, Carolina Osorio, Jose E. Campo Maldonado, Afzaal Jafri, Aaron D Chokka, Carlos Manuel Zapata Martín Del Campo, Zisis Kozlakidis, Allen Thayakumar Basanthakumar, Vinita Chittoor, Surabhi Dixit, Monal Sharma, Basanta Bhowmik, Duygu Koyuncu Irmak, Erdal Karaoz, Awaad Kadhim Al Sarkhi, Vasudeo Pandharinath Zambare, Rutuja Sunil Patankar, Tafirenyika Mafugu, Swapan Chatterjee, Gyaneshwer Chaubey Chaubey, Nikhil Srivastava, Kamalesh Sarkar, Bidisa Sarkar, Vugar Mammadov, Lala Jafarova, Ashok K Singh, Aakansha Singh, Ankit Kumar Dubey, Jean Pierre Doussoulin, Benoît Mougenot, Rayan Ahmed, Thakur Uttam Singh, Madhu Lingaraju, Subhashree Parida, Meemansha Sharma, Sweta Kamboj, Rohit Kamboj, Shikha Kamboj, Rohit Dutt, Reeva Chabbra, Priyanka Kriplani, Ashim Gupta, Hugo C. Rodriguez, Manu Gupta, Emilio Cavazos-Escobar, Enrique Montalvo, Saadiq El-Amin Iii, Zachary P Morehouse, Rodney Nash, Caleb Proctor, Gabriella Ryan, Saurabh Kumar, Chandra Devi, Subhabrata Sarkar, Vivek Kumar Garg, Priyanka Choudhary, Madhu Chopra, Vinit Sharma, Ravi Prakash, Nidhi Jyotsana, Evgeny Evsikov, Anielle C.A. Almeida Silva, Eliete A. Alvin, Anna Victória Bernardes E Borges, Rafaela M. Barbosa, Marcela Lemes, Rhéltheer De P. Martins, Carlo Oliveira, Diógenes Meneses, Bruno G. Lucca, Virmondes Rodrigues, Renata Balvedi, Fabiane Abreu, Marcos Silva, Noelio Oliveira Dantas, Moez Guettari, Ahmed El Aferni, Sandeep Kumar Vashist, Subramanian Murugan, Guiffo Djoko, Brandt Pence, Theodore Cory, Manish Sharma, Pargin Bangotra, Alok Sagar Gautam, Burcu Biterge Süt, Boopathy Ramasamy, Subhasmita Panda, Priyadatta Satpathy, Trupti Das, Ahmed R.G., Valeriy Ivanovich Vechorko, Oksana Alekseevna Baykova, Natalya Vadimovna Teplova, Dmitriy Aleksandrovich Doroshenko

First published in London, United Kingdom, 2022 by IntechOpen
IntechOpen is the global imprint of INTECHOPEN LIMITED, registered in England and Wales, registration number: 11086078, 5 Princes Gate Court, London, SW7 2QJ, United Kingdom
Printed in Croatia

British Library Cataloguing-in-Publication Data
A catalogue record for this book is available from the British Library

Additional hard and PDF copies can be obtained from orders@intechopen.com

Biotechnology to Combat COVID-19
Edited by Megha Agrawal and Shyamasri Biswas
p. cm.
Print ISBN 978-1-83968-626-9
Online ISBN 978-1-83968-627-6
eBook (PDF) ISBN 978-1-83968-628-3

For EU product safety concerns:
IN TECH d.o.o. Prolaz Marije Krucifikse Kozulić 3, 51000 Rijeka, Croatia, info@intechopen.com or visit our website at intechopen.com.

A collaborative project with Biotechnology Kiosk

Meet the editors

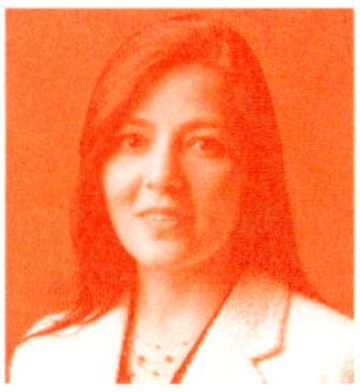

Dr. Megha Agrawal is a co-founder, executive publisher, and chief editor of *Biotechnology Kiosk*, an international journal in biotechnology. She is recognized as one of the world's leading neuroscientists and biotechnologists. Dr. Agrawal's research has been well cited. She has published more than 100 articles and edited several books in prestigious scientific journals in the field of biotechnology, neuroscience, molecular biology, and biochemistry. She was a faculty member and principal investigator at the University of Illinois Chicago and an associate editor for *Frontiers in Molecular Diagnostics and Therapeutics*. Dr. Agrawal is an invited columnist and contributing editor in biotechnology for a leading high-tech trade journal, *Vacuum Technology & Coating Magazine*, for which she writes a monthly column on vacuum advances in biotechnology.

Megha Agrawal
Biotechnology Kiosk, Gainesville, Florida
United States of America

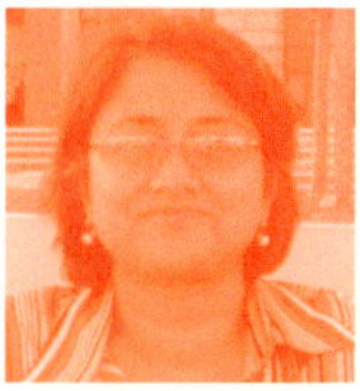

Dr. Shyamasri Biswas is a co-founder, executive publisher, and chief editor of *Biotechnology Kiosk*, an international journal in biotechnology. She is an internationally recognized structural and molecular biologist, protein chemist, and biotechnologist and is well known worldwide for her works in solving challenging protein crystal structures of therapeutic relevance. She has published more than 100 articles in reputed journals. She received her Ph.D. in Biotechnology under the prestigious DAAD sandwich fellowship program jointly from the University of Potsdam, Germany and Banaras Hindu University, India. She was a senior scientist at UMass Worcester, North Carolina State University, and University of Florida Gainesville. She is a senior editorial board member of *Proteins and Peptide Letters* and a contributing editor for *Vacuum Technology & Coating Magazine*.

Shyamasri Biswas
Biotechnology Kiosk, Gainesville, Florida
United States of America

Contents

Preface

This milestone book, *Biotechnology to Combat COVID-19*, includes contributions by authors from the United States, India, France, Azerbaijan, Russia, Chile, Peru, Turkey, Saudi Arabia, Egypt, Brazil, South Africa, Zambia, New Zealand, Tunisia and Mexico. We thank all contributors for making this book a comprehensive and inclusive platform on COVID-19 that covers almost all topics related to the pandemic and mitigation strategies to combat the disease.

With respect to discussions on the biology and science of SARS-CoV-2, this book has plenty to offer. For example, it includes topics ranging from transmission, epidemiology, genomic structures, and sequencing of the virus to diagnostics, antiviral drugs, repurposing of drugs, vaccines, and co-morbidity, just to name a few. This book also presents authoritative descriptions of the effects of COVID-induced lockdowns and public health measures on the meteorological and climatic aspects in big, industrialized cities in countries with high population density, such as India. It also discusses the societal impact of COVID-related government and public health measures. In addition, the book assesses the roles of media and governments in handling the pandemic.

This book is for a diverse and wide audience, including virologists, epidemiologists, biologists, pharmacists, biomaterial scientists and engineers, medical professionals, clinicians, therapists, public health and government professionals, and all global citizens who have endured and battled against the pandemic.

Dr. Megha Agrawal, PhD and Dr. Shyamasri Biswas, PhD
Biotechnology Kiosk,
Gainesville, Florida, USA

Section 1

Transmission Epidemiology Pathogenesis and Genome Sequencing

Chapter 1

Epidemiology, Pathogenesis, and Healing Strategies of COVID-19

Basanta Bhowmik

Abstract

In the present chapter, some notable features (epidemiology, pathogenesis, and clinical characteristics) regarding recent outbreak COVID-19 have been reviewed. Most significant features related to COVID-19 such as (i) roots of infection and disease manifestation, (ii) shape and structure of viral S-protein, (iii) genome sequence study and replication in host cell, (iv) role of environmental factors, (v) diagnosis tools and (vi) role of biosensor have been critically investigated. The biological and behavioral risk factors for pregnant women before and after child birth have been dictated clearly. Pulmonary abnormalities due to COVID-19 of the patient having diabetes, cancer etc. history have been clarified with help of CT imaging. Finally, prevention and cure strategies adopted by many health professionals based on the existing drugs are mentioned with their side effects.

Keywords: COVID-19, transmission, genome, prevention, cure strategies

1. Introduction

Emergence of COVID-19 threatens human health and economy around the globe. Possibly, world populations have ever faces such crisis and will remain the witness of such incident. Each new day experiences number of new cases with increasing death toll since its first identification. However, suggested name of corona virus comes from Latin word corona, signifies crown or halo. Electron microscopy of corona virus reveals encapsulation of crown like fringe at outer surface [1]. Novel Corona virus known as different name such as COVID-19, HCoV-19 was outbreak in Wuhan, Capital of Hubei province, China in month of December-2019 and later become pandemic by quick spreading into the major countries in the globe [2, 3]. Outbreak has very high risk with potentiality of human to human transmission. Experts around the globe suggest that, the average incubation period of COVID-19 is ~5 days with a range of 2–14 days [2]. Symptom includes high fever, dry cough to severe respiratory acute disease and death (in some cases) [2]. Average fatality rate reported to be ~1–2% [1, 2]. Scientific community and researchers are at the midst of COVID-19 pandemic and have struggling to find out how much similarity with SARS-CoV. The study reveals that, COVID-19 is similar like SARS corona virus which is believed to be originated from either bats or civet cats or raccoon dogs [2, 3]. However, due to lack of evidence many scientific communities ruled out such report. As per WHO officials, COVID-19 is ten times more infectious than the 2009 pandemic H1N1 influenza virus. There is no effective drug or vaccine against the corona virus or similar infectious agents so far and it is still unknown how many more month require to develop. However, one needs to understand the priority and treatment protocol based on the severity of the disease.

2. Transmission and cellular mechanism of COVID-19

COVID-19 is the seventh coronavirus which infect humans like earlier reported coronavirus SARS-CoV, MERSCoV, HKU1, NL63, OC43 and 229E. [4]. For an enveloped virus, primary mode of transmission is close contact with the infected individual. Transmission is appeared to be silently enter into the host body and no immediate onset symptoms have been evident. Therefore, before infected host tested positive, he/she already transmitted virus to many others (provided infected person does not maintaining isolation/social distancing). In most cases, human to human transmission occurs, though human to human transmission has been ruled out at the very early stage of the outbreak. However, probability of getting infectious becomes higher when an infected person or person in incubation stage comes closer to the healthy person. Alternative transmission medium might be via contact surfaces i.e. skin to skin touching or touching objects having COVID-19 particles. Then direct or indirect entrance of that surface particles into one's body through mouth, nose, or eyes. The other forms of transmission possibly through inhalation of particle aerosols emanated from exhaled breathe of infected person or via droplet due to cough/sneezes [4]. A recent study reveals that, COVID-19 may survive in aerosols (size <5 μm) for at least three long hour in an open air ambient [1, 2]. Relative humidity, fomite material, and air temperature possibly are the factors for prolonging virus life. Long time survival at the outside of its host organism (surfaces such as aluminum, sterile sponges, or latex surgical gloves) will increase the opportunity to produce new host via touching or breathing [2, 4]. Facal transmission is another transmission path where COVID-19 has been found in stool specimen like aluminum, sterile sponges, or latex surgical gloves etc. [2]. The surface stability of S-protein of COVID-19 found to be more on plastic, stainless steel than the copper and card board [2]. It is worth mentioning that, some positive COVID-19 cases were also reported due to the nosocomial transmission. Recent study of Wang et al. reflects 29% health professionals and 12% hospitalized patient (associated with other disease history) becomes infectious due to nosocomial transmission [5]. It is worth to mention that, urine of infected one does not contain any COVID-19 particles and therefore does not have any role for transmission [6]. Study of Casanova et al. suggest that, corona virus may remain active even in pure water and pasteurized settled sewage for few days to one week [7]. Airborne dust particles or microorganisms or particulate matter (PM) are the potential transmitter [6]. Some study finds the virus can transmit through air up to 1 m whereas another recent study find virus particles can transmit up to 13 ft. [6]. However, COVID-19 particles combined with airborne dust particles or microorganisms or particulate matter (PM) enters into the deeper alveolar and tracheobronchial regions of the host.

3. Role of environmental factors

The transmission, survival and characteristics of COVID-19 directly influenced by environment factors like temperature, pressure, pollution level [8]. In addition, outbreak further involved with the reproduction number (R0). The reproduction number (R_0) defined as the number of healthy people getting infected from a single infectious living in a susceptible populated environment. Reproduction no (R_0)

mainly governed by the factors like (i) stage of infection, (ii) transmissible strength of the pathogen, and (ii) the number of susceptible contacts. It is meaningless to set the exact value of R_0 until otherwise the surrounding environment clearly specified. For example, Li et al. reported R_0 value for COVID-19 as 2.2 (95% confidence interval, 1.4–3.9) [9]. However, in reality R_0 for COVID-19 might be very higher than expected if one does not obey the rule of social distancing or home quarantine. Few governing factor are crucial for reproduction rate or newly infected cases in a particular area viz.; (i) isolation of infected person from the day of infection, (ii) availability of general needs for ones to remain in isolation like food and other necessities and (iii) availability of sufficient diagnosis tools in the area. Based on the above facts, a mathematical model proposed by Tang et al. [10] determines the reproduction rate or spreading rate by individual infected host per day. If the above factors favor in a particular region, then contact rate $C(t)$ (assuming reproduction rate proportional to the number of new contact) in a certain period of time follows Eq. (1) leading to decreasing reproduction rate [10].

$$C(t)=(C_0-C_b)e^{-r_1 t}+C_b \tag{1}$$

Where C_0 initial contact rate, C_b is minimum contact rate under current control strategies, r_1 is coefficient of contact factor, t is investigated time period. However, reproduction rate further depends on the diagnosis rate as shown in Eq. (2) [10].

$$\frac{1}{\delta_I(t)}=\left(\frac{1}{\delta_{I0}}-\frac{1}{\delta_{If}}\right)e^{r_2 t}+\frac{1}{\delta_{If}} \tag{2}$$

Where $\delta_I(t)$ diagnosis rate and, δ_{I0} is initial diagnosis rate with $\delta_I(0)=\delta_{I0}$, δ_{If} is fastest diagnosis rate with $\lim_{t\to\infty}\delta_I(0)=\delta_{I0}$, and r_2 is exponential decreasing contact rate factor and the value depends the recourses available in the infected region. However, if the aforementioned factors are not favorable in the investigated region, then it is expected that, the new infected cases (induced by individual infected host) will begin to rise. A time dependent (30 days lockdown period) contact rate $C(t)$ and diagnosis rate $\delta_I(t)$ simulation study (from somewhere in Wuhan) have been reported based on adaptive Metropolis-Hastings (M-H) algorithm and Markov Chain Monte Carlo (MCMC) procedure and the result is shown

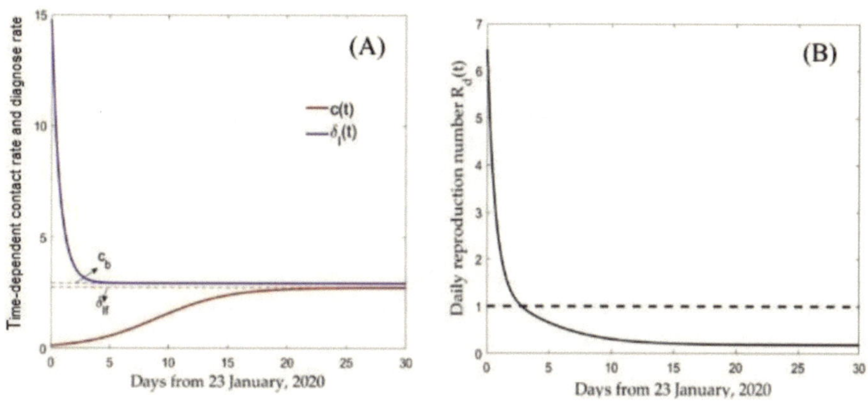

Figure 1.
Showing simulation data of (A) contact rate C (t) and diagnosis rate (B) effective daily reproduction ratio for the period of 30 days somewhere in Wuhan [10].

in **Figure 1** [10]. The model shows how self isolation (decrease in contact rate) and increase in diagnosis rate in a region can stop community spreading significantly.

4. Symptoms

Many infectious remains asymptomatic and silently affected so many. Most of the mild cases symptoms such as, fever (83–100%), myalgia (11–35%), diarrhea (2–10%), fatigue, headache (7–8%) and cough (59–82%), and dyspnoea have been found predominantly [11]. However, severe infection outcome includes drastic reduction in average circulating lymphocyte and platelet counts etc. Other abnormalities are on chest radiographic imaging, lymphopenia, leukopenia, and thrombocytopenia [2]. Respiratory system is highly affected. Though age is still not be a proven critical risk factor for COVID-19 infection, but it was observed that, mortality rate were prominent for elderly having some previous disorder like hypertension, chronic obstructive pulmonary disease, diabetes, cardiovascular disease. Such prior disorder with COVID-19 particles in body quickly developed some dangerous malfunction like coagulation dysfunction, septic shock, metabolic acidosis and acute respiratory distress syndrome which are hard to correct eventually leading to the death. Further, few other malfunction like decrease in neutrophil count, D-dimer, blood urea, and creatinine levels etc. were prominent in severe infected patient [2]. However, all effects (including inhaled particulate matter combined with an immune response or cytokine storm induced by COVID-19 infection) together exacerbate severe ill effect on respiratory system and increase the risk of patient life. In order to investigate the different organ disorder due to COVID-19, human protein database and distribution of antigiotensin converting enzyme 2 (ACE2) has been correlated. It would be appropriate to mention that, an ACE2 is a transmembrane enzyme, act as a receptor function in host body and help to enter COVID-19 in host cell [8–11]. **Figure 2(b)** and **(c)** shows the detection of ACE2 receptors over neurons and glial cells, further, how COVID-19 binds to ACE2 receptor in brain cell. **Figure 2(a)** and **(e)**, ensure presence of COVID-19 in general blood circulation with abundant number of virus in cerebral circulation. The presence of such virus possibly is the reason of slowing the blood circulation mechanism in capillary endothelium which results in higher interaction probability of COVID-19 spike protein with the ACE2 [3]. Hence, there is a possibility of neuronal damage or endothelial rupture of cerebral capillaries in association with bleeding in cerebral tissue which increases the life risk of patient infected with COVID-19. Few evidence of neurotropic mortality caused by COVID-19 has been reported but proper explanation is yet to be established [12]. A study of 218 patients from recent outbreak reveals 78 patient (36.4%) having neurological malfunctions due to the COVID-19. Rest of the patients is either losing control over breathing or suffering from acute respiratory failure [3, 12]. However, evidence of virus in cerebrospinal fluid is still under debate. Apart from blood circulation, entry of COVID-19 through cribriform plate close to the olfactory bulb can be an alternative pathway to the brain. Further, indirect consequences of multi organ failure (pulmonary, renal, cardiac, and circulatory damage) caused in patient having COVID-19 appears to be more dangerous than expected. The study reveals that COVID-19 severely damages leucocytes which possibly are the reason of multi organ failure [13]. Older infected people having diabetes mellitus-2 are at more risk to mortality due to the uncontrolled glycaemia [14]. COVID-19 infection in diabetes patient raises the stress level and hence blood glucose levels and abnormal glucose variability. Increase in blood glucose possibly due to the release of hyperglycemic hormones (glucocorticoids and catecholamines) [14].

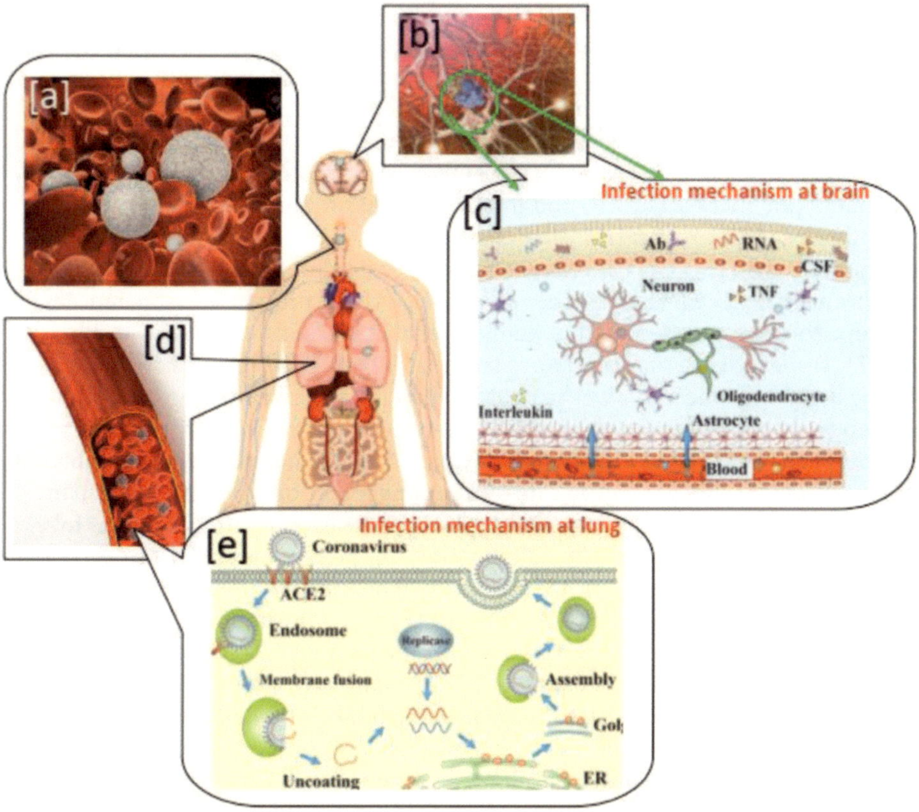

Figure 2.
Showing possible targets of COVID-19 (lungs, heart, kidneys, intestines, brain, and testicles); (a) COVID-19 distribution and ACE2 receptor in human, (b) COVID-19 transmission to brain through upper nasal trancribrial path (c) inset image shows binding mechanism of spike protein at the site of neuron (d) showing COVID-19 distribution through blood circulation at lungs and (e) inset image showing bind of COVID-19 with ACE2 receptor at lungs cell (reproduced with permission ref. [3, 12]).

5. Protein structure of COVID 19

The COVID-19 in the infected human body consists of critical virion which is a spike type glycoprotein known as S-protein [15]. The characteristics of spike protein or S-protein solely determine whether host cell is infected by corona virus or not. The spike protein has two subunit referred as S1 and S2 respectively. S1 is responsible for virus-host range and cellular tropism with the help of receptor binding domain (RBD) whereas S2 expedite the virus-cell membrane fusion with help of heptad repeats 1 (HR1) and heptad repeats 2 HR2 [16]. However, a polybasic cleavage site (RRAR) in between S1 and S2 influence the viral infectivity and host range with the effect of furin and other proteases [4]. O-linked glycans created by the proline, which possibly flank the cleavage site and shields epitopes or key residues on the SARS-CoV-2 spike protein [4]. However, the outermost part of critical virion cell is full of spike protein which helps to binding and subsequent fusion of antigiotensin converting enzyme 2 (ACE2) membranes in host cell. ACE2 is a transmembrane enzyme, act as a receptor function in human body and help to enter COVID-19 in host cell [1–9]. ACE2 exist at almost each organ of the body including arterial smooth muscle cells in the lungs, lymph nodes, stomach, colon, skin, liver bile ducts small intestine, kidney parietal epithelial cells, and the brain [14, 15].

The genome sequence of COVID-19 contains ~ 27 no of protein and almost ~30000 nucleotides in length as shown in **Figure 3(a)** [17]. Open reading frames (ORFs) are found to be variable in COVID-19 gene. In first ORFs (ORF1a/b), almost 2/3 viral RNA have been found which encodes 16 non-structural protein (NPS) and translates two polyproteins (pp1a and pp1ab). Accessory and structural proteins encoded by remaining 1/3 ORFs. Most essential proteins are RNA dependent polymerase (RdRP) and four structural proteins viz.; matrix protein (M), nucleocapsid protein (N), small envelope protein (E) and spike surface glycoprotein (S) [17]. The function of S protein is to binding and fusion of ACE2 membrane in host cell. On the other hand, M, N and E protein helps to budding, envelope formation, assembled, pathogenesis and RNA encasing in host cell [15–17]. Upper part of the respiratory tract has lower ACE2 results in less infection by S-protein whereas lower parts of the lungs have more amount of ACE2 consequently higher tendency of getting infected by S-protein as confirmed by higher opacity in CT image as shown in **Figure 4**. ACE2 has high binding capability with COVID-19 spike protein and its initiates the infection process as shown in **Figure 3(b)** [5]. The interaction of S-protein and ACE2 in the host cell is as follows; COVID-19 genome encodes many structural protein (glycosylated spike (S) protein) and non-structural protein (RNA-dependent RNA polymerase (RdRp), protease (3CLpro), and papain-like protease (PLpro)) for inducing host immune response [19]. 3CLpro and PLpro are responsible for COVID-19 genome replication in host cell by proteolytic processing of non-structural proteins. As per National Center for Biotechnology1 (NCBI) database, with ID NC_045512, the COVID-19 genome structure is 29,903 bp single-stranded RNA (+ss-RNA) coronavirus [3]. COVID-19 genome at the host cell releases it outer encapsulation and remain as single-stranded positive RNA (having 5′-cap structure and 3′-poly-A tail). RNA translated into viral polyproteins with help of host antigiotensin converting enzyme 2 (ACE2). Cleaving of polyproteins turns it to an effector protein by viral proteinases 3CLpro and PLpro [19]. Such mechanism reduces the host immune response drastically. Monte Carlo simulations by convolution contact maps suggest, receptor binding domain (RBD) area of spike protein shows various conformations with respect to the remaining portion of the protein structure [20]. The identified RBD area were then reassembled using pipeline method which produces a complex structure of spike trimer and the extracellular domain of human ACE2. Cryo-EM

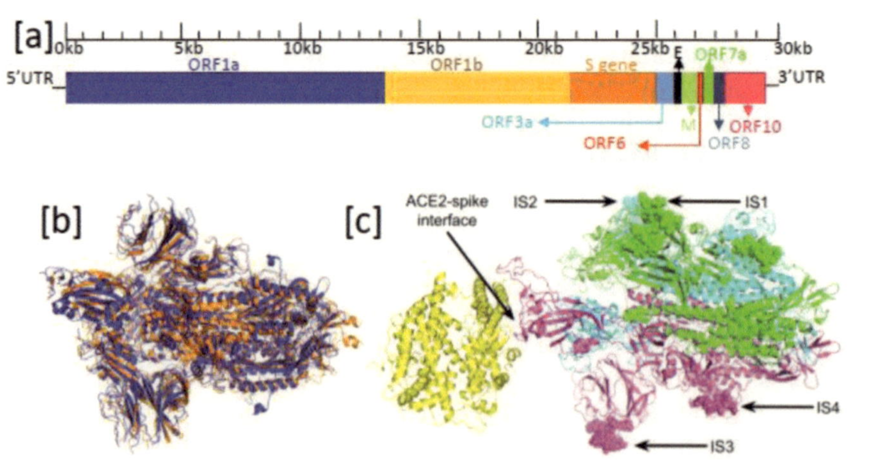

Figure 3.
(a) Genome structure of COVID-19, (b) spike protein structure of COVID-19 constructed from C-I-TASSER, and (c) human antigiotensin converting enzyme 2 (ACE2) (yellow color) and spike protein trimmer (right side multicolor (magenta, cyan and blue)).(reproduced with permission [1]).

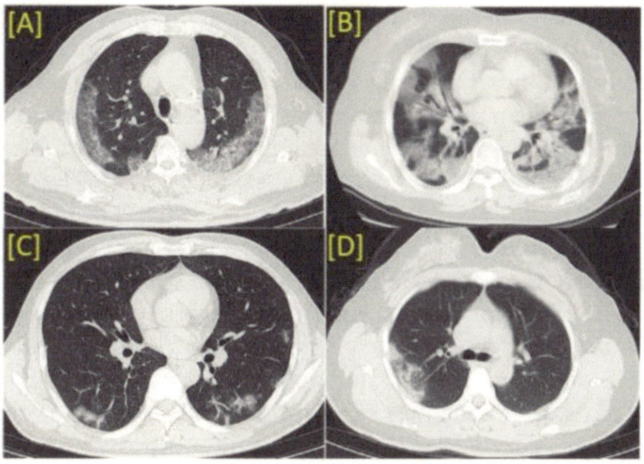

Figure 4.
CT image of (A) 75 year male patient having fever and cough since 5 days (B) 55 year female patient having fever and cough since 7 days (C) 43 year male patient having fever and cough since 7 days [D] 43 year female patient having fever and cough since 5 days; the abnormalities in axial CT were [a] bilateral subpleural CGO [B] extensive CGO with consolidations [C] small bilateral areas of peripheral CGO with minimal consolidation [d] peripheral consolidation in right lung (reproduced with permission from ref. [18]).

structure analysis reveals that, the binding affinity of ACE2 with the S protein of COVID-19 spike protein is 10–20 times higher than that of the SARS CoV spike protein [3]. However, corona virus genome sequence study suggests that, RBD in spike protein is the most variable part and determines probability of getting infected based on the binding efficiency with host receptor. From reports of Wan et al. six RBD amino acid of COVID-19 viz; L455, F486, Q493, S494, N501 and Y505 found to have high binding affinity with ACE2 receptor of human [21]. Possibly high binding capability of RBD with human ACE2 results in high rate of natural infection in human species.

6. Diagnostic tools

Diagnostics measure can play a major role for the screening of COVID-19 patient from the healthy ones. Initial identification of the COVID-19 have been carried out through molecular diagnostic approach viz.; metagenomic next generation sequencing (m-NGS), reverse-transcription PCR (RT-PCR) procedure and CRISPR. Rapid DNA alteration/genome structure of COVID-19 makes it difficult to detect by any specific method. Therefore, specific DNA sequence must be developed for early stage detection and subsequent alarming. A paper-based colorimetric assay for DNA detection based on pyrrolidinyl peptide nucleic acid (acpcPNA)-induced nanoparticle aggregation has been reported by Teengam et al. [22]. The oligonucleotide targets were detected by investigating different color measurement of silver nanoparticles (AgNP) with detection limit down to 1.53. Chen et al. followed real-time polymerase chain reaction (RT-PCR) using nucleic acid analysis for detection of COVID-19 [4]. Measurement accuracy reported to be about 71% [4]. Pathogens from bronchoalveolar lavage (BAL) fluid analysis found to be an alternative of finding genetic sequence of corona virus. Swab test possibly have higher accuracy but insufficient kits impose to go for other techniques. In this section few diagnosis process discussed elaborately.

Protein testing: Biomarker like viral protein antigens can be used for detection of infected COVID-19. Variation in infection stages make it hard to find a particular protein antigens or antibody pattern in host cell. Study of Wang et al., confirms viral increases in salivary in the first week of onset symptoms and then decreases gradually with progress in time [23]. Saliva testing possibly show shedding from salivary glands and the upper and lower respiratory tract [23]. Author tested posterior oropharyngeal (deep throat) saliva of 23 COVID-19 infected patients among which 13 were mild disease and 10 were severely affected. The findings reveals that, at initial stage of testing, posterior oropharyngeal saliva was 5·2 $\log_{10}$ copies per mL (IQR 4·1–7·0). The viral load decline to slope – 0·15, 95% CI –0·19 to –0·11; $R^2 = 0{\cdot}71$. Further, study finds relatively older aged patients having higher viral load of Spearman's $\rho = 0{\cdot}48$, 95% CI 0·074–0·75; $p = 0{\cdot}020$. Due to non-invasive and painless procedure, posterior oropharyngeal saliva testing is more acceptable to the patients. Similar study of nasopharyngeal swab or bronchoalveolar lavage fluid testing by CRISPR-nCoV method carried out by Hou et al. [24]. The finding reveals better accuracy of testing with lower turn-around time about ~40 minutes and does not require thermal cyclers. CRISPR-nCoV method composes recombinase polymerase amplification (RPA) step followed by T7 transcription and Cas13 detection step. In a typical process, a mixture of 2.5 µl of tested sample, primer (0.4 µM), reaction buffer, magnesium acetate (14 mM of) and the RT-RPA enzyme have been prepared [25]. The prepared sample was incubated at 42 °C for half an hour. Again mixture of amplification product, 166 nM of ssRNA, 66.7 nM of Cas13, 1 µl T7 RNA polymerase, 5 mM of each NTP, and 33.3 nM of gRNA allow to reacts in CRISPR. The temperature during reaction was maintained about ~42 °C. Finally, Fluorescent signals were collected. The sensitivity of CRISPR were found to be 100%. Results of 52 known infected sample showed positive COVID-19 with FC value ranging from 5–66.3 [25].

Metagenomic next-generation sequencing (mNGS): Study of Hou et al. demonstrated 52 confirm positive COVID-19 infected cases among 61 patients by mNGS method [25]. The rest are found to be negative. In this method, Qubit Fluorometer (Thermo Fisher Scientific, 99 Carlsbad, CA, USA) can be used to measure RNA concentrations and then transposase-based methodology with ribosomal RNA depletion approach might be useful for creating sequence libraries. 10 million single-end 75 bp reads must be generated for each sample followed by removal of read derived from host genome. The sequence libraries were generated by reverse-transcribed of RNA into cDNA. However, taxonomic classification and identification of sequence read may be performed by comparing with existing database of plasmid, bacteria, fungi, human, protozoa, univec, and virus sequences. It is worth mentioning that, a simultaneous testing of negative sample and its sequence generation must be carried out with each above sequence run for controlling contamination. Further, genetic similarity of all positive cases confirms Orf1ab and N gene are two potential sequences for identification of COVID-19 infection. The turnaround time ~ 20 hours (library preparation (8 hours), sequencing (10 hours) and bioinformatic analysis (2 hours)) and high cost makes this method limited use for COVID-19 detection.

Reverse-transcription PCR (RT-PCR): RT-PCR is widely used method using upper respiratory tract samples (including nasopharyngeal swabs, nasopharyngeal washes, nasal aspirates and oropharyngeal swabs) for COVID-19 testing. Probable test sample from lower respiratory tract might be sputum, BAL fluid and tracheal aspirates. However, BAL fluid and tracheal aspirates in general not used as sample for RT-PCR testing, because of aerosol formation from these samples. Mainly two steps followed in RT-PCR process; reverse transcription of viral RNA into cDNA and subsequent amplification of cDNA [26, 27]. Throughout RT-PCR diagnosis, crucial steps followed are sequence alignment, primer selection, optimization of assay (like reagent conditions, incubation times, and temperatures) and finally PCR testing. RNA-dependent RNA polymerase (RdRp) sequence and the open reading frame 1ab (ORF1ab) sequence has been used as gene target for COVID-19 detection. One step real time RT-PCR, where swab of the infected patient were mixed with following ingredients; reverse transcriptase, polymerase, magnesium, nucleotides, nuclease-free water, primers, a fluorophore-quencher probe [26, 27]. Whole mixture then transferred into PCR thermocycler which generates a fluorescent signal with help of fluorophore-quencher probe. Corman et al., uses three types of assay structure (RdRp gene, N gene and E gene) for testing 297 samples [27]. Result reveals that, detection probability ~97% for both assay RdRp gene and N-gene with 3.8 and 5.2 copies per reaction, respectively. The process turnaround time is about ~1.5 hours possibly due to the producing capability of many copies of specific gene sequence. Need of thermo cycler and use of sophisticated instruments hinders this method to use as diagnostic tool in limited resource setting. Accuracy of the method depends on sampling location, quality of RNA extraction and training of operators etc. However, still this method finds its application due to the faster nucleic acid amplification. Lower accuracy in RT-PCR results (negative result in infected sample sometimes) possibly due to the insufficient cellular material and improper extraction of nucleic acid from the specimen [27].

Computed Tomography (CT): Imaging technique like computed tomography offers easy capture of the cross sectional surface of the lung from many angles in non-invasive way. Analysis of such image modality by radiologist can offer insight about abnormal features that may come from COVID-19 infection. However, it should be noted that, abnormalities of pulmonary involvement may arise due to other viral disease as well. Note that, in some asymptomatic patients whose RT-PCR shows negative even he/she have travel history or closure contact to infected person, in that case CT imaging could be good approach of screening. Pattern change in peripheral ground-glass opacification (areas of hazy opacity), consolidations (i.e. fluid or solid material in compressible lung tissue), bilateral involvement, peripheral and diffuse distribution are found to be the responsible factor for abnormalities in pulmonary due to COVID-19 infection [28]. Further, it should be noted that, such marker may vary depending on the infected stages of COVID-19. For example, Bernheim et al. reported 56% pulmonary involvement after 2 days of onset symptoms whereas it researches to peak involvement on 10th day [29]. A CT imaging of asymptomatic patients reveals that, at the early stage of no symptoms only lesions in lungs and it gradually bilateral diffuse disease become prominent and then consolidation found on day of first or second week from onset of the symptoms [28]. Xie et al. reported five patients having negative RT-PCR result but their CT imaging confirms positive COVID-19 viral infection [30]. All the positive confirm cases does not had any prior abnormalities in pulmonary. However, same author also demonstrated 155 patients having positive RT-PCR which was found again positive by CT imaging method and 7 other patient who were positive in RT-PCR testing showed negative in CT imaging [30]. CT imaging of the five patients (who were tested RT-PCR negative) showed abnormalities in pulmonary like ground glass opacity (5 patients) and/or mixed CGO and mixed consolidations (2 patients) [30]. A series of 51 patients test by CT imaging and verification of the same by RT-PCR method resulted sensitivity about ~98% for CT and ~ 71% for RT-PCR study, respectively [18]. A CT image of four patients is shown in **Figure 4(a)–(d)** [18]. The CT investigation of 21 patients (among which 6 male 15 were male) from the onset of initial symptoms to recovery period were carried out by Pan et al. [28]. On an average, CT image capture and analysis of all the patients were carried out after every four days interval and all have been discharge after

17 ± 4 days. In most of the patients, maximum abnormalities were noted on or after 10th day since onset symptoms with R2 = 0.25 and $p < 0.001$. Based on the progress of infection level during complete hospital stay (~21 day) until recovery has been categorized into four stages viz.; stage 1(0–4 days), stage 2 (5–8 days), stage 3 (9–13 days), and stage 4 (>14 days). The most pulmonary abnormalities reported are (i) CGO in stage 1, in 17 among 24 (75%) patients (b) increased crazy paving pattern in stage 2, in 9 out of 17 (53%) patients (iii) consolidation in stage 3, in 19 out of 21 (91%) patients and (iv) gradual resolution of consolidation with decreased crazy paving pattern in stage 4, in 15 among 20 (75%) patients [28]. The governing factor (ground-glass opacification, bilateral involvement etc.) for detection of COVID-19 employing CT imaging, sometimes became imperceivable due to the low severity or few symptoms in patients making this method more challenging. Use of artificial intelligence for screening the infected patient by CT imaging possibly can increase the sensitivity of the method.

Nucleic Acid Testing. This testing does not require sophisticated laboratory instruments but dyes (malachite green, calcein and hydroxynaphthol blue) that utilize inherent by-products of the extensive DNA synthesis [31]. The testing based on the isothermal amplification at particular temperature for nucleic acid testing. The different isothermal techniques like polymerase amplification, helicase-dependent amplification, and loop-mediated isothermal amplification (LAMP) have been followed in nucleic testing [32]. Reverse transcription LAMP (RT-LAMP) is one of major techniques for detection of COVID-19 based on one-step nucleic acid amplification method [32]. In this method, few primer and DNA polymerase are essential to obtain insight about viral genome sequence. Yu et al. uses six primers to amplify the ORF1ab gene fragment [33]. The primer are as follows; forward inner primer (FIP), outer forward primer (F3), outer backward primer (B3), backward inner primer (BIP), loop forward primer (LF), and loop backward primer (LB) [34, 35]. In a typical process, the mixture of isothermic amplification buffer, dNTPs, manganese sulfate, FIP/BIP, F3/B3, FL/BL primers, Bst 2·0, antarctic thermolabile UDG, and Warm Start Reverse Transcriptase in ddH_20 were transferred in ice bath. The ice bath then kept in enclosed room and allows incubation at 63 °C for half an hour. RNA detection started with simultaneous occurrence of reverse transcription and amplification process. The detection can be confirmed by several identification like color change from orange to yellow or laddering pattern of bands after electrophoresis on a gel or by fluorescent light in response to UV excitation [32]. Loop mediated isothermal study of respiratory swabs employing pH-sensitive dyes and five primers for visual and colorimetric detection has been reported by Zhang et al. [31]. In conventional method, patient swabs were mixed with BSA (1%), amphotericin (15 µg/mL), penicillin G (100 units/mL), and streptomycin (50 µg/mL). The mixture sample then deactivated at 56 °C and finally COVID-19 RNA was extracted from the deactivated sample. Average detection sensitivity was ~100 copies in each five primer. All the samples were further confirmed through RT-PCR testing. Similar study by Yang et al. [36] reported detection of ORF1ab gene, E gene and N gene employing RT-LAMP method. Testing of 208 samples reveals sensitivity similar to RT-PCR method whereas specificity was 100%. RT-LAMP technique has high sensitivity and specificity. The turnaround time less than one hour and have flexibility to work at various pH level and temperature level. The cost of testing is relatively low compared to other techniques. However, optimum primer selection and producing suitable reaction environment are two major difficulties technician faces during sample testing.

Point-of-Care Testing: In point of care testing sample does not require to send in laboratory rather one can test with smaller device with turnaround time is less than one hour. One can either detect virus genetic content by nucleic acid based probes or by detection of toxin produced by pathogen or by epitopes of pathogen membrane [37]. In later two approaches, antibodies or antibody derivatives can be used for easy diagnosis. However, specificity of the later two (antibody based) approaches is lower than the former (nucleic acid based) approach. Some of reported point of care techniques are (i) biosensors, (ii) gold nanoparticles as antibody for binding virus protein (lateral flow assay), (iii) mirofluidic devices, (iii) electrochemical sensors, (iv) paper based systems, and (v) and surface-enhanced Raman scattering based systems [37]. Lab on chip point of care diagnosis offer portability, rapid detection time, and miniaturization. Further, testing require small sample volume [36–38]. The smart phone dongle attached with devices like mirofluidic device, electrochemical sensor or lab on chip can also be a point of care strategies for COVID-19 detection. Xiang et al. compared COVID detection by (i) ELISA test with IgG and IgM antibodies for 63 patients and (ii) colloidal gold-immunochromatographic assay (GICA) for 91 patients and the sensitivity were found to be 87.3% and 82.4% [37].

7. Influence of COVID-19 on pregnant women

COVID-19 outbreak converges existing reproductive health and economic stability of the women's and girl's. The crisis reduced the access of family planning, and increase the unsafe abortion, miscarriage, unintended pregnancies, post traumatic stress disorder, intimate partner violence etc. [39]. Limited resources available for illness prediction of COVID-19 infected pregnant women but provide some insight based on the effects one encounter from similar type of corona virus infection (SARS) and MERS). COVID-19 can increase the rate mortality for the case of pregnant women and enhances the chance of transmission to new born baby via vertical transmission. A study of 33 new born baby from infected mother reveals vertical COVID-19 transmission in 3 babies [39]. US Centers for Disease Control and Prevention (CDC) sets few rule and regulation for women having new born babies are (a) sanitize the hands before touching the baby, (b) wash feeding bottles before and after use, (c) women are allowed to breast feed until evidence suggest otherwise, (d) use mask during breast feeding, (e) use of dexamethasone as an alternative to betamethasone for fetal lung maturation etc. [24]. Study of Liu et al., from January 20, 2020, to February 10, 2020 gives a clear picture of different symptoms and subsequent treatment of infected women having different stage of pregnancies [40]. The entire clinical study reviewed by three radiologist for 15 pregnant infected women (diagnosis with reverse transcription–polymerase chain reaction (RT-PCR) at the time of admission) reveals that, 11 patient gave successful deliver of new born and 4 patient are still under observation (three are in second trimester and one in third trimester). They were not facing any natal asphyxia, neonatal death or abortion up to the end of the study. The CT imaging was carried out for infected women before and after delivery. All patients chest CT imaging shows pulmonary abnormalities. Similar chest diagnosis by CT scan and pulmonary abnormalities of all admitted patient has also been found in the report of Rasmussen et al. [41]. CT imaging reveals ground-glass opacity (GGO) in early stage of the infection and crazy paving pattern (denser, more profuse, and confluent) in patients having more infection than the images of healthy lungs [40, 41]. The most common symptoms were found to be fever (13 among 15 patients) and cough (9 among 15 patients). Lymphocytopenia was the most common abnormality found in 12 patients. CT scanning ensures no evidence of COVID-19 provocation after delivery. Among 11 patients. All were given antibiotic treatment before and after delivery whereas 4 patient who were still pregnant till end of the study period were treated only with antibiotics. Another study by Zhu et al., reported nine pregnant women with 10 new born (one twin) babies [42]. The report says onset symptoms of COVID-19 were evident in four patients before 1 to 6 day of delivery, in two patients on the same day of delivery and in three patients after 1to 3 day of delivery. Two among the nine mothers had intrauterine fetal distress and 6 babies were born preterm. No mortality was reported [42]. As far as respiratory acute failure is concern, 40% pregnant women were given mechanical ventilation whereas it was 13% for non-pregnant women [31]. However, what treatment is actually applied is still unknown. Pregnant women's are more likely to be affected due to the physical changes like diaphragm elevation, edema of respiratory tract mucosa, increased oxygen consumption etc. drive them to more complicated cases. What about the new born babies? Whether there is any vertical transmission of COVID-19 to new born or not? If transmission takes place, then in what mode and is it when fetal is in the mother womb or during delivery time (by means of surface contact)?. This question mark is still in dilemma. Because some evidence proofs that, there is no vertical transmission takes place [41]. On the other hand, few study ensure positive cases in new born babies [43]. Vertical transmission case study of four mother and their new born have been investigated by Chen et al. with different parameters variation in mother as well as in the new born babies [44]. All four mothers were admitted in hospital at their trimester with positive COVID-19. Initial health counseling of mothers was as follows; three among four have fever, two among four have myalgia or fatigue, two among four have cough. The fetal movement was normal except one mother who have dyspnea. Lymphocytes count ($<1.1 \times 109/L$) found to be lower than in normal case and C-response protein was found to be significantly increased in level for all four mothers. Chest CT imaging before delivery confirms abnormalities. However, after antiviral treatment, COVID-19 test found negative in three mother and they were released after 3–5 days. One who suffer with dyspnea takes more time to recover from COVID-19. The states of babies are as follows; all four babies were isolated upon birth from their mother. For prevention of COVID-19 perinatal and postnatal transmission, three mothers opted cesarean section and remaining one had vaginal delivery due to the sudden labor pain. The RT-PCR testing were carried out after 72 hour of their birth and only three babies were tested since one among four were not given consent for testing.

8. Adopted cure strategy

Worldwide scientist and physicians started major campaign to understand the emergence of the disease and its possible antiviral treatment by drug development or therapeutic agents or developing vaccines. As of now there is no specific therapeutics agent or vaccine approved to cure COVID-19 patient in clinical procedure. Due to limited clinical and basic research information, most of the clinical trial/manifestation follows basic symptomatic treatment protocol and supportive care which was followed for curing SARS and MERS patients [45]. The strategies of SARS-CoV and MERS-CoV therapy or antiviral drug have been extrapolated for the treatment of COVID-19 (**Table 1**). Most of the hospitalized infected patient have following status; (i) among the admitted patients, 23%–32% enters into ICU, (ii) 17%–29% feels critical respiratory failure (iii) ~7–8% were discharged and (iii) ~1% reported death. S-protein of COVID-19 has much similarity (in structural as well as replication procedure) with SARS and MERS protein and hence most of the articles reported broad spectrum antiviral activity of remdesivir, baricitinib, and chloroquine as the clinical trial antiviral drug [19] (**Figure 5**). Remdesivir demonstrated effectiveness for curing COVID-19 in USA [46]. Nucleotide type of remdesivir drug

Sr No	Target Protein	Possible Drug	Ref
1	Angiotensin-converting enzyme 2 (ACE2)	Arbidol	[34]
2	Viral spike glycoprotein (S-protein)	Arbidol	[34]
3	Transmembrane protease, serine 2 (TMPRSS2)	camostat mesylate	[50]
4	Coronavirus main protease 3CLpro (3CLpro)	lopinavir	[46]
5	Papain-like protease PLpro (PLpro)	lopinavir	[48]
6	RNA-dependent RNA polymerase (RdRp)	remdesivir, ribavirin, favipiravir	[47]
7	JAK kinas	baricitinib	[51]
8	Endosome/ACE2	Chloroquine, Hydroxychloroquine	[47]
8	RNA-dependent RNA polymerase (RdRp)	IDX-184	[35]

Table 1.
Target protein related to nCoV-19, SARS-CoV and MERS-CoV and possible drug proposed for prevention (data taken from reference [34–51]).

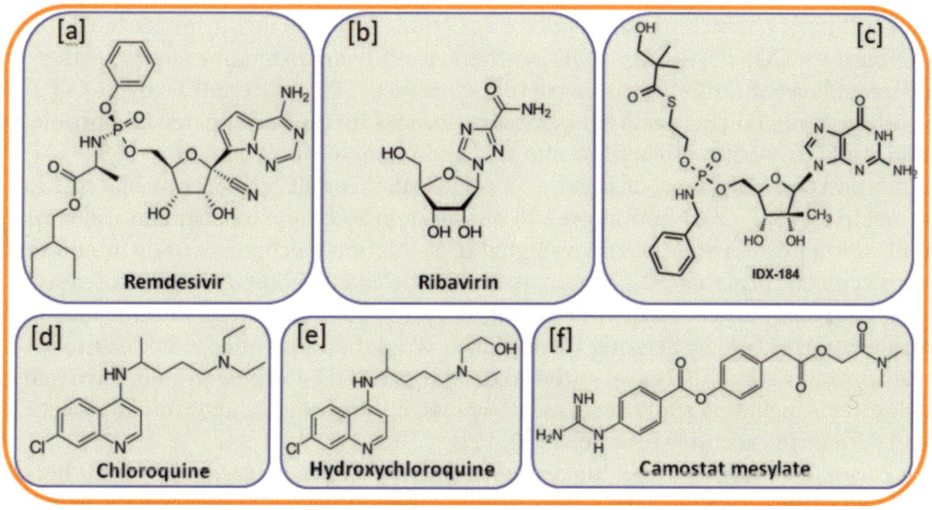

Figure 5.
structure of viral entry inhibitor (a) remdesivir, (b) ribavirin, (c) IDX-184, (d) chloroquine, (e) hydroxycholoroquine, and (f) camostat mesylate.

assisted to premature termination of RNA chain in host cell. On the other hand, ribavirin is a guanosine analogue mostly used for treating chronic hepatitis C [47]. However, study finds suitable dosage of ribavirin might stop the replication spike protein RNA [47]. Lopinavir (a viral protease inhibitor) with its pharmacological booster ritonavir (LPV/R) initially proved to be useful for HIV, SARS-CoV, MERS-CoV treatment with the action of protease inhibitors. Recently study in South Korea reveals significant decrease in COVID-19 viral load after treating with (LPV/R) [46, 48]. Similar reduction in viral loading (associated with pneumonia related symptoms) was also observed after treating with arbidol [34]. Chloroquine and its hydroxy-analogue hydroxychloroquine demonstrated to be relevant for patient having diabetes with infected COVID-19 [14]. Researcher and scientific community stress more on 3CLpro, PLpro and RdRp protein target than other target possibly due to the most responsible proteases for COVID-19 replication and hence attractive targets for antiviral therapies. Further, one needs to understand, the possible action mechanism of existing drug on COVID-19 before being used. For example, arbidol can be used for fusion of virus-host cells to prevent virus entry into the host. The clinical trial of arbidol is in process [34]. Clinically approved camostat mesylate a possible inhibitor used (to reduce activity of TMPRSS2) for blocking the COVID-19 entry into human body [35]. Combination of tocilizumab and hydroxychloroquine found to be very effective for curing COVID-19 patient underwent kidney transplant surgery [49].

9. Role of biosensor devices

Recently nanomaterial used for point of care diagnosis, therapeutics agent, or in vaccine development. Nanomaterial found to be the promising candidate for the modulation of viral infection cycle [4]. Especially, carbon quantum dots having size below 10 nm found to be a promising interferes for the viruses into the cells. Nanomaterial having different nanostructure offers multivalent character due to surface to volume ratio. Such multivalent properties facilitate several ligands to attach with virus. The viral-ligands interface blocks the entry of virus into the host cell [20]. Łoczechin et al. reported function of carbon quantum dot (CQD) as inhibitor for COVID-19 [52]. CQD synthesis itself from different precursor offer different level of inhibition strength to corona virus. Two different study of CQD synthesis from (i) citric acid/ethylenediamine and further conjugated by boronic acid, and (ii) 4-aminophenylboronic acid and phenylboronic acid offer 50% inhibition concentrations of EC50 = 52 ± 8 μg mL^{-1} and EC50 = 5.2 ± 0.7 μg mL^{-1}, respectively [52]. CQD inhibit growth of s-protein by fusion mechanism and stop replication process of S-protein by signal transduction mechanism or by interaction with cytosolic proteins [52]. Nanomaterial particles as therapeutic agent for stopping viral entry and subsequent replication of S-protein in host membrane may be an alternative of many existing treatment to avoid their side effects. For example, use of ribavirin and IFN as an antiviral drug for COVID-19 spike protein have many side effects including short-term memory loss, confusion, extrapyramidal effects and deficits in executive functions [20, 52].

Plasmonic biosensor working on the cumulative effect of plasmonic photothermal (PPT) and localized surface plasmon resonance (LSPR) transduction principle found to be another potential alternative diagnosis of COVID-19 [53]. Two dimensional (2D) gold nanoislands (AuNIs) functionalized with DNA receptors exploited as sensing of RNA gene sequence. Sensitivity of material can be enhanced to some order by direct thermoplasmonic heating to biosensor chip. The usable plasmonic heat to the chip has been generated by setting a particular plasmonic resonant frequency. Photon generated oscillation frequency modulated the electrons behavior on the surface of plasmon material which might be the crucial factor for detection of selective COVID-19 gene sequence from multi gene mixture. Enhanced plasmonic field at the nanostructures surfaces increases sensitivity of sensor by suppressing local variation like refractive index and molecular binding. Employing field effect transistor as biosensor for fast and accurate spike protein detection through nasopharyngeal swab has recently been reported by Seo et al. [54]. Graphene coated specific antibody has been used as sensing material for spike protein detection [54]. The spike protein directly not attached with graphene surfaces rather 1-pyrenebutyric acid N-hydroxysuccinimide ester was used as probe linker to conjugate protein structure on graphene surfaces. Such attachment of spike protein induced by 1-pyrenebutyric acid N-hydroxysuccinimide ester on graphene surface leading to changes in conductivity and subsequently in current through the FET structure

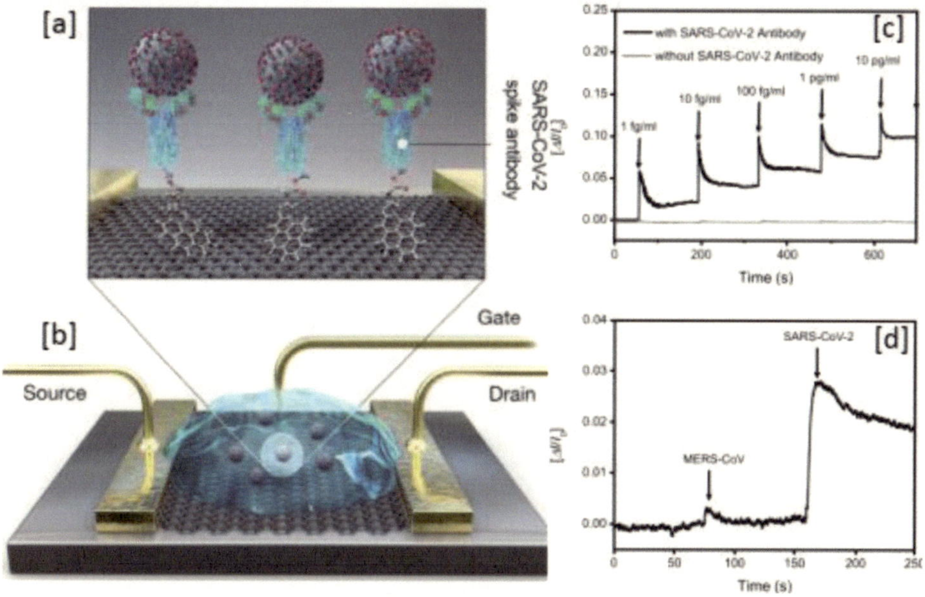

Figure 6.
(a) showing conjugation of spike protein on to the surface of graphene via 1-pyrenebutyric acid N-hydroxysuccinimide ester (b) model showing spike protein on the surface (covered with graphene) of field effect transistor (c) FET sensor sensitivity in presence of SARS-COV-2 antibody and in absence of SARS-COV-2 antibody and (d) FET sensor sensitivity in MERS-COV and SARS-COV-2 (reproduce with permission [32]).

(shown in **Figure 6 (a)** and **(b)**). The sensitivity which was measured by current fluctuation due to presence or absence of spike protein is shown in **Figure 6(c)** and **(d)**. The biosensor capable to detect down to 16 pfu/mL in cultural mode and 2.42 × 102 copies/mL in clinical sample [32]. The diagnosis method does not require sophisticated laboratory equipment and provide very high sensitivity with instantaneous measurements employing small volume of nasopharyngeal swab.

10. Conclusions

Like other epidemic, COVID-19 may also become seasonal, but at present one can only predicted about it not for sure. Meanwhile, to reduce the outbreak, it is required to have international collaboration with data sharing policies. Because, of the limited information, one can reuse the existing drugs as clinical trial for curing COVID-19 infection (based on the similarity of target protein with other coronavirus). Further, fight against COVID-19 requires the knowledge of computer science, medicine, health policy, environmental factors and risk management etc. Present situation imposes researcher and scientific community a number of research target viz.; (i) production of rapid point of care diagnosis (ii) enhancement in surveillance and monitoring (iii) design of new therapeutic agents and finally (iv) vaccine development. We can only reduce the transmission level up to certain extent but cannot be demolished completely. For complete cure one has to develop vaccine.

Conflict of interest

Author declares there is no conflict of interest.

Notes/thanks/other declarations

My sincere thanks to the doctor, nurses, and all other professionals for their continuous involvement directly or indirectly to fight against COVID-19.

Author details

Basanta Bhowmik
Thin Film Device Laboratory, Department of Electronics and Communication Engineering, National Institute of Technology, Jamshedpur, India

*Address all correspondence to: bb.cemk.ece@gmail.com

References

[1] Chengxin Z., Zheng W, Huang X, Bell EW, Zhou XZ, and Zhang Y., Protein Structure and Sequence Reanalysis of 2019-nCoV Genome Refutes Snakes as Its Intermediate Host and the Unique Similarity between Its Spike Protein Insertions and HIV-1. J. Proteome Res. 2019; 19:1351-1360

[2] Andersen K.G, Rambaut A, Lipkin W.I. et al. The proximal origin of SARS-CoV-2. Nat Med. 2020; 26: 450-452

[3] Baig AM, Khaleeq A, Ali U, Syeda H. Evidence of the COVID-19 Virus Targeting the CNS: Tissue Distribution, Host–Virus Interaction, and Proposed Neurotropic Mechanisms. ACS Chem. Neurosci. 2020; 11: 995-998.

[4] Szunerits S, Barras A, Khanal M, Pagneux Q, Boukherroub R. Nanostructures for the Inhibition of Viral Infections. Molecules. 2015; 20 14051-14081

[5] Wang D, Hu B, Hu C, et al. Clinical characteristics of 138 hospitalized patients with 2019 novel coronavirus-infected pneumonia in Wuhan. JAMA. 2020; 323(11) 1061-1069

[6] Wigginton KR, Boehm AB. Environmental Engineers and Scientists Have Important Roles to Play in Stemming Outbreaks and Pandemics Caused by Enveloped Viruses. Environ. Sci. Technol. 2020, 54: 3736-3739

[7] Casanova L, Rutala WA, Weber DJ, Sobsey MD. Survival of surrogate coronaviruses in water. Water Res. 2009, 43 (7): 1893-1898.

[8] Lu R, Zhao X, Li J, et al. Genomic characterization and epidemiology of 2019 novel coronavirus: implications for virus origins and receptor binding. Lancet 2020; 395:565-574

[9] Li Q, Guan X, Wu P, et al. Early transmission dynamics in Wuhan, China, of novel coronavirus-infected pneumonia. N Engl J Med, 2020; 382: 1199-1207

[10] Tang B, Bragazzi NL, Li Q, Tang S, Xiao Y, Wu J. An updated estimation of the risk of transmission of the novel coronavirus, Infectious Disease Modelling. 2020; 5: 248-255

[11] Qu G, Li X, Hu L, Jiang G. An Imperative Need for Research on the Role of Environmental Factors in Transmission of Novel Coronavirus (COVID-19). Environ. Sci. Technol. 2020; 54: 3730-3732

[12] Netland J, Meyerholz DK, Moore S, Cassell M, Perlman S. Severe acute respiratory syndrome coronavirus infection causes neuronal death in the absence of encephalitis in mice transgenic for human ACE2. J. Virol. 2008; 82 (15): 7264-75

[13] Wu Y, Xu X, Chen Z, Duan J, Hashimoto K, Yang L, Liu C, Yang C. Nervous system involvement after infection with COVID-19 and other coronaviruses, Brain, Behavior, and Immunity, https://doi.org/10.1016/j.bbi.2020.03.031

[14] Chen Y, Peng H, Wang L, Zhao Y, Zeng L, Gao H, Liu Y. Infants Born to Mothers with a New Coronavirus (COVID-19). Front. Pediatr. 2020; 8:104. doi: 10.3389/fped.2020.00104

[15] Du L, He Y, Zhou Y, Liu S, Zheng BJ, Jiang S. 2009. The spike protein of SARS-CoV - A target for vaccine and therapeutic development. Nat. Rev. Microbiol. 2009; 7 (3): 226-236. 23

[16] Xia S, Zhu Y, Liu M, Lan Q, Xu W, Wu Y, et al. 2020. Fusion mechanism of 2019- nCoV and fusion inhibitors targeting HR1 domain in spike protein.

Cell Mol Immunol. 2020, https://doi.org/10.1038/s41423-020-0374-2

[17] Li X, Geng M, Peng Y, Meng L, Lu S. Molecular immune pathogenesis and diagnosis of COVID-19. Journal of Pharmaceutical Analysis. 2020; 10: 102-108

[18] Fang Y, Zhang H, Xie J, Lin M, Ying L, Pang P, Ji W. 2020. Sensitivity of Chest CT for COVID-19: Comparison to RT-PCR. Radiology 2020, 200432 https://doi.org/10.1148/radiol.2020200432SectionsPDF.

[19] Liu C, Zhou Q, Li Y, Garner LV, Watkins SP, Carter LJ, Smoot J, Gregg AC, Daniels AD, Jervey S, Albaiu,D. Research and Development on Therapeutic Agents and Vaccines for COVID-19 and Related Human Coronavirus Diseases. ACS Cent. Sci. 2020; 6: 315-331

[20] Li YY, Zhang C, Bell EW, Yu DJ, Zhang Y. Ensembling multiple raw coevolutionary features with deep residual neural networks for contact-map prediction in CASP13. Proteins: Struct., Funct. Genet. 2019, 87 (12): 1082-1091

[21] Wan Y, Shang, J, Graham R, Baric RS. Li F. Receptor Recognition by the Novel Coronavirus from Wuhan: an Analysis Based on Decade-Long Structural Studies of SARS Coronavirus. J. Virol. 2020; 94 (7): e00127-20https://doi.org/10.1128/JVI.00127-20

[22] Teengam P, Siangproh W, Tuantranont A, Vilaivan T, Chailapakul O, Henry CS. Multiplex Paper-Based Colorimetric DNA Sensor Using Pyrrolidinyl Peptide Nucleic Acid-Induced AgNPs Aggregation for Detecting MERS-CoV, MTB, and HPV Oligonucleotides. Anal. Chem. 2017; 89: 5428-5435 DOI: 10.1021/acs.analchem.7b00255

[23] Wang KK et al. Temporal profiles of viral load in posterior oropharyngeal saliva samples and serum antibody responses during infection by SARS-CoV-2: an observational cohort study. Lancet Infect Dis, 2020; 20: 565-574 https://doi.org/10.1016/S1473-3099(20)30196-1

[24] Simbar RJMP, Goncé A, Villarreal AH, Figueras F. A Spanish-translated clinical algorithm for management of suspected SARS-CoV-2 infection in pregnant women. Lancet Infect Dis. ,2020, DOI: 10.1016/s1473-3099(20)30285-1

[25] Hou T, Zeng W, Yang M, Chen W, Ren L, Ai J, Ji W, Liao Y, Gou X, Li Y, Wang X, Su H, Gu B, Wang J, Xu T. Development and Evaluation of A CRISPR-based Diagnostic For 2019-novel Coronavirus. medRxiv preprint, 2020; doi: https://doi.org/10.1101/2020.02.22.20025460

[26] Freeman, WM., Walker SJ, Vrana KE, Quantitative RTPCR: Pitfalls and Potential. BioTechniques. 1999; 26 (1): 124-125

[27] Corman V, Bleicker T, Brünink S, Zambon M. 2020. Diagnostic Detection of Wuhan Coronavirus 2019 by Real-Time RT-PCR. World Health Organization: Geneva

[28] Pan F, Ye T, Sun P et al. Time course of lung changes on chest CT during recovery from 2019 novel coronavirus (COVID-19) pneumonia. Radiology, 2020, DOI:10.1148/radiol.2020200370

[29] Bernheim A, Mei X, Huang M, Yang Y, Fayad Z. A, Zhang N, Diao K, Lin B, Zhu X., Li K et al. Chest CT Findings in Coronavirus Disease-19 (COVID-19): Relationship to Duration of Infection. Radiology, 2020; https://doi.org/10.1148/radiol.2020200463

[30] Xie X, Zhong Z, Zhao W, Zheng C, Wang F, Liu J. 2020. Chest CT for Typical 2019-nCoV Pneumonia: Relationship to Negative RTPCR

Testing. Radiology 2020, 200343 https://doi.org/10.1148/radiol.2020200343

[31] Zhang Y, Odiwuor N et al. Rapid Molecular Detection of SARS-CoV-2 (COVID-19) Virus RNA Using Colorimetric LAMP, medRxiv. 2020 DOI: 10.1101/2020.02.26.20028373

[32] Lamb L. E, Bartolone SN, Ward E, Rapid Detection of Novel Coronavirus (COVID-19) by Reverse Transcription-Loop-Mediated Isothermal Amplification. medRxiv.2020; DOI: 10.1101/2020.02.19.20025155

[33] Yu L, Wu S et al. Rapid Colorimetric Detection of COVID- 19 Coronavirus Using a Reverse Tran-Scriptional Loop-Mediated Isothermal Amplification (RT-LAMP) Diagnostic Plat-Form: iLACO. medRxiv, 2020; DOI: 10.1101/2020.02.20.20025874

[34] Kadam RU, Wilson IA, Structural basis of influenza virus fusion inhibition by the antiviral drug Arbidol. Proc. Natl. Acad. Sci. U. S. A. 2017; 114 (2): 206-214

[35] Beauverd Y, Adam Y, Assouline B, Samii K. COVID-19 infection and treatment with hydroxychloroquine cause severe haemolysis crisis in a patient with glucose-6-phosphate dehydrogenase deficiency. Eur J Haematol. 2020; doi: 10.1111/ejh.13432.

[36] Yang W, Dang X et al. 2020. Rapid Detection of SARS-CoV-2 Using Reverse Transcription RT-LAMP Method. medRxiv, DOI: 10.1101/2020.03.02.20030130

[37] Xiang J, Yan M, Li H, Liu T, Lin C, Huang S, Shen C. Evaluation of Enzyme-Linked Immunoassay and Colloidal GoldImmunochromatographic Assay Kit for Detection of Novel Coronavirus (SARS-Cov-2) Causing an Outbreak of Pneumonia (COVID-19). medRxiv preprint, 2020 doi: https://doi.org/10.1101/2020.02.27.20028787

[38] Foudeh AM, Fatanat DT, Veres T, Tabrizian M. Microfluidic Designs and Techniques Using Lab-on-a-Chip Devices for Pathogen Detection for Point-of-Care Diagnostics. Lab Chip, 2012; 12(18): 3249-3266

[39] Hall KS, Samari G, Garbers S, Casey SE, Diallo DD, Orcutt M, Moresky RT, Martinez ME, McGovern T. Centring sexual and reproductive health and justice in the global COVID-19 response. The Lancet. 2020; 395: 1175-1177 https://doi.org/10.1016/S0140-6736(20)30801-1

[40] Liu D. Li L, Wu X, Zheng D, Wang J, Yang L, Zheng C. Pregnancy and Perinatal Outcomes of Women With Coronavirus Disease (COVID-19) Pneumonia: A Preliminary Analysis. American Journal of Roentgenology: 2020, 1-6. 10.2214/AJR.20.23072

[41] Rasmussen SA, Smulian JC, Lednicky JA, Wen TS, Jamieson DJ. Coronavirus Disease 2019 (COVID-19) and pregnancy: what obstetricians need to know. Am J Obstet Gynecol. 2020; 222(5):415-426 doi: 10.1016/j.ajog.2020.02.017.

[42] Zhu H, Wang L, Fang C, et al. Clinical analysis of 10 neonates born to mothers with 2019-nCoV pneumonia. Transl Pediatr. 2020; 9:51-60. 59

[43] D'Amore R. Can coronavirus pass from mother to baby? Maybe, but experts need more research. Global news. 2020; Available at: https:// globalnews.ca/news/6515302/coronavirus mother-baby-transmission/ Posted Feb. 7

[44] Netland J, Meyerholz DK, Moore S, Cassell M, Perlman S. Severe acute respiratory syndrome coronavirus infection causes neuronal death in the absence of encephalitis in mice transgenic for human ACE2. J. Virol. 2008; 82 (15): 7264-75.

[45] Hilgenfeld R, Peiris M. From SARS to MERS: 10 years of research on highly pathogenic human coronaviruses. Antiviral Res, 2013; 100: 286-295

[46] Sheahan TP, et al. Comparative therapeutic efficacy of remdesivir and combination lopinavir, ritonavir, and interferon beta against MERS-CoV, Nat. Commun. Ahead of Print. 2020; DOI: 10.1038/s41467-019-13940-6

[47] Guo, D. Old weapon for new enemy: drug repurposing for treatment of newly emerging viral diseases. Virol. Sin. 2020; DOI: 10.1007/s12250-020-00204-7. [Epub ahead of print]

[48] Maxmen A. More than 80 clinical trials launch to test coronavirus treatments. Nature, 2020; 578 (7795): 347-348

[49] Fontana F, Alfano G et al. Covid-19 pneumonia in a kidney transplant recipient successfully treated with Tocilizumab and Hydroxychloroquine, American Journal of Transplantation, 2020; doi:10.1111/AJT.15935

[50] Hoffmann M et al. SARS-CoV-2 Cell Entry Depends on ACE2 and TMPRSS2 and Is Blocked by a Clinically Proven Protease Inhibitor. Cell, 2020; DOI: 10.1016/ j.cell.2020.02.052. [Epub ahead of print].

[51] Richardson P. Baricitinib as potential treatment for 2019-nCoV acute respiratory disease. Lancet, 2020; 395: 30—e31.

[52] Łoczechin A et al, Functional Carbon Quantum Dots as Medical Countermeasures to Human Coronavirus. ACS Appl. Mater. Interfaces. 2020; 46: 42964-42974 DOI: 10.1021/acsami.9b15032

[53] Qiu G et al. Dual-Functional Plasmonic Photothermal Biosensors for Highly Accurate Severe Acute Respiratory Syndrome Coronavirus 2 Detection, ACS Nano, 2020; https://dx.doi.org/10.1021/acsnano.0c02439

[54] Seo G et al. Rapid Detection of COVID-19 Causative Virus (SARS-CoV-2) in Human Nasopharyngeal Swab Specimens Using Field-Effect Transistor-Based Biosensor. ACS Nano, 2020 14(4): 5135-5142 DOI: 10.1021/acsnano.0c02823

Chapter 2

Control of an Epidemic of SARS-CoV-2 by Assessing Transmissibility of Its Infected Cases in Absence of a Suitable Vaccine

Bidisa Sarkar and Kamalesh Sarkar

Abstract

SARS-CoV-2 or Covid 19 and it's pandemicity has been wreaking havoc in many countries worldwide. It is important to counter and contain the spread of Covid-19 using some effective infection control policies as we await an effective protection such as vaccine. Ahmedabad Model of Covid-19 Control could be used as an established epidemic management protocol for COVID 19 infection. It relies on the Cycle Threshold (Ct) Value, which was used as a proxy marker for assessing initial viral load. It was evident that cases with higher viral load spread the disease at much higher rate as compared to that of low viral load apart from population mobility and/or population density. Therefore, Ct value based segregation of infected cases with higher viral load along with contact tracing of them of previous 5 days is an effective epidemic control policy. It needs to be remembered that a section of infected cases is asymptomatic and capable of spreading infection in the community unknowingly. Hence, infection control practices must be accompanied with standard precautionary measures such as physical distancing, hand hygiene and wearing face mask. Community awareness is an integral part of it. Newer biotechnology based researches may be encouraged based on felt needs.

Keywords: SARS-CoV-2, epidemic, cycle threshold value, RT-PCR, transmissibility

1. Introduction

SARS-CoV-2 or COVID-19 is a newly discovered coronavirus representing the third coronavirus associated epidemic to emerge from a species leap i.e. from the wild animals to the humans, after severe acute respiratory syndrome (SARS) in 2003, and the Middle East Respiratory Syndrome (MERS) in 2012 [1]. COVID-19 transmission dynamics is yet to be understood thoroughly. Basic Reproduction Rate (R_0) is a term which is often used in an epidemic. It is the average number of secondary cases of an infectious disease that one case would generate in a completely susceptible population within its longest incubation period [2]. If $R_0 > 1$, then the number of infected cases is likely to rise, while if $R_0 < 1$ then the transmission will probably die out. The basic reproduction number is an important measurement in infectious disease epidemiology, indicating the risk of an infectious agent with respect to epidemic spread. Estimated basic reproductive number of COVID-19, declared by the WHO (dated January 23, 2020) ranges within 1.4–2.5 [3].

A recent review by Liu et al. found the average R_0 of COVID 19 infection to be 3.28 and median to be 2.79, which exceed the WHO estimates [4]. It was observed in SARS that a few of the infected people in the community spread most of the infection, whereas most people, although infected, spread it to only a handful [5–12]. In addition to R_0, scientists use a value called dispersion factor (K), a number that indicates the likelihood of a certain disease to spread in clusters [13]. Lower the K value, more is the transmission that occurs from a small number of people. In 2005, an article in Nature estimated that SARS had a K value of 0.16 [13]. In a recent publication, K value for COVID-19 was estimated to be as low as 0.1 [14] suggesting that probably about 10% of the total number of infected cases will be spreading to about 80% of the cases.

Apart from Basic Reproduction Rate, certain other terminologies are just as important to understand the transmission pattern of infected cases in a community or in a defined geographical area. The term epidemic is used when there is occurrence of large number of infected cases in a community or in a defined geographic area and in a particular period, clearly in excess than the expected number of cases during the same time of previous years. When the occurrence of cases is less than that of the expected number of cases compared to previous years, it is called endemic. Epidemic may be common source epidemic (all cases occurring simultaneously from a single source such as food poisoning following consumption of a meal at a marriage party) or propagated epidemic (when few cases occur from a source and then they further infect some other people, who in turn spread to another group). Certain factors are associated with transmission of infection such as virulence of organism, organisms' density in infectious material, lack of health seeking behaviour, population density, population movement, lack of awareness, lack of hygienic practices, etc. The infectiousness of an infectious disease is measured by Secondary Attack Rate (SAR) - defined as the occurrence of new cases among the susceptible population from the primary case within the longest incubation period of that disease. Usually it is expressed in percentage. Secondary Attack Rate depends on population density, population mobility, virulence of organism, organism density, behaviour of the individuals concerned, etc. in absence of any intervention such as vaccination or medication.

A review work was carried out by a group of researchers that raised several questions. COVID-19 via person-to-person contact had had spread like a wildfire, affecting almost every country in the world. In the past 100 years, the world never experienced a pandemic as cataclysmic as COVID-19. It is easily understood that both previous outbreaks of other members of the coronavirus family (severe acute respiratory syndrome (SARS-CoV) and middle east respiratory syndrome (MERS-CoV)) did not produce even 2% of the global harm which has already been inflicted by COVID-19. There are also four other CoVs capable of infecting humans (HCoVs), which circulate continuously in the human population, but their phenotypes are generally mild, and these HCoVs have received little attention. These dramatic differences between infection with HCoVs, SARS-CoV, MERS-CoV, and SARS-CoV-2 raise many questions, such as: How quick transmission occurs in COVID-19? Does viral structure play any role in it? Any specific human (host) factors are involved? Any environmental factors involved? A review work was done by a group of researchers with the aim of having possible logical answers to above questions [15].

Data collected in above mentioned review clearly indicated that SARS-CoV-2 uses multiple ways for efficient transmission. The virion structure is optimised to survive various environmental conditions, allowing this virus to use both respiratory and faecal-oral transmission modes. Its S protein has an amended structure for efficient interaction with the ACE2 receptor and is optimised for furin cleavage. Moreover, S protein could be primed with activation by TMPRSS2, furin, and multiple non-furin proteases (e.g., plasmin). In addition to ACE2, SARS-CoV-2 can interact with other cellular peptidase receptors, such as ANPEP and DPP4, and also can utilise non-peptidase receptors, such as DC-SIGN1, CLEC4G, and CLEC4M. SARS-CoV-2 utilises multiple ways for cellular entry (both non-endosomal and endosomal) and potentially uses various means of epigenetic control to inhibit the initiation of the host innate immune response. During pandemic period continuous genetic rearrangements occurs within the virus cell genetic structure, which enable the virus particles for immunological escape. SARS-CoV-2 is associated with intricate interplay involving various host genetic factors and pathways. Cytokine storm is the result of above interactions, which promotes cellular death programme of various cells, such as pyroptosis, apoptosis, and necrosis, which might contribute to the COVID-19 pathogenesis. This remarkably broad spectrum of means for the efficient SARS-CoV-2 transmission indicates that it is very unlikely that COVID-19 can be cured by targeting just one segment of this complex mosaic [15].

2. Recent experience from India

India had had witnessed a tremendous rise in the daily number of COVID-19 infected cases during its epidemic period. It started from January 2020 with single detected case in Kerala that reached its plateau in mid-September 2020 with almost 98,000 cases in a day during that period [16]. First Covid-related death was reported in March 2020 and on September 18 of the same year, 1195 reportedly died due to the very reason. Till September there was so sign of decline in the daily number of new cases. Reaching the plateau and subsequent decline then seemed to be a far-fetched dream in the absence of an effective vaccine or drug. On January 4th, 2021, a total of 16278 new cases were detected while 200 deaths were reported country wide. Various models of COVID-19 were put forward to predict the trend yet no estimate had turned out to be even close to the reality.

Officials had claimed that increasing the number of tests would have had helped control the epidemic [17, 18]. Yet they could not provide with any effective strategy for reducing new infections which would have had helped flattening of the national Covid-19 epidemic curve. Several survey results established that a small percentage of the people in the country have had developed herd immunity even though they were unaware of their infection. Thus controlling the epidemic through reaching an adequate amount of herd immunity is a remote possibility. Taking these situations into consideration, public health experts of the country opined and rooted for effective public health measures including evidence-based epidemic control policy to be undertaken unless some safe and effective vaccines were available. As per the suggestions of the authority, testing was increased manifold, resulting in detection of more cases and, increase in treatment and quarantine. But the problem was that all the tests were concentrated in the metropolitan cities and the urban areas. Also a sizable number of cases were asymptomatic or pre-symptomatic; they perhaps unknowingly had spread the infection to others.

An epidemiological study was conducted by ICMR-National Institute of Occupational Health, Ahmedabad, in western India, to assess the distribution of infected cases in the community and whether initial viral load of COVID-19-infected case indicated by cycle threshold (Ct) value of reverse transcription polymerase chain reaction (RT-PCR) could predict about transmission pattern in the community apart from population mobility and its density. The study revealed that only 7% of the infected ones carried high viral load, while another 9% of the infected population had moderate viral load and rest 84% were carrying low viral loads as per community distribution was concerned [19]. Viral load was categorised as high when cycle threshold value = <24, moderate = 24 to <31 and low = 31 & above (**Figure 1**).

Interestingly, most of the Covid-19 infected cases' clustering happened around the houses of cases, infected with with high viral load. Also, the number of secondary cases was directly related to the increase in viral load. Higher the viral load, more were the secondary cases (**Figure 2**). On an average, each index case with high viral load spread to 6.2 secondary cases, case with moderate viral load spread to 2.7 secondary cases and same with low vial load spread to 0.8 secondary case. Conclusion of the study was that viral load is an important determinant for transmission of Covid-19 infection in the community. It also advised, viral load based segregation of infected cases, with higher (high & moderate) viral load being quarantined away from their families along with contact tracing of all of them for previous 5 days and subsequent screening of the contacts, believing to be an effective strategy to combat the epidemic.

When the country was grappling in the dark, trying to come up with a suitable strategy to contain the epidemic, Ahmedabad COVID Control Model was developed based on previous study findings. The said model appears to be biologically plausible as the same holds true for other infectious diseases too, such as HIV, malaria, leprosy. Tuberculosis etc. Standing up to the expectations, execution of the Ahmedabad Model of Covid Control exhibited a reasonable reduction in the daily number of new cases within weeks of implementation in June 2020. This model of management did not add any extra cost to the existing health care delivery practices for managing COVID 19 cases. In it, Ct value obtained from the RT-PCR machine needed to be mentioned routinely on the all RT-PCR test reports; thereby indicating high, moderate & low viral load, that helped the healthcare personnel assess the transmissibility of the detected cases. It was assumed that on an average 50% reduction would happen which is largely dependent on dedication & motivation of grass root level community health workers, supportive & effective supervision, timely logistic supply of test facilities including contact tracing, timely referral for institutional quarantine etc. Fortunately, the model concerned had some extra added benefits. For instance, if the health care personnel are aware about who all the patients with high viral load are, they would take some extra precaution while dealing with the latter - thereby reducing the chances of infection among the health care providers. The following **Figures 3** and **4** depict the decline & ascent of daily cases in intervention as well as non-intervention areas following initiation of Ahmedabad Model for COVID 19 Control, which was published as an original

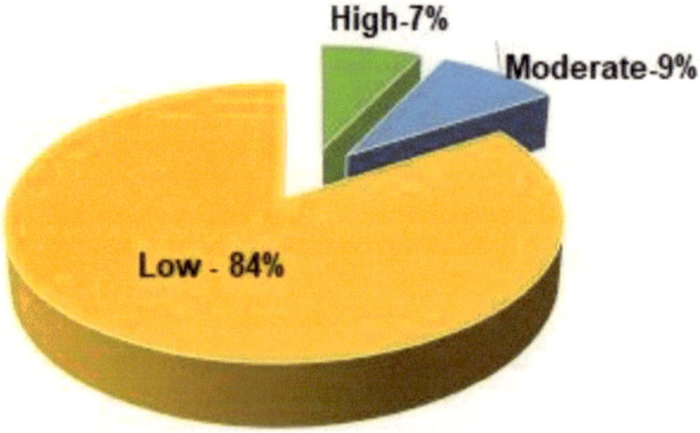

Figure 1.
Distribution of cases with viral load (n = 138) in the studied community.

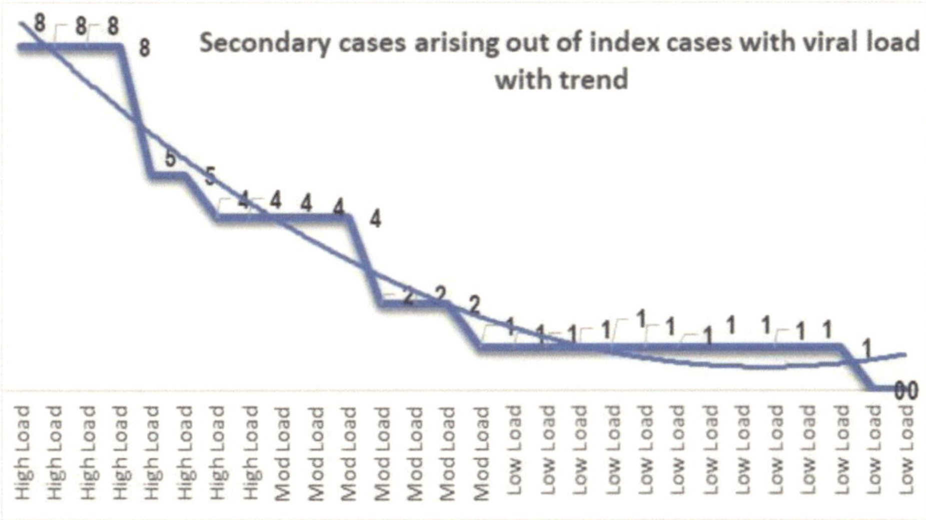

Figure 2.
Secondary cases observed in relation to index cases of high, moderate and low viral load with trend line.

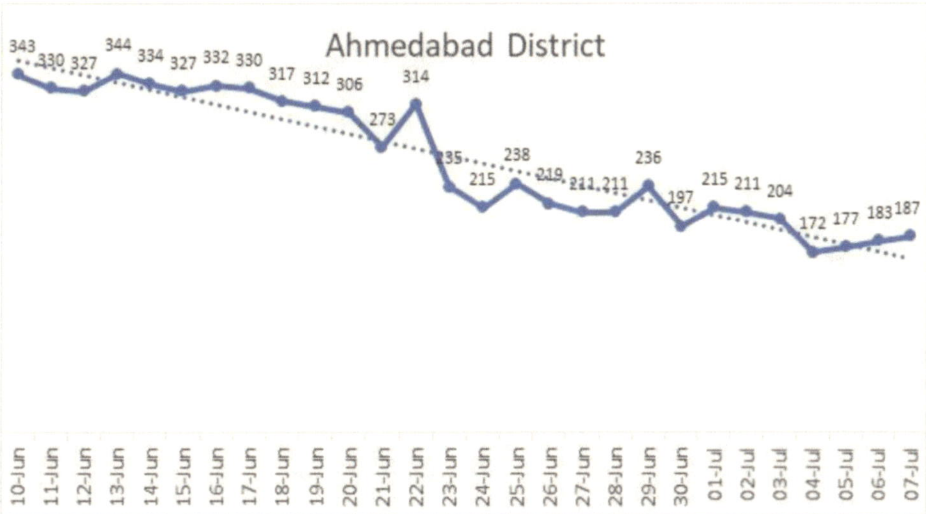

Figure 3.
Daily reported COVID-19 cases in Ahmedabad district 10 June till 07 July.

article titled COVID control strategy – is there any light at the end of the tunnel? in the journal of Family Medicine & Primary Care, 2020; 9:5502-5.

Because of continuous influx of people from UK to India during December 2020 & January 2021, resulting possible emergence of newly detected highly infectious viral strain of Britain in India, Indian Council of Medical Research (ICMR) has instructed various zone-wise Indian laboratories to search for the said infectious Covid 19 strain using cycle threshold (Ct) value of 30 or less considering the fact of their higher infectivity [20]. This again indicates that cycle threshold (Ct) value may be used as a marker of infectiousness or infectivity of Covid 19 transmission. If an appropriate measure is undertaken on time, it can reduce the transmission of cases as was observed in Ahmedabad based study (**Figure 3**), where it was implemented as a method of control.

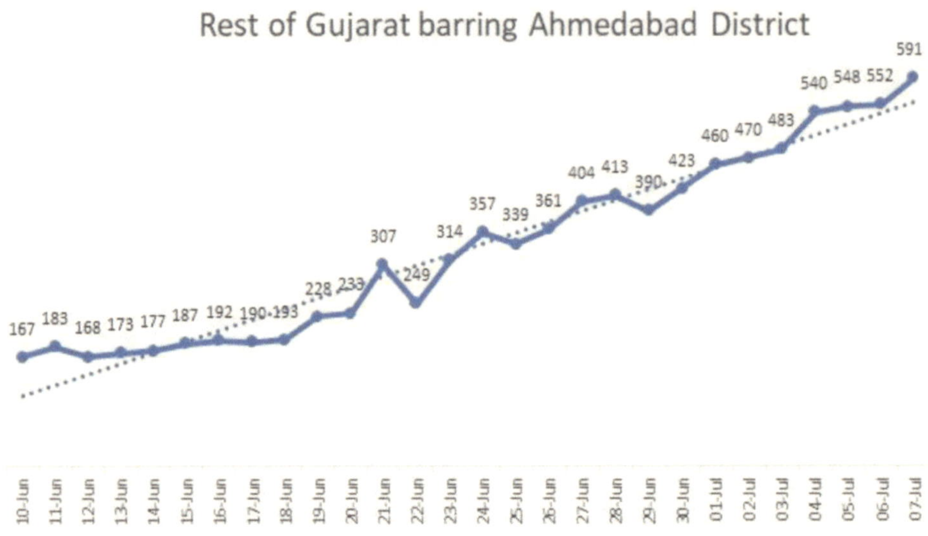

Figure 4.
Daily reported COVID-19 cases in rest of Gujarat State barring Ahmedabad district 10 June till 07 July.

Another study conducted by ICMR-National Institute of Occupational Health, India, showed that viral load is also an important determinant for fomites based transmission too [21]. The study was done on common surfaces such as packaging cardboard and stainless steel surfaces that were smeared with COVID 19 infected materials with known viral load. It showed that fomites contaminated with higher viral load remained infected for a longer period compared to that contaminated with low viral load material. So, viral load is a key factor for the presence of the infectious virus on the surfaces and possibly contributing to the transmission, even after a considerable duration. The viral RNA has higher chances of being identified post-90-min observation period on surfaces contaminated with higher viral load. Therefore surfaces with higher viral load are potentially contagious for longer period as compared to those with lower viral load. The study identified a positive relationship between the viral load of samples used for contaminating the surfaces and viral load of the surfaces post-90-min observation period. The relation was stronger among cardboard surfaces than stainless steel surfaces. A probable explanation can be acquired from the fact that the moist surface of the absorbent cardboard could provide a better harbouring site for viral particles than a non-absorbent surface like stainless steel. The results however partly corroborate with a similar study, where the cultured viral titre was measured over a duration on various surfaces [22]. This study could not suggest the viability of viral particles on the surface but it only assessed the presence of amplifiable viral RNA for specific genes (ORF1ab, in this case). The mentioned study, suggested the viability of these viral particles for over 3 days on these surfaces [21]. The said study was perhaps the earliest from India, to document the relationship between viral load and their detectability on common surfaces. In addition, surfaces with contaminated with relatively higher viral load and with higher absorbability (cardboard) are independently associated with higher risk of COVID-19 retention and transmission. Considering the rapidly evolving literature and experimental procedures, this study was limited by a single sample collection (post 90-minutes observation duration) and did not indicate the viability of viral particle/ virion. Further, the results might be extended to emphasise the need for sterilising such fomite surfaces to prevent viral transmission. Considering the positive relation between viral load and the disease contagiousness [19, 23, 24], the sources (spreader/positive subjects) with high viral load should be treated with great care, i.e., health care facility with possibly high viral load should adopt maximum precautionary measures. The study indicates that fomites could play an important role in the disease transmission in addition to human contact, particularly at COVID-19 care facilities, market places etc. Awareness on fomite-based COVID-19 transmission and the persistence of virion on these surfaces among the health care workers could reduce their risk of contracting COVID-19. Viral load on fomites and the potential role in disease transmission have potential implications in limiting transmission of the recent viral infectious respiratory disease. The above finding has far-reaching public health implications for educating the public in adopting safer behaviour to avoid transmission through fomites. About a fraction of the infected population harbour high viral load and are designated as super spreader which is a matter of great concern [25]. Apart from person to person transmission, the above population would also spread the infection at a much higher rate through fomites unless effective public health controls are undertaken. Similarly, infected cases with moderate vial load would spread the said infection at a moderate rate both by person to person as well as through fomites. Consequently, there should be an effective mass awareness programme using suitable mass awareness education tools by some experienced health care workers. This is more important in places like business areas, shopping malls, market places, tours and travelling, etc., where large gathering occurs with high population mobility and there is every possibility of transmission through fomites apart from person to person spread. So, respective authorities must pay adequate attention to minimise the spread in the above areas as mentioned already.

3. Other factors related to transmission

In Wuhan, China, a novel and alarmingly contagious primary atypical (viral) pneumonia broke out in December 2019. It had since been identified as a zoonotic coronavirus, similar to SARS coronavirus and MERS coronavirus and named COVID-19. As of 8 February 2020, 33738 confirmed cases and 811 deaths were reported in China. Scientists investigated the basic reproduction number (R_0) of the COVID-19 virus considering the fact that R_0 is an indication of the transmissibility of a virus among adjacent population, who are coming in contact to the primary case/s. This investigation found that the estimated mean R_0 for COVID-19 is around 3.28, with a median of 2.79 and IQR of 1.16, which is considerably higher than the WHO estimate of 1.95. The study concluded that the reproductive number of COVID-19 was higher compared to SARS coronavirus. These estimates of R_0 depended on the estimation method used as well as the validity of the underlying assumptions. Due to insufficient data and short onset time as mentioned by the authors, estimates of R_0 for COVID-19 were possibly biased as mentioned in a study [4].

Another study investigated the aerosol and surface stability of HCoV-19 and compared it with SARS-CoV-1, the most closely related human coronavirus. They also looked for the stability of HCoV-19 and SARS-CoV-1 in aerosols and on different surfaces and estimated their decay rates using a Bayesian regression model. The study found that the stability of SARS-CoV-2 was similar to that of SARS-CoV-1 under the experimental circumstances tested. The study concluded saying differences in the epidemiologic characteristics of these viruses probably arise from other factors, including high viral loads in the upper respiratory tract and the potential for persons infected with SARS-CoV-2 to shed and transmit the virus while asymptomatic. The study results indicated that aerosol and fomite transmission of SARS-CoV-2 is plausible, since the virus can remain viable and infectious in aerosols for hours and on surfaces perhaps for days (depending on the inoculum shed).

These findings echo those with SARS-CoV-1, in which these forms of transmission were associated with nosocomial spread and super-spreading events, and they provide information for pandemic mitigation efforts [26].

4. Basic requirements for controlling an epidemic in an area

4.1 Strengthening of inadequate Public Health System

Public Health is defined as a combined system of science & art of preventing diseases, promoting health and protecting lives in a defined geographic area through organised community based efforts. Primary health care is the backbone of public health. Primary health care is an essential health care that should be made available, accessible, acceptable and at a cost that every citizen of the country can afford. Primary health care is based on four principles – Equitable Distribution, Multi-sectoral Approach, Inter-sectoral Coordination and Appropriate Technology. This means resources for improvement of public health infrastructure need to be provided as per felt need of that area; underdeveloped area should receive more resources. In countries with weak public health infrastructure such as India, Bangladesh, Pakistan, Nepal, several African countries among others need their public health strengthened. This means increase of trained human resources (doctors, nurses, public health experts, field workers, etc.), construction of health establishments as per requirements, adequate supply of logistics, storage and transport facilities of vaccines maintaining appropriate temperature, strengthening of immunisation services, strengthening of maternal & child health services, improvement of malnutrition scenario, control of communicable and non-communicable diseases, improvement water and sanitation services etc. Improving all of the above together require an abundance of resources and appropriate planning for judicious usage. Most of the above mentioned countries are not in a position to afford them. Moreover, strong political will appears to be the most important determinant for the said improvement apart from having the resources. Mass awareness is another important issue that helps in generation of demand. Without demand generation by public, things do not move in right direction. A number of social activists, NGOs etc. work to mobilise people to be aware, understand their own needs and generate their demand. Policy makers of the country must be aware of major public health problems of the country so that they can prioritise while developing an appropriate policy for right place at right time. One wrong public health decision will incur heavy cost that the country could have had avoided altogether. Similarly, if an important public health decision is delayed particularly during a public health emergency situation, consequences are increased morbidity & mortality along with other indirect consequences such as loss of job, loss of economy as is being observed in recent COVID 19 epidemic.

4.2 Epidemic preparedness for control of epidemic

4.2.1 Epidemic preparedness team

An epidemic preparedness team comprising an experienced epidemiologist as the chairman, a clinician and a microbiologist as members, is needed to be formed to review the situation of their designated area at regular interval. They need to assess the situation of different regions (based on previous years' situation), the logistic supports needed by them and the services that are necessary for prevention & control of epidemics round the year. They ought to be responsible for arranging necessary training of subordinate staff that will be required for epidemic control. They should develop a set of guidelines/standard operating procedure including dos and don'ts for use by the health workers while dealing with an epidemic. They are also to be responsible for taking necessary measures for tackling any emerging and re-emerging epidemics well in advance such as establishing an effective surveillance system for early detection, creation of a reliable diagnostic services, constructing temporary shelters for emergency evacuation of affected population during public health emergency if needed etc.

4.2.2 Integrated Disease Surveillance Programme

Integrated Disease Surveillance Programme (IDSP) is an important activity for early detection of an epidemic. Surveillance is defined as the process of continuous collection of required information for necessary action such as prevention & control of diseases. Diseases under surveillance are usually classified into groups. Group A comprises diseases where immediate action is needed (within 24 hour), Group B diseases are less severe where necessary actions are taken usually within a week while Group C are diseases where actions are needed to be taken usually within a month. Continuous collection of information on occurrence of various cases from the entire area are sent promptly at the IDSP office to cover the designated geographical area. Based on the reported case/s from a particular area, necessary actions need to be taken by the designated staff as per need of the situation. This is to be done continuously 24-hour x 7 days, round the year to enable early detection of epidemic with necessary intervention. With the advent of newer technology, surveillance can be strengthened further with the help of drones, mobile phone based applications, electronic communication system etc. to collect information from the remote areas.

4.2.3 Regular analysis of data with epidemiological interpretation to assess the situation

Regular analysis of data with epidemiological interpretation is an essential component for early detection of epidemic in an area. Various soft wares are available and used for this purpose such as SPSS, Strata, Epi Info etc. If there is an evidence of existence of epidemic prone case(s) with tendency to increase compared to occurrence of them earlier, it must be brought to notice of IDSP authority/Epidemic Preparedness Team for immediate action/control measures. An all-time functional alert system needs to be generated to alert the authority whenever such a situation arises. This will help detect an epidemic at its early stage. Since timely intervention can reduce the damaging effect of an epidemic to a great extent, detection of an epidemic at its early onset is of utmost importance.

4.2.4 Early and prompt action for containment of epidemic immediately on detection

On receiving information, the epidemic investigation team must move to the spot immediately to verify the existence and magnitude of problem. Steps are needed initially towards controlling epidemic with verification of diagnosis and confirmation of epidemic. Diagnosis may be confirmed by isolating organism from the biological samples collected from the few cases from the affected area. If necessary, required assistance from a nearby laboratory may be sought for isolation of organism and confirmation of diagnosis with the help of microbiologist/virologist present in the epidemic investigation team. Confirmation of epidemic is done by comparing data of present situation with that of previous years. If it is clearly in excess (>2 standard Deviation of average number of cases of previous 3 years), epidemic is confirmed. Once epidemic is confirmed, rapid searching of cases is needed by house to house visit through health workers for further management. While visiting houses and identifying cases, relevant information is collected using a relevant questionnaire to assess the possible source of infection. Once the source(s) are identified, every attempt is to be made to break the chain of transmission, so that epidemic starts to subside. Searching of more number of cases should continue in the community till cases cease to occur. Whenever new cases are identified, they need referral to appropriate health centre for further management. Disposal of infectious material must be taken care of to avoid further spread.

4.2.5 Development of suitable strategy based on felt needs

An important action is making the community aware about the disease, its prevention measures, dos and don'ts, etc. Handling the media is an important aspect since rumours about the disease cause unnecessary panic. Epidemic team members will remain at the spot till epidemic subsides with regular communication to their coordination centre and higher management authority for necessary guidance and support.

4.3 Diagnostics, therapeutics and prophylactics using biotechnology for control of COVID 19

COVID 19 pandemic is complex problem, which needs trans-disciplinary studies. The development of medical biotechnology to produce pharmaceutical and diagnostic products is a need, which needs close collaboration with other disciplines. It should be emphasised that it has been clear that coronaviruses know no borders; therefore, border-less solutions are needed to fight COVID-19. Hopefully the lessons we learned from SARS-CoV-2 will help us to prevent possible pandemic in the near future. Regarding development of diagnostics, one of the crucial factors for control of epidemic is rapid and reliable detection of infected cases with some indication about assessment of its infectivity, if possible. A number of experts across the world have been trying to develop various kits, various machines for use of those kits for detection of causal organisms using various principles of biotechnology. Certain aspects need to be considered while developing kits & related items such as test results must have high sensitivity and high specificity apart from low cost, less time taken, user friendly technique that can be used by peripheral health workers without much fuss. Similarly, in therapeutics, one needs to develop low cost and efficacious drugs or other intervention agents targeting virus entry in the body, multiplication and rapid clearance from the body with minimum side effects.

Since it has been established that viral load is an important determinant for transmission of COVID 19 in the community, hence viral load may be considered an important factor of infectivity. Hence, rapid antigen detection kits that are being developed by various agencies for detection of COVID 19 may contain some indicator for assessing viral load or infectivity. Thanks to biotechnology, addition of indicators is possible and innovators must make sincere efforts towards that as it would help better control of epidemic caused by COVID 19, which was observed in Ahmedabad COVID control model.

4.3.1 Immunity

Following a natural infection, immunity develops through a series of processes that typically takes some time over 1 – 2 week. Human body normally responds to a viral infection immediately with a non-specific innate response in which macrophages, neutrophils, and dendritic cells slow the progress of virus and may even prevent it from causing symptoms. Non-specific response of this kind is usually followed by an adaptive response where the body makes antibodies that specifically bind to the virus. These antibodies are proteins called immunoglobulins. This is known as humoral immunity and B cells of our body are responsible for this process. Human body also makes another groups of cells called T-cells that recognise and eliminate other cells infected with the virus. This is called cellular immunity. Following this, virus may be cleared from the body by combined adaptive response, and if the response is strong enough, may prevent progression to severe illness or re-infection by the same virus. This process is often measured by the presence of antibodies in blood [27]. If a sizable portion of the community population (60 – 70% or more) get infected with COVID 19 infection, it is expected that most of them will develop antibody against COVID 19 infection. Some of the so called uninfected population will also develop antibody against COVID 19 virus, most likely due to subclinical or asymptomatic infection. If their antibody is able to prevent reinfection, it is known as herd immunity or community acquired immunity. Since the disease is new, community-based sero-survey for COVID 19 antibody and its titre can only tell us with certainty whether it is protective against reinfection or not. Similarly, if the cohort is followed up longitudinally with repeated sero-surveys for assessment of antibody titre, duration of protection would be ascertained. It is interesting to know that some of the naturally infected persons do not develop antibody following COVID infection.

4.3.2 Vaccination against COVID 19 Infection

Vaccination is a powerful tool for prevention/control of an epidemic provided it is safe, having a high protective efficacy and given in appropriate time. It is usually used for primary prevention which means it needs to be given before exposure to the infectious agent and occurrence of the disease. Across the world, several types of vaccines are being developed with the hope of combating the COVID-19 pandemic. Yet all the vaccines have the same primary impact - they stimulate the immunity system of the vaccinated individuals to grow memory B cells and T cells against the SARS-CoV-2 virus. These very memory B-cells and T-cells will protect the individuals against subsequent and serious Covid-19 infections.

Vaccination with the first dose will mimic a primary immune response similar to that of being exposed to the virus for the very first time. Mild symptoms of the infection may appear as the immune system gradually develops antibodies against the virus concerned. As a result, if the person is exposed to the virus again or if the subject receives a second dose of vaccine, his or her immunity will flare up and develop what we call a secondary immune response. Initial memory cells get activated. This secondary immune response is faster and much stronger when compared to that of the primary response. This manifests as elevated concentrations of antibodies and higher counts of T-cells. These together help in getting rid of the virus rapidly and thereby prevent occurrence of symptoms, severity and morbidity related to Covid-19. The individual, thus will have more memory B and T cells generated in his or her body; therefore, will have strong immune memory of the Covid-19 virus. It is this immune memory of the individual that will help him or her battle against the infection.

Vaccination and immunity development can be categorised into two types: ACTIVE IMMUNITY and PASSIVE IMMUNITY.

4.3.2.1 ACTIVE immunity

DNA Vaccines, RNA Vaccines, Viral Vectors, Viral Sub-units, Live Attenuated, Inactivated Virus, VLP or Virus-Like Particles, Split Virus Vaccines, RNP (Ribonucleoprotein) Vaccines.

4.3.2.2 PASSIVE Immunity

Antibodies (MONOCLONAL and POLYCLONAL), Convalescent Serum, mRNA induced Antibody.

Considering the chaos and the panic this pandemic has ensued, developing vaccines and immunising the population as soon as possible, is of immense importance - especially folks belonging to high risk groups, vulnerable groups and pockets that have been badly affected by this infection. This would help contain the disease and reduce not only spreading of the infection but also the morbidity and mortality associated with it. Thus vaccines happen to be an important tool in public health control of pandemic and epidemic. Substantial research is being undertaken to develop effective vaccines that would help check the disease spread adequately.

Since in a highly populous country or in resource poor setting, availability of vaccines may not be adequate compared to its number of recipients, particularly in the beginning, certain categories of people may be considered for immunisation on priority basis depending on country's situation:

a. Health care personnel

b. Essential workers such as law & order maintenance workers (police personnel)

c. Patients with comorbidities like Diabetes, Hypertension, Bronchial Asthma

d. Subjects over the age of 65 years

e. Street residents and slum dwellers

Manufacturing agency such as PFIZER and MODERNA have been working to develop mRNA Covid-19 vaccines where genetically sequenced spike proteins of COVID 19 virus is injected in body as vaccine and molecules of the virus' messenger RNA will be recognised and targeted by our immune systems as the antigen. Then the immunity system will get triggered enough to produce antibodies against the said virus [28].

Serum Institute of India, Pune has teamed up with British-Swedish OXFORD-ASTRAZENECA to launch *COVISHIELD* in India. It is a viral vector vaccine where viruses are being modified to hold the target pathogen and then these modified organisms are administered via the vaccines. These in the human body, will initiate and develop immunity against covid-19. Chimpanzee Adenovirus is being used to deliver the corona virus antigen in this SII vaccine. Participant enrolment and vaccination of Phase III Human Clinical Trial COMPLETED [29].

COVAXIN - Whole-Virion Inactivated SARS-CoV-2 Vaccine (BBV152) is India's indigenous Covid-19 vaccine and is being developed by India based manufacturing agency, BHARAT BIOTECH, in collaboration with ICMR - National Institute of Virology, Government of India. It is in its Phase III Human Clinical Trial. *ZyCoV-D* is a plasmid DNA vaccine being developed by ZYDUS CADILA, another Indian manufacturing agency and is on its Phase II Human Clinical Trial [29].

SPUTNIK V - DR. REDDY'S LABORATORIES LIMITED [Russian and Indian collaboration] and SPUTNIK LLC are jointly conducting Phase II Human Clinical Trial to assess safety and immunogenicity of Gam-COVID-Vac combined vector vaccine [29].

Biological E. Limited has developed a vaccine and is conducting studies to assess the safety, reactogenicity and immunogenicity of the vaccine containing Receptor Binding Domain of SARS-CoV-2 for protection against Covid-19 disease when administered to healthy volunteers on days 0 and 28, intramuscularly [29].

COVISHIELD has demonstrated efficacy of 70.4% against symptomatic Covid-19 and 100% efficacy against hospitalisation due to severe Covid-19. The Sputnik vaccine has demonstrated 92% efficacy. According to FDA, the Moderna vaccine was 94.1% effective at preventing symptomatic cases. The Pfizer vaccine has claimed 95% effectiveness.

The mentioned vaccines have undergone/are undergoing immunogenicity, efficacy and safety trials in 18 Years and above and hence will be allowed to be used in adults under "Emergency Use Authorisation." Only Pfizer's vaccine was authorised for people ages 16 and up in USA. Trials are underway for age group 12-18 and in due course of time the vaccines may be allowed to be used in this age group. Also no conclusive study in pregnant women have been conducted - so safety during pregnancy cannot be ascertained yet. Since surveys have not been conducted to establish the need or the lack of need for vaccines in individuals who already have had the disease, these recovered individuals may be considered last for vaccination.

As seen till now, one would require to get two shots of the same vaccine - 0.5 ml each dose, to attain a desired level of protection. The 2 doses Moderna and Covishield are to be taken 28 days apart while the 2 doses of Pfizer and Sputnik V are to be taken 21 days apart. Usually it takes about 14 days for the antibody formation but the mRNA vaccine of Pfizer has demonstrated response as early as 10 days after the 1st dose. One should remember two shots of the vaccine is not enough to protect one completely. Covid-19 is a brand new disease; the scientists, doctors, society and humankind are all learning more about it as days pass by. A vaccinated person most likely will not develop the disease or be severely ill but he may get infected if hand hygiene, respiratory hygiene, physical distancing and proper mask usage are not maintained. And if infected, chances of him spreading the infection will increase manifold. Therefore, it is important to follow the rules of the new normal even after vaccination.

4.4 Research to explore effective mechanisms to contain at an affordable cost

More operational and translational research works are needed to explore alternative control mechanisms such as newer diagnostics, therapeutic and prophylactic agents at an affordable cost. We also need to have various environmental measures where virus does not survive or virus transmission chain could be broken using bio-technology principles. Personal protective devices such face masks, various hand hygiene devices, disinfection devices may be made using novel techniques without major health hazards based on bio-technology principles. Disposal of used face masks, many of which are made of synthetic/non-bio-degradable materials is a threat to our environment. Hence suitable material that are bio-degradable and at the same time protects from virus without hampering oxygen supply to our body should be thought of. Suitable disinfection devices for disinfecting used non-disposable/re-usable items of health care personnel is needed particularly for rural health system of developing countries. Mobile van fitted with disinfection devices using engineering expertise along with bio-technology skill could be helpful as it could cover a number of health centres in a day for disinfecting their used items.

Necessity is the mother of invention – appears to be true as it is observed that many medical, engineering and bio-technology students are coming up with brilliant and innovative ideas for interrupting COVID virus transmission. Innovations of this kind must be encouraged.

5. Suggested measures for controlling an epidemic of COVID 19

One needs to understand about how an imported epidemic starts and progresses its course as time passes by. Based on our understanding it may be categorised as:

1. Stage I: Imported transmission - Initially cases occur only in people return from foreign countries, foreign visitors came to a country for business or tourism purpose etc. and their contacts.

2. Stage II: Cluster transmission – The disease spreads from above infected group to nearby local population usually confined to smaller geographic area where source of infection is by and large traceable.

3. Stage III: Community transmission – A large number of people are infected simultaneously in different parts of the area within a large geographic area and where source of infection is not identifiable for a large section of population

4. Stage IV: Declined and low level transmission – When epidemic curve declines after reaching plateau but cases still continue to occur in areas at much lower level involving relatively fewer populations.

It may be noted that incubation period of COVID 19 infection ranges between 2 to 14 days with an average incubation period of 5–7 days. Maximum colonisation of virus occurs in oropharynx and naso-pharynx on second or third day from the onset of symptoms of an infected person. Hence maximum chance of transmission of virus from an infected person in his/her early days following development of symptoms. As a result, chance of transmission is relatively higher following detection by RT-PCR (considering the fact that patient usually comes on second day following onset of symptoms), when there is an opportunity of intervention. If that opportunity is missed, infection will keep on spreading in nearby population. On the other hand, it is easily understood that an epidemic is easy to control if it is detected early when very few people are affected. In the event of any delay in detection and/or lack of required intervention at the beginning due to any reason, the community/ country needs to pay a heavy price for that. COVID 19 epidemic is the best example of it in recent time. Apart from direct consequences of high morbidity and mortality, indirect consequences are havoc such as downfall of country's economy, loss of jobs, loss of wages, poverty, starvation leading to malnutrition, increase of mental diseases etc. It may be kept in mind that because of high global population movement, any infectious disease with pandemic or high epidemic potential, it may spread to people of other parts of the world with the passage to time unless strict vigilance and control activities are undertaken rigidly.

COVID-19 test detects genetic material of the virus using a laboratory technique called real time RT-PCR reaction (Real-Time Reverse Transcription – Polymerase Chain Reaction). RT-PCR testing can tell us whether there is a detectable virus present in an individual. Still, it does not accurately tell us whether that individual is infectious or is capable of spreading the disease. Cell culture is the standard technique for determining whether a patient is contagious or not. In the absence of viral culture data, one can use viral load or cycle threshold (Ct) values derived from RT-PCR as a proxy for the likelihood of transmission. RT-PCR is a sensitive technique for mRNA detection and quantification currently available. It is a laboratory technique facilitating reverse transcription of RNA into DNA and amplification of specific DNA targets using polymerase chain reaction (PCR). It primarily wants to measure the quantity of a selected RNA. This is achieved by the amplification reaction using fluorescence, a way called real-time PCR or quantitative PCR (qPCR). Combined RT-PCR and qPCR are routinely used for analysis of organic phenomenon and quantification of viral RNA in research and clinical settings. Compared to the two other commonly used techniques for quantifying mRNA levels, Northern blot analysis and RNase protection assay, RT-PCR wants to quantify mRNA levels from much smaller samples. In fact, this system is sensitive enough to enable quantitation of RNA even from one cell. In a real time PCR assay a positive reaction is detected by accumulation of a fluorescent signal. The Ct (cycle threshold) is defined as the number of amplification cycles required for the fluorescent signal to cross the limit (i.e. exceeds set detection level). In other words, The Ct is the number of replication cycles required for a signal of RT-PCR product to cross a determined threshold. Ct values are inversely proportional to the quantity of target nucleic acid within the sample (i.e. the lower the Ct level the greater the quantity of targeted nucleic acid within the sample).

Considering above, it appears with reasonable certainty that viral load during early infection is an important determinant for transmission in the community by various routes including fomites based transmission. If viral load is high, chance of transmission is higher among nearby susceptible population with lack of proper precaution. Medical fraternity caring COVID 19 patients must take it seriously as many of the patients attended by them are with higher viral load with increased transmission potential and any lapse of precautionary measures on their part would make many of them infected as was observed in several countries. It is understood that virus multiplication occurs within first few days inside the body of an infected person. Antiviral agents such as Remdesevir may be beneficial not only for the patients but also for the attending health care personnel as it helps in reducing transmission to them by reducing viral load if given early in the disease. It is understood that there is hardly any benefit if anti-viral agents are given in late phase of the disease.

It is now evident that magnitude of viral load may be obtained easily from RT-PCR test of a COVID 19 positive case without any extra cost. More the cycle threshold (Ct) value, lower is the viral load (inversely related). Similarly, lower is the Ct value, higher is the viral load. Any Ct value of 35 and higher is considered as non-infectious although infected. Similarly, Ct value of 20 or below may be considered as highly infectious with higher transmission potential. Recently a number of qualitative COVID 19 detection kits are available in the market (such as rapid antigen detection kit) that does not indicate Ct value based viral load. Further studies are required to add viral load assessing facility in those rapid antigen detection kits for assessing infectivity of an infected case. Apart from viral load, it is now obvious that transmission will occur if favourable conditions are available such lack of protection measures, population density, population mobility, lack of awareness about the disease etc. So, mass awareness is an essential component of any public health control measures.

It is a fact that many countries in the world do not have an effective public health infrastructure such as required number of doctors, nurses, field workers, health technicians etc. as per WHO set guidelines, required number of various tiers of health establishments such as primary. Secondary and tertiary level of health establishments, diagnostics facilities, cold chain maintenance facilities and epidemic/infection control policy & strategies etc. Unless proper logistics supports are available, vaccination is not possible even if it is made available. Hence, prevention of occurrence of cases much before it turns to an epidemic proportion should be a better choice. Appropriate infection control policy with an effective infection control strategy must be made available with experienced public health experts.

To summarise, COVID control strategies may include (based on already established evidence) the followings:

1. Viral load indicated by Ct value could be used as an indicator of infectiousness of an infected person. Cases with high and moderate viral load must be kept away from the family/community even if they are asymptomatic or mildly symptomatic to avoid further transmission particularly in under-privileged areas, rural and slum areas.

2. Ct value based segregation identifying higher infectious cases along with contact tracing of them of previous 5 days appears to be an effective strategy as was observed in Ahmedabad Covid 19 infection Control programme.

3. Health care workers need to know their patients' Ct value on admission to hospital/health centre to enable them to remain more careful about the transmission potential of patients.

4. Effective implementation of it in primary health care set up would better utilise country's rural public health infrastructure.

5. Asymptomatic and mild symptomatic cases with low viral load may be kept at home with standard precaution.

6. Moderate and severe symptomatic cases need to be referred to Covid hospital for further management.

Home quarantine for cases with higher viral load is expected to facilitate intra-familial transmission of COVID 19 cases in other family members, hence it is not suggested. On the other hand, same with low viral load may be quarantined at home with standard physical distancing, hand hygiene and face mask. Presently COVID 19 epidemic is largely concentrated on cities & urban areas that are gradually approaching towards semi-urban/rural areas through population movement. More number of rural population are expected to become infected in coming days since 60 to 70% of developing country's population reside in villages. Considering above, primary health care physicians must prepare themselves on Ct value-based segregation of COVID 19 infected cases with contact tracing of cases with high & moderate viral load of previous five days to reduce transmission of cases in the community. This will also reduce hospitalisation of cases & deaths and help improving bed availability, thereby better utilisation of public health infrastructure would be possible. Extensive community awareness about prevention & control of COVID 19 infection along with role of viral load. Ct value is essential for that. One needs to remember that success of Ct value based segregation will largely depend on dedication and motivation of grass root level field workers. If they work sincerely with supportive supervision by their immediate supervisors and higher leaders, cases are expected to decline soon, leading to control of epidemic. Proper training of various categories of health workers as well as logistic support must be in place. Moderate to severe symptomatic persons need to be referred to nearby hospital/health centre for management of COVID 19 infection. Asymptomatic and mild symptomatic may be sent to home or institutional quarantine as per their reported viral load as mentioned already.

We need to understand that to control an epidemic with high transmission potential such as COVID 19, multiple strategy based attacks are needed to break the all possible transmission chains. Vaccines whenever possible must be considered in addition to other public health measures. Safety & protective efficacy must be assured of a vaccine before going for mass vaccination in a community. Since the disease is new and vaccine(s) are also new, continuous monitoring & supervision of the recipients of vaccines are needed. Cases with vaccines failure must be identified early for their alternative protection against this disease. Detailed epidemiological information may be collected about possible factor/s that are associated with vaccine failure. Since, COVID 19 is originated from RNA virus, frequent genetic mutation is possible over a period with consequent changes of its virulence and also its epidemic transmission potential. Herd immunity may be another important factor that develops from earlier infection or due to vaccination to a section of population of the community. Monitoring of above issues from time to time will be helpful for taking a judicious decision about vaccination strategy for a particular community. It may also be noted that most epidemics undergo a natural decline as time passes by, irrespective of intervention measures undertaken or not. That does not mean that intervention is not important as delay in intervention measure increases morbidity and mortality. Last but not the least, there is no single strategy or a straight forward pathway to control the epidemic. Rather it is a diversified and complex mechanism which is based on various situations and interplay of agent, host and environmental factors. A judicious planning, timely intervention and efficient management with required logistic support services can reduce human sufferings to a great extent.

Lastly, it was observed that an overall 35% (21 out of 60) asymptomatic infected cases got detected while doing contact tracing in a community based study in western India (unpublished data). The magnitude of asymptomatic cases was higher with cases of low viral load (46.6%), whereas it was about 20% with cases of high viral load. Asymptomatic cases of higher viral load would spread the disease at higher rate, similar to that of symptomatic cases. Hence, precautionary measures such as hand hygiene, face mask, physical distancing etc. are extremely important and required to be practiced by all considering the fact that everyone around us is potentially infected and could transmit the disease. So, community people need to be educated about transmissibility of asymptomatic infection and about ways of its prevention. Similarly, awareness about safe disposal of their used items considering the possibility of transmission from them is equally important too.

6. Continuous vigilance for variant of mutant strain of COVID 19 if any

Recently, mutation of SarsCov2, namely N501Y, has been reported in the United Kingdom and linking it to further increased transmissibility. It is a matter of great concern, especially at a time when the emergence of vaccines has brought joy and expectation for the mass population. The new UK strain designated as VUI2020/12/01 (variant under investigation, year 2020, month 12, variant type 01) has recorded over 20 mutations, mostly silent, causing no change in the protein. Biologically, mutations represent steps in virus evolution under selection pressure of the host immunity. Scientists view these as a process evolved by the virus to escape immunity or to enhance transmissibility. As the virus replicates, mutations happen in its genes continually through a process called "antigenic drift", causing minor changes in the surface protein. However, changes of this kind could accumulate over time, and result in newer viruses that could become antigenically different such that the existing antibodies mounted by the host immune system to the original virus fail to recognise and neutralise them [30].

Scientists wish to have the answer about mechanism of these mutations and whether there is a role for host immunity in driving them? More importantly, could antibody treatment or other therapies have an influence in the process? The preprint of a recently submitted paper to medRxiv portal by the group in Cambridge, UK, led by Dr. Ravinder Gupta, has focused exactly on these issues [31]. The above study is based on a single case report of an immune compromised individual with chronic SARSCoV-2 infection, lasting over 100 days and treated with three units of convalescent plasma, two on day 65 and one on day 95 in an effort to neutralise the virus and treat the chronic infection. The virus was detectable in all his nasal swab samples collected at least 23 times over a period of 101 days, despite the plasma therapy. The authors investigated the SARS-CoV-2 evolution and found important changes in its genome caused by two new mutations in the spike protein, one a deletion of AA Histidine and Valine at positions 69 and 70 and, two, one AA replacement at position 796 (D796H). The authors state that while the two mutations did not increase infectivity of the virus, these might have been responsible for decreased sensitivity of the patient to convalescent therapy. Since it is a single case report, the results of the study is not generalizable. But, it raises an important issue of generation of "escape mutants" of the virus in patients with persistent infection. The virus escaped attack by neutralising antibodies present in the convalescent plasma. Continuous vigilance of such newer strains is needed particularly for both their transmissibility and potential to evade vaccine-mediated immunity. The emergence of new mutants of the coronavirus further emphasises the need for observing infection-control practices even more strictly and until the protective herd immunity is developed.

Epidemiologically, continuous collection of pertinent information is required to look for evolution of any variant or mutant strains over a period particularly with higher virulence and more destructing effect to human. Investigation facilities such as ability to perform genetic sequencing for matching newer strain with original virus is needed to identify them. It is obvious that earlier the detection, better actions to control the epidemic is possible. Finally, we wish to conclude that Ahmedabad COVID Control Model appears to be an important evidence in documenting the purpose of this chapter [32].

Author details

Bidisa Sarkar[1] and Kamalesh Sarkar[2*]

1 Department of Community Medicine, Kalinga Institute of Medical Sciences, Odisha, India

2 ICMR-National Institute of Occupational Health, Gujarat, India

*Address all correspondence to: kamalesh.sarkar@gmail.com

References

[1] Guo YR, Cao QD, Hong ZS, Tan YY, Chen SD, Jin HJ, et al. The origin, transmission and clinical therapies on coronavirus disease 2019 (COVID-19) outbreak-An update on the status. Mil Med Res 2020; 7:11.

[2] Heesterbeek JA, Dietz K. The concept of Ro in epidemic theory. Stat Neerl 1996; 50:89-110.

[3] Stuart B, Martin C, Supamit C, Vladimir D, Didier H, Youngmee J, et al. Statement on the meeting of the international health regulations (2005) emergency committee regarding the outbreak of novel coronavirus (2019-nCoV). Geneva: World Health Organization (WHO); 2020.

[4] Liu Y, Gayle AA, Wilder-Smith A, Rocklöv J. The reproductive number of COVID-19 is higher compared to SARS coronavirus. J Travel Med. 2020:13;27: taaa021. doi: 10.1093/jtm/taaa021. PMID: 32052846; PMCID: PMC7074654.

[5] Bauch CT, Lloyd-Smith JO, Coffee MP, Galvani AP. Dynamically modeling SARS and other newly emerging respiratory illnesses: Past, present, and future. Epidemiology 2005; 16:791-801.

[6] Centers for Disease Control and Prevention (CDC). Severe acute respiratory Syndrome-Singapore, 2003. MMWR Morb Mortal Wkly Rep 2003; 52:405-411.

[7] Dye C, Gay N. Epidemiology. Modeling the SARS epidemic. Science 2003; 300:1884-1885.

[8] Kucharski AJ, Althaus CL. The role of super spreading in Middle East respiratory syndrome coronavirus (MERS-CoV) transmission. Euro Surveill 2015; 20:14-18.

[9] Lipsitch M, Cohen T, Cooper B, Robins JM, Ma S, James L, et al. Transmission dynamics and control of severe acute respiratory syndrome. Science 2003; 300:1966-1970.

[10] Riley S, Fraser C, Donnelly CA, Ghani AC, Abu-Raddad LJ, Hedley AJ, et al. Transmission dynamics of the etiological agent of SARS in Hong Kong: Impact of public health interventions. Science 2003; 300:1961-1966.

[11] Shen Z, Ning F, Zhou W, He X, Lin C, Chin DP, et al. Super spreading SARS events, Beijing, 2003. Emerg Infect Dis 2004; 10:256-260.

[12] Li Y, Yu IT, Xu P, Lee JH, Wong TW, Ooi PL, et al. Predicting super spreading events during the 2003 severe acute respiratory syndrome epidemics in Hong Kong and Singapore. Am J Epidemiol 2004; 160:719-728.

[13] Lloyd-Smith JO, Schreiber SJ, Kopp PE, Getz WM. Super spreading and the effect of individual variation on disease emergence. Nature 2005; 438:355-359.

[14] Endo A, Centre for the Mathematical Modelling of Infectious Diseases COVID-19 Working Group; Abbott S, Kucharski AJ, Funk S. Estimating the over dispersion in COVID-19 transmission using outbreak sizes outside China. Welcome Open Res 2020; 5:67.

[15] Elrashdy F, Redwan EM, Uversky VN. Why COVID-19 Transmission Is More Efficient and Aggressive Than Viral Transmission in Previous Coronavirus Epidemics? Biomolecules. 2020 Sep 11;10(9):1312. doi: 10.3390/biom10091312. PMID: 32933047; PMCID: PMC7565143.

[16] COVID scenario in India. [cited 2020 Jun 30]. Available from: https://www.covid19india.org/.

[17] Test, test, test: Eight Steps India must take to tackle the coronavirus epidemic by Indranil Mukherjee, published on April 3, 2020 [cited 2020 May 11]. Available from: https://scroll.in/pulse/958091/test-test-test-eight-steps-indiamust-take-to-tackle-the-coronavirus-epidemic.

[18] Letter to the PM addressing issues of scaling up access to free testing and treatment for COVID19 by PHMINDIA_JSA, published on March 25, 2020 [cited 2020 Apr 7]. Available from: http://phmindia.org/2020/03/25/letter-to-the-pmaddressing-issues-of-scaling-up-access-to-free-testing-andtreatment-for-covid19/

[19] Sarkar B, Sinha RN, Sarkar K. Initial viral load of a COVID-19-infected case indicated by its cycle threshold value of polymerase chain reaction could be used as a predictor of its transmissibility - An experience from Gujarat, India. Indian J Community Med 2020; 45:278-282.

[20] Article on THE TIMES OF INDIA, accessed on Dec 31, 2020 - available through: https://timesofindia.indiatimes.com/india/india-split-into-6-regions-in-massive-hunt-for-uk-strain/articleshow/80035844.cms

[21] Singh DP, Sahu MC, Pagdhune A, Viramgami A, Perumal S, Balachandar R, et al. Viral load could be an important determinant for fomites based transmission of viral infections. J Family Med Prim Care 2021 (in press)

[22] van Doremalen N, Bushmaker T, Morris DH, Holbrook MG, Gamble A, Williamson BN, et al. Aerosol and surface stability of SARS-CoV-2 as compared with SARS-CoV-1. N Engl J Med 2020;382:1564-1567

[23] Rao SN, Manissero D, Steele VR, Pareja J. A systematic review of the clinical utility of cycle threshold values in the context of COVID-19. Infect Dis Ther 2020; 9:573-586.

[24] Shrestha NK, Marco Canosa F, Nowacki AS, Procop GW, Vogel S, Fraser TG, et al. Distribution of transmission potential during non-severe COVID-19 illness. Clin Infect Dis 2020. doi: 10.1093/cid/ciaa886

[25] Paul J. High viral load: Only a few spread the most Covid-19 infections, reveals Ahmedabad's NIOH study, in Times of India. 2020, Times News Network: Ahmedabad.

[26] Neeltje van Doremalen, Trenton Bushmaker, Dylan H. Morris, Myndi G. Holbrook, Amandine Gamble, Brandi N. Williamson, Azaibi Tamin, Jennifer L. Harcourt, Natalie J. Thornburg, Susan I. Gerber, James O. Lloyd-Smith, Emmie de Wit, Vincent J. Munster. Aerosol and surface stability of HCoV-19 (SARS-CoV-2) compared to SARS-CoV-1; The New England Journal of Medicine doi: 10.1056/NEJMc2004973

[27] Immunity passports in the context of COVID 19. World Health Organisation; 24 April 2020; Available through: https://www.who.int/news-room/commentaries/detail/immunity-passports-in-the-context-of-covid-19 on 31 December 2020

[28] Online portal for Health News, accessed on Dec 29, 2020; available through https://www.health.com/condition/infectious-diseases/coronavirus/difference-between-pfizer-moderna-vaccine

[29] ICMR Website accessed on Dec 29, 2020; available through https://vaccine.icmr.org.in/covid-19-vaccine

[30] Prof. N.K. Mehra. The Hindustan Times, Thursday, 31 December 2020 Available through file:///C:/Users/admin/Downloads/Dr%20NK%20Mehra%20Sir_Mutant%20Strain..._HTDEL_31122020. pdf and accessed on 31.12.2020

[31] U.K. variant puts spotlight on immunocompromised patients' role in the COVID-19 pandemic. Science Magazine, UK, By Kai Kupferschmidt Dec. 23, 2020, 2:30 PM. Available through https://www.sciencemag.org/news/2020/12/uk-variant-puts-spotlight-immunocompromised-patients-role-covid-19-pandemic; accessed on 31.12.2020

[32] Sarkar B, Sarkar K, Sengupta P. COVID control strategy-is there any light at the end of the tunnel? J Family Med Prim Care 2020;9:5502-5

Chapter 3

Whole Genome Sequencing: A Powerful Tool for Understanding the Diversity of Genotypes and Phenotypes among COVID-19 Infected Patients to Help in Controlling Outbreaks

Rayan A. Ahmed

Abstract

In Wuhan, China (December 2019), viral pneumonia cases of uncertain origin have been reported. The emergency has drawn global attention. To determine the pathogenic potential, joint efforts were conducted by Chinese Multidisciplinary Task Forces. An integral component of wide range of research applications is not only determining the causative agent but also the nucleic acid bases order in biological samples. Research techniques determining genetic material features and its order is called "sequencing", classified into three generations. Moreover, the first sequencing attempt was conducted and a genetic link identified between samples isolated from China and other previously sequenced Coronaviruses. However, there was patient to patient diversity in terms of clinical and laboratory manifestations and diseases severity. After the genetic material of the causative agent was successfully sequenced, it was named the novel coronavirus causing COVID-19. Here, we review the genome sequences of novel coronavirus infected patients from different countries such as India, Bangladesh and Ecuador compared to China (first reported case), seeking not only to recognize similarities and differences between genome sequences of novel coronavirus, but also to compare them with other forms of coronaviruses family. Utilizing this data will assist in making right decisions minimizing negative consequences of the outbreak.

Keywords: whole genome sequencing (WGS), sequencing, sequencer genotype, phenotype, novel-coronaviruse, SARS-CoV-2, COVID-19

1. Introduction

A number of viral pneumonia cases of uncertain origin arose in late of December 2019 (Wuhan, Hubei Province of China). These cases have gained public attention and considered an emergency. The Public Health Emergency of International Concern and the World Health Organization (WHO) have declared "epidemic" [1]. Thereafter, the Multidisciplinary Task Forces under the organization of the National Health Commission of the People's Republic of China undertook collective efforts to define the causative agent. At the beginning, a group of researchers from the Chinese Academy of Medical Sciences has announced their study on the causative agent identification. Basically, they conducted a metagenomic study of specimens of the respiratory tract collected from five patients who had pneumonia. After they have successfully isolated the virus and carried out the genomic sequencing, the results have revealed that it belongs to the beta-coronavirus family [1, 2].

In more details, the results from their project showed that the genomic analysis of the specimens have approximately 79 percent homology to the Acute Respiratory Syndrome (SARS) Coronavirus (SARS-CoV) genome, approximately 52 percent similarity to the Middle East Respiratory Syndrome Coronavirus (MERS-CoV), and approximately 87 percent similarity to two bat-derived SARS-like coronavirus genomes (Zhoushan, 2015) [2]. Likewise, identical findings were published by a team from the Chinese Center for Disease Control and Prevention [3]. Such proof, the isolated virus was proposed to be a novel coronavirus and this novel coronavirus later dubbed the novel coronavirus 2019 (nCoV 2019), quickly recognized by the WHO as the pathogen accountable for this transmissible illness [1].

2. Sequencing

The arrangement of nucleic acids inside the chains of polynucleotides provides the details of inherited and biochemical characteristics of life. Determining the order of nucleic acid sequences in biomolecules is a crucial part of a wide range of research applications. Huge numbers of researchers have spent the last fifty years developing technological approaches to simplify sequencing of (DNA and RNA) molecules. During this time span, significant changes were being seen ranging from short to very long oligonucleotide sequencing, from struggling to deduct a single gene's coding sequence to quick and widely available sequencing of the whole genome [1]. In this section we will go over the several generations of the nucleic acids sequencing indicting the major discoveries, impact of researchers and the major characteristics of (first, second and third) generations sequencing technology.

2.1 First-generation nucleic acids sequencing

James D. Watson and Francis H.C. Crick are two scientists who were able to discover the three-dimensional structure of DNA (1953). Watson and Crick were working on crystallographic data provided by Maurice and Rosalind Franklin Wilkins, contributed to both DNA replication conceptual frameworks and the transcription of proteins in the nucleic acids. However, reading the sequence is not achieved yet [1, 2]. The initial efforts were concentrated on sequencing RNA molecule which is not as complicated as the DNA molecule.

Frederick Sanger said "knowledge of sequences could contribute much to our understanding of living matter." In a collaboration with other scientists, Sanger was able to create a new technology based on the determination of radiolabeled partial-digestion fragments after two-dimensional fractionation (1965) [3], allowing the scientists to continuously build on the growing pool of RNA (ribosomal and transfer) sequences [4–8]. In the same year, Robert Holley and colleagues generated, for the first time, the whole nucleic acid sequence of alanine transfer RNA isolated from *Saccharomyces cerevisiae* [9]. Utilizing these techniques enabled Walter Fiers and colleagues, in the period of 1972–1976, to produce the first complete protein coding gene sequence and then the whole genome of bacteriophage MS2 [10, 11]. In the mid of seventies, a strong impact was produced to get much greater resolution by replacing two steps two-dimensional fractionation with one step as single electrophoresis separation through polyacrylamide gel (considered the birth of 1st generation) [3, 12, 13]. Using this procedure, in 1977, Sanger and colleagues were able for the first time to sequence the bacteriophage X174 or (PhiX) genetic material, becoming a positive control in sequencing genome laboratories [14]. In the same year, establishment of Sanger's "chain-termination" or dideoxy method produced a huge advancement in DNA sequencing technology [15]. Subsequently, tremendous efforts were made to generate an automated DNA sequencing technology and the first commercially available machine was made for sequencing the highly complex species genome [1, 16–22].

One of the major drawbacks of the first-generation nucleic acids sequencing machines is reading short base pairs below a kilo base (kb); however, scientists tried to overcome this issue by techniques an example of which is Shotgun sequencing method in which individual cloning and sequencing of two parts of DNA will be carried out and then compiled into a long sequence [23, 24].

Nonetheless, many improvements were made to the sequencing of first-generation nucleic acids that eventually ended with new dideoxy sequencers an example of which is the ABI PRISM created by Applied Biosystems from Leroy Hood's research. This sequencer allowed hundreds of samples to be sequenced concurrently and was used in the generating the first draft of Human Genome Project completed years ahead of schedule [25–28].

2.2 Second-generation nucleic acids sequencing

The luminescent method for measuring pyrophosphate synthesis was the starting point for the second generation of DNA sequencers. Basically, it is a two-enzymes reaction where ATP sulphurylase converts pyrophosphate to ATP as a luciferase substrate. Light generation is thus proportional to the amount of pyrophosphate [29].

Pyrosequencing was later licensed to 454 Life Sciences, a Jonathan Rothburg-founded biotechnology corporation, which grew into the first major successful technology as a commercially available next-generation sequencing (NGS). The 454-sequence equipment, later bought via Roche, were a paradigm shift allowed sequencing reactions to be mass parallelized, considerably raising the amount of DNA sequenced in a single experiment [30].

The parallelization technique rises the yield of sequencing efforts by order of magnitudes, enabling scientists to fully sequence a whole human genome belonging to the developer of the DNA structure, James Watson, with much low-priced and faster than a similar effort exerted by the team of DNA sequencing entrepreneur Craig Venter exploitation Sanger sequencing method [31, 32]. The novel 454 machine, called the GS 20 later replaced by the 454 GS FLX which provides not only better-quality data but also higher numeral of readings attributed to having more wells in the pico-titer plate. Indeed, it was the first high-throughput sequencing machine (HTS) broadly accessible to customers. Moreover, the concept of having massive numbers of parallel sequencing reactions on a micrometer measure improves microfabrication and high-resolution imaging and this is actually what defined the second-generation of DNA sequencing [26, 33].

Furthermore, after the success of 454, there were several parallel sequencing methods suddenly emerged. Arguably, the most vital one is the Solexa technique of sequencing developed by Illumina [33]. The concept of this process based what they call bridge amplification. Basically, adapter-bracketed DNA molecules are passed over a complementary oligonucleotide attached to a flow cell. Then a solid phase PCR generates neighboring groups of clonal populations from each of the single original flow cell attached to the DNA strands [34–36]. Moreover, the HiSeq has emerged after the standard Genome Analyzer version (GAIIx). It is a machine characterized by its ability to huger read length and depth of a sequence. Then, the MiSeq was discovered. One of its drawbacks is having a lower-throughput. On the other hand, it is the lower price, quicker turnaround and longer read length instrument [37, 38].

Analogously to 454 sequencing, beads containing cloned DNA fragment populations produced by an emPCR are washed over a pico-well plate proceeded by each nucleotide in turn. Nevertheless, nucleotide integration is determined not by the production of pyrophosphate; however, the alteration in pH produced by the protons (H+ ions) production through polymerization facilitating a quick sequencing during the actual detection time [39, 40].

Alongside 454 and Solexa/Illumina, (SOLiD) system from Applied Biosystems was the third major choice at the early time of second-generation sequencing. Its sequencing concept is based on oligonucleotide ligation and detection. (SOLiD) system turn out to be Life Technologies following merged with Invitrogen [41, 42]. Even though the SOLiD platform is unable to manufacture Illumina system read length and depth and makes its assembly more difficult, it continued to be a cost-competitive instrument [39, 43].

One more important sequencing which utilizes the ligation technology was the DNA nanoballs method, in which sequences are similarly attained from probe-ligation. However, the generation of clonal DNA population is innovative. Instead of bead or bridge amplification, rolling circle amplification is used to produce extended DNA chains comprising of repetition units of the template sequence bordered by adapters. Then the sequence is self-assembled into nanoballs attached to a slide in order to be sequenced [44].

Lastly, an outstanding sequencing system of the second-generation sequencing is the one that Jonathan Rothburg created after leaving 454. It was the first so-called post-light sequencing technology "Ion Torrent" (another Life Technologies product), neither fluorescence nor luminescence is used in this technology [40].

The frequently mentioned "genomics revolution" has dramatically changed the cost and effort accompanying with DNA sequencing guided in large part by these extraordinary improvements in nucleotide sequencing technology. The Illumina sequencing platform; however, has been the most effective and valuable in recent years, and can therefore probably be considered having made the strongest impact to the second-generation of DNA sequencers [45].

2.3 Third-generation nucleic acids sequencing

There were substantial arguments to characterize the various generations of technology for DNA sequencing, particularly in regard to the division from the second to the third generation. However, a suggestive distinguishing characteristic of the third generation should be single molecule sequencing (SMS), real-time sequencing, and simply deviated from the earlier technologies [46–49].

The first SMS technology was developed in Stephen Quake's laboratory, later marketed by Helicos BioSciences, and worked broadly like Illumina does, but excluding bridge amplification step [50, 51]. Basically, the DNA templates are linked to a planar surface and then deoxyribonucleotide triphosphate (dNTPs) called virtual terminators, proprietary fluorescent reversible terminators [52]. Although it is relatively slow, costly and generating short reads, it was considered the first technology enabling non-amplified DNA to be sequenced evading biases and mistakes that might occur. Other businesses picked up the third-generation baton, as Helicos bankrupted early in 2012 [1, 46, 48]. Moreover, the most commonly used third-generation technology was possibly Pacific Biosciences single molecule real time (SMRT) platform (PacBio range) [53]. In a very brief period of time, this method sequences a single molecule. Some other beneficial features available in the PacBio range and not commonly shared by other commercially available machines are producing kinetic data, which enables the detection of changed bases, also capable of generating an extremely long read more than 10 kilo bases (KB) suitable for de novo genome assemblies [46, 53, 54].

Nanopore sequencing, an offshoot of a giant field of utilizing nanopores for the determination and quantification of all kinds of biological and chemical samples, is perhaps the most waited for area to develop of the third-generation DNA sequencing [55]. For example, Oxford Nanopore Technologies (ONT), the first corporation to deliver nanopore sequencers, created a lot of exuberance about their GridION and MinION nanopore platforms [56, 57]. MinION nanopore platforms is small, cell phone sized USB device, which was first launched in an early access trial in 2014 to end users [58]. In spite of the undoubtedly poor-quality data produced with GridION and MinION nanopore platforms, it is wished that such sequencers reflect an authentically disruptive DNA sequencing technology, delivering much cheaper, faster and extremely elongated, not-amplified reads of sequence data than previously possible [55, 57, 59].

To sum up, the value of DNA sequencing for biological research is hardly to overstate; however, it is the determination way of one of the vital features by which our lives forms can be identified and distinguished from one another. Hence, numerous investigators from all over the world have spent a countless time and money over the last half century just to improve and enhance the technologies of DNA sequencing and also to combine many features from different sequencers generations coming up with outstanding capabilities for new one. Using the experience of all generations of sequencers will offer new perspectives for future generations, as lessons learn from the prior generations guide the next generations' development.

3. Coronaviridae family: structure and classification

Coronaviridae family members are large, enveloped, single-stranded positive-sense RNA types of viruses. Their genomic material made up of nucleotide sets ranging from 25 to 32 kb and the virus diameter varies from 118–136 nm [30, 60]. The virus is roughly spherical in shape and has obvious proteins on its cell membrane such as the large spike (S) protein extended 16–21 nm from the virus envelope, membrane protein (M-protein) plays a major role in promoting membrane curvature, envelope protein (E-protein), in low quantity, and hemagglutinin-esterase (HE) as shown in **Figure 1** [27, 61].

Coronaviridae family divided into two subfamilies: the Coronavirinae and the Torovirinae. Coronavirinae is categorized into four geniuses, alpha-coronavirus, beta-coronavirus, gamma-corona-virus and delta-coronavirus. On the other hand, Torovirinae has only one genus which is Torovirus. In contrast to Coronavirinae subfamily, Toroviruses have a helical, doughnut-shaped nucleocapsid in their structure. Unlike Toroviruses, Coronavirinae subfamily is prevalent among mammals which cause mild respiratory illnesses such as Severe Acute Respiratory Syndrome 1–2 (SARS-1-2) and Middle East Respiratory Syndrome (MERS) or enteric infections [30, 64].

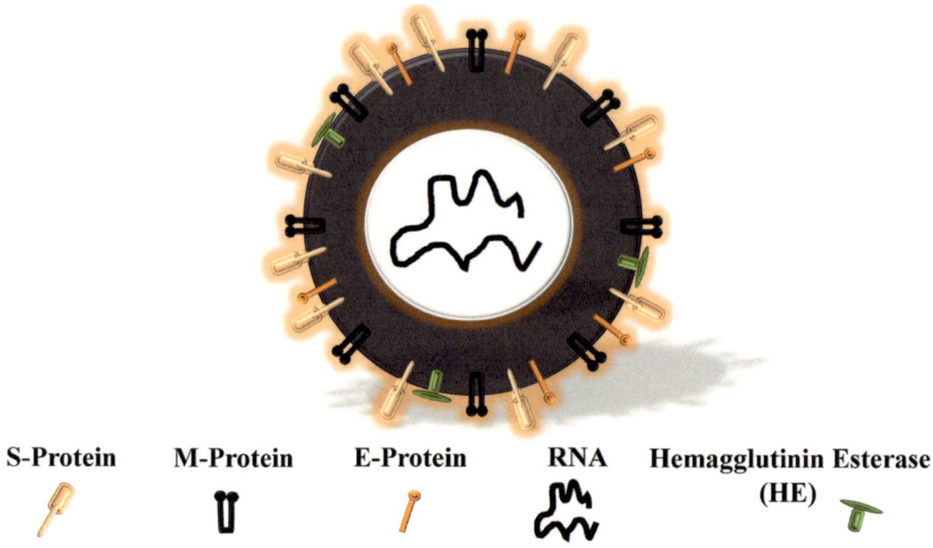

Figure 1.
Structural features shared by Coronaviridae family.

4. Coronavirinae: severe acute respiratory syndrome-2 (SARS-2) and corona virus disease-19 (COVID-19)

As mentioned before, Coronavirinae subfamily is categorized into four geniuses, known as alpha-coronavirus, beta-coronavirus, gamma-coronavirus and delta-coronavirus. The beta-coronavirus, in particular, has four lineages (A, B, C, and D) [62]. The lineage B of beta-coronavirus has a subgenus known as Sarbrcovirus under which SARS-CoV-2 goes [63]. Moreover, (novel coronavirus) or (Severe Acute Respiratory Syndrome Coronavirus-2) (SARS-CoV-2) is known as the causative microorganism associated with coronavirus disease-2019 (COVID-19). COVID-19-suffered patients are manifested with respiratory illnesses examples of which are pneumonia and breathing failure [61].

5. Country-wise genomic sequencing of SARS-CoV-2

Sequencing the genomic materials helps to discover the identity of the causative microorganism. Continues sequencing of the genomic materials is essential to discover changes that may happen during transcription and transmission process of the microorganism genomic materials. Utilizing this information helps in studying the nature of the causative agent whether it is altered or not and if these changes help determine severity of the infection and making right decisions to reduce the impact of the outbreak on several aspects of life consequently.

First of all, a case of pneumonia of unidentified cause has been registered in China, Hubei Province, Wuhan City (December 2019). Additional evaluation for these incidences was conducted to detect the pneumonia causal microorganism [64, 65]. The isolated virus identified and named as (SARS-CoV-2) after genomic characterization by next-generation sequencing (NGS) of the complete sequence has been carried out [66]. The genomic analysis of the virus showed that it is an enveloped RNA virus (sized of 29,903 bp). The phylogenetic sequence analysis displayed that the virus categorized under the subgenus Sarbecovirus of the genus beta-coronavirus and to the Coronaviridae family. Moreover, it was found that around 87.5 percent of genomic material was similar two bat-derived SARS-like CoV strains (bat-SL-CoVZC45 and bat-SL-CoVZXC21) commonly affected humans, including the virus that contributed to the outbreak of SARS-CoV-1 (2003) [62].

The Government of India has reviewed and introduced multi-sectoral initiatives to address this emerging public health problem following the first SARS-CoV-2 study from China. They started with monitoring country boarders at 21 international airports, strengthening state-level surveillance systems and preparedness in designated hospitals for the management of clinical cases. The reported and confirmed cases in India (January, 2020) were then sequenced (next-generation sequencing). The phylogenic analysis, compared with other published SARS-CoV-2 sequence in the database, were carried out to monitor and understand their relationships. The sequences of two out the first three confirmed cases in India were found to be high (about 99.98 percent) identity with Wuhan seafood market pneumonia virus (accession number: NC 045512). The phylogenetic analysis displayed that there were two distinct introductions to India. Therefore, continuous surveillance of the sequences and review shall be crucial to consider the genetic evolution and substitution rates of SARS-CoV-2 from the affected countries [60].

In Bangladesh, the first three cases were detected (March, 2020). However, the Bangladeshi complete genome sequence of novel coronavirus (SARS-CoV-2) isolate was accomplished by Illumina iSeq100 sequencer (April, 2020). Findings from these results showed that 9 mutations in the genome of this sample, compared to the Wuhan strain, reference genome (GenBank accession no. MN908947.3) [67].

In Ecuador, the first reported cases of COVID-19, which was on March, 2020 for a traveler came from Netherlands, and the three other confirmed cases were gnomically sequenced using the MinION platform (Oxford Nanopore Technologies) and ARTIC network protocols respectively. Results from these studies showed that the cases in Ecuador transmitted from three different European countries. The sequences of the confirmed cases in Ecuador were found to have high similarity (99.68 percent) with Wuhan strain reference case (GenBank accession number MN908947). The information discussed in this section is summarized in **Table 1** [68].

Numerous countries all over the world have also sequenced the viral genomic material of confirmed COVID-19 cases and have compared their results with reference cases sequence in China such as Nepal, Australia, USA and Turkey etc.

Country	Sequencer generation used for analysis	Sequence similarity (%)
China	Next-Generation Sequencing (NGS)	87.5% to bat-derived SARS-like CoV strains
India	Next-Generation Sequencing (NGS)	About 99.98% to the Wuhan strain
Bangladesh	Next-Generation Sequencing (NGS) -Illumina iSeq100 sequencer	9 mutations found compared to the Wuhan strain
Ecuador	Third-Generation Sequencing -MinION platform	99.68% to the Wuhan strain

Table 1.
Genomic analysis of COVID-19 confirmed cases from several countries.

6. Precautions and control measures globally taken by governmental authorities against COVID-19 outbreak

Several countries around the world have adopted precautionary and control measures (either registered COVID-19 cases centuries or not). These listed actions below, as examples, have been taken to avoid the introduction of SARS-CoV-2 to the countries or to limit the spread of the virus:

- Stopping domestic and international flights.
- Shifting schools and colleges to remote learning and virtual classrooms from in-person classes.
- Suspending all social and governmental gatherings and events.
- Activation online shopping and home delivery services for all shops and markets.
- Compulsorily wearing masks and gloves and using hand sanitizers.
- Issuing a lockdown on city to city and country to country levels.
- Implementing mass vaccination program

In this section, we will shed some light on the mass vaccination approach and logistics needed to implement such a program. In addition, its promising effects could end the pandemic of COVID-19 will be discussed. Mass vaccination during COVID-19 outbreaks or pandemics, against which (AstraZeneca, Moderna, BioNTech and Sputink V) vaccines are recently marketed, is a possible crucial public health intervention. The mass vaccination policy, as previously reported, was an important countermeasure against many infectious diseases, such as polio and smallpox [69]. Mass vaccination against COVID-19 is therefore an urgent option for the current emergency and rapidly spreading SARS-CoV-2, eventually might leading to herd immunity induction. The program is started with selection of the most susceptible groups of population such as immunocompromised patients due to underlying medical conditions and elderly people etc. [70].

In term of logistics, implementing this program requires huge mental and physical efforts starting with vaccine and locations availability, vaccinators and the unique roles and responsibilities taken by both private and public sectors partnership [71]. On one hand, the private sector must warrant compliance with CDC guidance and follow cold-chain management rules to ensure inoculation feasibility upon arrival, storage, and delivery [71]. On the other hand, the public sector ensures cold-chain management and CDC guidance too; in addition, to fill the gaps in delivery service particularly to those who live in nursing homes, assisted living facilities, etc. Furthermore, a facility is a place where clinical staff stay and need vaccine and consultation services to complete logistical requirements. Collectively, the public health sector in support to the private sector entity provide consultation, vaccinator training, and pandemic protocol guidance [71].

In fact, vaccine requests are more than certain to consume the resources available and necessitate the marshaling of resources to meet need. COVID-19 vaccine clinics, for example, include not only usual walk-through clinic sites at doctor's offices, pharmacies, departments of public health and big box stores, but also college campuses, worship houses, drive-through, public centers, and outdoor camps [71].

7. Conclusions

Even though the genetic diversity of SARS-CoV-2 is currently low, the combination of genetic, clinical, and epidemiological data is highly successful in generating outbreak management action plans. Genetic information, in particular, aids in tracking the viral introduction to countries, classifying the lineage of the ancestral origin of the virus, and recognizing the pattern of population spread during the outbreak. In addition, the information obtained from the genome sequencing tools of the SARS-CoV-2 virus identifies rates of substitution (mutation) that occurred in the viral genome.

Integration of genetic, clinical, and epidemiological information seems to be a vital step to understand the SARS-CoV-2 (genotype and phenotype) and contribute to the global landscape. The combination of this knowledge not only aids in decision-making process for the implementation of precautions and control measures, but also to the comprehension of virulence and severity, transmissibility of virus response to treatment, and effectiveness of vaccines for disease prevention.

Finally, it is doubtful that the current pandemic will be the last one, and it is therefore important to strengthen the responsiveness of our public health systems and to introduce and enhance ongoing scientific research programs combining preclinical, clinical and epidemiological information.

Conflict of interest

The authors declare no conflict of interest.

Author details

Rayan A. Ahmed
Department of Pharmacology and Toxicology, College of Pharmacy,
Jazan University, Jizan, Kingdom of Saudi Arabia

*Address all correspondence to: rayanahmed@jazanu.edu.sa

'Biotechnology to Combat COVID-19' is a collaborative project with Biotechnology Kiosk

References

[1] Heather JM, Chain B. The sequence of sequencers: The history of sequencing DNA. Genomics [Internet]. 2016;107(1):1-8. Available from: http://dx.doi.org/10.1016/j.ygeno.2015.11.003

[2] Zallen DT. Despite Franklin's work, Wilkins earned his Nobel. Nature. 2003.

[3] Sanger F, Brownlee GG, Barrell BG. A two-dimensional fractionation procedure for radioactive nucleotides. J Mol Biol. 1965;

[4] Brownlee GG, Sanger F. Nucleotide sequences from the low molecular weight ribosomal RNA of *Escherichia coli*. J Mol Biol. 1967;

[5] Cory S, Marcker KA, Dube SK, Clark BFC. Primary structure of a methionine transfer RNA from *Escherichia coli*. Nature. 1968

[6] Dube SK, Marcker KA, Clark BFC, Cory S. Nucleotide sequence of N-formyl-methionyl-transfer RNA. Nature. 1968;

[7] Goodman HM, Abelson J, Landy A, Brenner S, Smith JD. Amber suppression: A Nucleotide change in the anticodon of a tyrosine transfer RNA. Nature. 1968;

[8] Adams JM, Jeppesen PGN, Sanger F, Barrell BG. Nucleotide sequence from the coat protein cistron of R17 bacteriophage RNA. Nature. 1969;

[9] Holley RW, Apgar J, Everett GA, Madison JT, Marquisee M, Merrill SH, et al. Structure of a ribonucleic acid. Science (80-). 1965;

[10] Jou WM, Haegeman G, Ysebaert M, Fiers W. Nucleotide sequence of the gene coding for the bacteriophage MS2 coat protein. Nature. 1972;

[11] Fiers W, Contreras R, Duerinck F, Haegeman G, Iserentant D, Merregaert J, et al. Complete nucleotide sequence of bacteriophage MS2 RNA: Primary and secondary structure of the replicase gene. Nature. 1976;

[12] Sanger F, Coulson AR. A rapid method for determining sequences in DNA by primed synthesis with DNA polymerase. J Mol Biol. 1975;

[13] Maxam AM, Gilbert W. A new method for sequencing DNA. Proc Natl Acad Sci U S A. 1977;

[14] Sanger F, Air GM, Barrell BG, Brown NL, Coulson AR, Fiddes CA, et al. Nucliotide sequence of bacteriophage phi X174 DNA. Nature. 1977;

[15] Sanger F, Nicklen S, Coulson AR. DNA sequencing with chain-terminating inhibitors. Proc Natl Acad Sci U S A. 1977;

[16] Smith LM, Fung S, Hunkapiller MW, Hunkapiller TJ, Hood LE. The synthesis of oligonucleotides containing an aliphatic amino group at the 5′ terminus: Synthesis of fluorescent DNA primers for use in DNA sequence analysis. Nucleic Acids Res. 1985;

[17] Ansorge W, Sproat BS, Stegemann J, Schwager C. A non-radioactive automated method for DNA sequence determination. J Biochem Biophys Methods. 1986;

[18] Ansorge W, Sproat B, Stegemann J, Schwager C, Zenke M. Automated DNA sequencing: Ultrasensitive detection of fluorescent bands during electrophoresis. Nucleic Acids Res. 1987;

[19] Kambara H, Nishikawa T, Katayama Y, Yamaguchi T. Optimization

of parameters in a DNA sequenator using fluorescence detection. Bio/ Technology. 1988;

[20] Swerdlow H, Gesteland R. Capillary gel electrophoresis for rapid, high resolution DNA sequencing. Nucleic Acids Res. 1990;

[21] Luckey JA, Drossman H, Kostichka AJ, Mead DA, D'cunha J, Norris TB, et al. High speed DNA sequencing by capillary electrophoresis. Nucleic Acids Res. 1990;

[22] Hunkapiller T, Kaiser RJ, Koop BF, Hood L. Large-scale and automated DNA sequence determination. Science. 1991

[23] Staden R. A strategy of DNA sequencing employing computer programs. Nucleic Acids Res. 1979;

[24] Saiki RK, Scharf S, Faloona F, Mullis KB, Horn GT, Erlich HA, et al. Enzymatic amplification of β-globin genomic sequences and restriction site analysis for diagnosis of sickle cell anemia. Science (80-). 1985;

[25] Smith LM, Sanders JZ, Kaiser RJ, Hughes P, Dodd C, Connell CR, et al. Fluorescence detection in automated DNA sequence analysis. Nature. 1986;

[26] Ansorge WJ. Next-generation DNA sequencing techniques. New Biotechnology. 2009

[27] Lander ES, Linton LM, Birren B, Nusbaum C, Zody MC, Baldwin J, et al. Initial sequencing and analysis of the human genome. Nature. 2001;

[28] Craig Venter J, Adams MD, Myers EW, Li PW, Mural RJ, Sutton GG, et al. The sequence of the human genome. Science (80-). 2001;

[29] Nyrén P, Lundin A. Enzymatic method for continuous monitoring of inorganic pyrophosphate synthesis. Anal Biochem. 1985;

[30] Margulies M, Egholm M, Altman WE, Attiya S, Bader JS, Bemben LA, et al. Genome sequencing in microfabricated high-density picolitre reactors. Nature. 2005;

[31] Levy S, Sutton G, Ng PC, Feuk L, Halpern AL, Walenz BP, et al. The diploid genome sequence of an individual human. PLoS Biol. 2007;

[32] Wheeler DA, Srinivasan M, Egholm M, Shen Y, Chen L, McGuire A, et al. The complete genome of an individual by massively parallel DNA sequencing. Nature. 2008;

[33] Voelkerding K V., Dames SA, Durtschi JD. Next-generation sequencing:from basic research to diagnostics. Clinical Chemistry. 2009

[34] Shendure J, Ji H. Next-generation DNA sequencing. Nature Biotechnology. 2008

[35] Fedurco M, Romieu A, Williams S, Lawrence I, Turcatti G. BTA, a novel reagent for DNA attachment on glass and efficient generation of solid-phase amplified DNA colonies. Nucleic Acids Res. 2006;

[36] Bentley DR, Balasubramanian S, Swerdlow HP, Smith GP, Milton J, Brown CG, et al. Accurate whole human genome sequencing using reversible terminator chemistry. Nature. 2008;

[37] Balasubramanian S. Sequencing nucleic acids: From chemistry to medicine. Chem Commun. 2011;

[38] Quail MA, Smith M, Coupland P, Otto TD, Harris SR, Connor TR, et al. A tale of three next generation sequencing platforms: comparison of Ion Torrent, Pacific Biosciences and Illumina MiSeq sequencers. BMC Genomics. 2012;

[39] Glenn TC. Field guide to next-generation DNA sequencers. Mol Ecol Resour. 2011;

[40] Rothberg JM, Hinz W, Rearick TM, Schultz J, Mileski W, Davey M, et al. An integrated semiconductor device enabling non-optical genome sequencing. Nature. 2011;

[41] Luo C, Tsementzi D, Kyrpides N, Read T, Konstantinidis KT. Direct comparisons of Illumina vs. Roche 454 sequencing technologies on the same microbial community DNA sample. PLoS One. 2012;

[42] McKernan KJ, Peckham HE, Costa GL, McLaughlin SF, Fu Y, Tsung EF, et al. Sequence and structural variation in a human genome uncovered by short-read, massively parallel ligation sequencing using two-base encoding. Genome Res. 2009;

[43] Buermans HPJ, den Dunnen JT. Next generation sequencing technology: Advances and applications. Biochimica et Biophysica Acta - Molecular Basis of Disease. 2014

[44] Drmanac R, Sparks AB, Callow MJ, Halpern AL, Burns NL, Kermani BG, et al. Human genome sequencing using unchained base reads on self-assembling DNA nanoarrays. Science (80-). 2010;

[45] Stein LD. The case for cloud computing in genome informatics. Genome Biology. 2010

[46] Schadt EE, Turner S, Kasarskis A. A window into third-generation sequencing. Hum Mol Genet. 2010;

[47] Niedringhaus TP, Milanova D, Kerby MB, Snyder MP, Barron AE. Landscape of next-generation sequencing technologies. Analytical Chemistry. 2011

[48] Pareek CS, Smoczynski R, Tretyn A. Sequencing technologies and genome sequencing. Journal of Applied Genetics. 2011

[49] Gut IG. New sequencing technologies. Clin Transl Oncol. 2013;

[50] Braslavsky I, Hebert B, Kartalov E, Quake SR. Sequence information can be obtained from single DNA molecules. Proc Natl Acad Sci U S A. 2003;

[51] Harris TD, Buzby PR, Babcock H, Beer E, Bowers J, Braslavsky I, et al. Single-molecule DNA sequencing of a viral genome. Science (80-). 2008;

[52] Bowers J, Mitchell J, Beer E, Buzby PR, Causey M, Efcavitch JW, et al. Virtual terminator nucleotides for next-generation DNA sequencing. Nat Methods. 2009;

[53] Thermes C. Ten years of next-generation sequencing technology. Trends in genetics : TIG. 2014

[54] Flusberg BA, Webster DR, Lee JH, Travers KJ, Olivares EC, Clark TA, et al. Direct detection of DNA methylation during single-molecule, real-time sequencing. Nat Methods. 2010;

[55] Haque F, Li J, Wu HC, Liang XJ, Guo P. Solid-state and biological nanopore for real-time sensing of single chemical and sequencing of DNA. Nano Today. 2013

[56] Clarke J, Wu HC, Jayasinghe L, Patel A, Reid S, Bayley H. Continuous base identification for single-molecule nanopore DNA sequencing. Nat Nanotechnol. 2009;

[57] Eisenstein M. Oxford Nanopore announcement sets sequencing sector abuzz. Nature Biotechnology. 2012

[58] Loman NJ, Quinlan AR. Poretools: A toolkit for analyzing nanopore sequence data. Bioinformatics. 2014;

[59] Branton D, Deamer DW, Marziali A, Bayley H, Benner SA, Butler T, et al. The potential and challenges of nanopore sequencing. Nature Biotechnology. 2008

[60] Yadav P, Potdar V, Choudhary M, Nyayanit D, Agrawal M, Jadhav S, et al. Full-genome sequences of the first two SARS-CoV-2 viruses from India. Indian J Med Res. 2020;

[61] Nomier YA, Rao DS, Suhaqi AH, Ahmed RA. Distinctive therapeutic strategies against Corona Virus-19 (COVID-19): A pharmacological review. Syst Rev Pharm. 2020;11(9)

[62] Lu R, Zhao X, Li J, Niu P, Yang B, Wu H, et al. Genomic characterisation and epidemiology of 2019 novel coronavirus: implications for virus origins and receptor binding. Lancet. 2020;

[63] Letko M, Marzi A, Munster V. Functional assessment of cell entry and receptor usage for SARS-CoV-2 and other lineage B betacoronaviruses. Nat Microbiol. 2020;

[64] Lu H, Stratton CW, Tang YW. Outbreak of pneumonia of unknown etiology in Wuhan, China: The mystery and the miracle. Journal of Medical Virology. 2020

[65] Chen N, Zhou M, Dong X, Qu J, Gong F, Han Y, et al. Epidemiological and clinical characteristics of 99 cases of 2019 novel coronavirus pneumonia in Wuhan, China: a descriptive study. Lancet. 2020;

[66] Zhu N, Zhang D, Wang W, Li X, Yang B, Song J, et al. A Novel Coronavirus from Patients with Pneumonia in China, 2019. N Engl J Med. 2020;

[67] Saha S, Malaker R, Sajib MSI, Hasanuzzaman M, Rahman H, Ahmed ZB, et al. Complete Genome Sequence of a Novel Coronavirus (SARS-CoV-2) Isolate from Bangladesh. Microbiol Resour Announc. 2020;

[68] Marquez S, Prado-Vivar B, Guadalupe JJ, Gutierrez Granja B, Jibaja M, Tobar M, et al. Genome sequencing of the first SARS-CoV-2 reported from patients with COVID-19 in Ecuador. medRxiv Prepr Serv Heal Sci. 2020;

[69] Branton D, Deamer DW, Marziali A, Bayley H, Benner SA, Butler T, et al. The potential and challenges of nanopore sequencing. Nature Biotechnology. 2008

[70] Frederiksen LSF, Zhang Y, Foged C, Thakur A. The Long Road Toward COVID-19 Herd Immunity: Vaccine Platform Technologies and Mass Immunization Strategies. Front Immunol. 2020;11(July):1-26

[71] Russo T. Pandemic Policy and the Logistics of COVID -19 Mass Vaccination. Homel Secur Aff J [Internet]. 2020;16(13). Available from: www.hsaj.org/articles16514

Section 2

Spike Protein Receptor Epigenetic Regulation

Chapter 4

Glycan and Its Role in Combating COVID-19

Swapan Kumar Chatterjee and Snigdha Saha

Abstract

Newly identified beta-coronavirus i.e. the 2019 novel coronavirus is associated with a contagious transmittable respiratory disease called COVID-19. This disease has been declared as a "pandemic" by the World Health Organization (WHO). The entry of coronavirus in the human respiratory epithelial cells depends upon the interaction between host cell receptor ACE2 and viral S-glycoprotein. However, this type of molecular recognition in between cell surface receptors and envelope glycoproteins are mediated by specific glycan epitopes and attribute to viral entry through membrane fusion. Glycans are essential biomolecules made by all living organisms, have roles in serving structure, energy storage, and system regulatory purposes. The glycan shield plays a crucial role in concealing the surface S protein from molecular recognition. The immunomodulatory properties of Glycan-binding proteins (GBPs) like Lectins, build them as an attractive candidates for vaccine adjuvant. Investigations involving the complement system activation by the lectin pathway in COVID-19 and diseases are in need of the hour. The innate immune response involving complement system could have varied biological effects against an array of microbial infections. The advances in glycoprotein style methods especially immunomodulatory action of some lectins are necessary to boost the effectiveness of treatment of COVID-19 and other pandemics.

Keywords: Glycan, S-glycoprotein, ACE2 receptor, Glycan binding protein (GBP), COVID-19

1. Introduction

A new virus called the 2019 novel coronavirus (an enveloped beta-coronavirus) is identified in December 2019 and associated with a de novo contagious respiratory disease. The coronavirus disease 2019 (COVID-19) has been declared as a "pandemic" by the World Health Organization (WHO). Previous reports have recognized various human coronaviruses, like in 2003 SARS-CoV, in 2004 HCoVNL63, in 2005 HKU1, in 2012 MERS-CoV, and now in 2019 pathogenic SARS-CoV-2. In humans, the effects of these viruses are correlated with severe respiratory tract infections. COVID-19 disease has signs that are similar to a common cold. However, this infection can lead to serious respiratory failure, as well as compromised and harmful immune responses. Increased monocyte-neutrophil ratios and exacerbated release of inflammatory mediators particularly IL-6, characterize this condition, which can contribute to organ dysfunction. Given the fact that other coronavirus outbreaks have occurred, there is no known treatment or vaccination for COVID-19.

Another major problem is the urgent need for easy and fast instruments to detect viruses in clinical and environmental samples. Early identification of SARS-CoV-2 in asymptomatic and/or presymptomatic individuals is crucial for stopping the transmission chain [1]. Plasmapheresis is also essential for extracorporeal removal of SARS-CoV-2 from blood in order to present alternative therapies. These dynamic pictures have imposed a fight against time through numerous fields of knowledge such as biomedical research, biotechnology, drug production, and molecular analysis in order to find as many resolutions as possible to these and other complications presented by the pandemic.

Viral members of the CoVs family restrain a positive-sense, single-strand RNA genome, which are 26 to 32- kilo bases in length [1]. The infectivity and immeasurable distribution capacity of CoVs have been established them as an important pathogen. In addition to numerous avian hosts, various members of CoVs have been recognized in a range of mammals, like masked palm civets, bats, dogs, mice, camels, and cats are responsible for disease related to gastrointestinal systems, hepatic, respiratory, and nervous system in humans. The outer surface membrane (M), envelope (E), and spike (S) structural proteins are coupled within the envelope of coronavirus which consists of a lipid bilayer. It is believed that glycosylated SARS-CoV-2 spike (S) protein, mediates host cell entry by binding to the angiotensin- converting enzyme 2 (ACE2) and establish the host tropism. Similar to many other viral fusion proteins, the SARS-CoV-2 spikes also utilize a highly dense coating of non-immunogenic or weakly immunogenic complex carbohydrates - glycan shield to thwart the host immune response [2]. Glycans are carbohydrate-based polymers made by all living organisms. The heavily glycosylated SARS-CoV spike protein suppresses almost 23 putative *N*-glycosylation sites, amidst 12 of them are effectively glycosylated [3]. In viral fusion proteins presence of N-glycan coating is correlated with protein glycosylation and plays a decisive role in viral pathogenesis. The N-glycans expressed on the surface of viral envelope glycoproteins have very diverse biological roles and are all inextricably linked to their nature. However, molecular recognition in between cell surface receptors and envelope glycoproteins are mediated by specific N-glycan epitopes and attribute to viral entry through membrane fusion. Moreover, an extremely dense coating of non-immunogenic or feeble immunogenic complicated carbohydrates on otherwise perilously exposed viral proteins constitutes an ideal camouflage (or shield) to evade the system [4].

The glycan shield plays a crucial role in concealing the surface S protein from molecular recognition. However, to effectively perform, the spike has to acknowledge and bind to ACE2 receptors as the primary infection route. For this reason, the RBM should become absolutely exposed and accessible. During this situation, the glycan shield works as one with an outsized conformational modification that permits the RBD to emerge higher than the N-glycan coverage. Each the S-glycoprotein and ACE2 receptor are proverbial to be extensively glycosylated, i.e. they contain covalently linked complex oligosaccharides referred to as glycans. Recently published studies have shown that the spike glycoprotein contains sixty-six glycosylation sites with forty-four of them being enclosed within the model. Another recent study analyzed site-specific N-linked glycosylation of MERS and respiratory illness SARS S glycoproteins, indicating that every of those glycosylation sites is occupied by up to 10 totally different glycans (called glycoforms), which greatly extends epitope diversity [4, 5].

The synthesis, folding, and glycosylation (as alternative PTMs) of infectious agent proteins depend upon host organelles (ribosome, endoplasmic reticulum, and Golgi apparatus) and enzymes (glycosyltransferases and glycosidases). The present experimental knowledge relating to the glycosylation of viral proteins depends on the carbohydrate processing enzymes present within the biological systems accustomed to propagate the viral strain. During this sense, our data regarding the natural pattern of viral protein glycosylation is incredibly restricted. It's conjointly vital to think that viral proteins could follow totally different pathways than those discovered from host glycoproteins [5, 6]. Attribute to their chemical complexity and restricted sensitivity of existing analytical instruments, glycans are left neglected. This can be unfortunate as they verify a major part of the structure and performance of the many glycoproteins. This can be very true within the field of host/pathogen interactions, wherever glycan diversity is employed by each host to evade recognition by pathogens and therefore the pathogens to flee the system response. Moreover, glycans, and specifically their outmost components, have vital conformational flexibility. This contributes to the overall conformational dynamics of the molecule that may each generate novel potential drug binding sites or shield binding sites predicted mainly from polypeptide-only models [7].

Beyond a function in shielding the underlying proteins from recognition by antibodies, the glycans on infective proteins may additionally attenuate the flexibility of the host system to lift antibodies against any epitopes that embrace the glycan. In an exceedingly T-cell-dependent adaptative immune reaction, peptides from the infective agent are presented on antigen- presenting cells by major histocompatibility complex II molecules, conjointly referred to as human leukocyte antigen (HLA) complexes. HLA complexes have the most popular peptide antigen motifs, and supported data of those preferences it's doable to predict that peptides in exceedingly infective proteins are probably to be HLA antigens [8]. However, once that peptide contains a glycosylation site, the probability of the peptide to be presented in an HLA complex could also be compromised, if as an example the peptide cannot bind to the HLA molecule owing to the steric presence of the glycan. However, glycopeptides could also be presented in HLA complexes if the glycan is compact enough or if it's found on the end of the peptide antigen wherever it does not interfere with HLA binding. The glycan-mediated shielding of predicted HLA antigens derived from the S glycoprotein is conjointly containing a glycosite. Glycosylation systematically decreases the surface exposure of the residues proximal to the glycosites however conjointly junction rectifier to non-sequential changes in exposure, as a result of the 3D topology of the protein surface within the close proximity of every glycosite [8, 9].

The SARS-CoV-2 envelope glycoproteins are involved in the viral adhesion and entry processes. The presence of glycoproteins in the viral envelope opens up a world of possibilities for using carbohydrate-binding agents like lectins to fix some of the pandemic's most pressing issues. Lectins can recognize glycans, allowing them to be used in a number of biotechnological applications. The presence of glycoproteins on the viral envelope unfolds a large vary of prospects for the application of lectins to deal with some urgent issues concerned during this pandemic. The growing popularity of glycans enables the use of lectins for many biotechnological applications. Significantly, these agglutinins block the viral adhesion to the host cells by targeting the sugar moieties in surface proteins, and are considered as broad-spectrum inhibitors of viral invasion. The interaction with glycoproteins conjointly allows the use of lectins within the development of devices for identification and characterization of glycoproteins in a viral envelope or alterations in host glycoproteins throughout virus infection. Lectins are natural proteins that focus on the sugar moieties of a large vary of glycoproteins [10]. They are prevailing among higher plants and are divided into seven families of structurally and evolutionarily connected proteins. Over a decade ago, studies revealed that through inhibition of virus-cell fusion, plant lectins were reportable to inhibit HIV replication in lymphocyte cell cultures [9].

Sugar-binding proteins that are neither antibodies nor enzymes are known as lectins. To be labeled as a lectin, a glycoprotein must meet three distinct criteria. To begin, lectin is a carbohydrate-binding protein or glycoprotein (s). Second, lectins aren't the same as immunoglobulins (antibodies). Finally, lectins do not alter the biochemistry of the carbohydrates they bind. Plant lectins are a specific type of carbohydrate-binding proteins which are capable of specific recognition and reversible binding to carbohydrates. Since lectins can recognize specific carbohydrate structures such as proteoglycans, glycoproteins, and glycolipids, they can control various cells through glycoconjugates and their physiological and pathological phenomena via host-pathogen interactions and cell–cell communications.

Initially, it had been reported that plant lectins inhibit virus replication by forestalling virus adsorption however studies had been later shown that they prevent the fusion of HIV particles with their target cells. Additionally to the antiviral impact of mannose- and N-acetylglucosamine-specific agglutinins on HIV, the associate repressive impact of those plant lectins was reported on respiratory syncytial viral infection, CMV infection, and influenza A virus infection in vitro. Carbohydrate-binding agents are thought of as anti-CoV agents that focus on spike protein and restrain CoV entry [10]. They're proficient to bind specifically with the oligosaccharides on virus surfaces like HIV and S glycoprotein. In mouse model and additionally, in vitro condition they inhibit a large variety of CoVs, as well as SARS-CoV, HCoV NL63, HCoV 229E, and HCoV OC43. Plant lectins, such as those present in leeks, have been shown to be effective coronavirus inhibitors by interacting with two targets in the viral replication cycle. The first target was discovered early in the replication cycle, most likely during viral attachment, while the second was discovered toward the end of the infectious virus cycle. Depending on the nature of their sugar specificity, the antiviral activity spectrum of plant lectins varies considerably. In general, the plant lectins which were mannose-specific found to be highly effective against coronaviruses. Mannose-binding glycoprotein (MBL; additionally called mannan-binding lectin) could be a pattern-recognition molecule that plays a critical role in spacing and orientation of the carbohydrate-recognition domains [2, 10].

In several expression systems, glycosylation act as a live to gauge antigen quality. For styling appropriate immunogens for vaccine development, it is important to have basic understanding concomitant with the RBD domain of the SARS-CoV-2 spike protein which is able to incorporate complicated sialylated N-glycans and

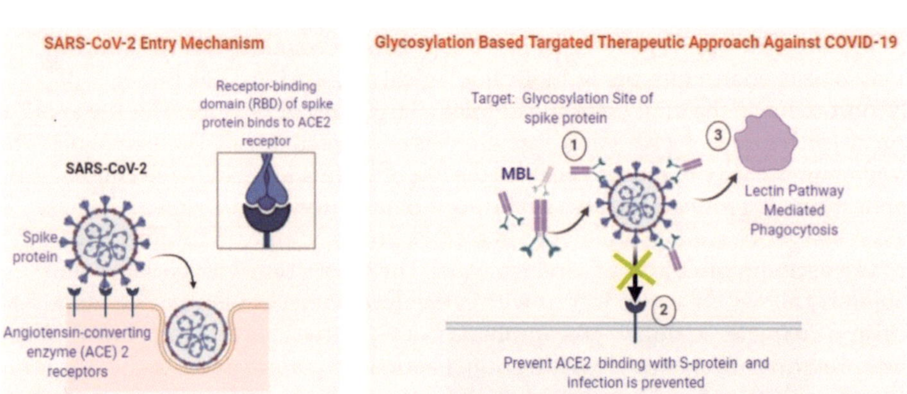

Figure 1.
Potential role of MBL in prevention of SARS-CoV2. 1. Attachment of MBL at the glycosylation site of spike protein by "Lock and Key" mode. 2. Prevent ACE2 mediated entry of viral pathogen. 3. Lectin pathway-mediated phagocytosis of intracellular pathogens (adapted from reference [2]).

sialylated glycoprotein O-glycans. The interaction with glycoproteins additionally permits the utilization of lectins within the development of devices for the identification and characterization of glycoproteins in infectious agent envelopes or alterations in host glycoproteins throughout virus infection. MBL could be a serum C-type glycoprotein, that is in a position to bind SARS-CoV intrinsically or infected cell and additionally capable to inhibit the infectivity of the virus. Hence, with this background knowledge, we could to anticipate that glycosylation of infectious agent peptides by "Lock and Key Technology" may be considerate as a novel therapeutic strategy against the current COVID-19 pandemic (**Figure 1**) [2, 10, 11].

2. Glycosylation and its role in onset of disease

The "glycome biology" or "glycobiology" studies the thorough repertoire i.e. the structure, biosynthesis, and biology of glycoconjugates composed of carbohydrate chains, or glycans, which are covalently, linked to lipid or protein molecules. The formation of glycoconjugates, differences in their glycan sequences, their length, and the connection between them depends upon on a process called glycosylation. Synthesis of glycoconjugate is a dynamic process that relies on the sugar precursors, the local milieu of enzymes, structures of organelle as well as cellular signals, and the cell types. Studies of rare genetic disorders that have an effect on glycosylation 1st highlighted the biological importance of the glycome, and technological advances have improved our understanding of its heterogeneousness and quality. However the replication process of secreted and cell-surface glycomes, overall cellular standing in health and sickness requires a detail research and assessment. In fact, changes in glycosylation will modulate inflammatory responses, alter viral immune escape, promote neoplastic cell metastasis, or regulate apoptosis; the composition of the glycome conjointly affects urinary organ operate in health and sickness. Easy and extremely dynamic protein-bound glycans also are well endowed within the nucleus and living substance of cells, wherever they exert restrictive effects. In fact, additionally to forming vital structural options, the sugar elements of glycoconjugates modulate or mediate a good form of functions in physiological and pathophysiological states. Glycoproteins and polysaccharides have vital functions in viral cells, and even glycoproteins have central roles within the biology of most viruses [10, 12]. Glycoconjugates are measured by the addition of sugars to proteins and lipids. A huge range of naturally occurring sugars will be combined to make a variety of distinctive glycan structures on lipid and protein molecules that modulate their activity. Multiple enzymatic site preferences, similarly because the use of stereochemical α or β conjugations, produce diversity in wherever and the way these sugars are linked to every alternative. In fact, altogether, these options imply the potential existence of ~1012 completely different branched glycan structures.

Protein glycosylation includes the addition of N-linked glycans, O-linked glycans, phosphorylated glycans, glycosaminoglycans, and glycosylphosphatidylinositol (GPI) anchors to amide backbones similarly to C-mannosylation of essential amino acid residues. Glycolipids are glycoconjugate which include glycosphingolipids (GSLs) formed through the addition of sugars to lipids. Glycosylation of proteins and lipids happens within the endoplasmic reticulum (ER) and with most of the terminal processing occurring within the cis-, medial- and trans-Golgi compartments. In these organelles, glycosidases, and glycosyltransferases form carbohydrate structures in a series of steps that are dominance by the availability of the enzyme activity, substrate, levels of gene transcription, and enzyme location. In fact, the glycome of a specific cell reflects its distinctive gene-expression pattern that controls the level of the enzymes responsible for glycoconjugation.

The glycome is created in a non-templated manner and is in an elaborate way controlled at multiple levels within the ER and cyst, unlike exome or proteome [12, 13].

3. Different type of glycosylation in human

3.1 N-linked glycosylation

The covalently N-linked glycans are superimposed co-translationally to native polypeptides within the endoplasmic reticulum (ER) as blocks of fourteen sugars (Glc3Man9GlcNAc2). These glycans are measure then subject to extensive modification throughout their transport through the ER and also the Golgi body before reaching their final destinations within or outside the cell. Within the ER and also the early secretory pathway, the sugar repertoire is still very little. Within the Golgi body, however, the glycans acquire complicated and extremely numerous structures by terminal glycosylation, which ends up in a very tremendous heterogeneity. Such diversity differs between cell sorts, tissues and species, and helps to additional increase microheterogeneity in the presence of the same genetic polypeptide background. This leads to the creation of new functionalities and specificities. The N-glycans may also have a very important role in correct macromolecule folding and degradation, and solubility, by avoiding the precipitation that's caused by lipophylic aminoacid stretches within the emergent polypeptide. The presence of a glycan protect on the peptides additionally allows the protection of the glycoproteins against degradation by proteases [13, 14].

3.2 O-linked glycosylation

Glycosylation will occur on amino acids with functional hydroxyl group teams, that is most frequently Ser and Thr. In humans, the foremost common sugars joined to Ser or Thr are GlcNAc and N-acetylgalactosamine (GalNAc)7. GalNAc-linked glycans usually referred to as mucin-type O-glycans, are abundant on various living things and secreted glycoproteins together with mucins, which type an important interface between animal tissue cells and the external tissue layer surfaces of the body. Mucins are characterized by a variable range of tandem repeats with Ser and Thr that create many sites for O-glycosylation. O-glycosylation performs various functions, such as providing resistance to proteolysis of stem regions of membrane proteins, creating specific recognition phenomena, and selection of ligands for selectins. Masking of immunogenic epitopes on the protein is in need to special mention [13, 14].

3.3 Glycosphingolipids

GSLs comprise a sphingolipid to which a glycan is connected at the C1 group position of a ceramide; they are one in every of the foremost plentiful glycolipids in humans are generally found within the lipid bilayers of cellular membranes. GSL glycosylation starts with the addition of glucose or galactose to the lipid moiety at the protoplasm facet of the ER or the Golgi body; however, the structure is then flipped to the luminal side for the additional process. The enzymes that initiate GSL glycosylation are specific for lipids, but an additional process of the sugar chain is performed by additional general glycosyltransferase [13, 14].

3.4 Proteoglycans and glycosaminoglycans

Proteoglycans are glycoproteins within the extracellular matrix that, in addition to containing canonical N-glycans and O-glycans, are characterized by the presence of long sugar repeats connected via O-linked glycosylation motifs [13, 14]. These extended sugar chains are termed glycosaminoglycans and contribute to a considerable proportion of the proteoglycan's molecular mass. Whereas N-glycans generally embrace 5–12 monosaccharides, a glycosaminoglycan motif will simply contain more than eighty sugars (for example, keratan salt is a poly-N-acetyl lactosamine chain that contains up to fifty oligosaccharide units). These long chains are constructed through oligosaccharide repeats fashioned by GlcNAc or GalNAc, combined with associate uronic acid (that is, glucuronic or iduronic acid) or brain sugar. Glycosaminoglycans are functionally various and include heparan salt, chondroitin salt, keratin sulfate, and hyaluronan. Glycosaminoglycans are crucial to the formation of the glycocalyx, an important structure for the upkeep of the cytomembrane that conjointly functions as a reservoir for sequestered growth factors [13–15].

3.5 Role of glycans in immunity and inflammation

Cells of the immune system, equally to any or all different cells, express cell surface-associated glycoproteins and glycolipids that, besides glycan-binding proteins and different molecules, sense environmental signals. Many immune receptors that are expressed on innate and adaptive immune cells acknowledge glycans found on the surface of microorganisms that are referred to as pathogen-associated molecular patterns. Examples of such glycan-containing molecules embrace bacterial lipopolysaccharides, peptidoglycans, teichoic acids, capsular polysaccharides, and fungal mannans. The recognition of those glycosylated microbial patterns by the immune system has been exploited for the vaccine's development, example diplococcus vaccines, are developed employing a mixture of capsular polysaccharides. The recent progress in HIV-1 immunogen development has conjointly been driven by a far better understanding of the HIV-1 envelope (Env) conjugated protein and the effects of its glycan composition on immune responses and immune evasion [15, 16].

Pro-inflammatory cytokines may contribute to inflammatory vascular diseases by inducing changes in cell-surface N-glycosylation of epithelial tissue cells. In the adaptive immune system, glycans even have crucial and multifarious roles in B lymphocyte and lymphocyte differentiation. These functions involve multiple cell-surface and secreted proteins (such as CD43, CD45, selectins, galectins, and siglecs), differing kinds of cell–cell interactions, and also the recognition of glycan-containing antigens. The regulation of cellular glycosylation and its impact on the molecules that perform as ligands and receptors throughout associate inflammatory response is controlled through numerous mechanisms and is dependent on the inflammatory insult. These mechanisms, that embrace ERK, and p65 signaling are vital to understanding the failure to regulate chronic inflammation in multiple disease states. Immunoglobulins, for instance, are crucial parts of humoral immunity, and altered glycosylation patterns of some antibody isotypes are known in chronic inflammatory reaction, and infectious diseases, like arthritis (RA), systemic lupus erythematosus (SLE), and HIV infection [16, 17].

The glycoproteins CD43 and CD45 are profusely expressed on the surface of B cells and T cells and contain each O-glycans and N-glycans. Glycosylation of those proteins is modulated throughout cellular differentiation and activation and regulates multiple T cell functions, as well as cellular migration, T cell receptor signaling, cell survival, and apoptosis. CD45 has an active receptor-like protein tyrosine phosphatase domain that interacts with Src family kinases in B cells and T cells to control the signaling threshold for the activation of B lymphocyte receptors (BCRs) and T cell receptors. CD45 additionally has non-catalytic functions, for instance, in modulating the function of the repressive co-receptor CD22 on B cells [17, 18].

Siglecs are sialic acid-binding proteins expressed on several cells of the system that perform varied functions, as well as the regulation of antigen-specific immune responses and cell homing. CD22 is one in all sixteen siglec proteins characterized in humans and is expressed on B cells, wherever it specifically binds α-2, 6-linked sialic acid-containing ligands; this interaction is crucial for the formation of nanoclusters within the cell wall that manage BCR signaling following antigen binding [17, 18].

The selectin family of proteins consists of E-selectin, P-selectin, and L-selectin that are chiefly expressed on epithelium cells, platelets, and leukocytes, respectively. These cell adhesion molecules are vital for white cells rolling on the epithelial tissue before tissue extravasations. Another study demonstrates that targeting selectins could be helpful in some inflammatory diseases. Immunoglobulin isotypes disagree within the variety of N-glycans present on their serious chains. Some immunoglobulin, such as IgA1 and immune globulin, additionally contain O-glycans, which are sometimes clustered within the hinge-region segments of these antibodies. Immunoglobulin glycans impact the effect or functions of antibodies counting on the branching of N-glycans and/or the terminal sugars of N-glycans or O-glycans that embody brain sugar and sialic acid. In fact, immunoglobulin glycosylation can verify glycoform is pro-inflammatory, like Ig with galactose-deficient N-glycans, or anti-inflammatory drug, like Ig with sialylated N-glycans [17–19].

3.6 Glycan and COVID-19

Coronavirus illness 2019 (Covid-19) has a broad clinical spectrum, not nevertheless absolutely delineate or understood, with a regarding the potential for severe respiratory illness, multiorgan involvement, and death. As a result of containment of the virus has verified to be very troublesome, mitigation efforts like mask-wearing, physical distancing, confinement, and quarantines are enforced worldwide leading to restricted exposures/contagious events with also a robust social, health, and economic burden [2]. Since ideal preventive ways like repurposing of known medication to treat Covid-19, and vaccines associated with inevitably long testing, development, and producing time emerges as an attractive approach to timely fulfill the continued need.

Glycoproteins of SARS-CoV-2 are concerned with cell adhesion and invasion, maturation, and modulation response processes. Though alternative SARS-CoV-2 proteins have foreseeable glycosylation sites (such as M-protein, E-protein), the bulk of experimental knowledge is presently accessible on the S-protein. This might be a trimeric protein that mediates viral adhesion through binding to the human angiotensin-converting accelerator two (hACE2) and conjointly interacts with the host immune defense [19, 20].

The S-protein from SARS-CoV-2 has 2 practical subunits (S1 and S2) with 23 potential sites for N-glycosylation and O-glycosylation. Some variations within the glycosylation sites repertoire and famed epitopes are rumored for the SARS-CoV-2 spike protein, despite it's similarity with the SARS-CoV spike (approximately 87.2%). The oligo mannose-type glycans were predominant in 2 sites (N234 and N709). Complex-type glycans were preponderantly exhibited in fourteen organic compound residues (N17, N74, N149, N165, N282, N331, N343, N616, N657, N1098, N1134, N1158, N1173, and N1194), whereas six sites showed a combination of oligomannose- and complex-type glycans (N1074, N801, N717, N603, N122, and N61). The foremost common configuration of oligomannose-type glycans was Man5GlcNAc2. Afucosylated and fucosylated hybrid-type glycans were detected in a minimum of 9 sites. Studies highlighted that the glycosylation profile of the

SARS-CoV-2 S-protein was completely different from those discovered for host glycoproteins or for alternative engulfed viruses. Another experimental study revealed the configuration of the N-glycosylation and O-glycosylation of spike protein subunits, even in the HEK293-based expression system. The authors have solved the structures of N-linked glycans in seventeen foretold sites and rumored the presence of three categories of N-glycans. Significantly, this study discovered O-glycosylation modifications on 2 residues (Thr323 and Ser325) present within the receptor-binding domain (RBD) of the S1 monetary unit. Recently, the characterization of the glycosylation profile of the S-protein expressed in BTI-Tn-5B1–4 insect cells was rumored to show the presence of high-mannose N-glycans altogether twenty two foretold sites. Apparently, these glycans cowl most of the RBD space [17, 20].

The glycan shield plays a vital role in hiding the S protein surface from molecular recognition. However, to effectively operate, the spike has to recognize and bind to ACE2 receptors as the primary host cell infection route. For this reason, the RBM should become totally exposed and accessible. During this state of affairs, the glycan shield works in concert with an oversized conformational amendment that permits the RBD to emerge on top of the N-glycan coverage. The glycans protect the RBD region that does not directly act with ACE2 by "up" and "down" conformations. Ultimately, this analysis shows that the RBM is often accessible once RBD is "up", whereas it's terribly well camouflaged when "down". This implies that the glycan shield of this vital domain is effectively paired with its "down-to-up" conformational amendment, allowing the RBM to transiently emerge from the glycan shield and bind to ACE2 receptors [16, 19, 20].

Protein glycosylation plays a crucial role in the infective agent pathological process, as incontestable by the characteristically thick N-glycan coating of the infective agent fusion proteins. Within the HIV-1 envelope spike (Env), as an example, the protein-accessible expanse is nearly entirely coated in N-glycans. These are thus densely packed that they account for quite half the protein's mass. The N-glycans present on the surface of viral envelope glycoproteins show terribly diverse type of biological roles. Infective agent entry through membrane fusion is initiated by envelope glycoproteins through molecular recognition events involving cell surface receptors, which are usually mediated by specific N-glycan epitopes. Furthermore, an extremely dense coating of nonimmunogenic or frail immunogenic advanced carbohydrates on otherwise perilously exposed infective agent proteins constitutes a perfect camouflage (or shield) to evade the immune system. To the current study, the HIV-1 Env glycan defends, which is essentially structured by oligomannose (Man5–9) N-glycans, has been shown to be quite effective in allowing the virus to thwart the system [16, 17, 19].

4. Therapeutic approach of glycomedicine

Developments within the field of glycobiology have enabled the development of a range of glycan-based medical specialties. As an example, envelope conjugated protein gp120 is expressed on the surface of HIV-1, and its variable glycosylation facilitates viral escape from immune detection. Adding new glycan-dependent epitopes to the recombinant gp120 used for vaccination inflated the ability of broadly speaking neutralizing being antibodies to recognize HIV-1, suggesting that this approach is used to optimize vaccination protocols and antigens. Moreover, HIV-1 envelope glycoproteins not solely differentiate HIV-1 clad however can even be wont to estimate the efficacy of vaccine regimens on the premise of protein binding to a panel of gp120 glycan-dependent epitopes 240. As printed antecedently, glycosylation plays an important role in regulating purposeful immune responses through complex receptor–glycan motif interactions. This site is currently being exploited in Ig therapies [20].

4.1 Role of lectins in COVID 19 and activation of complement pathway

Lectins, are glycan-binding proteins (GBPs) that are present in plants and lots of alternative species, are known to act with various glycan molecules either attached or released to a peptide backbone. This distinctive property has been explored within the development of analytics for glycan determination. Many relevant platforms are according to which lectin-based microarray has incontestable a utility in capturing glycan profiles of therapeutic compound glycoprotein [21].

As antecedently mentioned, the S-protein of SARS-CoV-2 encompasses a crucial role in infectious agent adhesion by binding to hACE2. Therefore, the disruption of this interaction is taken into account as a gorgeous target for antiviral medical care. Some non-mammalian-derived lectins (from plants and bacteria) are pointed as various antiviral agents against swallowed viruses thanks to their ability to acknowledge the glycans present within the structural proteins and to impair the initial steps of the infectious agent pathological process. Given the recent emergence of SARS-CoV-2, solely the glycoprotein isolated from Indian bean [Flt3 receptor-interacting glycoprotein (FRIL)] has been according up to now as an antiviral against this virus. FRIL may be a glucose/mannose glycoprotein conjointly called DLL-I. This protein molecule utterly inhibited the cytopathic result of SARS-CoV-2 (strain hCoV-19/Taiwan/NTU04/2020) toward Vero cells at higher concentrations [17, 21].

According to a study, evaluation of the in vitro antiviral activity of thirty three plant lectins toward coronaviruses (SARS-CoV and feline infectious redness virus). Mannose-binding agglutinins showed the best anti-SARS-CoV effects. Among the studied lectins, the upper selective indexes (SIs) were found for those isolated from alliaceous plant (APA; SI > 222.2), black mulberry (Morniga M II; SI > 62.5), and helleborine (EHA; SI > 55.5). Nettle (UDA) and common tobacco agglutinins (NICTABA), each specific for GlcNAc, conjointly showed promising activity. NICTABA and FTO have conjointly shown restrictive activity against different swallowed viruses as well as respiratory disease A/B, breakbone fever virus kind a pair of (DENV-2), herpes simplex virus varieties one and a pair of (HSV-1 and HSV-2) and human immunological disorder viruses (HIV-1/2). Other plant lectins are shown to exhibit restrictive action toward different coronaviruses. Some mannose-binding lectins: concanavalin A (Con A), amaryllis hybrid antibody (HHA), *Galanthus nivalis* antibody (GNA or GNL) one in every of these studies highlighted the importance of glycosylation within the sensibility of 2 kinds of coronaviruses (mouse liver disease virus and feline infectious redness virus) (**Figure 2**) [17, 21].

Non-plant-derived agglutinins also are pointed as promising agents against coronaviruses, e.g. the mannose-binding-lectins cyanovirin-N (from *Cyanobacterium protoctiste)* ellipsosporum and griffithsin (GRFT) (from red marine alga *Griffithsia* sp.) However, solely GRFT has been evaluated against SARS-CoV and MERS-CoV. This protein molecule binds to multiple sites of SARS-CoV and MERS-Cov glycoproteins with high affinity and inhibits infectious agent entry. In addition, this glycoprotein conjointly reduced the mortality and therefore the severity of fatal pneumonic infection iatrogenic by SARS-CoV in mice. This result is related to the decrease of pro-inflammatory cytokines in infected respiratory organ tissue [17–19, 21].

The mitogenicity and pro-inflammatory properties of lectins raise many queries relating to their worth to treat clinical conditions with severe inflammatory

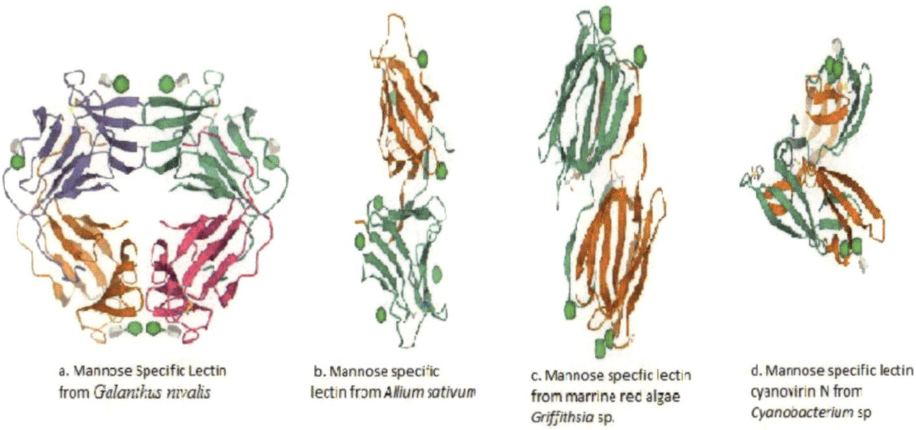

Figure 2.
Crystal structure of different mannose specific lectins (structures adapted from RCSB PDB).

elements, as seen in COVID-19. The broad-spectrum activity of those agents and therefore the techniques utilized in their style ought to be thought of within the hunt for anti-infective compounds toward SARS-CoV-2. These compounds ought to enhance the response iatrogenic by the immunogen, whereas keeping the equilibrium between body substance and cellular immune responses. Noteworthy to say that even the right induction of Th1-biased response, which is very important for defense against infectious agents, still remains a limitation for a few adjuvants.

Lectins are well-known to push the proliferation of lymphocytes and modulate the discharge of effectors molecules (cytokines and gas oxide) by immune cells. For example, many lectins are potent inducers of IL-12 and IFN-γ production that are key cytokines in the establishment of the Th1 axis. Some lectins may also bind to toll-like receptors and/or increase their expression levels, which can conjointly modulate the discharge of pro-inflammatory cytokines and increase the receptor's ability to acknowledge the pathogens. In fact, the improvement of Th1-based response is very important for protecting immunity against viruses and different intracellular pathogens thanks to the activation of cytotoxic cells (natural killer cells and TCD8 lymphocytes) and production of neutralizing antibodies concerned in immunologic memory. During this sense, the immunomodulatory properties of lectins build them attractive candidates for vaccine adjuvant. Some studies involving glycoprotein as an adjuvant for respiratory disease vaccines need special mention [21].

Innate immunity plays an essential role against numerous pathogens, in that, physical barriers complement components, coagulation cascade, antigen-presenting cells, and immunoglobulins synergistically regulate opsonisation, inflammation, and phagocytosis. Although the innate system might not determine each antigen getting into the host, it will acknowledge numerous microorganisms mainly based on pathogen-associated molecular patterns (PAMPs) present on the cell surface. The notable examples of PAMPs are bacterial peptidoglycan, lipopolysaccharides, mannans, lipoteichoic acids, bacterial DNA, double-stranded ribonucleic acid, glucans, and infective agent surface macromolecule. Duly, the complement system could be a wing of an innate immune response having varied biological effects against a good vary of bacteria, fungal, and infective agent infections [22].

The complement cascade consists of soluble factors and cell surface receptors which will sensitize and counteract against both invading and self-antigens. The complement system bridges the innate and accommodative reaction through humoral immunity, and by modulating T- and B-cell functions. Complement pathways, which, once activated, lead to consecutive protein reactions, breakdown of complement components C3 and C5, and end in by-products formation (C3a and C5a). These anaphylatoxins elicit an excessiveness of physiochemical responses that successively activate phagocytic cells, and release cytokines, chemokines, reactive element species (ROS), adhesion molecules, and inflammation at the site of infection. Immunoglobulin and cytokines are essential parts of antiviral immunity. In fact, there are 3 main phases of complement activation - (1) foreign molecule recognition, (2) convertase enzyme formation which will cleave C3 and C5, and (3) fabrication of MAC for cell lysis. The alternative, classical, and mannose-binding lectin (MBL) pathways are activation cascades of assorted host-pathogen interaction conditions, joining at the juncture C3, from wherever the central complement cascade proceeds. Among the 3 pathways of complement activation, the MBL pathway is primary in infective agent infections to induce a pro-inflammatory response. Detail Investigations involving the complement system activation by the lectin pathway in COVID-19 and diseases are in need of the hour [22, 23].

5. Conclusion

Glycosylation could be a common modification of proteins and lipids that involves non-template dynamic and complex processes. Glycans have multiple crucial roles in cellular responses to environmental stimuli likewise as cellular growth and differentiation; specific changes in glycan composition are directly joined to several diseases. Technological advances are commencing to overcome many of the challenges display by the complexities of glycoconjugates, improving our understanding of the physiological and pathological processes that are regulated by glycans.

The application of lectins to unravel differing types of issues involved in viral infections like COVID-19 depends upon the presence of glycoproteins within the viral envelope. Within the therapeutic space, the lectins can be thought-about leading molecules for the event of the latest antiviral approaches because of their ability to inhibit microorganism entry within the host cell. The advances in glycoprotein style methods are necessary to spice up the clinical application of those agents thought-about for the treatment of SARS-CoV-2 and alternative microorganism infections. The immunomodulatory action of some lectins may also be exploited to boost the effectiveness of immunization schemes for microorganism infections.

On the opposite hand, lectin–carbohydrates interactions will be accustomed style devices for diagnosing targeting microorganism glycoproteins or host glycoproteins alterations throughout microorganism infections. This kind of apparatuses hold the promise of producing sensitive, quick, and cost-effective identification of infected people and are of important would like throughout the pandemic things, as obligatory for COVID-19.

Author details

Swapan Kumar Chatterjee* and Snigdha Saha
Molecular Pharma Pvt. Ltd., Kolkata, West Bengal, India

*Address all correspondence to: swapan1chatterjee@gmail.com

References

[1] Furukawa, N. W., Brooks, J. T., & Sobel, J. (2020). Evidence Supporting Transmission of Severe Acute Respiratory Syndrome Coronavirus 2 While Presymptomatic or Asymptomatic. *Emerging infectious diseases*, *26*(7), e201595. https://doi.org/10.3201/eid2607.201595.

[2] Chatterjee, S. K., Saha, S., & Munoz, M. (2020). Molecular Pathogenesis, Immunopathogenesis and Novel Therapeutic Strategy Against COVID-19. *Frontiers in molecular biosciences*, *7*, 196. https://doi.org/10.3389/fmolb.2020.00196.

[3] Lu R, Zhao X, Li J, Niu P, Yang B, Wu H, Wang W, Song H, Huang B, Zhu N, Bi Y, Ma X, Zhan F, Wang L, Hu T, Zhou H, Hu Z, Zhou W, Zhao L, Chen J, Meng Y, Wang J, Lin Y, Yuan J, Xie Z, Ma J, Liu WJ, Wang D, Xu W, Holmes EC, Gao GF, Wu G, Chen W, Shi W, Tan W. (2020). Genomic characterisation and epidemiology of 2019 novel coronavirus: implications for virus origins and receptor binding. Lancet. 395(10224):565-574. doi: 10.1016/S0140-6736(20)30251-8. Epub 2020 Jan 30. PMID: 32007145; PMCID: PMC7159086.

[4] Tortorici, M. A., & Veesler, D. (2019). Structural insights into coronavirus entry. *Advances in virus research*, *105*, 93-116. https://doi.org/10.1016/bs.aivir.2019.08.002.

[5] Xiong X, Tortorici MA, Snijder J, Yoshioka C, Walls AC, Li W, McGuire AT, Rey FA, Bosch BJ, Veesler D. (2018). Glycan Shield and Fusion Activation of a Deltacoronavirus Spike Glycoprotein Fine-Tuned for Enteric Infections. J Virol. 92(4):e01628-17. doi: 10.1128/JVI.01628-17. PMID: 29093093; PMCID: PMC5790929.

[6] Doores K. J. (2015). The HIV glycan shield as a target for broadly neutralizing antibodies. *The FEBS journal*, *282*(24), 4679-4691. https://doi.org/10.1111/febs.13530.

[7] Pereira, M. S., Alves, I., Vicente, M., Campar, A., Silva, M. C., Padrão, N. A., Pinto, V., Fernandes, Â., Dias, A. M., & Pinho, S. S. (2018). Glycans as Key Checkpoints of T Cell Activity and Function. *Frontiers in immunology*, *9*, 2754. https://doi.org/10.3389/fimmu.2018.02754.

[8] Zhang, S., Zhou, P., Wang, P., Li, Y., Jiang, L., Jia, W., Wang, H., Fan, A., Wang, D., Shi, X., Fang, X., Hammel, M., Wang, S., Wang, X., & Zhang, L. (2018). Structural Definition of a Unique Neutralization Epitope on the Receptor-Binding Domain of MERS-CoV Spike Glycoprotein. *Cell reports*, *24*(2), 441-452. https://doi.org/10.1016/j.celrep.2018.06.041.

[9] Grant, O. C., Montgomery, D., Ito, K., & Woods, R. J. (2020). Analysis of the SARS-CoV-2 spike protein glycan shield: implications for immune recognition. *bioRxiv : the preprint server for biology*, 2020.04.07.030445. https://doi.org/10.1101/2020.04.07.030445.

[10] Luís Cláudio Nascimento da Silva, Juliana Silva Pereira Mendonça, Weslley Felix de Oliveira, Karla Lílian Rodrigues Batista, Adrielle Zagmignan, Isabelle Freire Tabosa Viana, Maria Tereza dos Santos Correia. (2020). Exploring lectin–glycan interactions to combat COVID-19: Lessons acquired from other enveloped viruses, *Glycobiology*, cwaa099, https://doi.org/10.1093/glycob/cwaa099.

[11] Bagdonaite I, Wandall HH. (2018). Global aspects of viral glycosylation.

Glycobiology. 28(7):443-467. doi: 10.1093/glycob/cwy021. PMID: 29579213; PMCID: PMC7108637.

[12] Bagdonaite I, Vakhrushev SY, Joshi HJ, Wandall HH. (2018). Viral glycoproteomes: technologies for characterization and outlook for vaccine design. FEBS Lett. 592(23): 3898-3920. doi: 10.1002/1873-3468.13177. Epub 2018 Jul 12. PMID: 29961944.

[13] Reily C, Stewart TJ, Renfrow MB, Novak J. (2019). Glycosylation in health and disease. Nat Rev Nephrol. 15(6):346-366. doi: 10.1038/s41581-019-0129-4. PMID: 30858582; PMCID: PMC6590709.

[14] Wong NA, Saier MH Jr. (2021). The SARS-Coronavirus Infection Cycle: A Survey of Viral Membrane Proteins, Their Functional Interactions and Pathogenesis. Int J Mol Sci. 22(3):1308. doi: 10.3390/ijms22031308. PMID: 33525632; PMCID: PMC7865831.

[15] Schnaar RL. (2016). Glycobiology simplified: diverse roles of glycan recognition in inflammation. J Leukoc Biol. 99(6):825-38. doi: 10.1189/jlb.3RI0116-021R. Epub 2016 Mar 22. PMID: 27004978; PMCID: PMC4952015.

[16] Crispin M, Ward AB, Wilson IA. (2018). Structure and Immune Recognition of the HIV Glycan Shield. Annu Rev Biophys. 47:499-523. doi: 10.1146/annurev-biophys-060414-034156. Epub 2018 Mar 29. PMID: 29595997; PMCID: PMC6163090.

[17] Clark MC, Baum LG. (2012). T cells modulate glycans on CD43 and CD45 during development and activation, signal regulation, and survival. Ann N Y Acad Sci. 1253:58-67. doi: 10.1111/j.1749-6632.2011.06304.x. Epub 2012 Jan 30. PMID: 22288421; PMCID: PMC4190024.

[18] Ohmi Y, Ise W, Harazono A, Takakura D, Fukuyama H, Baba Y, Narazaki M, Shoda H, Takahashi N, Ohkawa Y, Ji S, Sugiyama F, Fujio K, Kumanogoh A, Yamamoto K, Kawasaki N, Kurosaki T, Takahashi Y, Furukawa K. (2016). Sialylation converts arthritogenic IgG into inhibitors of collagen-induced arthritis. Nat Commun. 7:11205. doi: 10.1038/ncomms11205. PMID: 27046227; PMCID: PMC4822049.

[19] de Haas P, Hendriks WJAJ, Lefeber DJ, Cambi A. (2020). Biological and Technical Challenges in Unraveling the Role of N-Glycans in Immune Receptor Regulation. Front Chem. 8:55. doi: 10.3389/fchem.2020.00055. PMID: 32117881; PMCID: PMC7013033.

[20] Shimada M, Yoshizaki S, Jounai N, Kondo A, Ichino M, Ryo A, Okuda K. (2010). DNA vaccine expressing HIV-1 gp120/immunoglobulin fusion protein enhances cellular immunity. Vaccine. 28(31):4920-7. doi: 10.1016/j.vaccine.2010.05.035. Epub 2010 Jun 3. PMID: 20566393.

[21] Malaquias MAS, Gadotti AC, Motta-Junior JDS, Martins APC, Azevedo MLV, Benevides APK, Cézar-Neto P, Panini do Carmo LA, Zeni RC, Raboni SM, Fonseca AS, Machado-Souza C, Moreno-Amaral AN, de Noronha L. (2020). The role of the lectin pathway of the complement system in SARS-CoV-2 lung injury. Transl Res. S1931-5244(20)30259-0. doi: 10.1016/j.trsl.2020.11.008. Epub ahead of print. PMID: 33221483; PMCID: PMC7677075.

[22] Ram Kumar Pandian S, Arunachalam S, Deepak V, Kunjiappan S, Sundar K. (2020). Targeting complement cascade: an alternative strategy for COVID-19. 3 Biotech. 10(11):479. doi: 10.1007/

s13205-020-02464-2. Epub 2020 Oct 19. PMID: 33088671; PMCID: PMC7571295.

[23] Casalino L, Gaieb Z, Goldsmith JA, Hjorth CK, Dommer AC, Harbison AM, Fogarty CA, Barros EP, Taylor BC, McLellan JS, Fadda E, Amaro RE. (2020). Shielding and Beyond: The Roles of Glycans in SARS-CoV-2 Spike Protein. bioRxiv [Preprint]. 2020.06.11.146522. doi: 10.1101/2020.06.11.146522. Update in: ACS Cent Sci. 2020 Oct 28;6(10):1722-1734. PMID: 32577644; PMCID: PMC7302197.

Chapter 5

Epigenetic Regulation Mechanisms in Viral Infections: A Special Focus on COVID-19

Burcu Biterge Süt

Abstract

The outbreak of Coronavirus Disease-2019 (Covid-19), caused by a novel and highly pathogenic coronavirus (severe acute respiratory syndrome coronavirus-2, SARS-CoV-2), is a persisting global health concern. Research so far has successfully identified the molecular mechanisms of viral entry, alterations within the host cell upon infection, and the stimulation of an immune response to fight it. One of the most important cellular regulatory machineries within the host cell to be affected by the SARS-CoV-2 infection is epigenetic regulation, which modulates transcriptional activity by DNA sequence-independent factors such as DNA-methylation, RNA interference and histone modifications. Several studies in the literature have previously reported epigenetic alterations within the host due to infections of the Coronaviridae family viruses including SARS-CoV and MERS-CoV that antagonized immune system activation. Recent studies have also identified epigenetic dysregulation of host metabolism by SARS-CoV-2 infection, linking epigenetic mechanisms with the pathophysiology and illness severity of Covid-19. Therefore, this book chapter aims to provide a comprehensive overview of the epigenetic regulation mechanisms in viral infections with a special focus on SARS-CoV-2 infection.

Keywords: Coronavirus infection, Covid-19, epigenetic regulation, host repression, immune evasion, cytokine storm, susceptibility

1. Introduction

Coronavirus Disease-2019 (COVID-19), which is caused by a newly emerged, highly pathogenic coronavirus (severe acute respiratory syndrome coronavirus-2, SARS-CoV-2), has been one of the gravest global health concerns of the last century. Previous infections of *Coronaviridae* family, including MERS-CoV and SARS-CoV resulted in human diseases and were associated with the spread of MERS (Middle East respiratory syndrome) and SARS, respectively. SARS-CoV-2 is an enveloped, positive-sense RNA virus. It has a large genome, which consists of six major open reading frames encoding four structural proteins S (spike), E (envelope), M (membrane), N (nucleoprotein) and sixteen non-structural proteins (Nsp1–16).

Epigenetic mechanisms are vital for the regulation of transcriptional activity. Alterations within the epigenetic landscape affect gene expression via influencing chromatin accessibility rather than changing the underlying DNA sequence. Therefore, epigenetic modifications provide a reversible and flexible mechanism of directing cellular function in response to environmental stimuli. Viral infections

IntechOpen

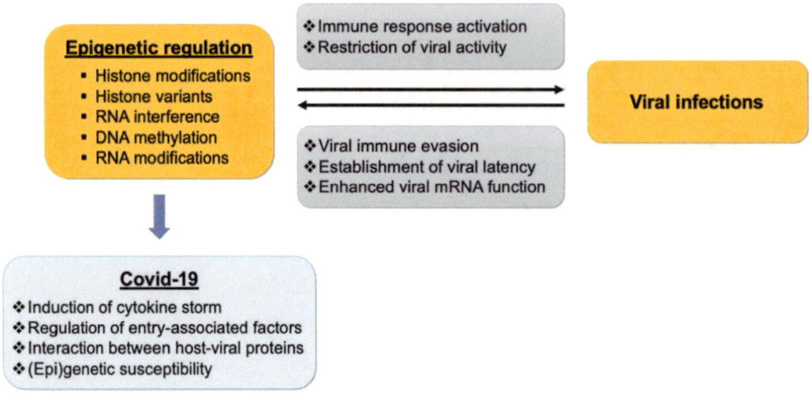

Figure 1.
Summary of the interplay between the host epigenetic regulation machinery and viral infections.

are important sources of such stimuli that cause drastic changes in the gene expression patterns of the host. While epigenetic reprogramming ensures transcriptional activation that is required for the induction of a proper immune response against viral infections, factors of the epigenetic regulation mechanisms are also hijacked by viruses to subvert the host antiviral defense machinery. This establishes a bidirectional relationship between the host cell and the virus, as depicted in **Figure 1**, controlling the viral life cycle and the dysregulation of the host gene expression [1].

Herein, we unfold the complex regulatory pathways of epigenetic mechanisms affecting the host cell and the virus. Particularly, we discuss the epigenetic basis of viral entry and cytokine storm induction in relation to SARS-CoV-2 infection, as well as epigenetic susceptibility to Covid-19 from a molecular point of view.

2. Epigenetic regulation mechanisms

Epigenetics was first introduced to the scientific community as a term to describe the molecular mechanisms that cause heritable phenotypic changes, which are independent of the genetic material [2]. Since then, regulation of DNA accessibility through chromatin condensation has been identified as the main mechanism of epigenetic regulation, implicating them in several cellular processes like cell cycle, cellular proliferation, transcriptional memory, and DNA damage repair [3]. The level of chromatin compaction in a given genomic locus determines its transcriptional activity as genes within the loosely packaged euchromatin regions are actively transcribed and the highly condensed heterochromatin regions are transcriptionally silent [4]. The interplay between euchromatin and heterochromatin enables the establishment of differential gene expression patterns and is essentially regulated by epigenetic mechanisms involving DNA methylation, non-coding RNAs and RNA interference (RNAi), DNA replication-independent incorporation of histone variants and histone post-translational modifications (**Figure 2**).

In eukaryotic cells, chromatin condensation is achieved by packaging the DNA into chromatin by wrapping the naked DNA onto octamers of core histones H2A, H2B, H3, and H4 [5]. Deposition of the linker histone H1 leads to the formation of higher-order chromatin and is associated with transcriptional silencing [6]. Histones can be covalently modified by the post-translational addition of a variety of functional groups including but not limited to methyl-, acetyl-, phosphoryl-, ubiquitin and ADP-ribose that altogether constitute an epigenetic signature of transcriptional activity [7]. Histone acetylation is generally associated with an

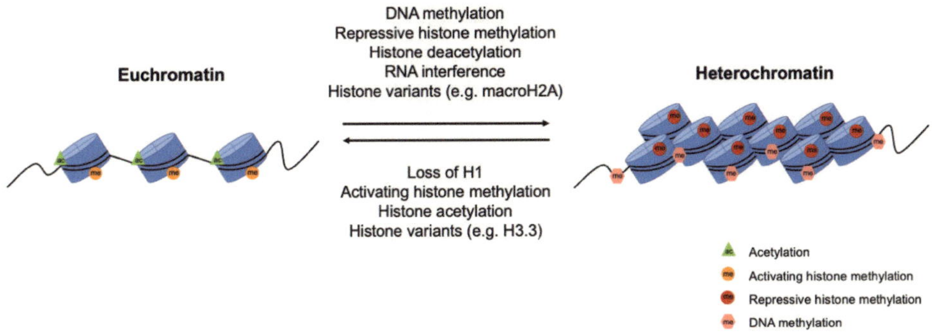

Figure 2.
The conformational transition between euchromatin and heterochromatin is mediated by epigenetic mechanisms.

open chromatin conformation and active gene expression. H3K9ac, H4K16ac and H3K27ac are the most abundant histone acetylations found at the promoters and enhancers of actively transcribed genes [8, 9]. On the other hand, the impact of histone methylations on gene expression strictly depends on their degree and location. For instance, H3K4me1–2-3 and H3K9me are marks of active transcription sites, while H3K9me2–3 and H3K27me2–3 are found in heterochromatin and are indicators of repressed gene state [10].

The main constituents of nucleosomes are canonical histones and share only a certain level of similarity with their corresponding "replacement" variants. These differences in amino acid sequence affects gene expression both by causing conformational alterations of chromatin and disruption of existing interactions between histones and their chaperons, while establishing new ones (reviewed in [11]). Histone variants are involved in several chromatin-related processes such as transcriptional regulation (H3.3 and macroH2A), DNA damage signaling (H2A.X), nucleosome positioning (H2A.Z) and the formation of centromeres (CENP-A).

RNA interference (RNAi) is another mechanism of epigenetic regulation that facilitates heterochromatin formation and transcriptional silencing by the action of non-coding RNAs. X chromosome inactivation is a significant example of RNAi mediated transcriptional repression, which results in the random heterochromatinization and silencing of one of the X chromosomes in females to provide dosage compensation [12]. X-inactivation is initiated by the long non-coding RNA Xist (X-inactive specific transcript) and via the recruitment of histone modifiers and corepressor complexes, an inactive gene state throughout the X chromosome is achieved [13]. Furthermore, small non-coding RNAs including micro-RNAs (miRNAs), small interfering-RNAs (siRNAs) and Piwi-interacting RNAs (piRNAs) are important contributors of transcriptional regulation mediated by RNAi [14–17].

DNA methylation is a reversible post-translational modification of DNA that cause repression of gene expression when present at CpG islands in promoter regions. CpG denotes cytosine residues followed by a guanine nucleotide, where the methyl-group is covalently attached to the 5th carbon of cytosine, giving rise to 5-methylcytosine (5mC). DNA methylation is catalyzed by DNMT enzymes in mammals. 5mC marks that the *de novo* DNA methyltransferases DNMT3A and DNMT3B set during embryonic development are inherited in every cell division semi-conservatively [18] and the maintenance DNA methyltransferase DNMT1 methylates the newly synthesized, hemi-methylated strand [19]. Heterochromatin exhibits high levels of 5mC that correlates with lower levels of gene expression led by transcriptional silencing [20, 21].

Recent studies identified a number of RNA modifications that play a wide range of regulatory roles in various cellular processes and embryonic development.

The list of RNA modifications comprises of N7-methylguanosine (m7G), 2′-O-methylation (Nm), 5-methyl cytosine (m5C), N1-methyladenosine (m1A), N6-methyladenosine (m6A), and 3-methylcytidine (m3C). All these epigenetic modifications of RNA constitute a complex regulatory network over several aspects of mRNA metabolism such as translation efficiency, mRNA splicing and nuclear export [22].

3. Epigenetic regulation during viral infections

As intracellular parasites that lack critical cellular components for replication, protein synthesis, metabolism, and energy production, viruses are incapable of self-maintenance. Therefore, they strictly rely on the cellular machineries of the host cell for their propagation, including the host's epigenetic factors [23]. Viruses hijack the epigenetic regulation mechanisms for multiple reasons. Firstly, several molecular processes such as viral genome replication, transcription of viral proteins and the packaging of new viral particles may simultaneously take place within a single host cell. The existence and coordination of distinct viral genome states allowing these molecular processes are often orchestrated by the machineries of epigenetic regulation [1]. Secondly, as key regulators of gene expression, epigenetic factors are required for the transcription of viral proteins. Especially for viruses encompassing large genomes such as Herpesviruses, epigenetic regulation ensures that only the relevant set of genes are expressed in accordance with the stage of infection [24]. Lastly, the genetic material of DNA viruses is either found in a eukaryotic chromatin-like state in the viral particle or gets packaged within the host cell, making it a target for epigenetic regulation. For instance, the DNA of polyomaviruses (such as Simian Virus 40 – SV40) exists as chromatin throughout their life cycle and is regulated by histone modifications, RNAi, and nucleosome positioning [25, 26]. Similarly, the linear DNA of adenoviruses is packaged by viral proteins that are similar to histones, namely protein VII, which then get replaced by histones upon viral entry into the host [27].

There are three main outcomes of viral exploitation of epigenetic mechanisms, which are the restriction of viral replication by the host immunity and its evasion, regulation of viral latency and the enhancing of viral mRNA function.

3.1 Epigenetic mechanisms of host repression and viral immune evasion

Epigenetic mechanisms can alter gene expression patterns in the cell in response to environmental stimuli, enabling them to quickly adapt to external changes. As important external stimuli that induce cellular response, viral infections are often confronted by epigenetic alterations within the host cell to repress viral replication and gene expression [28]. Upon entry into the host cell, viral DNA rapidly gets packaged and heterochromatinized, inhibiting viral gene transcription. The epigenetic restriction of viral activity is considered as an innate immune response, which further participates in inducing adaptive immunity and apoptosis in the infected cells [23]. On the other hand, viruses have also developed epigenetic strategies to counteract and evade the cellular antiviral response both by suppressing host immunity and by creating a suitable environment for viral replication [28].

Viral DNA is distinguished and targeted for epigenetic repression by two main mechanisms involving pro-myelocytic leukemia nuclear bodies (PML-NBs) and interferon-inducible protein 16 (IFI16). PML-NBs consist of PML proteins and several epigenetics factors such as transcriptional co-repressors and histone chaperons, which constitute a regulatory hub for gene expression. In alpha-herpes virus HSV-1, histone variant H3.3 carrying repressive histone modifications (e.g. H3K9me3) is incorporated into the viral DNA via PML-NB-associated histone chaperons HIRA, Daxx and ATRX [29, 30]. In hepatitis B virus, Smc5/6 proteins, together with PML-NBs, provide viral inhibition. In overcoming host repression, both herpesviruses and the hepatitis B virus target PML-NBs for degradation and dispersion of the effector proteins. In herpesviruses, the viral protein VP16 interacts with host proteins HCF-1 and Oct-1 to recruit histone demethylases LSD1 and JMJD2 for the removal of previously established repressive H3K9me3 marks [31, 32]. Next, activating H3K4me3 marks are deposited by histone methyltransferases Set1 and MLL1 to allow the transcription of viral immediate early protein ICP0 [33]. As an E3 ubiquitin ligase, ICP0 targets PML-NB for ubiquitylation and degradation, which subsequently releases Daxx and ATRX from the vicinity of viral DNA [34]. Likewise, pp71 protein in beta-herpesvirus HCMV, BNRF1 protein in Epstein–Barr virus and HBx protein in hepatitis B virus exert similar functions in disassembling the PML-NBs and avoiding the repressive mechanisms of the host [35–37].

Foreign DNA is recognized by several factors in the host cell, which trigger the induction of innate immunity and the secretion of cytokines and chemokines. IFI16 acts as an innate immune DNA sensor for viral DNA and induces inflammasome activation [38]. In addition to its key role in stimulating interferon-β secretion, IFI16 contributes to the restriction of viral propagation via deposition of repressive histone marks to the viral DNA and displacing transcription factors from viral gene promoters [39, 40]. Similar to the viral evasion of PML-NB-mediated host repression, IFI16 can be degraded by the ICP0 protein in HSV-1 and its repressive activity can be blocked by HCMV proteins [41, 42]. Furthermore, IFI16 itself is subjected to epigenetic regulation, in which its acetylation by p300 may provide another layer of modulating transcriptional activity [43].

Another viral mechanism that provides escape from recognition and elimination by the host immune system makes use of viral miRNAs that share sequence homology with cellular mRNAs and miRNAs. By specifically targeting and silencing transcripts for host proteins that might function as inhibitors of viral replication, such as regulators of antiviral immunity, viruses can avoid host repression [44]. Viral miRNAs have also been attributed additional roles in regulating viral protein expression and controlling viral replication [45]. The biogenesis of viral miRNAs relies solely on the cellular machineries of the host; whereby the host RNA polymerases, ribonucleases and endonucleases act in cohort to transcribe and process the viral miRNA precursors into mature viral miRNAs [46]. Viral miRNAs are detected in several types of viruses, including but not limited to the frequent human infectors such as Epstein Barr virus, herpes B virus, human cytomegalovirus, human immunodeficiency virus 1, herpes simplex virus 1 and 2, Kaposi sarcoma-associated herpesvirus and simian virus 40. Currently, there are more than 300 viral miRNA precursors and more than 500 mature viral miRNAs available in the miRBase collection [47].

Lastly, viral infections can induce global alterations in histone modifications or the chromatin composition of the host, resulting in distinct epigenetic landscapes. For instance, E1A protein in adenoviruses interacts with lysine acetyltransferases p300/CBP to preferentially block histone acetylation and to repress a set of genes that would normally inhibit infection [48]. Likewise, protein VII can act as a histone mimic due to its structural resemblance to histones and change the host chromatin composition. It also binds to high-mobility group proteins (HMGBs) and tethers them to chromatin, inhibiting their release that typically acts as a danger signal to activate immune system in response to inflammatory stimulus [49].

3.2 Epigenetic regulation of viral latency

Viral invasions often fail to achieve successful propagation and production of infectious progeny due to several reasons such as host repression, deficiency in host resources and failure to replicate the viral genome properly [50]. In contrast to the lytic infections that produce and release infectious progeny via host cell lysis, latent infections result in the stable maintenance of viral genome within the host cell without expression of viral antigens and production of viral particles. When viruses infect non-permissive cells, they repurpose the epigenetic mechanisms of host repression to enter a dormant state, which would allow establishment of long-term infections while avoiding the host adaptive immune response [51]. The majority of viruses that can achieve latency belongs to the families of herpesviruses and retroviruses. While herpesviruses accomplish latency by means of epigenetic repression, retroviruses reverse transcribe their RNA genome into DNA and integrate it to the host genome for viral persistence.

Latent infections are reversible, as it is possible to reactivate viral replication and switch to lytic infection under permissive conditions. The decision between a lytic and a latent infection requires the expression of distinct sets of genes, indicating epigenetic regulation [1]. During the establishment of latency, viral gene expression is tightly controlled in a temporal manner, in which the latency genes are first turned on and then partially turned off to limit the production of viral antigens while the lytic gene foci are heterochromatinized for transcriptional repression [23]. The silencing of lytic gene expression in latent infections is mainly orchestrated by the action of transcriptional corepressor complex Co-REST and the Polycomb complex [52–54]. Consequently, the viral genome is enriched in repressive histone marks such as H3K27me3 and H3K9me3, which are excluded from the latency related genes [50]. Likewise, activating histone methylations (e.g. H3K4me3) are found at the transcript start sites and the regulatory regions of latency genes [55]. Interestingly, viral genomes can harbor bivalent chromatin states consisting of both activating and repressive histone marks that enable transition between latent and lytic phases [56]. Formation of higher-order chromatin structures via chromatin organizing factor CTCF is implicated in the regulation of latency as well [57]. In addition to the host-driven mechanisms, viral proteins BNRF1, HCF1 and VP16 participate in the recruitment of histone chaperons and histone deacetylases to prevent lytic gene expression [58, 59].

In order to be stably maintained within the host cell through several rounds of cell division, the viral genome forms minichromosomes (episomes) and segregates along the host chromosomes following replication [1]. For this purpose, the viral episome is tethered to the host metaphase chromatin via viral proteins, replicated by the host replication machinery and the newly synthesized episomes are equally divided between the daughter cells prior to the completion of cell division [50]. The cellular targets of viral episome tethering includes AT-rich DNA, histones and other chromatin associated factors [60–62]. The formation of episomes also serves to protect viral genome integrity via formation of "endless" i.e., circular genomes [50].

3.3 Enhanced viral mRNA function

Viral RNAs are heavily modified by the covalent addition of functional groups that are similar to cellular mRNAs; however, some of these modifications are found in significantly higher levels in viruses than eukaryotes. Recent studies attributed important roles for RNA modifications in promoting viral replication, through enhanced stability of viral transcripts, increased efficiency of translation and escaping immune recognition [1]. N_6-methyladenosine (m^6A) constitutes a major source of RNA modifications, which is deposited by METTL3 and recognized by the YTH domain of YTHDC1, YTHDC2, YTHDF1, YTHDF2 and YTHDF3 proteins [63]. m^6A has been shown to promote viral gene expression and replication, as well as to enhance immune evasion [64–66]. Mutations that alter m^6A deposition sites and thereby reduce m^6A levels result in a substantial decrease in viral pathogenicity, suggesting a novel strategy that could be used in engineering vaccines based on attenuated viruses [65]. 5-methylcytidine (m^5C) is another abundant RNA modification. It is catalyzed mainly by NSUN2 and its loss causes decreased translation efficiency of HIV-1 transcripts [67]. N4-acetylcytidine (ac^4C) is set by NAT10 and is found both in viral and cellular RNAs. Previous reports have established a link between ac^4C and improved stability and translation efficiency of viral transcripts and indicated that its loss at even 3′-untranslated regions of viral mRNAs leads to reduced levels of viral transcription and protein synthesis [23]. 2′O-methylation is a distinct type of RNA modification, in the sense that it can be deposited by the nucleolar protein FTSJ3 on either one of the three types of ribonucleotides (A, U and G) and on cytidine residues possibly by an unknown mechanism. Viruses that lack 2′O-methylation due to depletion of FTSJ3 activity trigger the cytoplasmic viral RNA sensor MDA5, implicating 2′O-methylation as a viral mechanism of escaping recognition by the host immune system [68].

4. Epigenetic regulation in relation to Covid19

4.1 Role of epigenetic mechanisms in the induction of cytokine storm

As detailed in the previous section, epigenetic regulation plays a significant role during viral infections. Viruses of the *Coronaviridae* family that previously caused MERS (Middle East respiratory syndrome, MERS-CoV) and SARS (SARS-CoV) have previously been shown to dysregulate the host immune system by inducing epigenetic changes that antagonize antigen presentation or activate interferon-stimulated genes (ISGs) [69, 70]. These viruses have also been implicated in blocking pathogen recognition and immune system signaling [71]. Due to this tight link with the host immune response, patients suffering from infections of coronaviruses, including SARS-CoV-2, are characterized by an abnormal induction of acute inflammation, namely cytokine storm. The excessive secretion of proinflammatory cytokines and recruitment of immune cells at the site of infection often leads to tissue damage and organ failure, which are hallmarks of Covid-19-related deaths [72].

The transcriptional regulation of cytokine production is under tight control of epigenetic mechanisms. Promoters of interferons (IFNs), tumor necrosis factors (TNFs) and ISGs that are drastically upregulated in Covid-19 patients are enriched by histone marks of open chromatin in activated macrophages and dendritic cells [71, 73, 74]. In addition to the common histone modifications, Covid-19 patients exhibit elevated levels of arginine citrullination on histone H3 [75]. Citrullination, which is a marker of a specific type of immune response to infection, namely neutrophil extracellular traps (NETs), is associated with chromatin decondensation and transcriptional activation [76]. Induction of NETosis is hypothesized to lead to sustained inflammation during SARS-CoV-2 infection and the subsequent cell death due to cytokine storm [77].

4.2 Regulation of SARS-CoV-2 entry-associated factors by epigenetic mechanisms

The novel coronavirus SARS-CoV-2 interacts with and requires the action of multiple host proteins for viral entry. Spike (S) protein, which is anchored into the viral envelope, binds to angiotensin converting enzyme 2 (ACE2) on the host cell surface [78]. ACE2 is a membrane protein found in a wide variety of cell types. The interaction between ACE2 and the receptor binding domain (RBD) within the S1 subunit of the spike protein initiates entry, while S2 subunit triggers direct membrane fusion or endocytosis upon cleavage and activation by host proteases FURIN and TMPRSS2 [79]. Two members of the cathepsin family, namely CTSB and CTSL are also involved in the viral glycoprotein processing and the fusion between viral and endosomal membranes [80].

Among all SARS-CoV-2 entry-associated host factors, ACE2 is the best characterized protein in terms of epigenetic regulation. ACE2 is located on the X-chromosome, which typically gets heterochromatinized and undergoes X-inactivation in females to achieve dosage compensation. In line with this, higher ACE2 expression was observed in males than in females, accompanied by marks of open chromatin [81]. The heterozygosity of ACE2 alleles, hence the lower levels of ACE2 expression in females is considered as a significant advantage in counteracting SARS-CoV-2 infection [82]. However, X-inactivation is often incomplete, and a significant proportion of X-linked genes, including ACE2, escape silencing [81]. Therefore, ACE2 seems to show a rather heterogeneous sex bias [83].

Several epigenetic factors such as DNA methyltransferase DNMT1, histone acetyltransferases p300 and HAT1, histone deacetylases HDAC2 and SIRT1, histone methyltransferase EZH2 and histone demethylase KDM5B have been reported as potential regulators of ACE2 expression [84, 85]. Accordingly, histone marks H3K27ac, H3K27me3, H3K4me1 and H3K4me3 were detected within the ACE2 locus. Furthermore, studies have shown that ACE2 is under tight regulation of DNA methylation. In all tissues tested, lung epithelial cells exhibited the lowest levels of DNA methylation in ACE2 promoter, which positively correlated with high expression [86]. It was also claimed that the CpG methylation pattern of ACE2 promoter is associated with age and gender, suggesting a possible explanation for increased mortality in elderly men during SARS-CoV-2 infection [84, 86].

Other SARS-CoV-2 entry-associated factors are subject to epigenetic regulation as well. A recent study identified a regulatory region upstream of FURIN gene that is heavily occupied by the histone acetyltransferase p300 in T cells [87]. Also, DNMT1-mediated hypermethylation of TMPRSS2 was associated with its down-regulation [88]. Moreover, loss of DNA methylation was implicated in increased levels of CTSL/CTSB in pancreatic adenocarcinoma, which could cause greater susceptibility to SARS-CoV-2 infection [89]. In accordance with this finding, silencing of CTSL/CTSB was shown to inhibit SARS-CoV-2 replication and virally induced apoptosis [90]. Additionally, significant hypomethylation of CTSL promoter was observed in chronic myeloid leukemia [91].

4.3 Interaction between the host epigenetic factors and viral proteins

Interactome analysis of SARS-CoV-2 proteins has provided experimental evidence of physical interaction between several viral proteins and human factors, implicating them in a variety of cellular processes such as epigenetic regulation of gene expression, RNA processing, DNA replication, trafficking and transport of proteins, mitochondrial function, cellular structure, and cell signaling pathways [92]. Viral envelope protein E interacts with bromodomain proteins BRD2 and BRD4 via its C-terminal end that mimics the N-terminal tail of histone H3. As specific binders and readers of histone acetylation, bromodomain-containing proteins are associated with transcriptional activity [93]. By disrupting BRD2/4 binding to histone H3, protein E can induce genomic alterations that affect host gene expression. Another inhibitory link with histone acetylation was established between

Nsp5 and HDAC2, which could potentially influence the host immune response against SARS-CoV-2. HDACs are commonly classified as transcriptional repressors since their main task is the removal of histone acetylation, a mark of active chromatin. However, HDAC2 plays an activating role during the transcriptional elongation of ISG expression via regulating BRD4 availability at newly activated promoters [94]. Similarly, Nsp8 was identified as a binding partner of histone lysine methyltransferase NSD2, which sets H3K36me3 at the gene bodies of actively transcribed genes [95]. H3K36me3 is suggested as an epigenetic mark of transcriptional memory in ISGs, indicating another layer of innate immune response regulation [96]. Viral proteins Nsp13 and Orf10 interact with ubiquitin specific peptidase USP13 and the components of the Cullin-RING E3 ubiquitin ligase complex, respectively. USP13 has previously been attributed significant immune response-related roles in interferon-induced signaling by STAT1 targeting and deubiquitination [97] and increased immune cell infiltration in several types of cancers [98]. Interestingly, USP13 antagonizes antiviral response via ubiquitination of STING, an important effector of innate immune signaling in response to viral infections [99]. Likewise, Cullin-RING E3 ubiquitin ligase complex members are often hijacked by viruses, inducing the proteasomal degradation of host restriction factors, and promoting viral replication [100]. Nsp13 also interacts with TLEs and TBK1/TBKBP1 proteins which are modulators of NF-kB-dependent inflammatory response and IFN signaling [101].

The list of interactions between SARS-CoV-2 and the epigenetic factors of the host cell that are based on experimental evidence has also been extended by in silico approaches that identified p53 as a binding partner of spike (S) protein [102] and several human miRNAs targeting SARS-CoV-2 transcripts [103]. Conversely, an interplay between SARS-CoV-2 miRNAs and the immune signaling pathways of the host was suggested, which could contribute to the prolonged latency of the virus leading to asymptomatic individuals.

4.4 (Epi)genetic susceptibility to Covid-19

Certain risk groups have been associated with increased susceptibility and disease severity since the emergence of the SARS-CoV-2 outbreak. Age is one of the main risk factors for Covid-19, as evident by its high occurrence and mortality rates in elderly patients [104]. Epigenetic machineries often become defective during the process of aging as well, which results in increased genomic instability, altered gene expression profiles and loss of resilience [105]. These age-related epigenetic changes could hamper the activation of innate and adaptive immune responses, which could also be manipulated by viruses to evade host repression. Coronaviruses have previously been linked with accelerated rate of host immune system aging through epigenetic mechanisms such as DNA methylation and transcriptional silencing that impede with host antigen presentation and the expression of major histocompatibility complexes [70]. Moreover, age-dependent fluctuations in the levels of glycosylation and NAD+, which have epigenetic associations, are implicated in predisposition to SARS-CoV-2 infection [106, 107].

There is a growing body of evidence pointing towards the role of DNA methylation in Covid-19 severity. Analysis of genome-wide DNA methylation profiles of severe COVID-19 cases revealed increased methylation of IFN-related genes while inflammatory genes were hypomethylated [108]. Likewise, a genome-wide association study identified a total of 44 CpG sites, most of which were located to coding genes including the components of the inflammasome complex and the major histocompatibility complex HLA-C as potential markers of COVID-19 severity and respiratory failure [109]. Furthermore, in lupus patients, loss of DNA methylation in ACE2 and interferon/cytokine-regulated genes, together with enhanced NF-kB expression were defined as contributors of severe COVID-19 [110]. Lastly, SARS-CoV-2 can demethylate and activate the expression of Syncytin-1 and Syncytin-2 genes of the host that are required for the creation of giant multinucleated cells, a process known as syncytium formation [111]. Syncytin genes are normally methylated and silenced during development, except for the mammalian placenta, where induction of multinucleated cells provides tissue impermeability in aid of immune tolerance between mother and child [112]. Syncytium formation followed by extensive cell death is suggested as an underlying cause of the detrimental effects of cytokine storm in COVID-19 patients [113].

5. Clinical implications and future perspectives

Until the successful development of the first Covid-19 vaccine in December 2020, one of the greatest challenges in fighting the disease was the lack of specific medication and vaccination. To this end, epigenetic mechanisms have been considered as promising targets for novel therapeutic approaches due to the important role of epigenetic regulation during viral infections including viruses of the *Coronaviridae* family. Several epigenetic modifier enzymes such as DNMTs, HATs, HDACs, HMTs and KDMs are proposed as candidate targets for the treatment of Covid-19. For instance, histone demethylase KDM5B could be targeted for the prevention of Covid-19 as its inhibition stimulates interferon production and provides resistance to viral infections [84]. Targeting epigenetic modifiers could open up a new revenue for the inhibitors against these enzymes, which are already in the market for therapeutic purposes, as potential antiviral agents to be used in drug repurposing attempts. In line with this, Decitabine, an inhibitor of DNA methylation (NCT04482621) and Dipyridamole, an inhibitor of NET formation (NCT04391179) are currently in clinical trials for Covid-19 therapy [28, 114]. Other clinical trials based on epigenetic markers aim to study microRNAs and DNA methylation patterns in relation to Covid-19 (NCT04403386 and NCT04411563) [28].

In conclusion, it is critical to characterize the molecular pathways that take part in SARS-CoV-2 infections to the best of our knowledge to have a better understanding of Covid-19 and to develop better therapies and vaccines for treatment. Epigenetic regulation machineries are involved in several virus-related cellular processes, suggesting epigenetic factors as promising targets for therapy. In this book chapter, we provided a comprehensive overview of epigenetic mechanisms in viral infections with a special focus on SARS-CoV-2 infection, which we believe will be useful for future studies.

Conflict of interest

The author declares no conflict of interest.

Author details

Burcu Biterge Süt
Department of Medical Biology, Faculty of Medicine, Niğde Ömer Halisdemir University, Niğde, Turkey

*Address all correspondence to: bbitergesut@ohu.edu.tr

'Biotechnology to Combat COVID-19' is a collaborative project with Biotechnology Kiosk

References

[1] Balakrishnan L, Milavetz B. Epigenetic Regulation of Viral Biological Processes. Viruses. 2017 Nov 17;9(11):346. doi: 10.3390/v9110346.

[2] Waddington CH (1939) An introduction to modern genetics/by C. H. Waddington. George Allen & Unwin, London

[3] Kouzarides T. Chromatin modifications and their function. Cell 2007; 6(4): 693-705.

[4] Huisinga KL, Brower-Toland B & Elgin SC. (2006) The contradictory definitions of heterochromatin: transcription and silencing. Chromosoma 115, 110-122

[5] Luger K, Mäder AW, Richmond RK, Sargent DF, Richmond TJ. (1997) Crystal structure of the nucleosome core particle at 2.8 A resolution. Nature, 18;389(6648):251-60

[6] Robinson PJ and Rhodes D. (2006) Structure of the '30 nm' chromatin fibre: a key role for the linker histone. Curr. Opin. Struct. Biol. 16, 336e343

[7] Strahl BD, Allis CD. (2000) The language of covalent histone modifications. Nature, 403(6765):41-5

[8] Pasini D, Malatesta M, Jung HR, Walfridsson J, Willer A, Olsson L, Skotte J, Wutz A, Porse B, Jensen ON, Helin K. (2010) Characterization of an antagonistic switch between histone H3 lysine 27 methylation and acetylation in the transcriptional regulation of Polycomb group target genes. Nucleic Acids Research:1-12

[9] Wang Z, Zang C, Rosenfeld JA, Schones DE, Barski A, Cuddapah S, Cui K, Roh TY, Peng W, Zhang MQ, Zhao K. (2008) Combinatorial patterns of histone acetylations and methylations in the human genome. Nat Genet 40:897-903

[10] Black JC, Van Rechem C, Whetstine JR. (2012) Histone lysine methylation dynamics: establishment, regulation, and biological impact. Mol Cell. 48(4):491-507

[11] Biterge B, Schneider R. Histone variants: key players of chromatin. Cell Tissue Res. 2014 Jun;356(3):457-66. doi: 10.1007/s00441-014-1862-4.

[12] Penny GD, Kay GF, Sheardown SA, Rastan S & Brockdorff N. (1996) Requirement for Xist in X chromosome inactivation. Nature 379, 131-137

[13] Galupa R, Heard E. X-chromosome inactivation: a crossroads between chromosome architecture and gene regulation. Annu Rev Genet. 2018;52:535-566.

[14] Mochizuki K, Fine NA, Fujisawa T, et al. Analysis of a piwi-related gene implicates small RNAs in genome rearrangement in tetrahymena. Cell. 2002;110(6):689-699.

[15] Reinhart BJ, Bartel DP. Small RNAs correspond to centromere heterochromatic repeats. Science. 2002;297(5588):1831.

[16] Cam HP, Sugiyama T, Chen ES, et al. Comprehensive analysis of heterochromatin- and RNAi-mediated epigenetic control of the fission yeast genome. Nat Genet. 2005;37(8): 809-819.

[17] Saetrom P, Snøve O, Rossi JJ. Epigenetics and microRNAs. Pediatr Res. 2007;61(5 Pt 2):17R–23R.

[18] Okano M, Bell DW, Haber DA, Li E. (1999) DNA methyltransferases Dnmt3a and Dnmt3b are essential for de novo

methylation and mammalian development. Cell, 99(3):247-57

[19] Li E, Bestor TH, Jaenisch R. (1992) Targeted mutation of the DNA methyltransferase gene results in embryonic lethality. Cell, 69(6):915-26

[20] Grewal SI, Jia S. (2007) Heterochromatin revisited. Nat Rev Genet. 8(1):35-46

[21] Deaton AM, Bird A. CpG islands and the regulation of transcription. Genes Dev. 2011 May 15;25(10):1010-22. doi: 10.1101/gad.2037511.

[22] Roundtree IA, Evans ME, Pan T, He C. Dynamic RNA Modifications in Gene Expression Regulation. Cell. 2017 Jun 15;169(7):1187-1200. doi: 10.1016/j.cell.2017.05.045.

[23] Tsai, K., Cullen, B.R. Epigenetic and epitranscriptomic regulation of viral replication. Nat Rev Microbiol 18, 559-570 (2020). https://doi.org/10.1038/s41579-020-0382-3

[24] Lieberman PM. Epigenetics and Genetics of Viral Latency. Cell Host Microbe. 2016 May 11;19(5):619-28. doi: 10.1016/j.chom.2016.04.008.

[25] Milavetz B, Kallestad L, Gefroh A, Adams N, Woods E, Balakrishnan L. Virion-mediated transfer of SV40 epigenetic information. Epigenetics. 2012 Jun 1;7(6):528-34. doi: 10.4161/epi.20057.

[26] Balakrishnan L, Milavetz B. Epigenetic Analysis of SV40 Minichromosomes. Curr Protoc Microbiol. 2017 Aug 11;46:14F.3.1-14F.3.26. doi: 10.1002/cpmc.35.

[27] King CR, Tessier TM, Mymryk JS. Color Me Infected: Painting Cellular Chromatin with a Viral Histone Mimic. Trends Microbiol. 2016 Oct;24(10):774-776. doi: 10.1016/j.tim.2016.08.005.

[28] Sen R, Garbati M, Bryant K, Lu Y. Epigenetic mechanisms influencing COVID-19. Genome. 2021 Apr;64(4):372-385. doi: 10.1139/gen-2020-0135.

[29] Cohen C, Corpet A, Roubille S, Maroui MA, Poccardi N, Rousseau A, Kleijwegt C, Binda O, Texier P, Sawtell N, Labetoulle M, Lomonte P. Promyelocytic leukemia (PML) nuclear bodies (NBs) induce latent/quiescent HSV-1 genomes chromatinization through a PML NB/Histone H3.3/H3.3 Chaperone Axis. PLoS Pathog. 2018 Sep 20;14(9):e1007313. doi: 10.1371/journal.ppat.1007313.

[30] Placek BJ, Huang J, Kent JR, Dorsey J, Rice L, Fraser NW, Berger SL. The histone variant H3.3 regulates gene expression during lytic infection with herpes simplex virus type 1. J Virol. 2009 Feb;83(3):1416-21. doi: 10.1128/JVI.01276-08.

[31] Liang Y, Vogel JL, Arbuckle JH, Rai G, Jadhav A, Simeonov A, Maloney DJ, Kristie TM. Targeting the JMJD2 histone demethylases to epigenetically control herpesvirus infection and reactivation from latency. Sci Transl Med. 2013 Jan 9;5(167):167ra5. doi: 10.1126/scitranslmed.3005145.

[32] Liang Y, Vogel JL, Narayanan A, Peng H, Kristie TM. Inhibition of the histone demethylase LSD1 blocks alpha-herpesvirus lytic replication and reactivation from latency. Nat Med. 2009 Nov;15(11):1312-7. doi: 10.1038/nm.2051.

[33] Narayanan A, Ruyechan WT, Kristie TM. The coactivator host cell factor-1 mediates Set1 and MLL1 H3K4 trimethylation at herpesvirus immediate early promoters for initiation of infection. Proc Natl Acad Sci U S A. 2007 Jun 26;104(26):10835-40. doi: 10.1073/pnas.0704351104.

[34] Lee JS, Raja P, Knipe DM. Herpesviral ICP0 Protein Promotes Two Waves of Heterochromatin Removal on an Early Viral Promoter during Lytic Infection. mBio. 2016 Jan 12;7(1):e02007-15. doi: 10.1128/mBio.02007-15.

[35] Lukashchuk V, McFarlane S, Everett RD, Preston CM. Human cytomegalovirus protein pp71 displaces the chromatin-associated factor ATRX from nuclear domain 10 at early stages of infection. J Virol. 2008 Dec;82(24):12543-54. doi: 10.1128/JVI.01215-08.

[36] Tsai K, Thikmyanova N, Wojcechowskyj JA, Delecluse HJ, Lieberman PM. EBV tegument protein BNRF1 disrupts DAXX-ATRX to activate viral early gene transcription. PLoS Pathog. 2011 Nov;7(11):e1002376. doi: 10.1371/journal.ppat.1002376.

[37] Decorsière A, Mueller H, van Breugel PC, Abdul F, Gerossier L, Beran RK, Livingston CM, Niu C, Fletcher SP, Hantz O, Strubin M. Hepatitis B virus X protein identifies the Smc5/6 complex as a host restriction factor. Nature. 2016 Mar 17;531(7594):386-9. doi: 10.1038/nature17170.

[38] Unterholzner L, Keating SE, Baran M, Horan KA, Jensen SB, Sharma S, Sirois CM, Jin T, Latz E, Xiao TS, Fitzgerald KA, Paludan SR, Bowie AG. IFI16 is an innate immune sensor for intracellular DNA. Nat Immunol. 2010 Nov;11(11):997-1004. doi: 10.1038/ni.1932.

[39] Johnson KE, Bottero V, Flaherty S, Dutta S, Singh VV, Chandran B. IFI16 restricts HSV-1 replication by accumulating on the hsv-1 genome, repressing HSV-1 gene expression, and directly or indirectly modulating histone modifications. PLoS Pathog. 2014 Nov 6;10(11):e1004503. doi: 10.1371/journal.ppat.1004503.

[40] Gariano GR, Dell'Oste V, Bronzini M, Gatti D, Luganini A, De Andrea M, Gribaudo G, Gariglio M, Landolfo S. The intracellular DNA sensor IFI16 gene acts as restriction factor for human cytomegalovirus replication. PLoS Pathog. 2012 Jan;8(1):e1002498. doi: 10.1371/journal.ppat.1002498.

[41] Li T, Chen J, Cristea IM. Human cytomegalovirus tegument protein pUL83 inhibits IFI16-mediated DNA sensing for immune evasion. Cell Host Microbe. 2013 Nov 13;14(5):591-9. doi: 10.1016/j.chom.2013.10.007.

[42] Orzalli MH, DeLuca NA, Knipe DM. Nuclear IFI16 induction of IRF-3 signaling during herpesviral infection and degradation of IFI16 by the viral ICP0 protein. Proc Natl Acad Sci U S A. 2012 Oct 30;109(44):E3008-17. doi: 10.1073/pnas.1211302109.

[43] Li T, Diner BA, Chen J, Cristea IM. Acetylation modulates cellular distribution and DNA sensing ability of interferon-inducible protein IFI16. Proc Natl Acad Sci U S A. 2012 Jun 26;109(26):10558-63. doi: 10.1073/pnas.1203447109.

[44] Fruci D, Rota R, Gallo A. The Role of HCMV and HIV-1 MicroRNAs: Processing, and Mechanisms of Action during Viral Infection. Front Microbiol. 2017 Apr 21;8:689. doi: 10.3389/fmicb.2017.00689.

[45] Imperiale MJ. Polyomavirus miRNAs: the beginning. Curr Opin Virol. 2014;7:29-32. doi:10.1016/j.coviro.2014.03.012

[46] Zhuo Y, Gao G, Shi JA, Zhou X, Wang X. miRNAs: biogenesis, origin and evolution, functions on virus-host interaction. Cell Physiol Biochem. 2013;32(3):499-510. doi: 10.1159/000354455.

[47] Griffiths-Jones S, Saini HK, van Dongen S, Enright AJ. miRBase: tools for

microRNA genomics. Nucleic Acids Res. 2008 Jan;36(Database issue):D154-8. doi: 10.1093/nar/gkm952.

[48] Ferrari R, Gou D, Jawdekar G, Johnson SA, Nava M, Su T, Yousef AF, Zemke NR, Pellegrini M, Kurdistani SK, Berk AJ. Adenovirus small E1A employs the lysine acetylases p300/CBP and tumor suppressor Rb to repress select host genes and promote productive virus infection. Cell Host Microbe. 2014 Nov 12;16(5):663-76. doi: 10.1016/j.chom.2014.10.004.

[49] Avgousti DC, Herrmann C, Kulej K, Pancholi NJ, Sekulic N, Petrescu J, Molden RC, Blumenthal D, Paris AJ, Reyes ED, Ostapchuk P, Hearing P, Seeholzer SH, Worthen GS, Black BE, Garcia BA, Weitzman MD. A core viral protein binds host nucleosomes to sequester immune danger signals. Nature. 2016 Jul 7;535(7610):173-7. doi: 10.1038/nature18317.

[50] Lieberman PM. Epigenetics and Genetics of Viral Latency. Cell Host Microbe. 2016 May 11;19(5):619-28. doi: 10.1016/j.chom.2016.04.008.

[51] Speck SH, Ganem D. Viral latency and its regulation: lessons from the gamma-herpesviruses. Cell Host Microbe. 2010 Jul 22;8(1):100-15. doi: 10.1016/j.chom.2010.06.014.

[52] Du T, Zhou G, Khan S, Gu H, Roizman B. Disruption of HDAC/CoREST/REST repressor by dnREST reduces genome silencing and increases virulence of herpes simplex virus. Proc Natl Acad Sci U S A. 2010 Sep 7;107(36):15904-9. doi: 10.1073/pnas.1010741107.

[53] Cliffe AR, Coen DM, Knipe DM. Kinetics of facultative heterochromatin and polycomb group protein association with the herpes simplex viral genome during establishment of latent infection. mBio. 2013 Jan 15;4(1):e00590-12. doi: 10.1128/mBio.00590-12.

[54] Toth Z, Brulois K, Lee HR, Izumiya Y, Tepper C, Kung HJ, Jung JU. Biphasic euchromatin-to-heterochromatin transition on the KSHV genome following de novo infection. PLoS Pathog. 2013;9(12):e1003813. doi: 10.1371/journal.ppat.1003813.

[55] Tropberger P, Mercier A, Robinson M, Zhong W, Ganem DE, Holdorf M. Mapping of histone modifications in episomal HBV cccDNA uncovers an unusual chromatin organization amenable to epigenetic manipulation. Proc Natl Acad Sci U S A. 2015 Oct 20;112(42):E5715-24. doi: 10.1073/pnas.1518090112.

[56] Purushothaman P, Uppal T, Verma SC. Molecular biology of KSHV lytic reactivation. Viruses. 2015 Jan 14;7(1):116-53. doi: 10.3390/v7010116.

[57] Bloom DC, Giordani NV, Kwiatkowski DL. Epigenetic regulation of latent HSV-1 gene expression. Biochim Biophys Acta. 2010 Mar-Apr;1799(3-4):246-56. doi: 10.1016/j.bbagrm.2009.12.001.

[58] Tsai K, Chan L, Gibeault R, Conn K, Dheekollu J, Domsic J, Marmorstein R, Schang LM, Lieberman PM. Viral reprogramming of the Daxx histone H3.3 chaperone during early Epstein-Barr virus infection. J Virol. 2014 Dec;88(24):14350-63. doi: 10.1128/JVI.01895-14.

[59] Roizman B, Zhou G, Du T. Checkpoints in productive and latent infections with herpes simplex virus 1: conceptualization of the issues. J Neurovirol. 2011 Dec;17(6):512-7. doi: 10.1007/s13365-011-0058-x.

[60] Frappier L. EBNA1. Curr Top Microbiol Immunol. 2015;391:3-34. doi: 10.1007/978-3-319-22834-1_1.

[61] Ballestas ME, Kaye KM. The latency-associated nuclear antigen,

a multifunctional protein central to Kaposi's sarcoma-associated herpesvirus latency. Future Microbiol. 2011 Dec;6(12):1399-413. doi: 10.2217/fmb.11.137.

[62] McBride AA. The papillomavirus E2 proteins. Virology. 2013 Oct;445 (1-2):57-79. doi: 10.1016/j.virol.2013.06.006.

[63] Wu F, Cheng W, Zhao F, Tang M, Diao Y, Xu R. Association of N6-methyladenosine with viruses and related diseases. Virol J. 2019 Nov 11;16(1):133. doi: 10.1186/s12985-019-1236-3.

[64] Kennedy EM, Bogerd HP, Kornepati AV, Kang D, Ghoshal D, Marshall JB, Poling BC, Tsai K, Gokhale NS, Horner SM, Cullen BR. Posttranscriptional m(6)A Editing of HIV-1 mRNAs Enhances Viral Gene Expression. Cell Host Microbe. 2016 May 11;19(5):675-85. doi: 10.1016/j.chom.2016.04.002.

[65] Xue M, Zhao BS, Zhang Z, Lu M, Harder O, Chen P, Lu Z, Li A, Ma Y, Xu Y, Liang X, Zhou J, Niewiesk S, Peeples ME, He C, Li J. Viral N6-methyladenosine upregulates replication and pathogenesis of human respiratory syncytial virus. Nat Commun. 2019 Oct 9;10(1):4595. doi: 10.1038/s41467-019-12504-y.

[66] Lu M, Zhang Z, Xue M, Zhao BS, Harder O, Li A, Liang X, Gao TZ, Xu Y, Zhou J, Feng Z, Niewiesk S, Peeples ME, He C, Li J. N6-methyladenosine modification enables viral RNA to escape recognition by RNA sensor RIG-I. Nat Microbiol. 2020 Apr;5(4):584-598. doi: 10.1038/s41564-019-0653-9.

[67] Courtney DG, Tsai K, Bogerd HP, Kennedy EM, Law BA, Emery A, Swanstrom R, Holley CL, Cullen BR. Epitranscriptomic Addition of m5C to HIV-1 Transcripts Regulates Viral Gene Expression. Cell Host Microbe. 2019 Aug 14;26(2):217-227.e6. doi: 10.1016/j.chom.2019.07.005.

[68] Ringeard M, Marchand V, Decroly E, Motorin Y, Bennasser Y. FTSJ3 is an RNA 2'-O-methyltransferase recruited by HIV to avoid innate immune sensing. Nature. 2019 Jan;565(7740):500-504. doi: 10.1038/s41586-018-0841-4.

[69] Menachery VD, Eisfeld AJ, Schäfer A, Josset L, Sims AC, Proll S, Fan S, Li C, Neumann G, Tilton SC, Chang J, Gralinski LE, Long C, Green R, Williams CM, Weiss J, Matzke MM, Webb-Robertson BJ, Schepmoes AA, Shukla AK, Metz TO, Smith RD, Waters KM, Katze MG, Kawaoka Y, Baric RS. Pathogenic influenza viruses and coronaviruses utilize similar and contrasting approaches to control interferon-stimulated gene responses. mBio. 2014 May 20;5(3):e01174-14. doi: 10.1128/mBio.01174-14.

[70] Menachery VD, Schäfer A, Burnum-Johnson KE, Mitchell HD, Eisfeld AJ, Walters KB, Nicora CD, Purvine SO, Casey CP, Monroe ME, Weitz KK, Stratton KG, Webb-Robertson BM, Gralinski LE, Metz TO, Smith RD, Waters KM, Sims AC, Kawaoka Y, Baric RS. MERS-CoV and H5N1 influenza virus antagonize antigen presentation by altering the epigenetic landscape. Proc Natl Acad Sci U S A. 2018 Jan 30;115(5):E1012-E1021. doi: 10.1073/pnas.1706928115.

[71] Schäfer A, Baric RS. Epigenetic Landscape during Coronavirus Infection. Pathogens. 2017 Feb 15;6(1):8. doi: 10.3390/pathogens6010008.

[72] Ragab D, Salah Eldin H, Taeimah M, Khattab R, Salem R. The COVID-19 Cytokine Storm; What We Know So Far. Front Immunol. 2020 Jun 16;11:1446. doi: 10.3389/fimmu.2020.01446.

[73] Costela-Ruiz VJ, Illescas-Montes R, Puerta-Puerta JM, Ruiz C,

Melguizo-Rodríguez L. SARS-CoV-2 infection: The role of cytokines in COVID-19 disease. Cytokine Growth Factor Rev. 2020 Aug;54:62-75. doi: 10.1016/j.cytogfr.2020.06.001.

[74] Wilk AJ, Rustagi A, Zhao NQ, Roque J, Martínez-Colón GJ, McKechnie JL, Ivison GT, Ranganath T, Vergara R, Hollis T, Simpson LJ, Grant P, Subramanian A, Rogers AJ, Blish CA. A single-cell atlas of the peripheral immune response in patients with severe COVID-19. Nat Med. 2020 Jul;26(7):1070-1076. doi: 10.1038/s41591-020-0944-y.

[75] Zuo Y, Yalavarthi S, Shi H, Gockman K, Zuo M, Madison JA, Blair C, Weber A, Barnes BJ, Egeblad M, Woods RJ, Kanthi Y, Knight JS. Neutrophil extracellular traps in COVID-19. JCI Insight. 2020 Jun 4;5(11):e138999. doi: 10.1172/jci.insight.138999.

[76] Leshner M, Wang S, Lewis C, Zheng H, Chen XA, Santy L, Wang Y. PAD4 mediated histone hypercitrullination induces heterochromatin decondensation and chromatin unfolding to form neutrophil extracellular trap-like structures. Front Immunol. 2012 Oct 4;3:307. doi: 10.3389/fimmu.2012.00307.

[77] Cicco S, Cicco G, Racanelli V, Vacca A. Neutrophil Extracellular Traps (NETs) and Damage-Associated Molecular Patterns (DAMPs): Two Potential Targets for COVID-19 Treatment. Mediators Inflamm. 2020 Jul 16;2020:7527953. doi: 10.1155/2020/7527953.

[78] Walls AC, Park YJ, Tortorici MA, Wall A, McGuire AT, Veesler D. Structure, Function, and Antigenicity of the SARS-CoV-2 Spike Glycoprotein. Cell. 2020 Apr 16;181(2):281-292.e6. doi: 10.1016/j.cell.2020.02.058.

[79] Bestle D, Heindl MR, Limburg H, Van Lam van T, Pilgram O, Moulton H, Stein DA, Hardes K, Eickmann M, Dolnik O, Rohde C, Klenk HD, Garten W, Steinmetzer T, Böttcher-Friebertshäuser E. TMPRSS2 and furin are both essential for proteolytic activation of SARS-CoV-2 in human airway cells. Life Sci Alliance. 2020 Jul 23;3(9):e202000786. doi: 10.26508/lsa.202000786.

[80] Bittmann S, Weissenstein A, Villalon G, Moschuring-Alieva E, Luchter E. Simultaneous Treatment of COVID-19 With Serine Protease Inhibitor Camostat and/or Cathepsin L Inhibitor? J Clin Med Res. 2020;12(5):320-322. doi: 10.14740/jocmr4161.

[81] Tukiainen T, Villani AC, Yen A, Rivas MA, Marshall JL, et al. Landscape of X chromosome inactivation across human tissues. Nature. 2017 Oct 11;550(7675):244-248. doi: 10.1038/nature24265.

[82] Gemmati D, Bramanti B, Serino ML, Secchiero P, Zauli G, Tisato V. COVID-19 and Individual Genetic Susceptibility/Receptivity: Role of ACE1/ACE2 Genes, Immunity, Inflammation and Coagulation. Might the Double X-chromosome in Females Be Protective against SARS-CoV-2 Compared to the Single X-Chromosome in Males? Int J Mol Sci. 2020 May 14;21(10):3474. doi: 10.3390/ijms21103474.

[83] Chlamydas S, Papavassiliou AG, Piperi C. Epigenetic mechanisms regulating COVID-19 infection. Epigenetics. 2021 Mar;16(3):263-270. doi: 10.1080/15592294.2020.1796896.

[84] Pinto BGG, Oliveira AER, Singh Y, Jimenez L, Gonçalves ANA, Ogava RLT, Creighton R, Schatzmann Peron JP, Nakaya HI. ACE2 Expression Is Increased in the Lungs of Patients With Comorbidities Associated With Severe COVID-19. J Infect Dis. 2020 Jul

23;222(4):556-563. doi: 10.1093/infdis/jiaa332.

[85] Li Y, Li H, Zhou L. EZH2-mediated H3K27me3 inhibits ACE2 expression. Biochem Biophys Res Commun. 2020 Jun 11;526(4):947-952. doi: 10.1016/j.bbrc.2020.04.010.

[86] Corley MJ, Ndhlovu LC (2020). DNA methylation analysis of the COVID-19 host cell receptor, angiotensin I converting enzyme 2 gene (ACE2) in the respiratory system reveal age and gender differences. Preprints. 10.20944/preprints202003.0295.v1

[87] Ortutay Z, Grönholm A, Laitinen M, Keresztes-Andrei M, Hermelo I, Pesu M. Identification of Novel Genetic Regulatory Region for Proprotein Convertase FURIN and Interferon Gamma in T Cells. Front Immunol. 2021 Feb 18;12:630389. doi: 10.3389/fimmu.2021.630389.

[88] Ragia G, Manolopoulos VG. Assessing COVID-19 susceptibility through analysis of the genetic and epigenetic diversity of ACE2-mediated SARS-CoV-2 entry. Pharmacogenomics. 2020 Dec;21(18):1311-1329. doi: 10.2217/pgs-2020-0092.

[89] Li H, Xie L, Chen L, Zhang L, Han Y, Yan Z, Guo X. Genomic, epigenomic, and immune subtype analysis of CTSL/B and SARS-CoV-2 receptor ACE2 in pan-cancer. Aging (Albany NY). 2020 Nov 20;12(22):22370-22389. doi: 10.18632/aging.104147.

[90] Wei J, Alfajaro MM, DeWeirdt PC, Hanna RE, Lu-Culligan WJ, Cai WL, Strine MS, Zhang SM, Graziano VR, Schmitz CO, Chen JS, Mankowski MC, Filler RB, Ravindra NG, Gasque V, de Miguel FJ, Patil A, Chen H, Oguntuyo KY, Abriola L, Surovtseva YV, Orchard RC, Lee B, Lindenbach BD, Politi K, van Dijk D, Kadoch C, Simon MD, Yan Q, Doench JG, Wilen CB. Genome-wide CRISPR Screens Reveal Host Factors Critical for SARS-CoV-2 Infection. Cell. 2021 Jan 7;184(1):76-91.e13. doi: 10.1016/j.cell.2020.10.028.

[91] Samaiya M, Bakhshi S, Shukla AA, Kumar L, Chauhan SS. Epigenetic regulation of cathepsin L expression in chronic myeloid leukaemia. J Cell Mol Med. 2011 Oct;15(10):2189-99. doi: 10.1111/j.1582-4934.2010.01203.x.

[92] Gordon DE, Jang GM, Bouhaddou M, Xu J, Obernier K, et al. A SARS-CoV-2 protein interaction map reveals targets for drug repurposing. Nature. 2020 Jul;583(7816):459-468. doi: 10.1038/s41586-020-2286-9.

[93] Josling GA, Selvarajah SA, Petter M, Duffy MF. The role of bromodomain proteins in regulating gene expression. Genes (Basel). 2012 May 29;3(2):320-43. doi: 10.3390/genes3020320.

[94] Marié IJ, Chang HM, Levy DE. HDAC stimulates gene expression through BRD4 availability in response to IFN and in interferonopathies. J Exp Med. 2018 Dec 3;215(12):3194-3212. doi: 10.1084/jem.20180520.

[95] Tanaka H, Igata T, Etoh K, Koga T, Takebayashi SI, Nakao M. The NSD2/WHSC1/MMSET methyltransferase prevents cellular senescence-associated epigenomic remodeling. Aging Cell. 2020 Jul;19(7):e13173. doi: 10.1111/acel.13173.

[96] Kamada R, Yang W, Zhang Y, Patel MC, Yang Y, Ouda R, Dey A, Wakabayashi Y, Sakaguchi K, Fujita T, Tamura T, Zhu J, Ozato K. Interferon stimulation creates chromatin marks and establishes transcriptional memory. Proc Natl Acad Sci U S A. 2018 Sep 25;115(39):E9162-E9171. doi: 10.1073/pnas.1720930115.

[97] Yeh HM, Yu CY, Yang HC, Ko SH, Liao CL, Lin YL. Ubiquitin-specific

protease 13 regulates IFN signaling by stabilizing STAT1. J Immunol. 2013 Sep 15;191(6):3328-36. doi: 10.4049/jimmunol.1300225.

[98] Biterge Süt B. Molecular profiling of immune cell-enriched Severe Acute Respiratory Syndrome Coronavirus 2 (SARS-CoV-2) interacting protein USP13. Life Sci. 2020 Oct 1;258:118170. doi: 10.1016/j.lfs.2020.118170.

[99] Sun H, Zhang Q, Jing YY, Zhang M, Wang HY, Cai Z, Liuyu T, Zhang ZD, Xiong TC, Wu Y, Zhu QY, Yao J, Shu HB, Lin D, Zhong B. USP13 negatively regulates antiviral responses by deubiquitinating STING. Nat Commun. 2017 May 23;8:15534. doi: 10.1038/ncomms15534.

[100] Becker T, Le-Trilling VTK, Trilling M. Cellular Cullin RING Ubiquitin Ligases: Druggable Host Dependency Factors of Cytomegaloviruses. Int J Mol Sci. 2019 Apr 2;20(7):1636. doi: 10.3390/ijms20071636.

[101] Ramasamy S, Saez B, Mukhopadhyay S, Ding D, Ahmed AM, Chen X, Pucci F, Yamin R, Wang J, Pittet MJ, Kelleher CM, Scadden DT, Sweetser DA. Tle1 tumor suppressor negatively regulates inflammation in vivo and modulates NF-κB inflammatory pathway. Proc Natl Acad Sci U S A. 2016 Feb 16;113(7):1871-6. doi: 10.1073/pnas.1511380113.

[102] Singh N, Bharara Singh A. S2 subunit of SARS-nCoV-2 interacts with tumor suppressor protein p53 and BRCA: an in silico study. Transl Oncol. 2020 Oct;13(10):100814. doi: 10.1016/j.tranon.2020.100814

[103] Khan MA, Sany MRU, Islam MS, Islam ABMMK. Epigenetic Regulator miRNA Pattern Differences Among SARS-CoV, SARS-CoV-2, and SARS-CoV-2 World-Wide Isolates Delineated the Mystery Behind the Epic Pathogenicity and Distinct Clinical Characteristics of Pandemic COVID-19. Front Genet. 2020 Jul 10;11:765. doi: 10.3389/fgene.2020.00765.

[104] Cortis D. On Determining the Age Distribution of COVID-19 Pandemic. Front Public Health. 2020 May 15;8:202. doi: 10.3389/fpubh.2020.00202.

[105] Oberdoerffer P, Michan S, McVay M, Mostoslavsky R, Vann J, Park SK, Hartlerode A, Stegmuller J, Hafner A, Loerch P, Wright SM, Mills KD, Bonni A, Yankner BA, Scully R, Prolla TA, Alt FW, Sinclair DA. SIRT1 redistribution on chromatin promotes genomic stability but alters gene expression during aging. Cell. 2008 Nov 28;135(5):907-18. doi: 10.1016/j.cell.2008.10.025.

[106] Blanco-Melo D, Nilsson-Payant BE, Liu WC, Uhl S, Hoagland D, Møller R, Jordan TX, Oishi K, Panis M, Sachs D, Wang TT, Schwartz RE, Lim JK, Albrecht RA, tenOever BR. Imbalanced Host Response to SARS-CoV-2 Drives Development of COVID-19. Cell. 2020 May 28;181(5):1036-1045.e9. doi: 10.1016/j.cell.2020.04.026.

[107] Saksena N, Bonam SR, Miranda-Saksena M. Epigenetic Lens to Visualize the Severe Acute Respiratory Syndrome Coronavirus-2 (SARS-CoV-2) Infection in COVID-19 Pandemic. Front Genet. 2021 Mar 22;12:581726. doi: 10.3389/fgene.2021.581726.

[108] Corley MJ, Pang APS, Dody K, Mudd PA, Patterson BK, Seethamraju H, Bram Y, Peluso MJ, Torres L, Iyer NS, Premeaux TA, Yeung ST, Chandar V, Borczuk A, Schwartz RE, Henrich TJ, Deeks SG, Sacha JB, Ndhlovu LC. Genome-wide DNA methylation profiling of peripheral blood reveals an epigenetic signature associated with severe COVID-19. J Leukoc Biol. 2021 Jan 19:10.1002/JLB.5HI0720-466R. doi: 10.1002/JLB.5HI0720-466R.

[109] Castro de Moura M, Davalos V, Planas-Serra L, Alvarez-Errico D, Arribas C, Ruiz M, et al. Epigenome-wide association study of COVID-19 severity with respiratory failure. EBioMedicine. 2021 Apr;66:103339. doi: 10.1016/j.ebiom.2021.103339.

[110] Sawalha AH, Zhao M, Coit P, Lu Q. Epigenetic dysregulation of ACE2 and interferon-regulated genes might suggest increased COVID-19 susceptibility and severity in lupus patients. Clin Immunol. 2020 Jun;215:108410. doi: 10.1016/j.clim.2020.108410.

[111] Pruimboom L. Methylation Pathways and SARS-CoV-2 Lung Infiltration and Cell Membrane-Virus Fusion Are Both Subject to Epigenetics. Front Cell Infect Microbiol. 2020 May 26;10:290. doi: 10.3389/fcimb.2020.00290.

[112] Alsaadi EAJ, Neuman BW, Jones IM. A Fusion Peptide in the Spike Protein of MERS Coronavirus. Viruses. 2019 Sep 5;11(9):825. doi: 10.3390/v11090825.

[113] Huang C, Wang Y, Li X, Ren L, Zhao J, Hu Y, Zhang L, Fan G, Xu J, Gu X, Cheng Z, Yu T, Xia J, Wei Y, Wu W, Xie X, Yin W, Li H, Liu M, Xiao Y, Gao H, Guo L, Xie J, Wang G, Jiang R, Gao Z, Jin Q, Wang J, Cao B. Clinical features of patients infected with 2019 novel coronavirus in Wuhan, China. Lancet. 2020 Feb 15;395 (10223):497-506. doi: 10.1016/S0140-6736(20)30183-5.

[114] Atlante S, Mongelli A, Barbi V, Martelli F, Farsetti A, Gaetano C. The epigenetic implication in coronavirus infection and therapy. Clin Epigenetics. 2020 Oct 21;12(1):156. doi: 10.1186/s13148-020-00946-x.

Section 3

Stem Cells Extracellular Vesicles Ex-Vivo and 3D Models

Chapter 6

Mesenchymal Stem Cells and Extracellular Vesicles: An Emerging Alternative to Combat COVID-19

Hugo C. Rodriguez, Manu Gupta, Emilio Cavazos-Escobar, Enrique Montalvo, Saadiq F. El-Amin III and Ashim Gupta

Abstract

The global SARS-CoV-2 outbreak has been accompanied with severe socio-economic and health burdens that will ripple through history. It is now known that SARS-CoV-2 induces a cytokine storm that leads to acute respiratory distress syndrome and systemic organ damage. With no definitive nor safe therapy for COVID-19 as well as the rise of viral variants the need for an urgent treatment modality is paramount. Mesenchymal stem cells (MSCs) and their extracellular vesicles (EVs) have long been praised for their anti-viral, anti-inflammatory and tissue regenerative capabilities. MSCs and their EVs are now being studied for their possible use as a treatment modality for COVID-19. In this review we explore their capabilities and outline the evidence of their use in ALI, ARDS and COVID-19.

Keywords: COVID-19, Coronavirus, SARS-CoV-2, Mesenchymal stem cells, Extracellular vesicles, Exosomes, Regenerative medicine

1. Introduction

Over the past several months, the world has had to endure another global outbreak, the likes of which have not been seen since the Spanish flu pandemic of 1918 [1]. Coronavirus disease 2019 (COVID-19) caused from the virus now known as severe acute respiratory syndrome coronavirus 2 (SARS-CoV-2) is understood to undergo human-to-human transmission by respiratory droplets and known to cause a broad range of symptoms contributing to its rapid spread [2]. As of February 14, 2021, there have been over 109 million reported cases and over 2.39 million deaths worldwide, with the United States having over 27.6 million reported cases along with over 484,000 deaths [3]. As cases continue to accumulate and cause significant strain on medical resources and society, the need for an urgent, effective and safe treatment is paramount. Current measures to curb the COVID-19 pandemic revolve around a broad range of pharmaceutical remedies and the distribution of a vaccine [4]. With vaccines being a prophylactic measure, current treatment options being unproven, non-definitive and suboptimal, and the emergence of new viral strains, attention needs to be placed on alternatives.

IntechOpen

Investigations have identified that the majority of Intensive Care Unit (ICU) patients with COVID-19 have high plasma levels of granulocyte colony-stimulating factor (GCSF), tumor necrosis factor-alpha (TNF-α), interferon gamma inducible protein-10 (IP-10), monocyte chemoattractant protein-1 (MCP1) and macrophage inflammatory protein 1-alpha (MIP1A) [5]. These factors have been shown to be interconnected with the recruitment of proinflammatory cells and the production of a cytokine storm. A cytokine storm is a large and abrupt increase in proinflammatory cytokines that is suggested to be the main cause of acute respiratory distress syndrome (ARDS) and other severe pathophysiological effects seen in COVID-19 patients [6]. The cytokine storm induces a vast signaling cascade that recruits immune cells such as humoral B-cells, T-cells, and macrophages (MOs) as well as shifts most of these cells into a proinflammatory state [7]. Interestingly, clinicians have found that through the attenuation of the cytokine storm with mesenchymal stem cells (MSCs) patients have been able to recover even in severe cases [6].

MSCs have been successfully and safely used to treat pneumonia, acute lung injury (ALI), and ARDS in the past [8, 9]. Their effectiveness has been attributed to their ability to be directly antiviral, immunomodulate, induce tissue regeneration, inhibit apoptosis/fibrosis and clear alveolar fluid [10]. MSCs have also been shown to aggregate within the lung microvasculature when intravenously (IV) administered, affecting the local environment in an efficient manner [11]. MSCs are able to be so affective by inhibiting the function, recruitment and activation of MOs, dendritic cells (DCs), T-cells and B-cells, subsequently reducing proinflammatory cytokines such as interleukin-6 (IL-6) and TNF-α among others [12]. MSCs have also been shown to differentiate into a multitude of tissues, and secrete cytokine (CKs), growth factors (GFs) and extracellular vesicles (EVs), all of which play an integral part in their mechanism of action [13, 14]. MSCs can be derived from various types of tissues from both allogenic and autogenic sources. These tissues include: adipose, bone marrow, placenta, amniotic fluid, umbilical cord, and umbilical cord-derived Wharton jelly [15–18].

Extracellular vesicles (EVs) are composed of hypoimmunogenic properties that resemble amphipathic structures such as the lipid bilayer that allow the vesicles to migrate rapidly as well as harmlessly towards the target organs, without the occurrence of blood flow coagulations [19]. EVs can be obtained from any MSC source and act in a paracrine manner delivering enclosed biological molecules such as DNA, RNA, proteins, and lipids [20]. These EVs include microvesicles (MVs) and exosomes and provide microenvironment that further decreases inflammation, promotes tissue regeneration, and overall enhance the effects of MSCs [21].

In the face of the COVID-19 pandemic, scientists rush to generate and successfully distribute viable therapeutics and vaccines. Due to the urgent need and limitations with the current options, MSCs and their EVs may be a viable option. The cooperative mechanism of actions of MSCs and their EVs that include their ability to be directly antiviral, immunomodulate, induce tissue regeneration, inhibit apoptosis/fibrosis and clear alveolar fluid as well as sequester into the lung microvasculature make them an exciting alternative therapy.

2. Current treatments and therapeutic status

The scientific and medical community have been quick to adapt and have explored a plethora of therapeutic approaches. Treatments originally known for their efficacy against prior viral infections such as corticosteroids, and convalescent plasma (CP) have been repurposed for SARS-CoV-2 [22–24]. Recent novel treatments and vaccines have emerged such as the monoclonal antibodies casirivimab and imdevimab (REGN-COV2) and the Pfizer and Moderna mRNA vaccines [4]. Unfortunately, these current treatments have limitations and potentially dangerous adverse effects and although vaccinations are an effective preventive measure, they do not treat COVID-19 [4]. Considering these limitations and emergence of new viral strains there is an urgent need for a safe and effective therapeutic option [25].

Corticosteroids have long been used due to their immunomodulation and they have been a therapeutic option in many autoimmune diseases and in conditions such as ARDS [26]. Although they have a long history, their use in COVID-19 still remains controversial. Data from their prior use in viral infections indicated that they were associated with increased mortality, longer hospitalizations and increased tendency for mechanical ventilation [27–29]. In addition, observational studies in patients with SARS and MERS suggested that the use of corticosteroids delayed viral clearance, increased rates of secondary infections and had somewhat severe adverse effects of psychosis, hyperglycemia, and avascular necrosis [27, 30, 31]. Thus, similar adverse effects and outcomes can be expected in pateitns with COVID-19. Passive immunity with convalescent plasma has also been used and has been shown to improve the survival rate of patients with prior viral epidemics [32]. CP is a therapy that utilizes artificial passive immunity from pooled plasma of patients with resolved SARS-CoV-2 infections [32, 33]. Although the science is sound, there are several limitations associated with CP [34]. The efficacy of CP is highly reliant on the time of its administration, as it seems to only be beneficial to patients a week after infection when viremia is at its highest [35]. Additionally, the effect of CP on SARS-CoV-2 is highly dependent on the neutralizing antibody titer which has to be >1:160, seen 12 weeks after onset of disease [34].

CP infusions can also have severe adverse effects such as anaphylaxis, transfusion-related ALI and cardiac overload. Additionally, there are several limitations to the collection of CP such as age, weight, state of health, and informed consent all of which make CP a limited treatment option to the current pandemic [34].

Recently attention have been geared towards novel treatments such as REGN-COV-2, which is a cocktail of two human antibodies (casirivimab and imdevimab) using both transgenic mice and B cells from recovered COVID-19 patients [36]. REGN COV-2, although approved by the FDA, has specific criteria that have to be met before a patient can receive it. REGN-COV-2 is authorized for use in mild to moderate COVID-19 in adults, pediatric patients (12 years or older) with a weight of 40 kg and who have had a positive SARS-CoV-2 test with a high risk of progressing to severe COVID-19. Patients are not indicated for treatment if they are hospitalized, require supplemental O2, and/or currently using chronic supplemental O2 due to another underlying condition [37].These criteria are limitations and important obstacles associated with REGN-COV-2.

Currently, the emergence of new vaccines against SARS-CoV-2 have drawn much excitement. There are several vaccine candidates that are subdivided into five general categories: protein subunit, virally vectored, nucleic acid (mRNA), inactivated and live attenuated [23]. The Pfizer and Moderna vaccines utilize nucleic acids (mRNA) and are composed of a lipid particle with nucleoside-modified RNA, encoding for the S protein [38]. These two vaccines have the most data and have been the most widely used [4]. Although the data suggest that these vaccines are 95% effective at preventing SARS-CoV-2 infections they fail to actively treat disease once patients develop symptoms leaving a substantial amount of the population without a safe and efficacious treatment [38, 39].

Considering the limitations and adverse effects associated with current treatments as well as vaccines being only a preventative measure the need to develop a safer and more efficacious therapy is vital. MSCs and their EVs lack severe adverse effects and studies suggest they have high efficacy making them a potential candidate for COVID-19 treatment. MSCs and their EVs immunomodulatory effects and regenerative capabilities make them an exciting new option combating COVID-19 [12].

3. Mesenchmal stem cells (MSCs)

3.1 Origins of MSCs

In 1968, Friedenstein et al. isolated stem cells from the bone marrow (BMSCs) of mice [40]. The study showed that BM contained clonogenic progenitor cells and adherent cells similar to fibroblasts, termed as a colony forming unit-fibroblast [40]. These cells were found to have the ability to differentiate into chondrocytes, osteocytes, osteoblasts and adipocytes *in vitro* [40]. In 1991, Arnold Caplan changed the terminology to "Mesenchymal Stem Cell", due to their similarities with stem cells from mesodermal origins in embryonic tissues [41]. Later in 2017 Caplan suggested that the name MSC be alerted to "medicinal signaling cells" to accurately reflect their *in vivo* abilities of acting as an in situ medication [42]. Currently, "Mesenchymal Stem Cell" is the most common nomenclature, however Caplan did manage to emphasize their function.

With the variations in nomenclature as well as controversy surrounding their characteristics, the need for an official and concise criterion was needed. In 2006, The International Society of Cellular Therapy (ISCT) established parameters with four minimum criteria should be used to define MSCs. The criteria were quickly accepted by the medical community and are the status quo currently [43, 44].

The ISCT criteria for MSCs: 1) Plastic adherence in standard culture condition, 2)Positive expression (≥95%) of CD105, CD90, CD73 cell surface antigens, 3) Low expression (≤ 2%) of CD45, CD34, CD14, CD11b, CD79, CD19 and HLA-DR cell surface antigens, 4)Potential to differentiate into osteoblasts, adipocytes and chondrocytes in vitro.

3.2 MSC sources

MSCs can be differentiated by either being totipotent, pluripotent, multipotent, or unipotent [45, 46]. Totipotent MSCs for example, can form both embryonic and extraembryonic structures and proliferate indefinitely into cell types from all three embryonic germ layers [45]. Multipotent MSCs or adult stem cell are the most widely used and can differentiate into cell types from their respective source tissue [46]. MSCs can then be further subdivided by their source tissue. Two of the most common sources of MSCs are BM and adipose tissue. These are autologous sources that have been studied substantially and have the most associated data. Both of these sources require the patient to undergo an invasive procedure and are considered the first and second most reputable sources respectively for MSCs [47, 48]. Allogenic birth derived tissues such as umbilical cord (UC), UC-derived Wharton's jelly, amniotic fluid and placenta are also viable sources for MSCs. These sources have advantages in relation to their availability, lack of invasiveness, and presence of more pluripotent cells [12, 49, 50]. However, these sources have less data and do not have such an extensive history of use in comparison with allogenic sources.

3.3 MSC's mechanisms of action

MSCs have a long history of use in the treatment of viral lung infections, pneumonia, ALI and ARDS [6, 12]. This prior literature has been used to support their current use in COVID-19. Studies have showed that when IV administered, MSCs have specific and optimal mechanisms of action for the treatment of COVID-19. MSCs are able to evade the body's immune system and accumulate within the lung microvasculature enabling them to act locally [51, 52]. They have direct anti-viral activity, as well as anti-inflammatory, anti-apoptotic, and anti-fibrotic properties [47]. MSCs have also been touted for their ability to induce tissue regeneration, transdifferentiate into cells and produce EVs [53].

IV infusion is the one of the most commonly used route for MSC delivery with hundreds of clinical trials showing evidence of its safety [54]. A systematic review and meta-analysis by Lalu et al. summarized the results of IV administered MSCs in over 1000 patients [55]. The review indicated that there were no associated adverse events within any of the studies and no patient developed any organ system complications, infusion related toxicity, infections nor death [55]. In a study by Hwa Lee et al. IV infused MSCs were shown to accumulate into emboli within the lungs with no negative physiological effects [51]. In fact, the cells were noted to secrete TSG-6, a potent anti-inflammatory, the effects of which were amplified due to the sequestration within the lung [51]. As immune privileged cells, MSCs can be used either allogenically or autologously, due to their low levels of class I major histocompatibility complex (MHC) and class II MHC [52]. MSCs have also been shown to lack the associated co-stimulatory molecules (B7–1, B7–2, CD40, CD80 and CD86) needed to activate antigen presenting cells and the inflammatory process [52]. With these factors in mind MSCs are primed to act locally within the lungs to effectively and efficiently carry out their functions.

3.4 MSCs and immunomodulation

3.4.1 Innate immune response

In addition to the therapeutic potential of MSCs in regenerative medicine, for which they been most known for, they have also shown promising results in the regulation of immune responses [47]. MSCs through their ability to secrete various soluble factors are able to suppress both the innate and adaptive immune responses [47].

NOs and MOs both play a vital role in the innate immune response with DCs being the gate keeper to the adaptive response [56]. MOs can be subdivided into M1 or M2 subtypes each with their own distinct functions [57]. The M1 subtype are well known to be classically activated and responsible for phagocytosis, antigen presentation to DCs and secretion of pro-inflammatory cytokines such as TNF-α, IL-1α, IL-β, IL-6, IL-12 ultimately promoting a Th1 response [57]. The M2 subtype are known for their high secretion of IL-10 promoting an anti-inflammatory Treg and Th2 response along with inducing tissue remodeling and wound repair [57]. MSCs have been shown to secrete prostaglandin E2 (PGE2) and induce a switch in the MO population into an M2 subtype as well as substantially decreasing levels of IL-1β and IL-6 [58]. Wahnon et al. further elucidated this anti- inflammatory switch by reporting that the transcription factor signal transducer activators of transcription-3 (STAT3) activated in MSCs through cell to cell interactions between MOs produced IL-10 and promoted an M2 phenotypic switch [59]. NO activation and function have also been shown to be inhibited by MSCs. NOs are known to be a key component of the innate immune response and in pathophysiology of ARDS. NOs when activated release harmful reactive oxygen species, superoxide anions, peroxidases and proteases that lead to diffuse alveolar damage, and accumulation of alveolar fluid that underlie ARDS [60]. MSCs have been shown to secrete a potent antioxidant enzyme, SOD3 that has been shown to decrease the release of peroxidases, proteases and the oxidative burst of NOs [61]. They have also able to directly engulf dead NOs through ICAM-1 thereby further inhibiting release of their toxic contents [61]. Secretion of tumor necrosis factor-inducible gene 6 protein (TSG-6) via MSCs has also been shown to bind to IL-8 and CXCL8, inhibiting further migration, extravasation and recruitment of NOs [62].

Immature DCs patrol peripheral tissues for foreign antigens and are activated by cytokines (TNF-α, IL-1β, and IL-6) from M1 MOs [63]. Once immature DCs are activated they mature into conventional DCs and present their cleaved epitopes on their HLA complexes, inducing a pro-inflammatory Th1 and Th17 response [63]. PGE2 from MSCs has been shown to decrease CD38, CD80, CD86, IL-6, and IL-12 thereby decreasing DC function and pro-inflammatory T cell responses [64]. Preventing the maturation of these conventional DCs is vital in order to prevent this T cell response and the associated pro inflammatory state. Furthermore, DC maturation was inhibited by the inactivation of MAPK and NF-κB signaling cascades via the secretion of the TSG-6 [65]. In a study by Chen et al. DC maturation was induced from a conventional (pro-inflammatory) DC into a plasmacytoid DC population by PGE2 from MSCs, shifting the T cell population into a Th2 (anti-inflammatory) subset [66]. In addition, specific miRNAs (miR-21-5p, miR-142-3p, miR-223-3p, miR-126-3p) within EVs of MSCs have shown to further attenuate the DC maturation process [67].

3.4.2 Adaptive immune response

MSCs role in modulating T and B cell responses begins with their attenuation of MO and DC functions and continues with PGE2 from MSCs. PGE2 has been proven to increase the production of cAMP in T cells down regulating IL-2, and the IL-2 receptor as well as inhibiting the release of intracellular Ca2+ resulting in the direct inhibition of T cell activation [68]. PGE2 has also been shown to inactivate T cells via the hydrolysis of phosphatidylinositol, diacylglycerol and inositol phosphate [68]. In addition, PGE2 promotes a Th2 and a T reg shift in the T cell population overall influencing immunosuppression and an anti-inflammatory response [13, 69]. MSCs through their secretion of IDO, PGE2, TGF-β1, and Hepatocyte growth factor (HGF) have also been shown to induce G0/G1 cell cycle arrest in T cells and B cells [70, 71]. Nitric oxide (NO) from MSCs has shown to play a role in this by suppressing the phosphorylation of signal transducer and activator of transcription 5, thereby inhibiting TCR activated T cell proliferation and production of cytokines [72]. Studies have also suggested that MSCs can induce T cell and B cell apoptosis through direct cell to cell contact. Utilizing their interactions with the Fas/Fas ligand, TNF-related apoptosis-inducing ligand/death receptor signaling and programed death ligand-1/programmed death-1 pathways have shown to promote T and B cell apoptosis [73, 74]. This process was especially seen in CD4+, CD8+ and Th17 cells with a synergistic increase in T reg cells [75]. The down regulation of CXCR4, and CXCR5 via MSCs has shown further evidence of inhibiting B cell migratory abilities towards chemoattractant agents such as CXCL12 and CXClL13 [74]. Lastly, GM-CSF from MSCs have been recognized as having inhibitory actions on the production of CXCR4, CXR5, IL-6, and IL-7 while having no negative effects on IL-4 and IL-10 from B cells with a net anti-inflammatory affect [74].

3.5 MSC's additional mechanisms of action

Studies have shown that MSCs have been effective in inhibiting the viral replication of influenza, hepatitis B, herpes simplex, cytomegalovirus and the measles virus [76–79]. In a study by Khatri et al. MSCs had the ability to inhibit viral replication, shedding and lung damage in a porcine model with influenza induced pneumonia [76]. MSC-derived EVs were shown to be the key players in this process via their transfer of RNAs to virus infected epithelial cells. Lung epithelial cell apoptosis, hemagglutination and viral shedding were all significantly reduced in the study [76]. MSC-derived EVs have also demonstrated to decrease pro-inflammatory cytokine while increasing IL-10 and increase T regs [76]. IDO via MSCs has also been shown to directly decrease viral replication in most of the viruses that have been studied [76–79].

The secretion of various CKs, GFs and EVs have been reported to promote tissue regeneration and inhibit apoptosis, tissue fibrosis and alveolar fluid accumulation. As previously elucidated, M2 MOs promote anti-inflammatory Treg and Th2 responses while inducing tissue remodeling and wound repair [57]. Direct tissue regeneration from MSCs has been attributed to keratinocyte growth factor (KGF), vascular endothelial growth factor (VEGF), and hepatocyte growth factor (HGF) all of which have also been known to contribute to the in decrease collagen build up and fibrosis [80, 81]. In an in vivo bleomycin-induced pulmonary fibrosis model, Aguilar et al. noted that KGF was the key factor in the inhibition of collagen accumulation, promoting endogenous type II pneumocyte proliferation and overall attenuation of lung damage [82]. Previous studies have also further characterized KGF as being a potent factor in lung epithelial cell proliferation, while simultaneously being capable to increase matrix metalloproteinase-9 (MMP-9), IL-1RA and promoting clearance of apoptotic cells and inhibiting fibrosis [82, 83]. Gazdhar et al. used an in vivo bleomycin induced lung injury model in which he found that MSC-derived HGF was able to inhibit lung fibrosis and induce alveolar epithelial repair by decreasing TGF-B and α-smooth muscle actin expression [84]. The positive effects of HGF was further studied by Wang et al. who showed that MSC-derived HGF was responsible for increasing endothelial cell proliferation, intercellular junction proteins (VE-cadherin and occludin), and IL-10 while decreasing IL-6 and overall apoptosis [85]. MSC-derived VEGF and HGF have also shown to be able to stabilize Bcl-2 and inhibit pro-apoptotic factors hypoxia-inducible factor-1α protein, Bnip3 and CHOP contributing to their anti-apoptotic and anti-fibrotic effects [86]. In addition to the intracellular stabilization via these aforementioned GFs, factors such as MSC derived aniopoietin 1, and EVs have shown to induce alveolar fluid clearance within the lungs adding in their therapeutic benefits in ARDS [87]. In a study by Zhu et al. using an E.coli endotoxin-induce ALI model, MSC-derived EVs showcased their ability to transfer mRNA encoding for KGF inhibiting NOs, pulmonary edema and lung permeability [88].

4. Extracellular vesicles

Extracellular vesicles (EVs) are currently being studied as potential therapeutic agents for immune related pathologies due to their immunomodulatory and regenerative properties [89]. Interest in EVs has grown due to their ability to have similar therapeutic effects as MSCs as a cell free therapy [89]. What was once viewed as cellular waste products, may now have the potential to treat one of the largest natural disasters in modern history that is the COVID-19 pandemic.

The field of EVs has grown significantly in the recent years leading to the formation of the International Society for Extracellular Vesicles (ISEV) [89]. ISEV defines EVs as particles naturally released from a cell that are delimited by a lipid bilayer and cannot replicate [90]. EVs are further subclassified as exosomes (40-120 nm), microvesicles (50-1000 nm), and apoptotic bodies (500-2000 nm). Both microvesicles and apoptotic bodies bud-off directly from the cellular membrane and participate in two distinct cellular pathways: apoptotic bodies are products of cell mediated death whereas microvesicles are involved in paracrine communication [89, 91]. Exosome biogenesis, however, differs greatly in that it involves cell membrane invagination and formation of an intraluminal vesicles that undergoes modification in what is called a multivesicular body (MVB) [92]. Once modifications are performed, the MVB fuses with the cell membrane and the ILV's are secreted into the extracellular space as exosomes [92].

Once secreted, EV's carry a variety of nucleic acids, proteins, and lipids that can regulate or alter a plethora of biological processes through effects on cell receptors, adhesion molecules, cytokines, and other cell signaling molecules [89, 93–96]. They have attracted significant attention for their ability to inhibit tumorigeneses, suppress immune responses, promote tissues repair, and have therapeutic effects on neurological disease [96]. A recent study by Schultz et al. performed bioinformatic analysis of mRNA and miRNA cargo of EV's using Gene Expression Omnibus (GEO) database and miRWalk 3.0 servers. The study found that 266 miRNA's within exosomes have the ability to attenuate cell death by inhibiting TNF-a, IFN-y, JAK2, and JAK1 among others. Similarly, 148 miRNA's were identified with 1 or 2 targets of molecules involved in the intrinsic and extrinsic coagulations cascade pathways [97]. Continually, EV's also have the capability of replenishing glycolytic enzymes such as glyceraldehyde 3-phosphate dehydrogenase (GAPDH), phosphoglycerate kinase (PGK), phosphoglucomutase (PGM), enolase (ENO), and pyruvate kinase m2 isoform (PKm2), and phosphorylated PFKFB3, all of which are involved in the production of glycolytic ATP. It was proposed that secretions of these enzymes can reduce levels of reactive oxygen species and consequently halt cellular death [96]. In addition, matrix metalloproteinase (MMP)-9, vascular endothelial growth factor (VEGF), extracellular and matrix metalloproteinase inducer (EMMPRIN) have also been found within exosomes further postulating their regenerative effects through angiogenesis stimulation and tissue repair [96].

In preclinical trials, EV's have already demonstrated their immunomodulatory capabilities. In a study by Monsel et al. [98] on pneumonia induced mice, EV's reduced neutrophils and macrophages by 73% and 49% respectively, while decreasing edema and permeability of the endothelial-epithelial barrier to protein [99]. In fact, a recent study demonstrated that EV's reduce levels of inflammatory interleukins: IL-8, IL-6, IL-17 and TNF-α, when transferring anti-apoptotic miR-21-5p to target cells which resulted in reduced edema and lung dysfunction [100]. Additionally, EV's have also demonstrated their efficacy against acute lung injury (ALI) through downregulation of TLR/NF-κB signaling in rat models [101]. A recent study assessed the safety and efficacy of EVs on patients with severe COVID-19 infections. 24 patients were recruited under the specified trial criteria and followed for 14 days [102]. In addition to not having any notable adverse effects to the 15 mL IV dose of exosomes, the experimental group exhibited lower neutrophil count, c-reactive protein, ferritin, and D-dimer indicating an immunomodulatory effect [102]. Additionally, the overall survival rates were 83% with 17/24 patients fully recovered and 3/24 in stable conditions [102]. The study actively demonstrated EVs ability to safely attenuate the cytokine storm associated with severe COVID-19 infections. To fully appreciate the impact of EVs on COVID-19, further studies should be developed. As of February 18, 2021, applying the search word "exosomes" or "extracellular vesicles" and "COVID-19" on clinicaltrials.gov, results in 9 and 5 listed clinical trials, respectively. One of these trials, (NCT04491240) evaluated the safety and efficacy of exosome inhalation in SARS-CoV-1 pneumonia. Although results are published in c linicaltrails.gov, publication of the article is pending. The same experiment, however, has been approved for phase 2 and is currently enrolling participants (NCT04602442).

The field of EV's continues to show increasing promise as a therapeutic in the battle against COVID-19 based on their ability to carry a variety of cellular and nuclear components in a stable and hypoimmunogenic bilayer [6, 19].

5. MSCs and COVID-19

Due to the mechanisms of action of MSCs as well as their success as a therapy in ALI and ARDS, MSCs have attracted the attention now for their possible use in COVID-19. Leng et al. conducted one of the first studies exploring the case for MSCs in COVID-19 [103]. Ten adult patients with a positive real-time reverse transcription polymerase chain reaction assay and that meet the clinical classification for COVID-19 by the National Health Commission of China were enrolled in the study. Of the ten patients seven patients were in the treatment group, of those seven one was categorized as critically severe type, four were severe, and two were common types. MSCs were administered via IV infusion with 1 x 106 cells per kilogram and patients were assessed for a 14 day period. Two-four days after infusion all patients with symptoms of a high fever, weakness, shortness of breath and low oxygen saturation resolved. None of the patients experienced any infusion-related nor allergic reactions with no delayed hypersensitivity reactions or infections. Three of the patients that subsequently recovered were discharged 10 days after treatment with one of them being characterized as a severe subtype. In regard to the patient having a critically severe type of COVID-19, their C-reactive protein (CRP) decreased from 19.0 g/L to 10.1 g/L, and their oxygen saturation (SaO2) increased from 89–98% without supplemental O2. The critically severe patient also had significant improvements in lymphopenia, as well as in indicators of liver, myocardial and kidney damage/disease (aspartic aminotransferase, creatine kinase and myoglobin). Chest CT imaging with the characteristic ground-glass opacity and pneumonia infiltration were also reduced by the 9th day after MSC infusion. Overall levels of pro-inflammatory CD4+/CD8+ T cells, TNF-α and conventional DCs all decreased while IL-10, VEGF, HGF and TGFβ increased, promoting a tissue regeneration state. It was also concluded that MSCs were ACE2R and TMPRSS2 negative, theoretically making them immune from possible SARS-COV-2 infection [103]. Additionally, evidence by Sanches-Guijo et al. indicated similar results [104]. Adipose-derived MSCs were used as a treatment for 13 COVID-19 patients. There were no adverse events in the MSC treatment group with no worsening of respiratory or hemodynamic parameters. Clinical improvement was seen in 70% of the patients, seven of them extubated and discharged, and two showing signs of improvement in their ventilatory and radiological parameters, two resulting in fatalities and the rest of the patients in stable condition. Overall levels of CRP, IL-6, ferritin, and D-dimer were decreased [104].These positive effects of MSCs in COVID-19 were further elucidated by Tang et al., the study included two patients with COVID-19 which received three separate IV infusions of menstrual blood derived MSCs [105]. The first patient (Patient 1) was a 37 year old woman with a past medical history of hypertension. Patient 1's levels of CRP, TNF-α, and IL-6 decreased while their SaO2 dramatically increased from 98%

on 100% fraction of inspired O2 (FiO2) to 97% SaO2 on 55% FiO2. Initial CXR findings revealed large, patches of high density lesions in bilateral lungs that resolved with treatment along with viral RNA testing. Patient 2 was a 71 year old male that similar improvements in inflammatory markers, SaO2 and CXR findings [105].

Recently, a study conducted by Shi et al. used UC-derived MSCs as a therapeutic in 101 patients diagnosed with severe COVID-19 [106]. The study was a double-blind, placebo-controlled phase 2 trial with 101 patients randomized in a 2:1 ratio with sixty six patients, with one patient withdrawing, in the treatment group and 35 in the placebo group. Overall chest CTs, age, sex, BMI, and onset of symptoms matched between the groups. The occurrence of adverse events during the study was similar between the treatment (55.38%) and the placebo group (60%) with none directly related to the MSCs. Three IV infusions of UC-derived MSCs with 4 x 107 cells per infusion were administered. High resolution chest CT images were assessed using both radiologist and artificial intelligence software to estimate the total lesion proportion (TLP) via the Hodges-Lehmann estimator of the entire lung. The median change in the TLP was −19.40% in the treatment group −7.30% in the placebo group with the overall difference of −13.31%. Solid lesions were found to decrease by −57.70% in the treatment group with an overall decrease in the ground-glass lesions. A 6-minute walk test (6-MWT) was used to assess the restoration of lung function and reserve capability in both groups. The median 6-MWT was 420 meters in the MSC treatment group in comparison with 403 meters in the placebo group [106]. In a similar study using UC-MSCs for COVID-19, Lanzoni et al. conducted a double-blind, phase 1/2a, randomized controlled trial [107]. Twenty-four patients hospitalized for COVID-19 were randomized 1:1 into either the treatment or control group. Two infusions of UC-derived MSCs with 100 ± 20 x 106 MSCs in each were administered. There were two serious adverse events (SAEs) observed in the treatment group while the control group had 16 SAEs, the intervention was deemed safe as it did not lead to an increase in specified infusion related AEs. Overall, the survival rate in the treatment group was far greater than in the control group with 91% of subjects in the treatment group surviving 31 days post first infusion in comparison with 42% in the control group. The time of recovery was also shorter for the MSC group, with a hazard ratio for recovery in the control group vs. the MSC group of 0.29 indicating a lower rate of recovery in the control group. Concentrations of GM-CSF, IFN- γ, IL-5, IL-6, IL-7, TNF-α, TNF-β, were also statistically decreased in the MSC treatment group in comparison with control [107].

With the current supporting data surrounding the use of MSCs in COVID-19 as well as their historical efficacy in lung injury models the case for their use on a compassionate basis can be made. In the future more randomized, controlled, multi-centered clinical trials are needed in order to increase the knowledge of the use of MSCs in COVID-19.

6. Ongoing clinical trials

Clinical trials that utilize MSCs and EVs and that are registered on ClinicalTrials.gov can be seen in **Tables 1** and **2** respectively. The data from current studies are promising and promotes the use of MSCs and EVs as a possible treatment for COVID-19. However, more multi-center, controlled, randomized clinical trias are needed to further solidify the use of MSCs and EVs in COVID-19.

Study Identifier	Stem Cell Source	Study Phase; Estimated Enrollment (N)	Primary Outcome Measure(s)	Recruitment Status	Country
NCT04313322	Wharton's Jelly Mesenchymal stem cells	Phase I; N = 5	Clinical outcome (Time Frame: 3 weeks); CT Scan (Time Frame: 3 weeks); RT-PCR results (Time Frame: 3 weeks)	Recruiting	Jordan
NCT04473170	Autologous Non-Hematopoietic Peripheral Blood Stem Cells	Phase I/II; N = 146	Adverse reactions incidence (Time Frame: Day 0–28); Rate of mortality within 28-days (Time Frame: Day 0–28); Time to clinical improvement on a seven-category ordinal scale (Time Frame: Day 0–28)	Completed	United Arab Emirates
NCT04428801	Autologous adipose-derived stem cells	Phase II; N = 200	Tolerability and acute safety of AdMSC infusion by assessment of the total number of AEs/SAEs related and non-related with the medication (Time Frame: 6 months); The overall proportion of subjects who develop any AEs/SAEs related and non-related with the AdMSC infusions as compared to the control group (Time Frame: 6 months); COVID-19 incidence rates in both the study and control groups (Time Frame: 6 months)	Not yet recruiting	USA
NCT04444271	Bone marrow derived Mesenchymal stem cells		Overall survival (Time Frame: 30 days post intervention)	Recruiting	Pakistan
NCT04416139	Umbilical Cord Mesenchymal stem cells	Phase II; N = 10	Functional Respiratory changes: PaO2/FiO2 ratio (Time Frame: 3 weeks); Clinical cardiac changes: Heart rate per minute (Time Frame: 3 weeks); Clinical Respiratory Changes: Respiratory rate per minute (Time Frame: 3 weeks); Changes in body temperature (Time Frame: 3 weeks)	Recruiting	Mexico
NCT04486001	Adipose-derived allogeneic Mesenchymal stem cells	Phase I; N = 20	Frequency of all adverse events (Time Frame: Through study completion, an average of three months); Frequency of infusion related serious adverse events (Time Frame: 6 hours post infusion); Frequency of serious adverse events (Time Frame: Through study completion, an average of three months)	Recruiting	USA
NCT04336254	Allogeneic human dental pulp mesenchymal stem cells	Phase I/II; N = 20	Time to Clinical Improvement (Time Frame: 1–28 days)	Recruiting	China

Study Identifier	Stem Cell Source	Study Phase; Estimated Enrollment (N)	Primary Outcome Measure(s)	Recruitment Status	Country
NCT04565665	Cord Blood-Derived Mesenchymal stem cells	Phase I; N = 70	Incidence of composite serious adverse events (Pilot) (Time Frame: Within 30 days of the first mesenchymal stem cell (MSC) infusion); Patients alive without grade 3, 4 infusional toxicity (Phase II) (Time Frame: At day 30 post MSC infusion); Patients alive with grade 3 or 4 infusional toxicity (Phase II) (Time Frame: At day 30 post MSC infusion); Patients not alive (Phase II) (Time Frame: At day 30 post MSC infusion)	Recruiting	USA
NCT04429763	Umbilical cord derived Mesenchymal stem cells	Phase II; N = 30	Clinical deterioration or death (Time Frame: 4 weeks)	Not yet recruiting	Colombia
NCT04315987	Mesenchymal stem cells (source not defined)	Phase II; N = 90	Change in Clinical Condition (Time Frame: 10 days)	Not yet recruiting	Brazil
NCT04456361	Mesenchymal stem cells derived from Wharton Jelly of Umbilical cords	Early Phase I; N = 9	Oxygen saturation (Time Frame: Baseline, and at days 2, 4 and 14 post-treatment)	Active, not recruiting	Mexico
NCT04366323	Allogenic and Expanded Adipose Tissue-Derived Mesenchymal stem cells	Phase I/II; N = 26	Safety of the administration of allogeneic mesenchymal stem cells derived from adipose tissue assessed by Adverse Event Rate (Time Frame: 12 months); Efficacy of the administration of allogeneic mesenchymal stem cells derived from adipose tissue assessed by Survival Rate (Time Frame: 28 days)	Active, not recruiting	Spain
NCT04348435	Allogeneic Adipose-derived Mesenchymal stem cells	Phase II; N = 100	Incidence of hospitalization for COVID-19 (Time Frame: week 0 through week 26); Incidence of symptoms associated with COVID-19 (Time Frame: week 0 through week 26)	Enrolling by invitation	USA
NCT04611256	Adipose tissue derived-Mesenchymal stem cells	Phase I; N = 20	Change form baseline in Arterial oxygen saturation (Time Frame: up to 25 days); Change form baseline in Arterial oxygen saturation (Time Frame: up to 25 days); Days to clinical improvement (Time Frame: up to 25 days)	Recruiting	Mexico

Study Identifier	Stem Cell Source	Study Phase; Estimated Enrollment (N)	Primary Outcome Measure(s)	Recruitment Status	Country
NCT04625738	Wharton's Jelly Mesenchymal stem cells	Phase II; N = 30	PaO2/FiO2 ratio (Time Frame: day 10)	Not yet recruiting	France
NCT04252118	Umbilical cord derived Mesenchymal stem cells	Phase I; N = 20	Size of lesion area by chest radiograph or CT (Time Frame: At Baseline, Day 3, Day 6, Day 10, Day 14, Day 21, Day 28); Side effects in the MSCs treatment group (Time Frame: At Baseline, Day 3, Day 6, Day 10, Day 14, Day 21, Day 28, Day 90 and Day 180)	Recruiting	China
NCT04273646	Human Umbilical Cord Mesenchymal stem cells	Not Applicable; N = 48	Pneumonia severity index (Time Frame: From Baseline (0 W) to 12 week after treatment); Oxygenation index (PaO2/FiO2) (Time Frame: From Baseline (0 W) to 12 week after treatment)	Not yet recruiting	China
NCT04349631	Autologous Adipose-derived Mesenchymal stem cells	Phase II; N = 56	Incidence of hospitalization for COVID-19 (Time Frame: Week 0 through week 26); Incidence of symptoms for COVID-19 (Time Frame: week 0 through week 26)	Active, not recruiting	USA
NCT04346368	Bone Marrow-derived Mesenchymal stem cells	Phase I/II; N = 20	Changes of oxygenation index (PaO2/FiO2) (Time Frame: At baseline, 6 hour, Day 1, Day 3, Week 1, Week 2, Week 4, Month 6); Side effects in the BM-MSCs treatment group (Time Frame: Baseline through 6 months)	Not yet recruiting	China
NCT04382547	Allogenic-pooled olfactory mucosa-derived Mesenchymal stem cells	Phase I/II; N = 40	Number of cured patients (Time Frame: 3 weeks)	Enrolling by invitation	Belarus
NCT04288102	Umbilical cord derived Mesenchymal stem cells	Phase II; N = 100	Change in lesion proportion (%) of full lung volume from baseline to day 28. (Time Frame: Day 28)	Completed	China
NCT04629105	Mesenchymal stem cells (source not defined)	Phase I; N = 70	Incidence of Treatment-Emergent Serious Adverse Events (Time Frame: Within 4 weeks after treatment); Number of Participants with Abnormal Clinical Significant Laboratory Values in Hematology (Time Frame: Baseline to 6 Months); Number of Participants with Changes in Echocardiography Overall Assessment (Time Frame: Baseline to 6 Months);	Recruiting	USA

Study Identifier	Stem Cell Source	Study Phase; Estimated Enrollment (N)	Primary Outcome Measure(s)	Recruitment Status	Country
			Number of Participants with Changes to overall assessment of Electrocardiogram (Time Frame: Baseline to 6 Months); Time to recovery of Sp02 (Time Frame: Baseline to 6 Months); Number of Participants with Abnormal Clinical Significant Lab Values in the Blood Chemistry testing (Time Frame: Baseline to 6 months); Number of Participants with Abnormal Clinical Significant Lab Values in the Coagulation (Time Frame: Baseline to 6 months); Number of Participants with Abnormal Clinical Significant Lab Values in the Urinalysis (Time Frame: Baseline to 6 months)		
NCT04527224	Allogenic adipose tissue derived Mesenchymal stem cells	Phase I/II; N = 10	Treatment related adverse events (Time Frame: From baseline to Week 12); Number of subjects with treatment related abnormal variation of vital signs, physical examination and laboratory test values (Time Frame: From baseline to Week 12)	Not yet recruiting	South Korea
NCT04366063	Mesenchymal stem cells (source not defined)	Phase II/III; N = 60	Adverse events assessment (Time Frame: From baseline to day 28); Blood oxygen saturation (Time Frame: From baseline to day 14)	Recruiting	Iran
NCT04573270	Mesenchymal stem cells derived from human umbilical cords	Phase I; N = 40	Survival Rates (Time Frame: 30 Days); Contraction Rates (Time Frame: 30 Days)	Completed	USA
NCT04302519	Dental pulp mesenchymal stem cells	Early Phase I; N = 24	Disappear time of ground-glass shadow in the lungs (Time Frame: 14 days)	Not yet recruiting	China
NCT04437823	Umbilical cord derived Mesenchymal stem cells	Phase II; N = 20	Safety and efficacy assessment of infusion associated adverse events (Time Frame: Day 01 to Day 30); Chest Radiograph or Chest CT Scan (Time Frame: Day 01 to Day 30)	Recruiting	Pakistan
NCT04494386	Umbilical Cord Lining Stem Cells	Phase I/II; N = 60	Incidence of Dose Limiting Toxicity (DLT) (Time Frame: 24 hours); Incidence of Dose Limiting Toxicity (DLT),	Recruiting	USA

Study Identifier	Stem Cell Source	Study Phase; Estimated Enrollment (N)	Primary Outcome Measure(s)	Recruitment Status	Country
			suspected adverse reaction (SAR), or serious adverse event (SAE) (Time Frame: 1 week); Treatment-emergent adverse events (AE) and serious adverse events (SAE) (Time Frame: 1 month); Treatment-emergent adverse events (AE) and serious adverse events (SAE) (Time Frame: 12 months)		
NCT04457609	Umbilical Cord Mesenchymal stem cells	Phase I; N = 40	Clinical improvement: Presence of dyspnea (Time Frame: 15 days); Clinical improvement: presence of sputum (Time Frame: 15 days); Clinical improvement: fever (Time Frame: 15 days); Clinical improvement: ventilation status (Time Frame: 15 days); Clinical improvement: blood pressure (Time Frame: 15 days); Clinical improvement: heart rate (Time Frame: 15 days); Clinical improvement: respiratory rate (Time Frame: 15 days); Clinical improvement: oxygen saturation (Time Frame: 15 days)	Recruiting	Indonesia
NCT04339660	Human umbilical cord-derived Mesenchymal stem cells	Phase I/II; N = 30	The immune function (TNF-α IL-1β IL-6 TGF-β IL-8 PCT CRP) (Time Frame: Observe the immune function of the participants within 4 weeks); Blood oxygen saturation (Time Frame: Monitor blood oxygen saturation of the participants within 4 weeks)	Recruiting	China
NCT04392778	Umbilical Cord-derived Mesenchymal stem cells	Phase I/II; N = 30	Clinical improvement (Time Frame: 3 months)	Recruiting	Turkey
NCT04490486	Umbilical Cord Tissue Derived Mesenchymal stem cells	Phase I; N = 21	Percent of participants with treatment related Serious Adverse Events (SAE) (Time Frame: 12 months)	Not yet recruiting	USA
NCT04355728	Human umbilical cord derived Mesenchymal stem cells	Phase I/II; N = 24	Incidence of pre-specified infusion associated adverse events (Time Frame: Day 5); Incidence of Severe Adverse Events (Time Frame: 90 days)	Completed	USA
NCT04522986	Adipose-derived Mesenchymal stem cells	Phase I; N = 6	Safety: Adverse Event (Time Frame: 12 weeks)	Not yet recruiting	Japan

Study Identifier	Stem Cell Source	Study Phase; Estimated Enrollment (N)	Primary Outcome Measure(s)	Recruitment Status	Country
NCT04371601	Umbilical Cord-derived Mensechynmal stem cells	Early Phase I; N = 60	Changes of oxygenation index (PaO2/FiO2), blood gas test (Time Frame: 12 months)	Active, not recruiting	China
NCT04362189	Allogeneic Adipose-derived Mesenchymal stem cells	Phase II; N = 100	Interleukin-6 (Time Frame: screening, day 0, 7, 10); C Reactive protein (Time Frame: screening, day 0, 7, 10); Oxygenation (Time Frame: screening, day 0, 7, 10); TNF alpha (Time Frame: screening, day 0, 7, 10); IL-10 (Time Frame: screening, day 0, 7. 10); Return to room air (RTRA) (Time Frame: Day 0, 3, 7, 10, 28)	Active, not recruiting	USA
NCT04390152	Wharton's Jelly derived Mesenchymal stem cells	Phase I/II; N = 40	Intergroup mortality difference with treatment (Time Frame: 28 days)	Not yet recruiting	Colombia
NCT04461925	Placenta-Derived MMSCs; Cryopreserved Placenta-Derived Multipotent Mesenchymal Stromal Cells	Phase I/II; N = 30	Changes of oxygenation index PaO2/FiO2, most conveniently the P/F ratio. (Time Frame: up to 28 days); Changes in length of hospital stay (Time Frame: up to 28 days); Changes in mortality rate (Time Frame: up to 28 days)	Recruiting	Ukraine
NCT04299152	Human cord blood stem cells	Phase II; N = 20	Determine the number of Covid-19 patients who were unable to complete SCE Therapy (Time Frame: 4 weeks)	Not yet recruiting	USA
NCT04348461	Allogeneic and expanded adipose tissue-derived mesenchymal stromal cells	Phase II; N = 100	Efficacy of the administration of allogeneic mesenchymal stem cells derived from adipose tissue assessed by Survival Rate) (Time Frame: 28 days); Safety of the administration of allogeneic mesenchymal stem cells derived from adipose tissue assessed by Adverse Event Rate (Time Frame: 6 months)	Not yet recruiting	Spain
NCT04535856	Allogeneic Mesenchymal stem cells (source not defined)	Phase I; N = 9	Incidence of TEAE* in Treatment group (Time Frame: 28 days)	Active, not recruiting	Indonesia
NCT04393415	Cord blood stem cells	Not Applicable; N = 100	The number of patients with positive covid 19 who will improve after receiving stem cells (Time Frame: 2 weeks)	Recruiting	Egypt

Study Identifier	Stem Cell Source	Study Phase; Estimated Enrollment (N)	Primary Outcome Measure(s)	Recruitment Status	Country
NCT04447833	Allogenic bone marrow derived Mesenchymal Stromal Stem Cells	Phase I; N = 9	The incidence of pre-specified treatment related adverse events of interest (TRAEIs). (Time Frame: From drug administration to day 10 post-infusion)	Recruiting	Sweden
NCT04397796	Allogenic Bone Marrow derived Mesenchymal stem cells	Phase I; N = 45	Incidence of AEs (Time Frame: 30 days); Mortality (Time Frame: 30 days); Death (Time Frame: 30 days); Number of ventilator-free days (Time Frame: 60 days)	Recruiting	USA
NCT04452097	Human umbilical cord Mesenchymal stem cells	Phase I/II; N = 39	Incidence of infusion-related adverse events (Time Frame: Day 3); Incidence of any treatment-emergent adverse events (TEAEs) and treatment emergent serious adverse events (TESAEs) (Time Frame: Day 28)	Not yet recruiting	USA
NCT04377334	Allogeneic bone marrow-derived human mesenchymal stem (stromal) cells	Phase II; N = 40	Lung injury score (Time Frame: day 10)	Not yet recruiting	Germany
NCT04331613	Differentiated cells obtained from human embryonic stem cells	Phase I/II; N = 9	Adverse reaction (AE) and severe adverse reaction (SAE) (Time Frame: Within 28 days after treatment); Changes of lung imaging examinations (Time Frame: Within 28 days after treatment)	Recruiting	China
NCT04345601	Bone Marrow Mesenchymal Stromal Cells	Early Phase I; N = 30	Treatment-related serious adverse events (tSAEs) (Time Frame: 28 days post cell infusion); Change in clinical status at day 14 (Time Frame: 14 days post cell infusion)	Not yet recruiting	USA
NCT04390139	Wharton-Jelly mesenchymal stromal cells	Phase I/II; N = 30	All-cause mortality at day 28 (Time Frame: Day 28)	Recruiting	Spain
NCT04398303	Allogenic human umbilical derived Mesenchymal stem cells	Phase I/II; N = 70	Mortality at day 30 (Time Frame: 30 days post treatment)	Not yet recruiting	USA
NCT04400032	Bone Marrow derived Mesenchymal Stromal Cells	Phase I; N = 9	Number of Participants With Treatment-Related Adverse Events as Assessed by CTCAE v4.0 (Time Frame: At time of infusion until one year post-infusion)	Recruiting	Canada

Study Identifier	Stem Cell Source	Study Phase; Estimated Enrollment (N)	Primary Outcome Measure(s)	Recruitment Status	Country
NCT04537351	Induced Pluripotent stem cells derived mesenchymoangioblasts	Phase I/II; N = 24	Trend in trajectory of PaO2/FiO2 ratio (P/F ratio) between groups (Time Frame: 7 days)	Recruiting	Australia
NCT04467047	Allogenic Bone Marrow Mesenchymal Stromal Cells	Phase I; N = 10	Overall survival (Time Frame: 60 days)	Not yet recruiting	Brazil
NCT04365101	Natural Killer (NK) cells derived from human placental hematopoietic stem (CD34+) cells	Phase I/II; N = 86	Phase 1: Frequency and Severity of Adverse Events (AE) (Time Frame: Up to 12 months); Phase 1: Rate of clearance of SARS-CoV-2 (Time Frame: Up to 12 months); Phase 1: Rate of clinical improvement (Time Frame: Up to 12 months); Phase 2: Time to Clearance of SARS-CoV-2 (Time Frame: Up to 28 days); Phase 2: Time to Clinical Improvement by NEWS2 Score (Time Frame: Up to 28 days)	Recruiting	USA
NCT03042143	Human umbilical cord derived CD362 enriched Mesenchymal stem cells	Phase I/II; N = 75	Oxygenation index (OI) (Time Frame: Day 7); Incidence of Serious Adverse Events (SAEs) (Time Frame: 28 days)	Recruiting	United Kingdom
NCT04269525	Umbilical cord derived Mesenchymal stem cells	Phase II; N = 16	Oxygenation index (Time Frame: on the day 14 after enrollment)	Recruiting	China
NCT04361942	Allogenic Mesenchymal stem cells (source not defined)	Phase II; N = 24	Proportion of patients who have achieved withdrawal of invasive mechanical ventilation (Time Frame: 0–7 days); Rate of mortality (Time Frame: 28 days)	Recruiting	Spain
NCT04333368	Umbilical cord Wharton's jelly-derived mesenchymal stromal cells	Phase I/II; N = 47	Respiratory efficacy evaluated by the increase in PaO2/FiO2 ratio from baseline to day 7 in the experimental group compared with the placebo group (Time Frame: From baseline to day 7)	Active, not recruiting	France
NCT04371393	Allogenic Bone Marrow derived mesenchymal stem cells	Phase III; N = 223	Number of all-cause mortality (Time Frame: 30 days)	Active, not recruiting	USA
NCT04367077	Multipotent adult progenitor cells (source not defined)	Phase II/III; N = 400	Ventilator-Free Days (Time Frame: Day 0 through Day 28); Safety and Tolerability as measured by the incidence of	Recruiting	USA

Study Identifier	Stem Cell Source	Study Phase; Estimated Enrollment (N)	Primary Outcome Measure(s)	Recruitment Status	Country
			treatment-emergent adverse events as assessed by CTCAE v5.0. (Time Frame: Day 28)		
NCT04524962	Allogenic mesenchymal stem cells (source not defined)	Phase I/II; N = 30	To assess the safety of Descartes-30 in patients with moderate-to-severe ARDS (Time Frame: 2 years)	Recruiting	USA
NCT04445220	Allogenic Bone Marrow derived Mesenchymal stromal cells	Phase I/II; N = 22	Safety and tolerability as measured by incidence of IP-related serious adverse events (Time Frame: Outcomes and Serious Adverse Events through Day 180)	Recruiting	USA
NCT04466098	Mesenchymal stromal cells (source not defined)	Phase II; N = 30	Incidence of grade 3–5 infusional toxicities and predefined hemodynamic or respiratory adverse events related to the infusion of mesenchymal stem cells (Time Frame: Within 6 hours of the start of the infusion)	Recruiting	USA

Table 1.
Clinical trials registered on ClinicalTrials.gov till January 5, 2021 utilizing sem cells for the treatment of COVID-19.

Study Identifier	Exosome Source	Study Phase; Estimated Enrollment (N)	Primary Outcome Measure(s)	Recruitment Status	Country
NCT04602442	Mesenchymal stem cells	Phase II; N = 90	Number of participants with non-serious and serious adverse events during trial (Time Frame: through study, an average of 2 months); Number of participants with non-serious and serious adverse during inhalation procedure (Time Frame: 10 days during inhalation procedures)	Enrolling by invitation	Russia
NCT04491240	Mesenchymal stem cells	Phase I/II; N = 30	Number of participants with non-serious and serious adverse events during trial (Time Frame: 30 days after clinic discharge); Number of participants with non-serious and serious adverse during inhalation procedure (Time Frame: after each inhalation during 10 days)	Completed	Russia
NCT04389385	T cell derived exosomes	Phase I; N = 60	Adverse reaction (AE) and severe AE (SAE) (Time Frame: 28 days); Efficacy Assessment – Time to Clinical Recovery (Time Frame: 28 days); The rate of recovery without Mechanical Ventilator (Time Frame: 28 days)	Active, not recruiting	Turkey
NCT04384445	Human Amniotic Fluid	Phase I/II; N = 20	Incidence of any infusion associated adverse events (Time Frame: 60 days); Incidence of Severe Adverse Events (Time Frame: 60 days)	Recruiting	USA
NCT04493242	Bone Marrow	Phase II; N = 60	All-cause mortality (Time Frame: 28 days); Median days to recovery (Time Frame: 28 days)	Not yet recruiting	USA
NCT04276987	Allogenic adipose Mesenchymal stem cells	Phase I; N = 24	Adverse reaction and severe adverse reaction (Time frame: up to 28 days); time to clinical improvement (Time frame: up to 28 days)	Completed	China
NCT04657458	Bone marrow Mesenchymal stem cells	Expanded Access	N/A	Expanded Access Available	USA

Table 2.
Clinical trials registered on ClinicalTrials.gov till January 5, 2021 utilizing extracellular vesicles and/or exosomes for the treatment of COVID-19.

7. Conclusion

The current pandemic we are encountering has placed an unprecedented burden upon the world and is likely to leave an everlasting impact for generations to come. With the lack of definitive and safe treatment along with the congruent rise in unknown viral variants the demand for a safe source of mitigation is urgently needed. Clincial studies have specified tht patients who suffer from SARS-CoV-2 related ARDS have an indued cytokine storm composed of a large and rapid surge in pro-inflammatory cytokines and inflammatory cells. MSCs and their EVs have a long been touted for their safty and effectiveness in the treatment of immune related diseases, ALI and ARDS. MSCs and EVs have are now being repourposed for COVID-19 due to their antiviral, anti-inflammatory and tissue regenerative capabilities. Data from clinical trials using MSCs and EVs have shown promising results that warrant their use on a compassionate basis for COVID-19. Eventually more pre-clinical and clinical trials are needed to further establish the safety and efficacy of MSCs and their EVs as a potential treatment for COVID-19.

Conflict of interest

The authors declare no conflict of interest.

Author details

Hugo C. Rodriguez[1,2,3,4], Manu Gupta[1], Emilio Cavazos-Escobar[4,5], Enrique Montalvo[4,6], Saadiq F. El-Amin III[7,8] and Ashim Gupta[1,2,8]*

1 Future Biologics, Lawrenceville, Georgia, USA

2 South Texas Orthopedic Research Institute, Laredo, Texas, USA

3 School of Osteopathic Medicine, University of the Incarnate Word, San Antonio, Texas, USA

4 Future Physicians of South Texas, San Antonio, Texas, USA

5 University of Texas Medical Branch at Galveston, Galveston, Texas, USA

6 Texas A&M International University, Laredo, Texas, USA

7 El-Amin Orthopaedic and Sports Medicine Institute, Lawrenceville, Georgia, USA

8 BioIntegrate, Lawrenceville, Georgia, USA

*Address all correspondence to: ashim6786@gmail.com

'Biotechnology to Combat COVID-19' is a collaborative project with Biotechnology Kiosk

References

[1] Munnoli PM, Nabapure S, Yeshavanth G. Post-COVID-19 precautions based on lessons learned from past pandemics: a review. J Public Health (Berl.). 2020;1-9. DOI: 10.1007/s10389-020-01371-3

[2] Lai CC, Shih TP, Ko WC, Tang HJ, Hsueh PR. Severe acute respiratory syndrome coronavirus 2 (SARS-CoV-2) and coronavirus disease-2019 (COVID-19): The epidemic and the challenges. Int J Antimicrob Agents. 2020;55:105924. DOI: 10.1016/j.ijantimicag.2020.105924

[3] COVID-19 Dashboard by the Center for Systems Science and Engineering (CSSE) at Johns Hopkins University (JHU) [Internet]. [cited 2021 Feb 14]. Available from: https://coronavirus.jhu.edu/map.html

[4] Chung JY, Thone MN, Kwon YJ. COVID-19 vaccines: The status and perspectives in delivery points of view. Adv Drug Deliv Rev. 2020;170:1-25. DOI: 10.1016/j.addr.2020.12.011

[5] Chen Y, Wang J, Liu C, Su L, Zhang D, Fan J, Yang Y, Xiao M, Xie J, Xu Y, Li Y, Zhang S. IP-10 and MCP-1 as biomarkers associated with disease severity of COVID-19. Mol Med. 2020; 26:97. DOI: 10.1186/s10020-020-00230-x

[6] Gupta A, Kashte S, Gupta M, Rodriguez HC, Gautam SS, Kadam S. Mesenchymal stem cells and exosome therapy for COVID-19: current status and future perspective. Hum Cell. 2020; 33:907-918. DOI: 10.1007/s13577-020-00407-w

[7] Channappanavar R, Perlman S. Pathogenic human coronavirus infections: causes and consequences of cytokine storm and immunopathology. Semin Immunopathol. 2017;39:529-539. DOI: 10.1007/s00281-017-0629-x

[8] Yun JW, Ahn JH, Kwon E, Kim SH, Kim H, Jang JJ, Kim WH, Kim JH, Han SY, Kim JT, Kim JH, Kim W, Ku SY, Do BR, Kang BC. Human umbilical cord-derived mesenchymal stem cells in acute liver injury: Hepatoprotective efficacy, subchronic toxicity, tumorigenicity, and biodistribution. Regul Toxicol Pharmacol. 2016;81:437-447. DOI: 10.1016/j.yrtph.2016.09.029

[9] Wilson JG, Liu KD, Zhuo H, Caballero L, McMillan M, Fang X, Cosgrove K, Vojnik R, Calfee CS, Lee JW, Rogers AJ, Levitt J, Wiener-Kronish J, Bajwa EK, Leavitt A, McKenna D, Thompson BT, Matthay MA. Mesenchymal stem (stromal) cells for treatment of ARDS: a phase 1 clinical trial. Lancet Respir Med. 2015;3:24-32. DOI: 10.1016/S2213-2600(14)70291-7

[10] Rogers CJ, Harman RJ, Bunnell BA, Schreiber MA, Xiang C, Wang FS, Santidrian AF, Minev BR. Rationale for the clinical use of adipose-derived mesenchymal stem cells for COVID-19 patients. J Transl Med. 2020;18:203. DOI: 10.1186/s12967-020-02380-2

[11] Fischer UM, Harting MT, Jimenez F, Monzon-Posadas WO, Xue H, Savitz SI, Laine GA, Cox CS Jr. Pulmonary passage is a major obstacle for intravenous stem cell delivery: the pulmonary first-pass effect. Stem Cells Dev. 2009;18:683-692. DOI: 10.1089/scd.2008.0253

[12] Rodriguez HC, Gupta M, Cavazos-Escobar E, El-Amin SF 3rd, Gupta A. Umbilical cord: an allogenic tissue for potential treatment of COVID-19. Hum Cell. 2021;34:1-13. DOI: 10.1007/s13577-020-00444-5

[13] Duffy MM, Ritter T, Ceredig R, Griffin MD. Mesenchymal stem cell effects on T-cell effector pathways. Stem Cell Res Ther. 2011;2:34. DOI: 10.1186/scrt75

[14] Zhou Y, Yamamoto Y, Xiao Z, Ochiya T. The Immunomodulatory Functions of Mesenchymal Stromal/Stem Cells Mediated via Paracrine Activity. J Clin Med. 2019;8:1025. DOI: 10.3390/jcm8071025

[15] Harrell CR, Sadikot R, Pascual J, Fellabaum C, Jankovic MG, Jovicic N, Djonov V, Arsenijevic N, Volarevic V. Mesenchymal Stem Cell-Based Therapy of Inflammatory Lung Diseases: Current Understanding and Future Perspectives. Stem Cells Int. 2019;2019:4236973. DOI: 10.1155/2019/4236973

[16] Potty AGR, Gupta A, Rodriguez HC, Stone IW, Maffulli N. Intraosseous Bioplasty for a Subchondral Cyst in the Lateral Condyle of Femur. J Clin Med. 2020;9:1358. DOI: 10.3390/jcm9051358

[17] Main BJ, Valk JA, Maffulli N, Rodriguez HC, Gupta M, Stone IW, El-Amin SF 3rd, Gupta A. Umbilical cord-derived Wharton's jelly for regenerative medicine applications in orthopedic surgery: a systematic review protocol. J Orthop Surg Res. 2020;15:527. DOI: 10.1186/s13018-020-02067-w

[18] Gupta A, Maffulli N, Rodriguez HC, Lee CE, Levy HJ, El-Amin SF 3rd. Umbilical cord-derived Wharton's jelly for treatment of knee osteoarthritis: study protocol for a non-randomized, open-label, multi-center trial. J Orthop Surg Res. 2021;16:143. DOI: 10.1186/s13018-021-02300-0

[19] Gattinoni L, Coppola S, Cressoni M, Busana M, Rossi S, Chiumello D. COVID-19 Does Not Lead to a "Typical" Acute Respiratory Distress Syndrome. Am J Respir Crit Care Med. 2020;201:1299-1300. DOI: 10.1164/rccm.202003-0817LE

[20] Kumar L, Verma S, Vaidya B, Gupta V. Exosomes: Natural Carriers for siRNA Delivery. Curr Pharm Des. 2015;21:4556-4565. DOI: 10.2174/138161282131151013190112

[21] Harrell CR, Jovicic N, Djonov V, Arsenijevic N, Volarevic V. Mesenchymal Stem Cell-Derived Exosomes and Other Extracellular Vesicles as New Remedies in the Therapy of Inflammatory Diseases. Cells. 2019;8:1605. DOI: 10.3390/cells8121605

[22] Dyall J, Gross R, Kindrachuk J, Johnson RF, Olinger GG Jr, Hensley LE, Frieman MB, Jahrling PB. Middle East Respiratory Syndrome and Severe Acute Respiratory Syndrome: Current Therapeutic Options and Potential Targets for Novel Therapies. Drugs. 2017;77:1935-1966. DOI: 10.1007/s40265-017-0830-1

[23] Won JH, Lee H. The Current Status of Drug Repositioning and Vaccine Developments for the COVID-19 Pandemic. Int J Mol Sci. 2020;21:9775. DOI: 10.3390/ijms21249775

[24] Pandey S, Pathak SK, Pandey A, Salunke AA, Chawla J, Sharma A, Sharma S, Thivari P, Ratna HVK. Ivermectin in COVID-19: What do we know? Diabetes Metab Syndr. 2020;14:1921-1922. DOI: 10.1016/j.dsx.2020.09.027

[25] van Oosterhout C, Hall N, Ly H, Tyler KM. COVID-19 evolution during the pandemic - Implications of new SARS-CoV-2 variants on disease control and public health policies. Virulence. 2021;12:507-508. DOI: 10.1080/21505594.2021.1877066

[26] Self WH, Semler MW, Leither LM, Casey JD, Angus DC, Brower RG, et al. Effect of Hydroxychloroquine on Clinical Status at 14 Days in Hospitalized Patients With COVID-19: A Randomized Clinical Trial. JAMA. 2020;324:2165-2176. DOI: 10.1001/jama.2020.22240 (PMID: 33165621)

[27] Arabi YM, Mandourah Y, Al-Hameed F, Sindi AA, Almekhlafi GA, Hussein MA, Jose J, Pinto R, Al-Omari

A, Kharaba A, Almotairi A, Al Khatib K, Alraddadi B, Shalhoub S, Abdulmomen A, Qushmaq I, Mady A, Solaiman O, Al-Aithan AM, Al-Raddadi R, Ragab A, Balkhy HH, Al Harthy A, Deeb AM, Al Mutairi H, Al-Dawood A, Merson L, Hayden FG, Fowler RA; Saudi Critical Care Trial Group. Corticosteroid Therapy for Critically Ill Patients with Middle East Respiratory Syndrome. Am J Respir Crit Care Med. 2018;197:757-767. DOI: 10.1164/rccm.201706-1172OC

[28] Stockman LJ, Bellamy R, Garner P. SARS: systematic review of treatment effects. PLoS Med. 2006;3:e343. DOI: 10.1371/journal.pmed.0030343

[29] Han K, Ma H, An X, Su Y, Chen J, Lian Z, Zhao J, Zhu BP, Fontaine RE, Feng Z, Zeng G. Early use of glucocorticoids was a risk factor for critical disease and death from pH1N1 infection. Clin Infect Dis. 2011;53: 326-333. DOI: 10.1093/cid/cir398

[30] Self WH, Semler MW, Leither LM, Casey JD, Angus DC, Brower RG, Chang SY, Collins SP, Eppensteiner JC, et al. Effect of Hydroxychloroquine on Clinical Status at 14 Days in Hospitalized Patients With COVID-19: A Randomized Clinical Trial. JAMA. 2020 Dec 1;324(21):2165-2176. doi: 10.1001/jama.2020.22240

[31] Russell CD, Millar JE, Baillie JK. Clinical evidence does not support corticosteroid treatment for 2019-nCoV lung injury. Lancet. 2020;395:473-475. DOI: 10.1016/S0140-6736(20)30317-2

[32] Marano G, Vaglio S, Pupella S, Facco G, Catalano L, Liumbruno GM, Grazzini G. Convalescent plasma: new evidence for an old therapeutic tool? Blood Transfus. 2016;14:152-157. DOI: 10.2450/2015.0131-15

[33] Zhu T, Xu A, Bai X, He Y, Zhang H. [Effect of convalescent plasma and immunoglobulin on patients with severe acute respiratory syndrome: a systematic review]. Zhonghua Wei Zhong Bing Ji Jiu Yi Xue. 2020;32: 435-438. Chinese. DOI: 10.3760/cma.j.cn121430-20200326-00240

[34] Zhao Q, He Y. Challenges of Convalescent Plasma Therapy on COVID-19. J Clin Virol. 2020;127: 104358. DOI: 10.1016/j.jcv.2020.104358 (PMID: 32305026)

[35] Cheng Y, Wong R, Soo YO, Wong WS, Lee CK, Ng MH, Chan P, Wong KC, Leung CB, Cheng G. Use of convalescent plasma therapy in SARS patients in Hong Kong. Eur J Clin Microbiol Infect Dis. 2005;24:44-46. DOI: 10.1007/s10096-004-1271-9

[36] Kaplon H, Reichert JM. Antibodies to watch in 2021. MAbs. 2021;13: 1860476. DOI: 10.1080/19420862.2020.1860476

[37] REGN-COV2 FDA Approval Status at Regeneron Pharmaceuticals, Inc. [Internet]. [cited 2021]. Available from: https://www.drugs.com/history/regn-cov2.html

[38] Polack FP, Thomas SJ, Kitchin N, Absalon J, Gurtman A, Lockhart S, Perez JL, Pérez Marc G, Moreira ED, Zerbini C, Bailey R, Swanson KA, Roychoudhury S, Koury K, Li P, Kalina WV, Cooper D, Frenck RW Jr, Hammitt LL, Türeci Ö, Nell H, Schaefer A, Ünal S, Tresnan DB, Mather S, Dormitzer PR, Şahin U, Jansen KU, Gruber WC; C4591001 Clinical Trial Group. Safety and Efficacy of the BNT162b2 mRNA Covid-19 Vaccine. N Engl J Med. 2020;383: 2603-2615. DOI: 10.1056/NEJMoa2034577

[39] Baden LR, El Sahly HM, Essink B, Kotloff K, Frey S, Novak R, COVE Study Group. Efficacy and Safety of the mRNA-1273 SARS-CoV-2 Vaccine. N Engl J Med. 2021;384:403-416. DOI: 10.1056/NEJMoa2035389

[40] Friedenstein AJ, Petrakova KV, Kurolesova AI, Frolova GP. Heterotopic of bone marrow. Analysis of precursor cells for osteogenic and hematopoietic tissues. Transplantation. 1968;6:230-247

[41] Caplan AI. Mesenchymal stem cells. J Orthop Res. 1991;9:641-650. DOI: 10.1002/jor.1100090504

[42] Caplan AI. Mesenchymal Stem Cells: Time to Change the Name! Stem Cells Transl Med. 2017;6:1445-1451. DOI: 10.1002/sctm.17-0051

[43] Horwitz EM, Le Blanc K, Dominici M, Mueller I, Slaper-Cortenbach I, Marini FC, Deans RJ, Krause DS, Keating A; International Society for Cellular Therapy. Clarification of the nomenclature for MSC: The International Society for Cellular Therapy position statement. Cytotherapy. 2005;7:393-395. DOI: 10.1080/14653240500319234

[44] Dominici M, Le Blanc K, Mueller I, Slaper-Cortenbach I, Marini F, Krause D, Deans R, Keating A, Prockop Dj, Horwitz E. Minimal criteria for defining multipotent mesenchymal stromal cells. The International Society for Cellular Therapy position statement. Cytotherapy. 2006;8:315-317. DOI: 10.1080/14653240600855905

[45] Morgani SM, Canham MA, Nichols J, Sharov AA, Migueles RP, Ko MS, Brickman JM. Totipotent embryonic stem cells arise in ground-state culture conditions. Cell Rep. 2013 Jun;3:1945-1957. DOI: 10.1016/j.celrep.2013.04.034

[46] Berebichez-Fridman R, Montero-Olvera PR. Sources and Clinical Applications of Mesenchymal Stem Cells: State-of-the-art review. Sultan Qaboos Univ Med J. 2018 Aug;18:e264-e277. DOI: 10.18295/squmj.2018.18.03.002

[47] Salem HK, Thiemermann C. Mesenchymal stromal cells: current understanding and clinical status. Stem Cells. 2010 Mar;28:585-596. DOI: 10.1002/stem.269

[48] Choudhery MS, Badowski M, Muise A, Pierce J, Harris DT. Donor age negatively impacts adipose tissue-derived mesenchymal stem cell expansion and differentiation. J Transl Med. 2014 Jan;12: 8. DOI: 10.1186/1479-5876-12-8

[49] Berebichez-Fridman R, Gómez-García R, Granados-Montiel J, Berebichez-Fastlicht E, Olivos-Meza A, Granados J, Velasquillo C, Ibarra C. The Holy Grail of Orthopedic Surgery: Mesenchymal Stem Cells-Their Current Uses and Potential Applications. Stem Cells Int. 2017;2017:2638305. DOI: 10.1155/2017/2638305

[50] Spitzhorn LS, Rahman MS, Schwindt L, Ho HT, Wruck W, Bohndorf M, Wehrmeyer S, Ncube A, Beyer I, Hagenbeck C, Balan P, Fehm T, Adjaye J. Isolation and Molecular Characterization of Amniotic Fluid-Derived Mesenchymal Stem Cells Obtained from Caesarean Sections. Stem Cells Int. 2017;2017:5932706. DOI: 10.1155/2017/5932706

[51] Lee RH, Pulin AA, Seo MJ, Kota DJ, Ylostalo J, Larson BL, Semprun-Prieto L, Delafontaine P, Prockop DJ. Intravenous hMSCs improve myocardial infarction in mice because cells embolized in lung are activated to secrete the anti-inflammatory protein TSG-6. Cell Stem Cell. 2009 Jul;5:54-63. DOI: 10.1016/j.stem.2009.05.003

[52] De Miguel MP, Fuentes-Julián S, Blázquez-Martínez A, Pascual CY, Aller MA, Arias J, Arnalich-Montiel F. Immunosuppressive properties of mesenchymal stem cells: advances and applications. Curr Mol Med. 2012 Jun;12:574-591. DOI: 10.2174/156652412800619950

[53] Ware LB, Matthay MA. Alveolar fluid clearance is impaired in the

majority of patients with acute lung injury and the acute respiratory distress syndrome. Am J Respir Crit Care Med. 2001 May;163:1376-1383. DOI: 10.1164/ajrccm.163.6.2004035

[54] Kabat M, Bobkov I, Kumar S, Grumet M. Trends in mesenchymal stem cell clinical trials 2004-2018: Is efficacy optimal in a narrow dose range? Stem Cells Transl Med. 2020 Jan;9:17-27. DOI: 10.1002/sctm.19-0202

[55] Lalu MM, McIntyre L, Pugliese C, Fergusson D, Winston BW, Marshall JC, Granton J, Stewart DJ; Canadian Critical Care Trials Group. Safety of cell therapy with mesenchymal stromal cells (SafeCell): a systematic review and meta-analysis of clinical trials. PLoS One. 2012;7:e47559. DOI: 10.1371/journal.pone.0047559

[56] Németh K, Leelahavanichkul A, Yuen PS, Mayer B, Parmelee A, Doi K, Robey PG, Leelahavanichkul K, Koller BH, Brown JM, Hu X, Jelinek I, Star RA, Mezey E. Bone marrow stromal cells attenuate sepsis via prostaglandin E (2)-dependent reprogramming of host macrophages to increase their interleukin-10 production. Nat Med. 2009;15:42-49. DOI: 10.1038/nm.1905

[57] Shapouri-Moghaddam A, Mohammadian S, Vazini H, Taghadosi M, Esmaeili SA, Mardani F, Seifi B, Mohammadi A, Afshari JT, Sahebkar A. Macrophage plasticity, polarization, and function in health and disease. J Cell Physiol. 2018;233: 6425-6440. DOI: 10.1002/jcp.26429

[58] Dayan V, Yannarelli G, Billia F, Filomeno P, Wang XH, Davies JE, Keating A. Mesenchymal stromal cells mediate a switch to alternatively activated monocytes/macrophages after acute myocardial infarction. Basic Res Cardiol. 2011;106:1299-1310. DOI: 10.1007/s00395-011-0221-9

[59] Gur-Wahnon D, Borovsky Z, Beyth S, Liebergall M, Rachmilewitz J. Contact-dependent induction of regulatory antigen-presenting cells by human mesenchymal stem cells is mediated via STAT3 signaling. Exp Hematol. 2007;35:426-433. DOI: 10.1016/j.exphem.2006.11.001

[60] Matthay MA, Zemans RL, Zimmerman GA, Arabi YM, Beitler JR, Mercat A, Herridge M, Randolph AG, Calfee CS. Acute respiratory distress syndrome. Nat Rev Dis Primers. 2019 Mar 14;5:18. DOI: 10.1038/s41572-019-0069-0

[61] Jiang D, Muschhammer J, Qi Y, Kügler A, de Vries JC, Saffarzadeh M, Sindrilaru A, Beken SV, Wlaschek M, Kluth MA, Ganss C, Frank NY, Frank MH, Preissner KT, Scharffetter-Kochanek K. Suppression of Neutrophil-Mediated Tissue Damage-A Novel Skill of Mesenchymal Stem Cells. Stem Cells. 2016;34:2393-2406. DOI: 10.1002/stem.2417

[62] Monsel A, Zhu YG, Gennai S, Hao Q, Liu J, Lee JW. Cell-based therapy for acute organ injury: preclinical evidence and ongoing clinical trials using mesenchymal stem cells. Anesthesiology. 2014;12:1099-1121. DOI: 10.1097/ALN.0000000000000446

[63] Liu YJ, Kanzler H, Soumelis V, Gilliet M. Dendritic cell lineage, plasticity and cross-regulation. Nat Immunol. 2001;2:585-589. DOI: 10.1038/89726

[64] van Megen KM, van 't Wout ET, Lages Motta J, Dekker B, Nikolic T, Roep BO. Activated Mesenchymal Stromal Cells Process and Present Antigens Regulating Adaptive Immunity. Front Immunol. 2019 Apr; 10:694. DOI: 10.3389/fimmu.2019.00694

[65] Liu Y, Yin Z, Zhang R, Yan K, Chen L, Chen F, Huang W, Lv B, Sun C, Jiang X. MSCs inhibit bone

marrow-derived DC maturation and function through the release of TSG-6. Biochem Biophys Res Commun. 2014; 450:1409-1415. DOI: 10.1016/j.bbrc.2014.07.001

[66] Chen L, Zhang W, Yue H, Han Q, Chen B, Shi M, Li J, Li B, You S, Shi Y, Zhao RC. Effects of human mesenchymal stem cells on the differentiation of dendritic cells from CD34+ cells. Stem Cells Dev. 2007;16: 719-731. DOI: 10.1089/scd.2007.0065

[67] Scalavino V, Liso M, Serino G. Role of microRNAs in the Regulation of Dendritic Cell Generation and Function. Int J Mol Sci. 2020;21:1319. DOI: 10.3390/ijms21041319

[68] Killeen PR. Markov model of smoking cessation. Proc Natl Acad Sci U S A. 2011 Sep;108 Suppl 3:15549-15556. DOI: 10.1073/pnas.1011277108

[69] Yagi H, Soto-Gutierrez A, Parekkadan B, Kitagawa Y, Tompkins RG, Kobayashi N, Yarmush ML. Mesenchymal stem cells: Mechanisms of immunomodulation and homing. Cell Transplant. 2010;19: 667-679. DOI: 10.3727/096368910X508762

[70] Franquesa M, Hoogduijn MJ, Bestard O, Grinyó JM. Immunomodulatory effect of mesenchymal stem cells on B cells. Front Immunol. 2012;3:212. DOI: 10.3389/fimmu.2012.00212

[71] Haddad R, Saldanha-Araujo F. Mechanisms of T-cell immunosuppression by mesenchymal stromal cells: what do we know so far? Biomed Res Int. 2014;2014:216806. DOI: 10.1155/2014/216806

[72] Ren G, Zhang L, Zhao X, Xu G, Zhang Y, Roberts AI, Zhao RC, Shi Y. Mesenchymal stem cell-mediated immunosuppression occurs via concerted action of chemokines and nitric oxide. Cell Stem Cell. 2008;2: 141-150. DOI: 10.1016/j.stem.2007.11.014

[73] Davies LC, Heldring N, Kadri N, Le Blanc K. Mesenchymal Stromal Cell Secretion of Programmed Death-1 Ligands Regulates T Cell Mediated Immunosuppression. Stem Cells. 2017; 35:766-776. DOI: 10.1002/stem.2509

[74] Asari S, Itakura S, Ferreri K, Liu CP, Kuroda Y, Kandeel F, Mullen Y. Mesenchymal stem cells suppress B-cell terminal differentiation. Exp Hematol. 2009;37:604-615. DOI: 10.1016/j.exphem.2009.01.005

[75] Luz-Crawford P, Noël D, Fernandez X, Khoury M, Figueroa F, Carrión F, Jorgensen C, Djouad F. Mesenchymal stem cells repress Th17 molecular program through the PD-1 pathway. PLoS One. 2012;7:e45272. DOI: 10.1371/journal.pone.0045272

[76] Khatri M, Richardson LA, Meulia T. Mesenchymal stem cell-derived extracellular vesicles attenuate influenza virus-induced acute lung injury in a pig model. Stem Cell Res Ther. 2018 Jan;9: 17. DOI: 10.1186/s13287-018-0774-8

[77] Mao R, Zhang J, Jiang D, Cai D, Levy JM, Cuconati A, Block TM, Guo JT, Guo H. Indoleamine 2,3-dioxygenase mediates the antiviral effect of gamma interferon against hepatitis B virus in human hepatocyte-derived cells. J Virol. 2011;85:1048-1057. DOI: 10.1128/JVI.01998-10

[78] Adams O, Besken K, Oberdörfer C, MacKenzie CR, Takikawa O, Däubener W. Role of indoleamine-2,3-dioxygenase in alpha/beta and gamma interferon-mediated antiviral effects against herpes simplex virus infections. J Virol. 2004;78:2632-2636. DOI: 10.1128/jvi.78.5.2632-2636.2004

[79] Obojes K, Andres O, Kim KS, Däubener W, Schneider-Schaulies J.

Indoleamine 2,3-dioxygenase mediates cell type-specific anti-measles virus activity of gamma interferon. J Virol. 2005;79:7768-7776. DOI: 10.1128/JVI.79.12.7768-7776.2005

[80] Li X, Yue S, Luo Z. Mesenchymal stem cells in idiopathic pulmonary fibrosis. Oncotarget. 2017;8: 102600-102616. DOI: 10.18632/oncotarget.18126

[81] Behnke J, Kremer S, Shahzad T, Chao CM, Böttcher-Friebertshäuser E, Morty RE, Bellusci S, Ehrhardt H. MSC Based Therapies-New Perspectives for the Injured Lung. J Clin Med. 2020;9: 682. DOI: 10.3390/jcm9030682

[82] Aguilar S, Scotton CJ, McNulty K, Nye E, Stamp G, Laurent G, Bonnet D, Janes SM. Bone marrow stem cells expressing keratinocyte growth factor via an inducible lentivirus protects against bleomycin-induced pulmonary fibrosis. PLoS One. 2009;4:e8013. DOI: 10.1371/journal.pone.0008013

[83] Shyamsundar M, McAuley DF, Ingram RJ, Gibson DS, O'Kane D, McKeown ST, Edwards A, Taggart C, Elborn JS, Calfee CS, Matthay MA, O'Kane CM. Keratinocyte growth factor promotes epithelial survival and resolution in a human model of lung injury. Am J Respir Crit Care Med. 2014; 189:1520-1529. DOI: 10.1164/rccm.201310-1892OC

[84] Gazdhar A, Grad I, Tamò L, Gugger M, Feki A, Geiser T. The secretome of induced pluripotent stem cells reduces lung fibrosis in part by hepatocyte growth factor. Stem Cell Res Ther. 2014;5:123. DOI: 10.1186/scrt513

[85] Wang H, Zheng R, Chen Q, Shao J, Yu J, Hu S. Mesenchymal stem cells microvesicles stabilize endothelial barrier function partly mediated by hepatocyte growth factor (HGF). Stem Cell Res Ther. 2017;8:211. DOI: 10.1186/s13287-017-0662-7

[86] Bernard O, Jeny F, Uzunhan Y, Dondi E, Terfous R, Label R, Sutton A, Larghero J, Vanneaux V, Nunes H, Boncoeur E, Planès C, Dard N. Mesenchymal stem cells reduce hypoxia-induced apoptosis in alveolar epithelial cells by modulating HIF and ROS hypoxic signaling. Am J Physiol Lung Cell Mol Physiol. 2018;314:L360-L371. DOI: 10.1152/ajplung.00153.2017

[87] Loy H, Kuok DIT, Hui KPY, Choi MHL, Yuen W, Nicholls JM, Peiris JSM, Chan MCW. Therapeutic Implications of Human Umbilical Cord Mesenchymal Stromal Cells in Attenuating Influenza A(H5N1) Virus-Associated Acute Lung Injury. J Infect Dis. 2019;219:186-196. DOI: 10.1093/infdis/jiy478 (PMID: 30085072)

[88] Zhu YG, Feng XM, Abbott J, Fang XH, Hao Q, Monsel A, Qu JM, Matthay MA, Lee JW. Human mesenchymal stem cell microvesicles for treatment of Escherichia coli endotoxin-induced acute lung injury in mice. Stem Cells. 2014;32:116-125. DOI: 10.1002/stem.1504. (PMID: 23939814)

[89] Zhao AG, Shah K, Cromer B, Sumer H. Mesenchymal Stem Cell-Derived Extracellular Vesicles and Their Therapeutic Potential. Stem Cells Int. 2020;2020:8825771. DOI: 10.1155/2020/8825771

[90] Witwer KW, Théry C. Extracellular vesicles or exosomes? On primacy, precision, and popularity influencing a choice of nomenclature. J Extracell Vesicles. 2019;8:1648167. DOI: 10.1080/20013078.2019.1648167

[91] D'Souza-Schorey C, Clancy JW. Tumor-derived microvesicles: shedding light on novel microenvironment modulators and prospective cancer biomarkers. Genes Dev. 2012;26: 1287-1299. DOI: 10.1101/gad.192351.112

[92] Schorey JS, Bhatnagar S. Exosome function: from tumor immunology to

pathogen biology. Traffic. 2008;9: 871-881. DOI: 10.1111/j.1600-0854.2008.00734.x

[93] Harding CV, Heuser JE, Stahl PD. Exosomes: looking back three decades and into the future. J Cell Biol. 2013;200: 367-371. DOI: 10.1083/jcb.201212113

[94] Ellwanger JH, Veit TD, Chies JAB. Exosomes in HIV infection: A review and critical look. Infect Genet Evol. 2017;53:146-154. DOI: 10.1016/j.meegid.2017.05.021

[95] Huang-Doran I, Zhang CY, Vidal-Puig A. Extracellular Vesicles: Novel Mediators of Cell Communication In Metabolic Disease. Trends Endocrinol Metab. 2017;28:3-18. DOI: 10.1016/j.tem.2016.10.003

[96] Cheng L, Zhang K, Wu S, Cui M, Xu T. Focus on Mesenchymal Stem Cell-Derived Exosomes: Opportunities and Challenges in Cell-Free Therapy. Stem Cells Int. 2017;2017:6305295. DOI: 10.1155/2017/6305295

[97] Schultz IC, Bertoni APS, Wink MR. Mesenchymal Stem Cell-Derived Extracellular Vesicles Carrying miRNA as a Potential Multi Target Therapy to COVID-19: an In Silico Analysis. Stem Cell Rev Rep. 2021:1–16. DOI: 10.1007/s12015-021-10122-0

[98] Monsel A, Zhu YG, Gennai S, Hao Q, Hu S, Rouby JJ, Rosenzwajg M, Matthay MA, Lee JW. Therapeutic Effects of Human Mesenchymal Stem Cell-derived Microvesicles in Severe Pneumonia in Mice. Am J Respir Crit Care Med. 2015;192:324-336. DOI: 10.1164/rccm.201410-1765OC

[99] Abraham A, Krasnodembskaya A. Mesenchymal stem cell-derived extracellular vesicles for the treatment of acute respiratory distress syndrome. Stem Cells Transl Med. 2020;9:28-38. DOI: 10.1002/sctm.19-0205

[100] Li JW, Wei L, Han Z, Chen Z. Mesenchymal stromal cells-derived exosomes alleviate ischemia/reperfusion injury in mouse lung by transporting anti-apoptotic miR-21-5p. Eur J Pharmacol. 2019;852:68-76. DOI: 10.1016/j.ejphar.2019.01.022

[101] Liu J, Chen T, Lei P, Tang X, Huang P. Exosomes Released by Bone Marrow Mesenchymal Stem Cells Attenuate Lung Injury Induced by Intestinal Ischemia Reperfusion via the TLR4/NF-κB Pathway. Int J Med Sci. 2019;16:1238-1244. DOI: 10.7150/ijms.35369

[102] Sengupta V, Sengupta S, Lazo A, Woods P, Nolan A, Bremer N. Exosomes Derived from Bone Marrow Mesenchymal Stem Cells as Treatment for Severe COVID-19. Stem Cells Dev. 2020 Jun;29:747-754. DOI: 10.1089/scd.2020.0080

[103] Leng Z, Zhu R, Hou W, Feng Y, Yang Y, Han Q, Shan G, Meng F, Du D, Wang S, Fan J, Wang W, Deng L, Shi H, Li H, Hu Z, Zhang F, Gao J, Liu H, Li X, Zhao Y, Yin K, He X, Gao Z, Wang Y, Yang B, Jin R, Stambler I, Lim LW, Su H, Moskalev A, Cano A, Chakrabarti S, Min KJ, Ellison-Hughes G, Caruso C, Jin K, Zhao RC. Transplantation of $ACE2^{-}$ Mesenchymal Stem Cells Improves the Outcome of Patients with COVID-19 Pneumonia. Aging Dis. 2020 Mar;11: 216-228. DOI: 10.14336/AD.2020.0228

[104] Sánchez-Guijo F, García-Arranz M, López-Parra M, Monedero P, Mata-Martínez C, Santos A, Sagredo V, Álvarez-Avello JM, Guerrero JE, Pérez-Calvo C, Sánchez-Hernández MV, Del-Pozo JL, Andreu EJ, Fernández-Santos ME, Soria-Juan B, Hernández-Blasco LM, Andreu E, Sempere JM, Zapata AG, Moraleda JM, Soria B, Fernández-Avilés F, García-Olmo D, Prósper F. Adipose-derived mesenchymal stromal cells for the treatment of patients with severe SARS-CoV-2 pneumonia

requiring mechanical ventilation. A proof of concept study. EClinicalMedicine. 2020;25:100454. DOI: 10.1016/j.eclinm.2020.100454.

[105] Tang L, Jiang Y, Zhu M, Chen L, Zhou X, Zhou C, Ye P, Chen X, Wang B, Xu Z, Zhang Q, Xu X, Gao H, Wu X, Li D, Jiang W, Qu J, Xiang C, Li L. Clinical study using mesenchymal stem cells for the treatment of patients with severe COVID-19. Front Med. 2020;14: 664-673. DOI: 10.1007/s11684-020-0810-9.

[106] Shi L, Huang H, Lu X, Yan X, Jiang X, Xu R, Wang S, Zhang C, Yuan X, Xu Z, Huang L, Fu JL, Li Y, Zhang Y, Yao WQ, Liu T, Song J, Sun L, Yang F, Zhang X, Zhang B, Shi M, Meng F, Song Y, Yu Y, Wen J, Li Q, Mao Q, Maeurer M, Zumla A, Yao C, Xie WF, Wang FS. Effect of human umbilical cord-derived mesenchymal stem cells on lung damage in severe COVID-19 patients: a randomized, double-blind, placebo-controlled phase 2 trial. Signal Transduct Target Ther. 2021;6:58. DOI: 10.1038/s41392-021-00488-5

[107] Lanzoni G, Linetsky E, Correa D, Messinger Cayetano S, Alvarez RA, Kouroupis D, Alvarez Gil A, Poggioli R, Ruiz P, Marttos AC, Hirani K, Bell CA, Kusack H, Rafkin L, Baidal D, Pastewski A, Gawri K, Leñero C, Mantero AMA, Metalonis SW, Wang X, Roque L, Masters B, Kenyon NS, Ginzburg E, Xu X, Tan J, Caplan AI, Glassberg MK, Alejandro R, Ricordi C. Umbilical cord mesenchymal stem cells for COVID-19 acute respiratory distress syndrome: A double-blind, phase 1/2a, randomized controlled trial. Stem Cells Transl Med. 2021. DOI: 10.1002/sctm.20-0472

Chapter 7

Application of Ex-Vivo/3D Organoid Models in COVID-19 Research

Allen Thayakumar Basanthakumar

Abstract

COVID-19 treatment methods based on 3D organoids and ex-vivo platforms are analyzed in this chapter. Initially, the platforms available for cell culture and its working characteristics are explained. Subsequently discusses the organoids with their definition and included their uses in various applications. Further, the chapter extends to describe the uses of different organoids with their use in different stages. Most of these methods utilized the 3D ex-vivo cell culture method to develop organoids and test them over infected tissues. Based on the study in this chapter, it is found that the demonstration of active replication of the human organoids culture system of lungs is found to be more helpful for COVID-19 treatment.

Keywords: COVID-19, 3D exvivo, 3D Organoid models, invivo, cell culture

1. Introduction

COVID-19 and SARS, such treatment drugs and vaccines, remains a challenge to predicting clinical reaction. Predicting clinical response to vaccines and drugs remains a challenge in any viral treatment such as COVID-19 and SARS. COVID-19, a sort of corona disease, created a pandemic danger situation caused due to newly raised virus. Predicting novel virus biology lies majorly in vitro models, as it permits viral replication. Animal and human organoids had raised their value in the experimental virology platform. COVID-19 is a killing disease that increased the death rate of human beings higher than influenza. The number of reported cases is more or less equal to the number of deaths. Similarly, the infection mortality rate tends to increase deaths to 1%. This disease was most leniently spread from person to person through contacts or even through the respiratory system. There are different approaches taken to solve this dreadful disease which took away the lives and livelihood of millions worldwide. One such research approach is by gearing towards the direction of 3D organoids and ex-vivo platforms. 3D organoid models and ex-vivo platforms are known to recreate the disease-specific and organ-specific microenvironment in the lab. These models are well studied in cancer research [1].

Studies indicated that using 3D organoid and ex vivo models at an early stage of virus research might help them from failure. Most organoids can be established from induced pluripotent stem cells (IPSC), commonly containing 3D structure. Also, it consists of cell types for the specific organ, and multipotent adult tissue stem cells can create an organoid. To predict tissue tropism of this emerged COVID-19, various research groups ought to get the help of an organoid approach for preventing gastric tract and kidney failure. COVID-19 directly infected capillary organoids and kidney organoids. This chapter describes 3D ex-vivo organoid enabled stem cell culture for prediction, helping to combat COVID-19. Using ex vivo platforms to predict the response for vaccines is important before it reaches clinical trials. Subsequently, treatment for tumors with an inhabitation induced activation, but all tumors failed to induce an antitumour response in a subset; likewise, COVID-19 drugs fail to give antiviral activity. Thus, it is important to use precision ex vivo models [2].

While new infection disease emerged, virologists expose indicator cell lines panel. From a typical human origin or monkey origin to patient materials and find for viral replication signs. Species barriers get complicated due to this trial-and-error approach. In the indicator panel, it was also done by the potential absence of a target. Recently severe acute respiratory syndrome due to coronavirus, organoids termed research emphasizes the value of more physiological in vitro models. In Wuhan city novel coronavirus disease 2019 (COVID-19) outbreak began that quickly transmitted everywhere china and to various parts of the domain in all countries. This spread of COVID-19 resulted in an extensive pandemic. Numerous treatment methods have been established for these diseases. As stated, earlier vaccines for this disease were not yet developed. Organoids are newly generated patterns developed from human stem cells, ex vivo duplicating process drug, and viral screening process for infection models. Self-categorized tissues are commonly seen in human organoids, which contain the different structure of cells. Cells that contain the same structure of cell functions as real organs for a human being. This pattern permitted viral infection efficiency and resulted in experimentation.

Areas unmet with COVID 19 research about leveraging this organoid method tends to help us predict the effect of this disease in tissues concerning organs. It will be an efficient tool for assisting researchers in predicting disease in the lab and helping to improve in development of a drug for COVID 19. It deciphers pathways for biomarker by keeping in mind that coronavirus is the fastest spreading disease, particularly for those with a weak immune system. Studying and understanding the effect of COVID 19 with the help of this platform in this increasing population is essential for regular therapeutics improvement in this field. They are focusing on miniature organ research at the lab to study coronavirus's progress in the human body. These organoids suggested that virus versatility for organs invading gut,

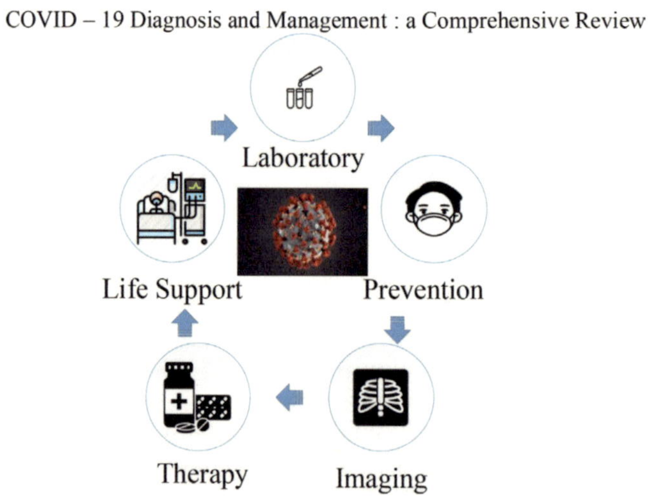

Figure 1.
COVID-19 diagnosis.

kidney, and lungs to the liver. Experiments are conducted using drugs with the help of these mini tissues for identifying the working of these therapies would be candidates for treating people. Experts understand that SARS-Cov-2 might have a side effect on organs in the human body from residing infected persons. Unfortunately, there is no proper statement about this damage directly affected by the virus to secondary complications of infection. Various groups with the help of organoid to represent in body virus, cell infects that cause damages [3, 4]. Splender of 3D ex vivo organoids recreates human microenvironment in true lab morphology of tissues. An overview of COVID-19 diagnosis and management is shown in **Figure 1**.

2. Nuts and bolts of 3D organoid and ex-vivo models

3D structures of organoids are placed from induced pluripotent stem cells, and also multipotent adult tissue stem cells are substituted. Organize themselves via spatially restricted for containing specific-organ cell types and cell sorting lineage commitment to creating cell assembly with permanent tissue architectural and functional characteristics. Typically, it consists of complement varied cell types that are present in interesting organs. Standardized organoid models since designed from cell sources that is extended from a wide amount of time. Organoids that depend on ipsc initially during cell population that permits certain extension. For generating organoids, given that ipsc permitted to form a human body and signals that takes through an execution developed to duplicate continuous improvement, brain or kidney organs are interested terms followed in vivo. Fully identified stem cells that taken straight from tissue, so the Establishment of ASC extracted organoids is complex. Smoothly design whole organoid structure several growth factors like tissues such as culturing and mouse gut in one cocktail. It involves active stem cells of relevant kinds of cells. Mainly organoids in other tissues are expanded by the proliferation of the progenitor cells and the ASCs in rich growth factors. The cell structure necessary to reduce the growth factor levels can be driven to adopt them [5].

3. Current approach on combat COVID 19

Some low-limit nations with similarly powerless wellbeing frameworks and restricted ability to balance the monetary and social expenses of populace level physical removal, incorporating a few nations with wellbeing framework delicacy and very weak populaces, presently announce inconsistent cases, bunches of cases, and network transmission. The window for control at the subnational and public level might be shut in many of these nations. Individuals living in aggregate destinations are powerless against COVID-19 to a limited extent as a result of the wellbeing hazards related to development or uprooting, stuffing, expanded climatic presentation because of the unacceptable sanctuary, and poor nourishing and wellbeing status among influenced populaces. Albeit, a few variations of site plans may not be achievable. Augmenting site getting ready for better removing among occupants and group the executives, adherence to contamination counteraction and control principles, solid danger correspondence and network commitment, and a decent observation framework to distinguish starting cases early can significantly decrease the inclination for COVID-19 to spread inside such settings. Proper case, the board can lessen mortality among those tainted with the infection. The Interim Guidance plots the essential strides to guarantee these limits are set up.

3.1 COVID-19 diagnosis

3.1.1 Saliva test

Samples of saliva often included more SARS-CoV-2 copies than swab samples, and up to 10 days after initial diagnosis, a larger fraction of Saliva samples were positive. And in 495 health care professionals' testing, two more asymptomatic cases were recognized as Swab's. The scientists concluded in their letter that these data confirm the potential for detecting SARS-CoV-2 infection are used saliva specimens. At least saliva seems comparable with nasopharyngeal swabs in regulated health care environments. However, COVID-19 is a global epidemic, with rural, disadvantaged or otherwise under deployed communities most afflicted. And such situations can affect the way saliva-based tests perform [6].

3.1.2 Polymerase chain reaction (PCR) test

PCR tests were also taken while affected by the Covid-19 virus. PCR accurately discover the occurrence of an antigen instead of bodily presence antibodies or immune responses. PCR test will find out at the initial stage of health patients has affected by virus based on recognizing the viral RNA, before antibodies generation, which will be available in the body illness signs occur. The general welfare authorities might better understand the transmission of disease, like Covid-19, among a population by using PCR testing to monitor huge bundles of Nasopharyngeal swab tests from within a populace.

3.1.3 Serologic testing

After Covid-19, how long immunity retro will be staying in the body is indeterminate. Previous numerous researches have illustrated, who survived the epidemic of SARS (Acute Rapid Air Syndrome) those peoples had antibodies in their body for long eons afterwards retrieval. In several cases, after affected diseases, immunity will be increased naturally. Still, if Covid-19 causes a comparable immunological reaction, it would be untimely to say that coronaviruses produce Covid-19 and SARS. Nowadays, specific patients again affected by covid-19. This represents that these patients did not get immunity in their body naturally, which was displayed in several kinds of research. For antibody tests, such as the PCR tests, which usually use swabs to identify Covid-19, blood samples are normally needed. There seems to be little coronavirus but substantial and quantifiable antibody presence, circulating throughout the blood linked with the respiratory tract.

3.2 Antibody treatment

A SARS-CoV-2 alteration that enables the virus to avoid detection using different COVID-19 therapies produced antibodies which are proved by much research. Modern medicines termed monoclonal antibodies are shown with immunological molecules that are naturally produced. Jesse Bloom and his team mapped all probable SARS-CoV-2 mutations at the Fred Hutchinson Cancer Research Laboratory in Seattle, Washington, that were likely to impede binding with three monoclonal antibodies. One was made by Indiana, Eli Lilly in Indianapolis, and the second was made in a cocktail prepared in Tarrytown, New York by Regeneron. The receptor-binding element is the Alterations that impair a protein fragment interacting and entering cells by the virus. The researchers detected an alteration that caused the virus to elude the identification of one of the three antibodies with Regeneron's antibodies cocktail. Not many of these changes are generally circling in tainted individuals. In every case, one is frequent in Europe and one in Denmark and Netherlands, where cases of mink and individuals working in mink ranching have been reported in SARS-CoV-2. The discoveries have not yet been peer-inspected.

3.3 Antiviral drugs

Fluvoxamine, Umifenovir, camostat, ritonavir, Famotidine, Nafamostat, Lopinavir, hydroxychloroquine and chloroquine are drugs that are testing for medication of COVID-19. The treatment for SARS-CoV-1 and the Covid, which induce respiratory disorders for the Middle East, was successfully proved in vitro tests. However, there was no testing that confirmed that equal SARS-CoV-2 activity component. Nafamostat and camostat are antagonists of serine proteases. Camostat was already reported to prevent SARS-CoV entrance by acting as a researcher and serine protease inhibitor TMPRSS2 suggest together camostat, and nafamostat may inhibit SARS-CoV-2. Russia and China have licensed for use only as Umifenovir, and this is a tiny prophylactic indole derivative compound for influenza A and B viruses. Thiazolidine is Nitazzoxanide used in parasitic, bacterial and viral contamination as a viable enemy of an infectious disease. Several bio-informatics approaches can be used in detecting the sequence of the virus [7]. Scientists are also working to counteract potential "cytokine storms" in some patients that cause lung harm and severe respiratory discomfort. As stated early, for covid-19, there is no vaccines or drugs for the treatment. Hence some methods may predict this disease and take treatments to reduce its severeness and stop spreading to other persons. Some of them are discussed below.

3.4 COVID-19 interferons

Interferons are anti-inflammatory proteins and natural broad-spectrum antiviral that induce signaling pathway followed by transformation of IFN-stimulated genes and bind to their receptors on the surface of various cells [8]. It includes an antiviral enzyme and also pro-inflammatory components. These are a group of cytokines and are primarily developed from infected cells and immune cells. These activated immune cells perform the killing of infected cells and also deactivate movement of the virus in the human body. This method is helpful during the early prediction of diseases, and hence treatment can happen with ease. While implementing interferon at the early-stage amount of infections in the beginning stage prompts decreases, disease duration is short. However, as mentioned earlier, there are no vaccines for Covid-19. Hence prevention is the only way to safeguard. Covering mouth during cough, wearing mask, washing hands rapidly, and a safe distance from each other might help. However, this method helps an average person with a better immune system and does not favor elderly persons and infants.

4. Combat COVID-19 using emerging organoids and ex vivo platforms

A human ex-vivo model affirmed the significance of NK cells in medication prompted demise under pressure in formerly led tests [9]. These discoveries focussed on an intermingling between drug-initiated obstruction and tumor-resistant contexture. Be that as it may, sympathetic to the science behindhand this viral reproduction, infection system medication disclosure endeavors are restricted because of the absence of an appropriate test model. Previously, single-cell RNA sequencing data of human organoids to explore explanations of ACE2 and

TMPRSS2, despite an assortment of RNA receptors to investigate their capacity in SARS-CoV-2 pathogenesis, were used. ACE2 is abundant in all organoids, besides the prostate and brain, and TMPRSS2 is omnipresent [1]. Natural, secure pathways in all organoids with the exception of the lungs are expanded in ACE 2(+) cells. Inquisitively, ACE2 (+) of the digestive tract, lung and retinal organoids have an extending low-thickness lipoprotein receptor with a more prominent joint in lung organoids. This investigation uncovers that organoids could be utilized for the review of this new pollution component and for the improvement of medications as a logical stage. General organoid application is shown in **Figure 2**.

4.1 3D organoids and virology

For acute gastroenteritis, human norovirus is the main cause. The primary drawback for the development of efficient therapy for norovirus is the absence of a powerful in vitro contamination model. Co-workers of Estes find the transfer of virus to gut enterocytes and its cell type is unavailable from cell lines intestine. Rather it was found in organoids. In ASC inferred enterocytes, little intestinal societies allowed development with different human norovirus strains. It ended up being an extra mind boggling factor. Mechanism of pathogenesis find organoids, where ipsc based organoids techniques are unique, and also it permits key aspect modeling for human brain development. While it happened during the Zika virus epidemic, it notably had an association between severe abnormalities and ZIKV infections. It does not affect the brain, and sequential studies used human cerebral organoids handled over causation proof. Replication of ZIKV in brain development and preferably affects and killed neural precursors.

It caused obstacles to microcephaly4 and cortical extension4. Similarly, organoids may be employed to reveal explicit species powerlessness differences. Pig H1N1 and Avian H7N2 flu infections mostly contaminate winged animals and pigs, separately, yet purported 'reassortant' flu infections. H1N1 virus (H1N1pdm) spread out speedily through human populaces. In the last periods, robust in vitro models are not available. The uses of ex vivo bronchus manipulating organizations to evaluate the seasonal infection of humans. The specimens of excision established

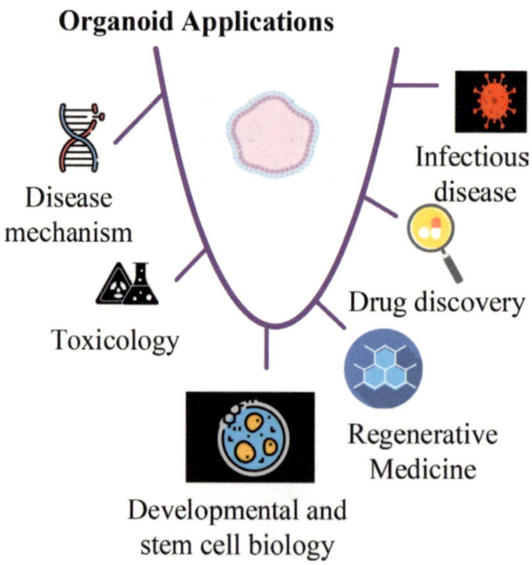

Figure 2.
Applications of organoids.

by these transitory bronchus explant cultures. Hui et al. [10] the expected replication capacity, tropism in the tissue and the generation of cytokines inducing bronchi- and human-aviation pathways organoids from human and avian strains of flu. These tests provide appropriate findings by using organoids and explants. Considering organoids may be enlarged over the eons and removed from airways and frozen, organoids were considered to be beneficial for assessing the pandemic risk of animal flu infections. This end was confirmed by an equal report. Zhou et al. [11] human aviation ways organoids generate wide tug cultures, here it involves a few considerable aviation ways epithelial cells categories such as club cells, basal cells, ciliated cells and flagon cells. Two sets of infections with a clearly identified infectiveness in individuals were provided to these organoids. The coordinated contagions that ineffectually infectious in peoples by imitated two infections of people were further comprehensive.

4.2 Organoid types

4.2.1 Gut organoids

Multiple organs are joined to generate the spinal tract, which arises from a rudimentary general tube that is elaborated between the mouth and the anus. The gut tube [10] has endodermal layer pillage, which has a three-region subdivision. Hindgut, midgut and Foreskin, where each location in the development of the embryonal layer produces certain organs throughout specific intervals. The Pancreas, stomach, liver, esophagus, Pharynx and part of the duodenum have also been raised by foregust. This portion is generated as 3D organoids from a mouse that depicts intestinal SC, which arise in a rich lamina madrigal from the structures of crypt-villus and all the primary cell types of the gut [12]. The biomedical platform uses Intestinal organoid technology for forskolin-induced human organoid, which permits the cellular structure of drug investigation. By isolating the colon, organoids grow superficially into a single-layer epithelium with notions of auto surgery that have injured the mouse colon [13, 14].

4.2.2 Organoids of liver

The liver comes from the extension of the foregut ventral wall that has been conceived to the structure of the liver bud. Hypoblasts described as hepatic endoderm cells formed from this bud, and both sinusoidal endothelial cells provide an estimate of the surrounding environment and mesenchyme. Hepatic vasculature is developed in conjunction with the development of liver bud, which forms a vasculogenesis and angiogenesis combination. It turns into a primary hematopoietic foetal organ. Therefore, the liver is designed based on the sensitive orchestration of signals between mesenchymal, endothelial and endodermal signals before the perfusion of the blood. 3D liver organoids designed for the treatment of liver failure are produced and assisted. The development of 3D organoids contributes to the development of epithelial liver bodies [15–17].

4.2.3 Organoids of kidney

Mesodermal origins are mostly in the metanephric kidney and generate the back of the trunk. The organogenesis starts with the defined intermediate mesoderm of the kidney precursor tissue, leading to mesonephric and epithelial mesenchyme and monitoring the rostral-caudal direction. Uteric bud is a new epithelial protrusion in the development of a branched collecting tube structure that invades and interacts with the neighboring MM. In the same way, mature nephrons and other MM derivatives cause MM differentiation, epithelization and condensation through progressive MM. The signals and branches are regulated. It is obvious before the other organs that the kidney tissue can be self-organized from previous research with reaggregation.

4.2.4 Organoids of brain

The neural ectoderm formed a neural plate system, which generates a flat lamina of ectodermal cells positioned in close contact with the embryo and gradually builds a cylindrical epithelial structure called a neural tube [11]. The stringent spatial–temporal gradient of morphogens allows for the epithelial tube to be separated into four prosencephalons, mesencephalon and rhombencephalon areas with rostral-caudal axes and ventral-dorsal axes. Here prosencephalon emerges from secondary vesicles and creates the diencephalon and telencephalon. Neural stem cells that are followed by organoids generate glia and CNS neurons. Rostro caudally resides in the neural tube, and symmetrical simulation also asymmetrical simulations are continually initialized. NSC also provides more segmented cell structures to self-renewing progenitors, which include interim progenitors and neurons. Mostly distinct cells move outside the NSC domain, creating multi-layered structures such as the cerebral cortex, optic tectum and the medulla [18–20].

4.2.5 Organoids of retina

The retina is a light open area of the eye and digests from neural ectoderm, and retinal primordia emerge from the diencephalon that evaginates along the side. This produces pseudo-stratified neuro-epithelia, called optical vesicles, which turns into a sensory neural retina in its distant section. Proximal segment offers to begin to cash layered tissue and melanin delivered retinal shade epithelium, and OVs go through invagination at their distal part that frames an optic cup with RPE and NR as its external and internal dividers as for one another. NR comprises PC that is isolated from ganglion cell design, cones and bars alongside strong cell types. This vertebrate retina is created as 3D organoids and utilized as a most remarkable reaggregation model in tissue designing for examining the neural layer at its fundamental. This examination was led in chick embryos and archived that supplanted retina performed with a surprising limit with respect to reassembling them as different round types with the entire plan [21–23].

Since COVID-19 has an extremely rapidly distributed worldwide channel for infection, it is still not favorable for pathogenic mechanisms. A disease model is essential for the study of the pathological characteristics of virus infection or drug prediction. In viral infection research, 2D models are most frequently utilized. However, in an ex vivo context, it was unable to imitate and search reliability was limited. The large distance between human beings and primates is a disadvantage for these species. Broncho-alveolar resections using lavage material are extracted from airway organoids. The procedure was helpful and can be modified for drug screening for beyond 1 year. The system includes mesenchymal cells, human-derived and endothelial. In the human liver environment, it was highly stimulated. For a consistent structure, intercellular interactions such as tight connections are needed. Additional organoids are notified that not only microvilli, bile capillaries and lipid droplets in hepatic cells are dedicated to more human organoids in LO. It is substantially more distinct from LO than in cells like the liver generated by human beings [24].

A precondition for suspect ability due to viral infection without considering as in vivo or in vitro. A prerequisite for questionable ability to develop in vivo or in vitro due to viral infection. Human pluripotent stem cell reveals lung markers, extracted from 3D LBO's ***EPCAM, KRT8, NKX2.1, FOXA1, FOXJ1, CC10, mucins, and P63***.

These LBOs showed growing, detachment and wretchedness tantamount to human lungs when the respiratory syncytial infection is contaminated. Contrasted with essential human hepatocytes, $Na+$ −taurocholate co-shipping polypeptide, an HBV section receptor, was higher in human iPSC-LOs, which showed high helplessness to HBV contamination. Factors also increase the efficiency of infection, such as ***GPC5, PPARA, and CEBPA,*** which were higher in human iPSC-Los. ***HBV, pgRNA, intercellularvDNA, cccDNA, and supernatantvDNA*** are the infection in human iPSC-LOs. It is present at a higher level than human iPSC-like cells [25].

During previous periods the improvement of organoids has shown as a revolution. Lung organoids, the invention of human intestinal organoids and human organs, are assent with the help of adult stem cell (ASC). The ASC also proved by the above-indicated organs. Once the separated intestinal organoids are produced, the multi-cellular structure and efficient complication of human intestine epithet are precisely mimicked for more than a year. The human gastrointestinal system is the widely used path of microbial attack. In vitro models for the study of intestinal illnesses have been shown to be popular in humans. In past studies, many studies were done to show an ASC culture of an intestine organoid epithelial bat. The possible source of SARS-CoV-2 is empirically linked to suggested bat organoids [26, 27]. The likelihood of enteric disease is investigated using SARS-CoV-2 in human intestinal organoids. The use of Crypts separated from the intestines in R Sinicus bats has been explored in SARS-CoV-2 and SARSr-breakout CoV's in fecal horseshoe bat species to evaluate high distinguishing features of SARS-CoV and SARSr-CoVs. It developed bat small bowel organoids (enteroids), which use the methodology to make human bowel organoids. In the environment expanding and in a ratio of 1:2 every seven days, the indistinguishable bat entereroids are grown. In order to facilitate separation, the expansion medium was converted into a differentiation media during which enteroids are incubated for 4 days. The developed enteroids in bat replicate the multicellular structure of the native bat's small intestinal epithelium. Employing electrical transmission microscopy, cells with typical characteristics of four important bat-enteroid intestinal cell kinds such as, enteroendocrine (EE) cells, paneth (P) cells, goblet (G), and including enterocytes (E) were found. Although one line of bat entereroids has been spread sequent for 12 weeks, the other lines, unlike human intestine organoids, stopped active production for at least 1 year following the passage for 4 or 5 weeks. It recognized the first bat intestinal organoid to imitate the bat intestinal epithelium cellular makeup [28].

4.3 Culturing of organic airways and isolation of human lung cells

The non-tumor lung tissue generated from patients in resection with pulmonary fluids was extracted from human lung stems. Human spherical organoids of 50 to 200 μm have been produced from pulmonary stem cells and lung parenchymatic cells. Rganoid and ex-vivo cultures belonged to the same 3 donors aged between 55 and 69 years. Every single donor was produced from a single line. Scalpel lung tissue with a laundry of 10 ml of DMEM, 10 mm HEPES and 1% of Glutamax media and F12 media penicillin–streptomycin solution. The ling tissue type 2 mg/mL ling tissue has been digested for one hour at 37°C on a shaking platform (St. Louis, MO, USA, Sigma-Aldrich).

The residual tissue parts and the Filter suspension were repeatedly sheared with Glutamax, 10 mM HEPES, and 1% penicillin streptomycin solution using a 100 μm filter with 10 mL complete DMEM and F12 media. The filtrate was then collected in a 50 mL bottle with 2% foetal serum bovine. Then the remaining volume is centrifuged for 5 minutes at 4°C at 600rcf. Lysis buffer Red blood cells lysed at room temperature for 5 min (Roche, Basel, Switzerland). Cut the whole DMEM/F12 media into a 10 mL cell pellet and centrifugate the pellet at 600rcf for 5 min. Matrigel will obtain human airway organoids during 14 days using cultivated. The Cultrex growth factor of cellular membrane type 2 matrix Culturex cell membrane (Gaithersburg, Trevigen, MD, United States) is reduced by the 40 μL droplet from cell membranic membrane extract cell suspension at 35°C for 15–30 min to solidify pre-heated 24-well suspension platforms with a 10 mg/mL lung cell. Each well was filled with 500 μL of organoid media and incubators with 5 percent CO2 at 37°C. The new organoid medium has taken on mechanical cutting with a 1000uL pipette and flamed Pasteur pipettes every four days. Every two weeks, the organoids were transported. The entire DMEM/F12 medium was added 10 mL, and organoids were centrifuged for 5 min at 450 rcf. The fragments are seeded in 1:1–1:6 proportions, and the fragmented organic fragmentation is replaced in a cold matrigel [29–31].

Human airway organoids are ready for infection at 37°C after 14 days at 5 percent CO2. Organoid matrigel with organoids comprising a number of organoids of the growth agent. Reactive substances and concentration for each growth factor. While less common than respiratory symptoms, gastrointestinal disorders have occurred in a considerable proportion of people with COVID-19. For a group of 73 COVID-19 patients, 53% had SARS-CoV-2 RNA in stool, with stool remaining positive even if breathing trials were negative with RNA viruses in 23% of patients. Viral NP-positive cells have been found in the gastrointestinal epithelial cells of these biopsy patients' tissues. Persistent fecal disposal was especially prominent in pediatric patients. Taken together, these clinical findings show that COVID-19 patients may get enteric infections. This shows, however, that a new pathway for the virus can be the human digestive system [32, 33].

5. Advantages and disadvantages of ex vivo and 3D platforms

Does not need animal care after operation in an ex-vivo instrument is valuable, permits more duplicability between lesions and gives the regeneration experiment a rigorously regulated artificial air [26]. Ex vivo models of the spinal cord include cultivation for up to three weeks of several hundred micron-sized crosspieces. Ex vivo methods specifically secluded perfused lung enjoys a benefit of generally controlled dosing complex multicellular reaction physiological openness productive utilization of material. It additionally shows certain restrictions. For example, it was, in fact, requesting, and it has a short perception time. Another method, to be specific accuracy cut lung cut, enjoys the benefit of controlled cell portion, complex multicellular reaction, and effective utilization of material. It additionally has certain weaknesses of non-physiological openness and short perception time. Impediments of ex vivo treatment incorporate incidental unite mass of numerous cell types like fibroblasts and astrocytes. One more prevalent constraint of ex vivo is that hereditary change is proper for secret modules that can digest cellularly information and does not help for remedial modules that assisted with entering objective cells. It is comparably huge not to make sham longings, and moreover to address two indispensable issues that swarm the majority of the current organoid systems: a shortfall of reproducibility and, coupled to this, our shortfall of cognizance of the cycles that deal with their development.

6. Future perspective of 3D culture, organoid models in COVID research

In its earliest phases, the creation of 3D organoid products from human PSCs has now advanced rapidly. Soon human organoids can be produced for organisms already developed in the mouse or when re-aggregation investigations have already demonstrated a source of self-orientation. The skin, mammary gland, muscle and bone are part of it [27]. Organ expansion models since organoids show a model approach that is plainly available and allow them to open up doors to increasingly complicated or unachievable issues that have been resolved through conventional approaches. This applies in particular to biological concepts specific to people. For particular, the particular class approach of human neural stem cells has already been studied with human brain organoids. Retinal organoids have also been used for testing changes between morphogenesis and timing of human and rodent tissue. In addition, GI tract organoids can also be employed to investigate the organized promotion of GI bodies, a method that shows crucial human change combined with animal laboratory. Organoids are also promising to model homosexuality for adults. The relevance of the crypt niche in stem-cell self-renovation and differentiation was previously studied by intestinal organoids. This applies primarily to organoids from adult progenitors such as the liver and stomach, which closely recreate regeneration processes seen in the adult organ. Although if numerous options of organoids are clear, it is important to remember their existing limitations. In the recapitulation of in vivo development, all organoid approaches that have been shown so far remain meticulously defined. For example, whereas retinal organoids finely show classical laminar composition, external parts do not shape; photoreceptors, for example, are short of being entirely developed to become light sensitive.

Consequently, brain organoids [34] recapitulate fast brain growth outcomes, but future features, for example, in cortical platelets, are not fully formed. The development issue appears to be a common impediment to organoid technologies and whether this will limit their research and therapeutic opportunities greatly is still to be explored. In the end, the lack of vascularization is usually an in vitro problem for organoids. Organoids have limited growth capacity, which may also impact their development because of nutrition supply restrictions. A whole subject of tissue engineering that has been tackled by the various techniques of vascularization. Spinners can provide healthier nutritional swaps with a size of up to a few millimeters in this example of organoids. Instead, endothelial cell co-culture can create systems like vascular systems. However, the transplantation of these tissues is possibly the most hopeful problem-solve, as was done with liver buds and kidney organoids that fosters hosts invasion [35, 36].

Organoids have significant potential as a way of drug testing and therapy for development and disease modeling. Potential initiatives will certainly get them closer to this prospect.

7. Conclusion/summary

In this chapter, a discussion about COVID-19 treatment methods based on 3D techniques was briefly analyzed. In the first section, platforms that are available for cell culture and its working characteristics were discussed. Later, it continuously discussed organoids, their definition, and their uses in different applications.

Further, its use as different organs is described with its use in different stages. Prediction, as well as treating COVID-19, was found to be crucial and also, research plays a major role to put forth hybridizing of any two methods for accurate curing of COVID-19 from a human body. This method utilized 3D exvivo cell culture method to develop organoids and replace them over infected tissues. 3D disease models are previously available invitro and invivo technologies. However, they showed certain limitations and hence, treating viral infection using any stem cell culture and 3D technologies are quite helpful. Summarizing this chapter is based on the demonstration of active replication of human organoids culture system of lungs are found to be more helpful in the treatment of COVID-19. An organoid culture system is previously proposed and then used in a variety of applications. Rather it implemented 3D technologies for the development of cell culture and then replaced defective cells for an effective cure of viral infection.

Author details

Allen Thayakumar Basanthakumar
Dana Farber Cancer Institute, Boston, MA, USA

*Address all correspondence to: allenthayakumar@gmail.com

'Biotechnology to Combat COVID-19' is a collaborative project with Biotechnology Kiosk

References

[1] Xinaris C, Brizi V, Remuzzi G. Organoid models and applications in biomedical research. Nephron. 2015.130:191-199.

[2] Munisha S, Siva K.N, Jayanta M, Douglas B, David G, Basavaraja S, Moriah P, Chinmayee D, Tanmoy S, Sachin K, Nithya R, Elliot O.E, Joshua L.S, Andrew B, Allen T, Mamunur R, Kazuya A, Mohammad K, Shiladitya S, Aaron G. Nano-Engineered Disruption of Heat shock protein 90 (Hsp90) Targets Drug-Induced Resistance and Relieves Natural Killer Cell Suppression in Breast Cancer. Cancer Research. 2020; 80: 5355-5466. DOI: 10.1158/0008-5472.CAN-19-4036.

[3] Boj S.F, Hwang C.I, Baker L.A, Chio I.I.C, Engle D.D, Corbo V, Jager M, Ponz-Sarvise M, Tiriac H, Spector M.S, Gracanin A. Organoid models of human and mouse ductal pancreatic cancer. Cell. 2015. 160:324-338.

[4] Gao D, Vela I, Sboner A, Iaquinta P.J, Karthaus W.R, Gopalan A, Dowling C, Wanjala J.N, Undvall E.A, Arora V.K, Wongvipat J. Organoid cultures derived from patients with advanced prostate cancer. Cell. 2014. 159:176-187.

[5] Dutta D, Heo I, Clevers H. Disease modeling in stem cell-derived 3D organoid systems. Trends in molecular medicine. 2017. 23:393-410.

[6] Wiersinga W.J, Rhodes A, Cheng A.C, Peacock S.J, Prescott H.C. Pathophysiology, transmission, diagnosis, and treatment of coronavirus disease 2019 (COVID-19): a review. Jama. 2020. 324:782-793.

[7] Starlin T, Prabha P.S, Thayakumar B.K.A, Gopalakrishnan V.K. Screening and GC-MS profiling of ethanolic extract of Tylophora pauciflora. Bioinformation. 2019. 15: 425- 429.

[8] Hui K.P, Cheung M.C, Perera R.A, Ng K.C, Bui C.H, Ho J.C, Ng M.M, Kuok D.I, Shih K.C, Tsao S.W, Poon L.L. Tropism, replication competence, and innate immune responses of the coronavirus SARS-CoV-2 in human respiratory tract and conjunctiva: an analysis in ex-vivo and in-vitro cultures. The Lancet Respiratory Medicine. 2020. 8: 687-695.

[9] Zhou H, Liu L.P, Fang M, Li Y.M, Zheng Y.W. A potential ex vivo infection model of human induced pluripotent stem cell-3D organoids beyond coronavirus disease 2019. Histology and Histopathology. 2020. 2020: 18223-18223.

[10] Andreatta F, Beccaceci G, Fortuna N, Celotti M, De Felice D, Lorenzoni M, Foletto V, Genovesi S, Rubert J. Alaimo A. The Organoid Era Permits the Development of New Applications to Study Glioblastoma. Cancers. 2020. 12:3303-3319.

[11] Broutier L, Mastrogiovanni G, Verstegen M.M, Francies H.E, Gavarró L.M, Bradshaw C.R, Allen G.E, Arnes-Benito R, Sidorova O, Gaspersz M.P. Georgakopoulos N. Human primary liver cancer–derived organoid cultures for disease modeling and drug screening. Nature medicine. 2017. 23:1424-1435.

[12] Zhou J, Li C, Liu X, Chiu M.C, Zhao X, Wang D, Wei Y, Lee A, Zhang A.J, Chu, H, Cai J.P. Infection of bat and human intestinal organoids by SARS-CoV-2. Nature medicine. 2020. 26:1077-1083.

[13] Krüger J, Groß R, Conzelmann, C, Müller J.A, Koepke L, Sparrer K.M, Weil T, Schütz D, Seufferlein T, Barth T.F, Stenger S. Drug inhibition of SARS-CoV-2 replication in human pluripotent stem cell-derived intestinal organoids. Cellular and Molecular

Gastroenterology and Hepatology. 2020. DOI: 10.1016/j.jcmgh.2020.11.003.

[14] Ji D.B, Wu, A.W. Organoid in colorectal cancer: progress and challenges. Chinese medical journal. 2020.133:1971-1977.

[15] Broutier L, Mastrogiovanni G, Verstegen M.M, Francies H.E, Gavarró L.M, Bradshaw C.R, Allen G.E, Arnes-Benito R, Sidorova O, Gaspersz M.P, Georgakopoulos N. Human primary liver cancer–derived organoid cultures for disease modeling and drug screening. Nature medicine. 2017. 23: 1424-1435.

[16] Broutier L, Andersson-Rolf A, Hindley C.J, Boj S.F, Clevers H, Koo B.K, Huch M. Culture and establishment of self-renewing human and mouse adult liver and pancreas 3D organoids and their genetic manipulation. Nature protocols. 2016. 11:1724-1766.

[17] Hu H, Gehart H, Artegiani B, LÖpez-Iglesias C, Dekkers F, Basak O, van Es J, de Sousa Lopes S.M.C, Begthel H, Korving J, van den Born M. Long-term expansion of functional mouse and human hepatocytes as 3D organoids. Cell. 2018. 175: 1591-1606.

[18] Zhang B.Z, Chu H, Han S, Shuai H, Deng J, Hu Y.F, Gong H.R, Lee A.C.Y, Zou Z, Yau T, Wu W. SARS-CoV-2 infects human neural progenitor cells and brain organoids. Cell research. 2020. 30:928-931.

[19] Jo J, Xiao Y, Sun A.X, Cukuroglu E, Tran H.D, Göke J, Tan Z.Y, Saw T.Y, Tan C.P, Lokman H, Lee Y. Midbrain-like organoids from human pluripotent stem cells contain functional dopaminergic and neuromelanin-producing neurons. Cell stem cell. 2016. 19:248-257.

[20] Yi S.A, Nam K.H, Yun J, Gim D, Joe D, Kim Y.H, Kim H.J, Han J.W, Lee J. Infection of brain organoids and 2D cortical neurons with SARS-CoV-2 pseudovirus. Viruses. 2020. 12:1004.-1015

[21] Tang H, Abouleila Y, Si L, Ortega-Prieto A.M, Mummery C.L, Ingber D.E, Mashaghi A. Human organs-on-chips for virology. Trends in Microbiology. 2020. 28: 934-946.

[22] Hui K.P, Cheung M.C, Perera R.A, Ng K.C, Bui C.H, Ho J.C, Ng M.M, Kuok D.I, Shih K.C, Tsao S.W, Poon L.L. Tropism, replication competence, and innate immune responses of the coronavirus SARS-CoV-2 in human respiratory tract and conjunctiva: an analysis in ex-vivo and in-vitro cultures. The Lancet Respiratory Medicine. 2020. 8:687-695.

[23] Majumder B, Baraneedharan U, Thiyagarajan S, Radhakrishnan P, Narasimhan H, Dhandapani M, Brijwani N, Pinto D.D, Prasath A, Shanthappa B.U, Thayakumar A. Predicting clinical response to anticancer drugs using an ex vivo platform that captures tumour heterogeneity. Nature communications. 2015. 6:1-14.

[24] Radhakrishnan P, Baraneedharan U, Veluchamy S, Dhandapani M, Pinto D.D, Thiyagarajan S, Thayakumar A, Prasath A, Kamal A, Velu A, Jain M. Inhibition of rapamycin-induced AKT activation elicits differential antitumor response in head and neck cancers. Cancer research. 2013.73:1118-1127.

[25] Lancaster M.A, Knoblich J.A. Organogenesis in a dish: modeling development and disease using organoid technologies. Science. 2014.345:1-25.

[26] Ji D.B, Wu A.W. Organoid in colorectal cancer: progress and challenges. Chinese medical journal. 2020.133:1971-1977.

[27] Le T.T, Andreadakis Z, Kumar A, Roman R.G, Tollefsen S, Saville M, Mayhew S. The COVID-19 vaccine development landscape. Nat Rev Drug Discov. 2020.19:305-306.

[28] Corey L, Mascola J.R, Fauci A.S, Collins F.S. A strategic approach to COVID-19 vaccine R&D. Science. 2020.368:948-950.

[29] Youk J, Kim T, Evans K.V, Jeong Y.I, Hur Y, Hong S.P, Kim J.H, Yi K, Kim S.Y, Na K.J, Bleazard T. Three-dimensional human alveolar stem cell culture models reveal infection response to SARS-CoV-2. Cell Stem Cell. 2020. 27: 905-919.

[30] Mahalingam R, Dharmalingam P, Santhanam A, Kotla S, Davuluri G, Karmouty-Quintana H, Ashrith G, Thandavarayan R.A. Single-cell RNA sequencing analysis of SARS-CoV-2 entry receptors in human organoids. Journal of cellular physiology. 2020. 1-9.

[31] Han Y, Yang L, Duan X, Duan F, Nilsson-Payant B.E, Yaron T.M, Wang P, Tang X, Zhang T, Zhao Z, Bram Y. Identification of Candidate COVID-19 Therapeutics using hPSC-derived Lung Organoids. bioRxiv. 2020. DOI: 10.1101/2020.05.05.079095.

[32] Duan X, Han Y, Yang L, Nilsson B, Wang P, Zhang T, Wang X, Xu D, Xiang J.Z, Huang Y, Chen H. Identification of Drugs Blocking SARS-CoV-2 Infection using Human Pluripotent Stem Cell-derived Colonic Organoids. bioRxiv. 2020. DOI: 10.1101/2020.05.02.073320.

[33] Han Y, Yang L, Duan X, Duan F, Nilsson-Payant B.E, Yaron T.M, Wang P, Tang X, Zhang T, Zhao Z, Bram Y. Identification of Candidate COVID-19 Therapeutics using hPSC-derived Lung Organoids. bioRxiv. 2020. DOI: 10.1101/2020.05.05.079095

[34] COVID-19: Organoid go viral

[35] Corey L, Mascola J.R, Fauci A.S, Collins F.S. A strategic approach to COVID-19 vaccine R&D. Science. 2020.368:948-950.

[36] Kim J, Koo B.K, Knoblich J.A. Human organoids: model systems for human biology and medicine. Nature Reviews Molecular Cell Biology. 2020. 21: 571-584.

Section 4

Diagnostics

Chapter 8

In Vitro Diagnostics for COVID-19: State-of-the-Art, Future Directions and Role in Pandemic Response

Sandeep Kumar Vashist, Subramanian Murugan and Guiffo Djoko

Abstract

There have been tremendous advances in *in vitro* diagnostics (IVD) for coronavirus disease 2019 (COVID-19) caused by severe acute respiratory syndrome coronavirus 2 (SARS-CoV-2). Although the confirmatory clinical diagnosis is made by real-time reverse transcriptase polymerase chain reaction (RT-PCR), lateral flow immunoassay (LFIA) based viral antigen (Ag) detection is used for mass population screening at point-of-care (POC) settings. The rapid RT-PCR tests (such as from Cepheid and Bosch) have an assay duration of less than 40 min, while most rapid Ag tests (such as Abbott's BinaxNOW™ COVID-19 Ag card) have an assay duration of about 15 min. Of interest is the POC molecular test (ID NOW™) from Abbott that takes less than13 min. Similarly, many immunoassays (IAs), i.e., automated chemiluminescent IA (CLIA), manual ELISA, and LFIA, have been developed to detect immunoglobulin G (IgG), immunoglobulin M (IgM), and immunoglobulin A (IgA) produced in subjects after SARS-CoV-2 infection. Many IVD tests have been approved by the United States Food and Drug Administration (FDA) under emergency use authorization (EUA), and almost all IVD tests are Conformité Européenne (CE) certified.

Keywords: COVID-19, pandemic, in vitro diagnostics, mobile healthcare, antigen, antibodies, molecular assays, CT scans

1. Introduction

SARS-CoV-2 is a positive-sense single-stranded ribonucleic acid (RNA) virus with characteristic spikes on its surface that provide its crown-like appearance. It comprises different structural proteins, namely nucleocapsid protein (NP), spike protein (SP), membrane protein (MP), and envelope protein (EP), which play an important role in the manifestation of SARS-CoV-2 infection (**Figure 1**). The World Health Organisation (WHO), on February 11, 2020, coined the term COVID-19 for the lung disease that SARS-CoV-2 causes. The WHO declared COVID-19 as a public health emergency of international concern (PHEIC) and a pandemic on January 30, 2020, and March 11, 2020, respectively. The pandemic's epicenter shifted from

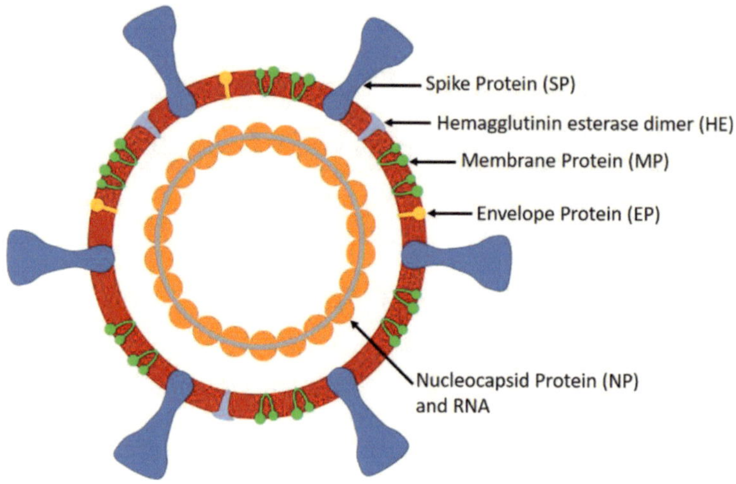

Figure 1.
Schematic of the SARS-CoV-2. Reproduced with permission from MDPI [1].

China to Europe and then to the United States of America (USA) and many countries during 2020.

SARS-CoV-2, discovered in the Hubei province of Wuhan city in China in December 2019, has spread to 219 countries and territories. The confirmed COVID-19 cases exceed 129 million [2], while global deaths exceed 2.82 million. USA accounts for the most COVID-19 cases, i.e., over 31 million, representing about 24% of global COVID-19 cases. With 12.6 and 12.2 million cases, Brazil and India have the subsequent highest incidence of COVID-19. Some nations, such as Singapore, New Zealand, and China, have effectively controlled the COVID-19 incidence by acting proactively and taking the desired measures at the right time.

The origin of SARS-CoV-2 is still unclear and contradictory, but the early reports mention its transmission to humans at the Wuhan's live animals market in December 2019 [3]. Some researchers claim its origin in bats, although the intermediate hosts are still not identified [4]. The genomic sequence of SARS-CoV-2 has ~82% homology with human SARS-CoV and ~ 89% homology with bat SARS-like CoVZXC21 [5]. The most vulnerable groups at higher risk of developing severe COVID-19 are persons over 65 years of age; persons with chronic diseases, such as diabetes mellitus, hypertension, cardiovascular diseases, lung disease; and decreased immunity. The intensive large-scale testing of the population to identify and quarantine COVID-19 infected persons is essential to avoid the spread of infection. Rapid LFIAs have played a phenomenal role here, and many of such tests have also been approved for self-use [6]. The use of face masks and social distancing measures has played a significant role in preventing COVID-19 infection [7–9]. There has been considerable improvement in the RT-PCR tests, which are the accepted gold standard for confirmatory COVID-19 clinical diagnosis. However, several deficiencies have also been reported where they were unable to detect COVID-19 during the early stages of infection and provided false negatives results to subjects [10, 11]. The false negative results could be due to the improper extraction of nucleic acid from clinical materials or insufficient cellular material for detection. The chest computerized tomography (CT) scan has further helped physicians detect COVID-19 infection in such RT-PCR false-negative subjects [12, 13]. The last year has also seen the emergence of many mutations in SARS-CoV-2 [14–17], which can only be diagnosed by next-generation sequencing (NGS). There are continuous efforts to develop POC biosensor devices for rapid diagnosis of COVID-19. Further, many IVD companies and researchers are working on new IVD approaches, such as detecting specific biomarkers that will enable the detection of COVID-19 infection at a very early stage. There is a need for continuous improvement in IVD assays to ensure reliable detection of SARS-CoV-2 infection without being impacted by the SP mutations.

2. Structure of SARS-CoV-2

SARS-CoV-2 has a characteristic crown-like appearance due to the spikes formed by a major glycoprotein (Mol. Wt. ~180 kDa), i.e., SP, which has two subunits, S1 and S2 [1] (**Figure 1**). S1 has the receptor binding domain (RBD) that recognizes and binds to angiotensin converting enzyme 2 receptor (ACE2) in the lower respiratory tract of SARS-CoV-2 infected subjects [18]. In contrast, S2 has other basic elements needed for membrane fusion. The amino-terminal region of S1 subunit is the most variable immunogenic antigen. SP is the most widely studied viral protein as it is responsible for the SARS-CoV-2 infection. It is the target of all SARS-CoV-2 neutralizing antibodies and COVID-19 vaccines. On the contrary, NP (Mol. Wt. ~40 kDa) is another viral structural protein, which is the most abundant viral phosphoprotein produced and shed during the first two weeks of SARS-CoV-2 infection, with peak shedding around 10 days after infection. It exhibits high immunogenicity and can be detected in either nasal/nasopharyngeal swabs, saliva, stool, serum or urine samples [19]. The sandwich ELISA is used for the detection of NP as it is a large protein with multiple epitopes. The other structural proteins of SARS-CoV-2 are the MP and EP. MP is the most abundant protein on SARS-CoV-2, while EP is the smallest structural protein of SARS-CoV-2 that plays a role in viral assembly, release of virions, and pathogenesis [1].

3. *In vitro* diagnostics for COVID-19

Various IVD assays have been developed for the detection of SARS-CoV-2 viral RNA, antibodies, and antigens, which encompass assays performed in certified COVID-19 diagnostic laboratories and rapid tests employed at POC settings. The various IVD assays, together with their characteristic features and bioanalytical performances, are specified in this section. Almost all the IVD assays for COVID-19 are CE IVD certified, while several are also approved by the FDA under the EUA. As shown in **Figure 2**, the RT-PCR is positive for about 3 weeks after the onset of symptoms in COVID-19 patients, while the rapid tests for viral antigen work best during the first week after the onset of symptoms [20]. On the contrary, the serology tests for detecting antibodies work best after seroconversion at the end of 3rd-week post onset of symptoms, when the COVID-19 patients enter convalescence [20, 21].

3.1 Molecular diagnostics

RT-PCR is the gold standard for the confirmatory clinical diagnosis of COVID-19 and the most used IVD assay globally. The first real-time RT-PCR assay, highly specific for SARS-CoV-2 RNA and no cross-reactivity to other coronaviruses, was developed by Tib-Molbiol, Germany, in January 2020 [22]. The assay involved the detection of SARS-CoV-2 RNA by employing envelope (E) and RNA-dependent RNA polymerase (RdRp) gene assays, where E-gene assay enabled the first-line screening and RdRp gene assay did the confirmatory

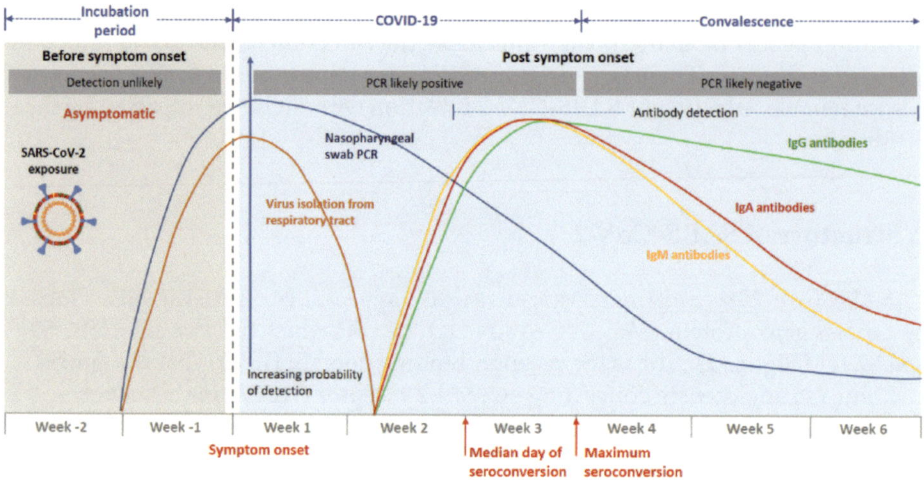

Figure 2.
An overview of the COVID-19 biomarkers' longitudinal response and the utility of various IVD tests at different stages of COVID-19.

testing. An alternative format, one-step RT-PCR assay, was developed to detect ORF1b and N regions of SARS-CoV-2 in less than 1.5 h [23]. It employed the N gene assay for screening and Orf1b gene assay for confirmatory analysis. But the assay could also detect SARS-CoV and other closely-related viruses as ORF1b and N regions are highly conserved among sarbecoviruses. The authors distinguished SARS-CoV-2 from SARS-CoV via sequence analysis of positive amplicons if the RT-PCR results are positive. A prospective development was the real-time RT-PCR assay to detect RdRp/helicase (H) genes of SARS-CoV-2 [24]. The assay has high sensitivity and detects COVID-19 in low viral load samples, saliva, plasma, and upper respiratory tract samples. Moreover, it showed no cross-reactivity with other human coronaviruses and respiratory viruses. Subsequently, many innovative RT-PCR assays were developed by many IVD companies and research groups.

A prominent test is the CE certified and FDA EUA approved rapid, real-time RT-PCR test, i.e., the Xpert® Xpress SARS-CoV-2 test, by Cepheid, USA [25]. The assay, requiring GeneXpert Dx or GeneXpert Infinity Systems, enables the qualitative detection of SARS-CoV-2 ribonucleic acid (RNA) in specimens collected from the upper respiratory tract [25]. These include nasopharyngeal, oropharyngeal, nasal, or mid-turbinate swab or nasal wash/aspirate specimens. The rapid RT-PCR test is run on GeneXpert Instrument Systems that have automated and fully integrated process steps, i.e., sample preparation, extraction of RNA, amplification of RNA, and detection of the target sequences. The systems employ single-use disposable cartridges, which have all the RT-PCR reagents together with a sample processing control (SPC) and a probe check control (PCC). SPC controls the sample processing and monitors the presence of potential inhibitors in the RT-PCR reaction. It ensures the presence of adequate RT-PCR reaction conditions for the amplification reaction and the proper working of RT-PCR reagents. On the other hand, PCC ensures reagent rehydration, filling of PCR tube, and the presence of all reaction components in the cartridge. It also monitors the integrity of the probe and the stability of the dye. The procedure involves the sample collection and its placement into a viral transport tube that contains 3 mL transport medium or 3 mL of saline. The specimen in the tube is mixed by rapidly inverting it 5 times, followed by transferring the sample to the sample chamber of the Xpert Xpress SARS-CoV-2 cartridge. The cartridge is then loaded onto the GeneXpert Instrument System for the automated sample processing and real-time RT-PCR. The kit comprises freeze-dried beads, lysis reagent, binding reagent, elution reagent, and disposable transfer pipettes, which are sufficient to process 10 specimens or quality control samples. The positive predictive agreement (PPA) and negative predictive agreement (NPA) of the test relative to the expected results were 97.8% and 95.6%, respectively. Cepheid has developed the same test on GeneXpert Xpress System, a POC system, with similar bioanalytical performance. The SARS-CoV-2 diagnosis is positive if the signal for the N2 nucleic acid target or signals from both nucleic acid targets (N2 and E) have a cycle threshold (Ct) within the valid range. But the diagnosis is presumptive positive if the signal for only the E nucleic acid target has a Ct within the valid range. It may require additional confirmatory testing. The overall assay duration is less than 45 min.

Cepheid has further developed another FDA EUA approved real-time multiplex RT-PCR test, Xpert® Xpress SARS-CoV-2/Flu/RSV, which is performed on GeneXpert Dx or GeneXpert Infinity Systems. It qualitatively detects and differentiates SARS-CoV-2, influenza A, influenza B, and respiratory syncytial virus (RSV) viral RNA in nasopharyngeal swab, nasal swab, or nasal wash/aspirate specimens. The principle of the assay is very similar to that of Cepheid's SARS-CoV-2 test. Cepheid recommends the use of external controls in the form of inactivated viruses that are provided by ZeptoMetrix, USA. They should be used to perform external quality control with each new lot and shipment of reagents. The PPA and NPA of the test relative to the predicate RT-PCR tests (FDA EUA approved) for SARS-CoV-2, Flu A, Flu B, and RSV were 97.9% and 100%; 100% and 100%; 100% and 99%; and, 100% and 100%, respectively. The company has developed the same test on GeneXpert Xpress System (a POC system) with similar bioanalytical performance.

The Simplexa™ COVID-19 real-time RT-PCR assay from DiaSorin Molecular, Italy, is another prospective assay for the qualitative detection of SARS-CoV-2 RNA in nasopharyngeal swabs, nasal swabs, nasal wash/aspirate, and bronchoalveolar lavage specimens from COVID-19 suspects. It contains reagents that are sufficient for 24 reactions. The assay targets the ORF1ab and S gene regions of the SARS-CoV-2 genome and is run on the LIAISON® MDX instrument using the Direct Amplification Disc and other accessories. It employs fluorescent probes together with corresponding forward and reverse primers for the amplification of SARS-CoV-2 RNA and internal control RNA. The company provides Simplexa™ COVID-19 Positive Control Pack, which may be used as an external control for quality control testing. The PPA and NPA in various sample matrices were both 100% w.r.t. an established comparator.

The cobas® SARS-CoV-2 is a real-time RT-PCR assay from Roche, which qualitatively detects SARS-CoV-2 RNA in clinically-collected nasal, nasopharyngeal, and oropharyngeal swabs specimens from COVID-19 suspects. The assay is also approved for clinically-instructed self-collected nasal swab specimens. It is performed on cobas® 6800/8800 Systems, which comprise a sample supply module, a transfer module, a processing module, and an analytical module. The cobas® SARS-CoV-2 employs fully automated sample preparation involving RNA extraction and purification, which is followed by PCR amplification and detection. It targets the ORF1 a/b and E gene regions of the SARS-CoV-2 genome. The company provides the assay controls, i.e., cobas® SARS-CoV-2 Control Kit and cobas® Buffer Negative Control Kit. The PPA and NPA determined in the clinical evaluation with nasopharyngeal swab samples were both 100%.

The Vivalytic COVID-19 test developed by Bosch, Germany, in collaboration with Randox Laboratories, UK is another prospective assay [26]. The fully-automated POC test can detect SARS-CoV-2 and nine respiratory viruses, including influenza A and B, within 2.5 h. The procedure involves sequentially taking the swab sample from the nose or throat of COVID-19 suspects, placing the swab inside a Vivalytic cartridge containing all the COVID-19 assay reagents, and plugging the cartridge into the Vivalytic analyzer.

The most prominent and rapid POC molecular test is the Abbott ID Now™ COVID-19 test [27], which qualitatively detects the viral RNA from SARS-CoV-2 specimens, i.e., throat, nasal, nasopharyngeal, or oropharyngeal swab samples, in just 5 min [27, 28]. It is a POC molecular test for the RdRp gene, which requires just a portable, touchscreen-operated, lightweight (6.6 pounds) and compact (the size of a small toaster) instrument called ID Now. It enables COVID-19 testing in hospitals, clinics, physicians' offices, or other POC settings. The test kit comprises 24 tests, positive and negative controls, pipettes, and swabs for sample collection.

3.2 Antigen detection

The LFIA-based rapid Ag tests for SARS-CoV-2 have played a phenomenal role in the COVID-19 pandemic response. They have been extensively used to screen a large population at POC settings as physician office laboratories, offices, schools, businesses, and homes. They have been approved for professional IVD use and self-testing by the FDA and several countries such as Germany. Germany has allowed the use of tens of rapid Ag tests for self-testing via approval provided by the Federal Institute for Drugs and Medical Devices (BfArM) [6]. The US FDA has granted EUA to several rapid Ag tests for SARS-CoV-2, which can be used for professional IVD use, home use, or both. Almost all the approved rapid Ag tests detect the NP of SARS-CoV-2 and have got good analytical performance. Although several reports have shown the contradictory analytical performance of rapid Ag tests, there is no doubt that such tests are of extreme importance as they have extended the outreach of SARS-CoV-2 testing enormously. The most widely used rapid Ag tests are those from Abbott, Becton Dickinson (BD), and Quidel, which have been further approved by FDA recently under EUA for the serial screening of COVID-19 suspects by testing them twice over 3 days with 24–48 h between tests.

The BinaxNOW™ COVID-19 Ag Card from Abbott Diagnostics is an LFIA that enables the qualitative detection of NP antigen from SARS-CoV-2 in direct anterior nasal (nares) swabs without viral transport media [29]. It is an immunochromatography membrane assay that employs highly sensitive and specific antibodies to detect NP from SARS-CoV-2. A test strip is constructed by immobilizing SARS-CoV-2 specific antibodies and a control Ab onto a membrane as two distinct lines and combining it with other reagents/pads. The COVID-19 Ag card is cardboard, book-shaped hinged card that has a well to hold nasal swab and the test strip mounted on opposite sides. The assay procedure involves taking the nasal swab specimen from the COVID-19 suspects and mixing it with the extraction reagent. The extraction agent disrupts the virus particles and exposes internal viral NP. It is followed by closing the card, which brings the extracted sample in contact with the test strip that starts the LFIA assay. The test results are detected visually by naked eyes after 15 min, where the presence of a pink/purple sample line shows the presence of NP in the sample. The test is intended for use in COVID-19 suspects who are within 7 days of symptoms onset. The PPA and NPA of the test were 97.1% and 98.5%, respectively, against the comparator method. FDA also approves it under EUA for the serial screening of COVID-19, where the individuals are tested twice over 3 days with at least 36 h between tests. However, the test does not differentiate between SARS-CoV-2 and SARS-CoV, and the positive results do not rule out bacterial infection or co-infection with other viruses. The negative test results should be treated as presumptive in patients beyond 7 days post onset of symptoms, where further confirmation with a molecular assay is required. It is essential that the results of the test should be read within 30 minutes, and the nasal swab specimens are used immediately after collection. Apart from the test cards, extraction reagent, and nasal swabs, the BinaxNOW™ COVID-19 Ag Card provides positive and negative control swabs. The positive control swab is a dried swab containing non-infectious recombinant SARS-CoV-2 NP, while the negative control swab has the sample matrix without any NP. It is recommended to test the positive and negative control swabs after each shipment of Ag tests and at least once for each untrained operator.

The BD Veritor™ System [30] for Rapid Detection of SARS-CoV-2 is another prospective rapid LFIA-based test that detects qualitatively the presence of SARS-CoV-2 NP in direct anterior nasal swabs from COVID-19 suspects within the first five days of the onset of symptoms. FDA also authorizes it under EUA for the serial screening of COVID-19 where the subjects are tested twice over 2 or 3 days with 24–48 h between tests. The swab specimens are placed in the extraction reagent tube for sample processing, and the processed sample is then added to the BD Veritor System test device. The SARS-CoV-2 NP in the sample form Ag-conjugate complexes by binding to antibodies conjugated to detector particles in the test strip. The complexes are then captured by the specific antibodies bound to the membrane at the test line. The BD Veritor™ System test device's test results are read after the completion of test in 15 min using the BD Veritor™ Plus Analyzer Instrument. The SARS-CoV-2 test kit includes BD Veritor™ System test devices, extraction reagent, nasal swabs, SARS-CoV-2 (+) Control Swab, and SARS-CoV-2 (−) Control Swab. Most of the assay characteristics in terms of interferences, specificity, and analysis are similar to that of Abbott's BinaxNOW™ COVID-19 Ag Card test. The specimens should be tested immediately after collection. The PPA and NPA of the test were 84% and 100%, respectively, against the RT-PCR method.

The QuickVue At-Home OTC COVID-19 Test from Quidel Corporation is another rapid test to detect SARS-CoV-2 NP qualitatively in direct anterior nasal swabs from COVID-19 suspects within the first six days of the onset of symptoms. FDA also authorizes it under EUA for the serial screening of COVID-19 suspects where they are tested twice over 2 or 3 days with 24–36 h between tests. The test procedure is very similar to that of the BD Veritor™ System for Rapid Detection of SARS-CoV-2 test except that the test strip is read visually by naked eyes after 10 min. The presence of a pink/purple-colored test line indicates the presence of SARS-CoV-2 NP in the specimen. Most assay characteristics are like that of Abbott's BinaxNOW™ COVID-19 Ag Card test. The PPA and NPA of the test were 83.5% and 99.2%, respectively, against the EUA molecular comparator assay.

All other SARS-CoV-2 rapid Ag tests detect the NP antigen qualitatively and have demonstrated good analytical performance. However, some SARS-CoV-2 rapid Ag tests, such as that from Sensing Self, Singapore, have also shown good analytical performance for the qualitative detection of SP antigens. But as most of these tests targeting the SP were developed last year, there is a need to demonstrate that they can work in subjects affected by various spike mutations. The preference for clinical decision-making is certainly the NP detection-based rapid Ag tests. Apart from nasal swabs, several companies have demonstrated the use of saliva, sputum, and stool samples to detect SARS-CoV-2 viral Ag.

3.3 Antibodies detection

Various IVD companies have developed serological IAs to detect anti-SARS-CoV-2 Ab in the serum, plasma, or whole blood samples. They enable identifying individuals with an adaptive immune response to SARS-CoV-2 either due to prior or recent infection [31]. Despite several reports stating the persistence of immunity after SARS-CoV-2 infection for several months [32, 33], it is still unclear how long the anti-SARS-CoV-2 Ab persists and whether they confer protective immunity. Therefore, serology tests are not used to diagnose acute SARS-CoV-2 infection. In the case of SARS-CoV-2, IgM, IgG, and IgA antibodies appear in the subjects at nearly the same time and have the seroconversion between 14 and 23 days post onset of symptoms. SARS-CoV-2 IgG and IgM antibodies may be below the detectable levels in COVID-19 patients who are within 14 days after the onset of symptoms. However, the COVID-19 samples should be handled with care as there is a possibility of detectable SARS-CoV-2 in samples even after seroconversion. Almost all assays have a poor PPA with RT-PCR in patient samples taken from subjects within 14 days from the onset of symptoms. But they have good PPA for samples taken from subjects more than 14 days post onset of symptoms. However, there is always a risk of false-positive results due to the presence of pre-existing antibodies or other possible causes. The most widely used IAs to detect anti-SARS-CoV-2 Ab are automated CLIA, manual ELISA, and rapid LFIA tests that are specified in more detail below.

3.3.1 Automated CLIA

The magnetic particles-based CLIAs are the gold standard in clinical diagnostics for the automated high-throughput analysis of many disease biomarkers on a random-access CLIA analyzer. The desired throughput can be customized from low- to high-throughput by selecting an appropriate CLIA analyzer. Many IVD companies have developed several SARS-CoV-2 serology tests for the detection of IgG and IgM. Most of these assays have an overall assay duration of less than 30 min and employ SP, NP, or both for the detection of anti-SARS-CoV-2 Ab.

The DiaSorin LIAISON® SARS-CoV-2 S1/S2 IgG assay [34, 35], used on the LIAISON® XL Analyzer, detects the anti-SARS-CoV-2 IgG qualitatively in human serum or plasma (sodium heparin, lithium heparin, and potassium EDTA). The assay employs the specific recombinant S1 and S2 antigens coated magnetic particles, which detect the anti-SARS-CoV-2 IgG in the patient sample. This is followed by subsequent binding to mouse monoclonal Ab to human IgG linked to an isoluminol derivative (isoluminol-Ab); adding the starter reagents to induce flash chemiluminescence (CL) reaction; and, measuring the CL signal of isoluminol-Ab conjugate via a photomultiplier. The assay employs two calibrators, one containing low and another having high anti-SARS-CoV-2 IgG levels. The assay has a PPA of 97.6% in samples taken from COVID-19 subjects ≥15 days after diagnosis by RT-PCR. DiaSorin also developed LIAISON® SARS-CoV-2 S1/S2 IgM assay for the qualitative detection of anti-SARS-CoV-2 IgM in human serum or plasma (sodium heparin, lithium heparin, and dipotassium EDTA). The assay principle is similar to that of IgG assay except that magnetic particles were coated with spike receptor-binding domain (RBD) antigen and mouse monoclonal IgG antibodies were linked to an isoluminol derivative, N-(4-Amino-Butyl)-N-Ethyl-Isoluminol (ABEI isoluminol-Ab conjugate). It employs two calibrators, one containing anti-SARS-CoV-2 human IgM monoclonal Ab while the other has no IgM. The PPA to PCR was 92.6% in samples taken from COVID-19 subjects between 15 and 30 days after PCR diagnosis.

The Elecsys anti-SARS-CoV-2 S cobas® [34, 36] is an electrochemiluminescent IA developed by Roche for the qualitative and semi-quantitative detection of Ab against the SP RBD in human serum and plasma (lithium heparin, dipotassium-EDTA (K_2-EDTA), tripotassium EDTA (K_3-EDTA), and sodium citrate). The IA is performed on cobas® e analyzers and has a total assay duration of just 18 min. It employs double-antigen sandwich principle, where the antigens present in the reagent capture mainly anti-SARS-CoV-2 IgG but also IgM and IgA. The assay procedure comprises of two incubations and a measurement step. The 1st incubation of the sample with biotinylated SARS-CoV-2 SP RBD-specific recombinant antigen and biotinylated SARS-CoV-2 SP RBD-specific recombinant antigen labeled with a ruthenium complex leads to the formation of a sandwich complex. It is followed by the 2nd incubation, during which the addition of streptavidin-coated magnetic particles binds to the sandwich complex via streptavidin-biotin interaction. Subsequently, the reaction mixture is aspirated into the measuring cell where the electrode magnetically captures the magnetic particles and the unbound substances are removed. Finally, a voltage is applied to the electrode, which induces the CL signal that is measured by a photomultiplier. The results are determined using a calibration curve with 2-point calibration and a master curve. The assay demonstrated a PPA to PCR of 96.6% in samples taken from COVID-19 subjects ≥15 days after PCR positive result and a NPA to PCR of 99.98%.

Another prospective assay is the IDS SARS-CoV-2 IgG assay developed by Immunodiagnostic Systems, United Kingdom (UK), which detects the anti-SARS-CoV-2 IgG antibodies qualitatively in human serum and plasma (lithium heparin, K_3-EDTA, and sodium citrate). The assay involves the incubation of magnetic particles coated with recombinant SARS-CoV-2 NP and SP antigens with the patient sample (4 μL), which is followed by a wash step and subsequent incubation with anti-SARS-CoV-2 Ab labeled with acridinium. The magnetic particles, having the specific immune complexes, are then captured by a magnet, and a wash step removes the unbound substances. Subsequently, the addition of trigger reagents induces the CL signal that is measured by a photomultiplier. The IA employs two calibrators, one calibrator having low anti-SARS-CoV-2 IgG level while other calibrator has high anti-SARS-CoV-2 IgG level. The assay demonstrated a PPA to PCR of 97.6% in samples taken from COVID-19 patients ≥15 days after symptoms onset and a PPA to PCR of 100% in samples taken from COVID-19 subjects ≥15 days after PCR method. The NPA to PCR was 99.6%.

Of interest is the SNIBE's MAGLUMI 2019-nCoV IgM/IgG assay [37], which employs the 2019-nCoV recombinant antigen, expressing the full-length SP and NP. The assay employs two separate cassettes; one cassette detects IgM via a capture CLIA while another cassette detects IgG via an indirect CLIA. The CL signal detection mechanism is similar to that of DiaSorin. It employs two calibrators and two controls both for the IgG as well as IgM assays. One calibrator and control have high anti-SARS-CoV-2 IgG/IgM levels, while another calibrator and control have low anti-SARS-CoV-2 IgG/IgM levels. The results are generated by a calibration curve generated by 2-point calibration for a specific SNIBE's analyzer and a master curve. The IgG and IgM assays demonstrated PPAs to PCR of 100% and 77.46%, respectively, in samples taken from COVID-19 patients ≥15 days post symptoms onset. The combined PPA to PCR was 93.94% in samples taken from COVID-19 patients ≥15 days post symptoms onset.

There are several other CLIAs developed by Siemens, Abbott, Beckman Coulter, Ortho Clinical Diagnostics, etc., which employ similar assay formats and have high analytical performance.

3.3.2 ELISA

Many IVD manufacturers have developed several CE-certified ELISA kits for the detection of anti-SARS-CoV-2 IgG and IgM antibodies. The most prominent ELISA kits from Euroimmun, InBios, Wantai, Epitope Diagnostics, and Thermo Fisher Scientific, have been approved by FDA under EUA.

The most widely used ELISA kit is the EUROIMMUN Anti-SARS-CoV-2 ELISA (IgG) kit [35, 38], which enables the qualitative detection of anti-SARS-CoV-2 IgG antibodies in human serum and plasma (K^+-EDTA, Li^+-heparin, and Na^+-citrate). The test kit contains microplate strips, where each strip has 8 break-off reagent wells that are pre-coated with S1 domain of SP of SARS-CoV-2, which is expressed recombinantly in the human cell line HEK 293. The assay procedure involves incubating reagent wells with diluted patient sample (diluted 1:101 in sample buffer), which leads to the binding of anti-SARS-CoV-2 IgG antibodies (and also IgA and IgM) with the coated viral Ag. It is followed by subsequent incubation with HRP labeled anti-human IgG detection Ab and TMB substrate reaction. The absorbance of the colored solution after stopping the enzyme-substrate reaction with a stop solution is measured at the wavelength of 450 nm with a reference wavelength of 620–650 nm. The provided two controls, i.e., a positive and a negative control, and calibrator must be used with each run. The overall assay duration is about 2 h and 15 min. The test is evaluated by calculating a ratio of the OD of the control/patient sample over the OD of the calibrator. The results are interpreted as negative, borderline, or positive if the ratio is <0.8, 0.8–1.1, or > 1.1, respectively. It is recommended to retest the patient after 1–2 weeks if he has a borderline result. The assay demonstrated a PPA to PCR of 100% in samples taken from COVID-19 patients ≥21 days post onset of symptoms and a PPA to PCR of 81.1% in samples taken from COVID-19 patients ≥11 days post PCR confirmation. The NPA to PCR was 98.6%. The independent validation study by Frederick National Laboratory for Cancer Research (FNLCR) determined the PPA to comparator method of 90% and NPA of 100%.

The SCoV-2 Detect™ IgG ELISA from InBios International, Inc., USA employs indirect ELISA for the qualitative detection of anti-SARS-CoV-2 IgG antibodies in diluted serum samples (diluted 1:100 in sample dilution buffer). The assay procedure and steps are similar to that of Euroimmun ELISA kit, and the overall assay duration is about 2 h. The kit has a positive and a negative IgG control and a cut-off IgG control. All the controls should be run whenever an assay is performed. The assay achieved a PPA to PCR of 100% in samples taken from COVID-19 subjects ≥22 days post onset of symptoms and a PPA to PCR of 100% in samples taken from COVID-19 subjects 0–28 days post PCR confirmation. The PPA to PCR was 95.45% in samples collected from suspects ≥15 days post onset of symptoms. The NPA to PCR was demonstrated to be 98.95%. The independent validation study by FNLCR showed both PPA and NPA to the comparator method to be 100%.

InBios has also developed the SCoV-2 Detect™ IgM ELISA that enables the qualitative detection of anti-SARS-CoV-2 IgM antibodies in human serum and plasma (K_2-EDTA) from individuals that are 7–64 days post symptoms onset. The assay procedure is similar to that of Euroimmun and InBios IgG kits, except that detection is done by HRP labeled anti-human IgM. The IA involves dilution of the patient sample, i.e., 1:100 in sample dilution buffer, and has an assay duration of about 2 h. It employs a positive and a negative IgM control, and a cut-off IgM control, which must be run for every assay. The assay achieved a PPA to PCR of 93.75% in samples taken from COVID-19 subjects ≥15 days post onset of symptoms. The NPA to PCR was demonstrated to be 98.95%. The independent validation study by FNLCR showed PPA and NPA to comparator method of 96.7% and 98.8%, respectively.

Bio-Rad has developed the Platelia SARS-CoV-2 Total Ab ELISA that enables the qualitative detection of total Ab (IgM/IgG/IgA) against SARS-CoV-2 in human serum and plasma (K_2-EDTA, K_3-EDTA, lithium heparin, acid citrate dextrose, or sodium citrate) [39, 40]. It is a one-step antigen capture format that employs the addition of pre-diluted patient samples to recombinant SARS NP coated wells, and the simultaneous addition of HRP labeled recombinant SARS NP. The mixture is incubated for 1 h at 37°C that leads to the formation of immune complex. Thereafter, the TMB substrate is added, and after 30 min, the colorimetric reaction is stopped by adding a stop solution. The optical density is read by a spectrophotometer at 450 nm with a reference wavelength of 620 nm. The assay employs a positive control, a negative control, and a cut-off control that should be run for each assay. The positive and cut-off controls comprise rabbit polyclonal anti-SARS NP antibodies in human serum and buffer, respectively, with other components. The analysis of results is similar to that of Euroimmun IgG ELISA. The assay has a PPA to PCR of 100% in samples taken from COVID-19 suspects ≥15 days post onset of symptoms while the NPA to PCR was 98.3%. A similar ELISA kit is the WANTAI SARS-CoV-2 Ab ELISA that enables the qualitative detection of total antibodies against SARS-CoV-2 in human serum and acid citrate dextrose plasma. The PPA to PCR was 98.72% in samples taken from COVID-19 suspects ≥15 days post onset of symptoms while the NPA to PCR was 98.3%. The FNLCR's independent validation showed PPA and NPA to comparator method of 96.7% and 97.5%, respectively.

A novel ELISA is the cPassTM SARS-CoV-2 Neutralization Activity Detection Kit from GenScript USA, Inc., which detects qualitatively the total anti-SARS-CoV-2 neutralization Ab in human serum and K_2-EDTA plasma (diluted 1:9 in sample dilution buffer) in just less than 1 h 15 min. The test mimics the virus-host interaction in a test tube or microplate by coating the surface of the well with human ACE2 and analyzing its specific binding to the purified recombinant SARS-CoV-2 SP RBD protein conjugated to HRP (HRP-RBD). The specific interaction between human ACE2 and HRP-RBD is blocked when the neutralization Ab against SARS-CoV-2 SP-RBD are present in the patient sample. The patient samples and controls are diluted and incubated with HRP-RBD so that the neutralization Ab could bind to HRP-RBD. It is followed by the addition of mixture to human ACE2 protein coated capture plate, where the unbound HRP-RBD and HRP-RBD bound to non-neutralizing Ab is captured on the plate. The neutralization Ab HRP-RBD immune complexes in the supernatant are removed during the washings. Subsequently, the TMB substrate is added, and the enzymatic reaction is stopped by adding a stop solution. The absorbance of the solution is read at 450 nm in a microplate reader. The assay employs a positive and a negative control that should be run for each assay. It has PPA and NPA of 100% with the comparator Plaque Reduction Neutralization Test at 50% viral neutralization ($PRNT_{50}$) and 90% viral neutralization ($PRNT_{90}$). The PRNTs employ the SARS-CoV-2 virus (WA01/2020 isolate).

3.3.3 Rapid LFIA

Numerous rapid LFIA-based POC tests have been developed to detect and differentiate anti-SARS-CoV-2 IgM and IgG antibodies produced in individuals after SARS-COV-2 infection. They provide the test results in less than 20 min using only a few microliters of the sample.

The COVID-19 IgG/IgM Rapid Test Cassette (Whole Blood/Serum/Plasma) test from Healgen Scientific LLC, USA, is rapid LFIA for the qualitative detection and differentiation of anti-SARS-CoV-2 IgM and IgG antibodies in human venous whole blood, serum, and plasma from anticoagulated blood (Li^+ heparin, K_2-EDTA, and sodium citrate) [41]. It employs anti-human IgG, anti-human IgM and rabbit IgG coated on a nitrocellulose strip at the test line IgG, test line IgM and control line C, respectively. The colloidal gold particles conjugated to recombinant SARS-CoV-2 S1 antigen (COVID-19 conjugates) are stored in the burgundy-colored conjugate pad. The assay procedure involves the addition of patient sample and assay buffer to the sample well. The presence of anti-SARS-CoV-2 IgM and/or IgG antibodies in the sample will lead to the formation of immune complex with COVID-19 conjugates, which will migrate through nitrocellulose membrane via capillary action and forms a burgundy-colored band at the test line IgM and/or IgG. The absence of colored test bands indicates a negative result. The control line C serves as a procedure control, which will change from blue to red if the proper volume of sample has been added and membrane wicking has occurred. The manufacturer recommends using positive and negative controls as a good laboratory practice to confirm the test result. These are not provided by the company but need to be identified by the laboratory themselves. The assay takes only 10 min and must be read visually within 15 min. The PPA and NPA for the detection of anti-SARS-CoV-2 IgG and IgM antibodies were 96.7% and 98%; and, 86.7% and 99%, respectively. The independent clinical study determined the overall PPA of 100% and NPA of 97.5%.

Another rapid test, the BIOTIME SARS-CoV-2 IgG/IgM Rapid Qualitative Test from Xiamen Biotime Biotechnology Co., Ltd., China, detects and differentiates anti-SARS-CoV-2 IgM and IgG antibodies in human serum, potassium EDTA venous whole blood and plasma (potassium EDTA) [35]. It takes only 20 min and must be read visually within 30 min. The company has SARS-CoV-2 IgG/IgM Control Set, which can be purchased separately by customers. The PPAs to PCR for the detection of anti-SARS-CoV-2 IgG and IgM antibodies in serum and plasma were 100% in samples collected from COVID-19 patients ≥15 days post onset of symptoms. The NPA to PCR for the detection of anti-SARS-CoV-2 IgG and IgM antibodies in serum and plasma were 98.46% and 100%, respectively. The FNLCR validation study demonstrated sensitivity and specificity for anti-SARS-CoV-2 IgM and IgG to be 100% and 98.8%; and, 96.7% and 97.5%, respectively. The combined sensitivity and specificity were 100% and 96.2%, respectively.

Of interest is the SGTi-flex COVID-19 IgG rapid LFIA from Sugentec, Inc., Korea, for the qualitative detection of anti-SARS-CoV-2 IgG antibodies in human serum, plasma (sodium heparin, lithium heparin, sodium citrate, and K_3-EDTA), and venous whole blood (sodium heparin, lithium heparin, sodium citrate, and K_3-EDTA). The assay principle is very similar to that of Healgen's test except that recombinant SARS-CoV-2 NP and SP RBD protein is used in the conjugate. The assay takes only 10 min, and must be read visually within 30 min. Sugentec also provides a separate SGTi-flex COVID-19 IgG Control, which contains a positive and a negative control that are prepared from processed human plasma or serum. The sensitivity (PPA) and specificity (NPA) of the test to PCR were 92.43% and 99.15%, respectively. The sensitivity (PPA) was 98.6% in samples taken from COVID-19 patients ≥15 days post onset of symptoms.

The INNOVITA 2019-nCoV Ab Test (Colloidal Gold) (IgM/IgG Serum/Plasma/ Venous whole blood Combo) from Innovita (Tangshan) Biological Technology Co., Ltd., China detects and differentiates anti-SARS-CoV-2 IgM and IgG antibodies in human serum, plasma (lithium heparin, sodium citrate, and K_2-EDTA), and venous whole blood (lithium heparin, sodium citrate, and K_2-EDTA) [36]. The assay duration is 10 min, and results must be read visually within 15 min. The test strip has two windows, with their distinct sample wells, to selectively detect anti-SARS-CoV-2 IgM and IgG antibodies. The assay principle is similar to that of Healgen's test except that recombinant SARS-CoV-2 NP and S1 antigen is used in the conjugate. The T lines in the IgM and IgG result windows are coated with mouse anti-human monoclonal IgM (μ chain) antibodies and mouse anti-human monoclonal IgG (γ chain) antibodies, respectively. The control C lines in both IgG and IgM result windows are coated with goat anti-mouse IgG antibodies. Innovita provides separate 2019-nCoV IgM Positive Control, 2019-nCoV IgG Positive Control, and 2019-nCoV IgM/IgG Negative Control, which can be purchased separately. The positive controls are lyophilized humanized anti-SARS-CoV-2 IgM and IgG antibody in negative control serum matrix while the negative control is lyophilized negative control matrix. The PPAs to PCR for detecting anti-SARS-CoV-2 IgG and IgM antibodies in K_2-EDTA plasma samples collected from COVID-19 patients ≥15 days post onset of symptoms were 97.78% and 97.67%, respectively. The NPA to PCR for the detection of anti-SARS-CoV-2 IgG and IgM antibodies was 100%. The FNLCR validation study showed sensitivity and specificity for anti-SARS-CoV-2 IgM and IgG w.r.t. the comparator method to be 93.3% and 98.8%; and, 93.3% and 98.8%, respectively. The combined sensitivity and specificity were 100% and 97.5%, respectively.

WANTAI SARS-CoV-2 Ab Rapid Test is a novel LFIA for the qualitative detection of total anti-SARS-CoV-2 Ab in human serum, venous whole blood, and plasma (K_2-EDTA, sodium citrate and lithium heparin). The assay format is similar to that of Healgen test except that SARS-CoV-2 SP RBD antigens are coated at the test (T) and control (C) zones, and colloidal gold particles are conjugated to recombinant SARS-CoV-2 SP RBD antigens. The company provides separate lyophilized positive and negative controls that can be bought separately. The positive control comprises monoclonal mouse anti-SP RBD antibodies in newborn calf serum buffer. The assay duration is 15 min, and results must be read visually within 20 min. The PPA and NPA to PCR were 94.7% and 98.89%, respectively. The PPA to PCR in samples collected from COVID-19 patients ≥15 days post onset of symptoms was 91.67%. The FNLCR validation study showed sensitivity (PPA) and specificity (NPA) to be 100% and 98.8%, respectively.

4. Challenges and future directions

Various novel IVD assay formats, based on reverse transcription loop-mediated isothermal amplification (RT-LAMP), lab-on-a-chip, microfluidics, biosensor, multiplex detection, and POC technologies, are being chased by many groups. An automated, fully integrated POC COVID-19 assay, which can perform molecular, Ag, and Ab testing on a single bioanalytical platform, would be a breakthrough. The smartphone-based POC electrochemical test for SARS-CoV-2 biomarkers, similar to the iHealth Align device developed by iHealth, USA, for blood glucose monitoring [42], would be a very useful test for pandemic response. The rapid and accurate early-stage diagnosis of people infected with the SARS-CoV-2 is critical to decreasing the spread of COVID-19.

Apart from the RT-PCR based IVD tests performed in central clinical laboratories, the rapid Ag tests have played a significant role in extending the outreach of COVID-19 diagnostics to remote, decentralized, and POC settings [43]. Many well-performing rapid Ag tests have been approved by FDA under EUA and many countries for the self-testing of COVID-19. There are concerns regarding the performance of rapid Ag tests and it has been shown that they are not as accurate as RT-PCR tests. But there is no doubt that they are still very useful in pandemic response as they have enabled the mass screening of the population and helped in identifying many COVID-19 positive cases. The serology tests to detect anti-SARS-CoV-2 Ab provide the desired information to the healthcare providers about the immune status of the COVID-19 patients and convalescent subjects.

The clinical accuracy of all COVID-19 tests needs to be stringently evaluated and constantly checked. The regulatory bodies and clinical authorities should analyze if the approved IVD tests are still working properly in all the patients or they are impacted by any specific SARS-CoV-2 mutation(s). Several safety alerts have been issued by the FDA where certain molecular tests impacted by SARS-CoV-2 mutations have been recalled from the market. Additionally, FDA has recalled a large number of COVID-19 tests due to the lacking clinical validation data or performance. The discovery and use of novel biomarkers for the diagnosis of SARS-CoV-2 infection at an early stage could further lead to a novel IVD assay that would be ideal for pandemic response.

There is a need for more extensive research so that novel rapid and highly sensitive diagnostic technologies for the POC detection of SARS-CoV-2 infection with good analytical performance could be developed. The early-stage detection of SARS-CoV-2 infection would enable the healthcare professionals to intervene early and prevent the spread of infection.

The sensitivity of rapid LFIA tests could be further enhanced by employing new nanomaterial labels [44], which could lead to much lower limit of detection for the detection of specific analytes in the patient sample. Colloidal gold nanoparticles (NPs) has been the most used in commercial LFIA rapid tests due to the availability of large number of conjugation and immobilization chemistries, easy synthesis and low cost. However, many prospective nanomaterial labels have been demonstrated to provide much higher sensitivity. These include quantum dots, up-conversion NPs, time-resolved fluorescence NPs, surface enhanced Raman scattering active NPs, magnetic NPs, carbon nanotubes and carbon NPs. In case of COVID-19, there is a need to detect very low concentrations of NP at pg/mL level, which is just at the limit of detection of conventional LFIA formats that are being used commercially in rapid tests. It is possible to increase the accuracy of detection at such low levels by employing such novel nanomaterial labels, which have been demonstrated by several researchers [44]. Several other biomarkers that are being investigated for the early-stage detection of COVID-19, such as cytokines, are also present at very low levels in the patient samples. Therefore, there is a requirement of very high sensitivity for analyte detection. Further, a large number of smartphone-based colorimetry, fluorescent and chemiluminescent readers for rapid LFIA have already been developed by many companies and groups [45–47], which would be ideal for POC readout of rapid tests and rapid transmission of test results to a dedicated healthcare server or Cloud. The current generation of smartphones have advanced imaging, processing, connectivity, and other characteristic features, which would be highly effective in the development of next generation of innovative IVD and healthcare technologies for pandemic response.

5. Conclusions

Several IVD assays have been developed for the diagnosis of COVID-19. The gold standard for the confirmatory clinical diagnosis is the RT-PCR assay, while the mass population screening has only been feasible with rapid Ag tests. The rapid molecular tests have further extended the RT-PCR based COVID-19 diagnosis at POC settings. The POC molecular test (ID NOW™) from Abbott is a breakthrough in IVD testing. A large number of serology IVD tests, such as automated CLIA, manual ELISA, and LFIA, have further enabled the detection of anti-SARS-CoV-2 Ab in COVID-19 patients and suspects. The ongoing research efforts and continuous advances in the field and complementary technologies will lead to improved IVD tests for COVID-19 in the near future.

Conflict of interest

The authors declare no conflict of interest.

Author details

Sandeep Kumar Vashist*, Subramanian Murugan and Guiffo Djoko
Pictor Pvt. Ltd., Auckland, New Zealand

*Address all correspondence to: sandeep.vashist@pictordx.com;
sandeep.vashist@yahoo.com

References

[1] Vashist SK. *In Vitro* Diagnostic Assays for COVID-19: Recent Advances and Emerging Trends. Diagnostics (Basel). 2020;10(4):202.

[2] COVID-19 coronavirus pandemic. https://www.worldometers.info/coronavirus/. 2020.

[3] Phelan AL, Katz R, Gostin LO. The Novel Coronavirus Originating in Wuhan, China: Challenges for Global Health Governance. JAMA. 2020;323(8):709-10.

[4] Zhou P, Yang XL, Wang XG, Hu B, Zhang L, Zhang W, et al. A pneumonia outbreak associated with a new coronavirus of probable bat origin. Nature. 2020;579(7798):270-3.

[5] Chan JF, Kok KH, Zhu Z, Chu H, To KK, Yuan S, et al. Genomic characterization of the 2019 novel human-pathogenic coronavirus isolated from a patient with atypical pneumonia after visiting Wuhan. Emerg Microbes Infect. 2020;9(1):221-36.

[6] Federal Institute for Drugs and Medical Devices (BfArM), Germany. Antigen tests for SARS-CoV-2 2021 [Available from: https://www.bfarm.de/EN/MedicalDevices/AntigenTests/_node.html.

[7] Chu DK, Akl EA, Duda S, Solo K, Yaacoub S, Schunemann HJ, et al. Physical distancing, face masks, and eye protection to prevent person-to-person transmission of SARS-CoV-2 and COVID-19: a systematic review and meta-analysis. Lancet. 2020;395(10242):1973-87.

[8] Klompas M, Morris CA, Sinclair J, Pearson M, Shenoy ES. Universal Masking in Hospitals in the Covid-19 Era. N Engl J Med. 2020;382(21):e63.

[9] Leung NH, Chu DK, Shiu EY, Chan K-H, McDevitt JJ, Hau BJ, et al. Respiratory virus shedding in exhaled breath and efficacy of face masks. Nature Medicine. 2020:1-5.

[10] Rothe C, Schunk M, Sothmann P, Bretzel G, Froeschl G, Wallrauch C, et al. Transmission of 2019-nCoV Infection from an Asymptomatic Contact in Germany. N Engl J Med. 2020;382(10):970-1.

[11] Bai Y, Yao L, Wei T, Tian F, Jin DY, Chen L, et al. Presumed Asymptomatic Carrier Transmission of COVID-19. JAMA. 2020;323(14):1406-7.

[12] Huang P, Liu T, Huang L, Liu H, Lei M, Xu W, et al. Use of chest CT in combination with negative RT-PCR assay for the 2019 novel coronavirus but high clinical suspicion. Radiology. 2020:200330.

[13] Xie X, Zhong Z, Zhao W, Zheng C, Wang F, Liu J. Chest CT for Typical Coronavirus Disease 2019 (COVID-19) Pneumonia: Relationship to Negative RT-PCR Testing. Radiology. 2020;296(2):E41-E5.

[14] Greaney AJ, Loes AN, Crawford KH, Starr TN, Malone KD, Chu HY, et al. Comprehensive mapping of mutations in the SARS-CoV-2 receptor-binding domain that affect recognition by polyclonal human plasma antibodies. Cell host & microbe. 2021.

[15] Li Q, Wu J, Nie J, Zhang L, Hao H, Liu S, et al. The Impact of Mutations in SARS-CoV-2 Spike on Viral Infectivity and Antigenicity. Cell. 2020;182(5):1284-94 e9.

[16] Liu Z, VanBlargan LA, Bloyet L-M, Rothlauf PW, Chen RE, Stumpf S, et al. Identification of SARS-CoV-2 spike mutations that attenuate monoclonal and serum antibody neutralization. Cell host & microbe. 2021.

[17] Rees-Spear C, Muir L, Griffith SA, Heaney J, Aldon Y, Snitselaar JL, et al. The impact of Spike mutations on SARS-CoV-2 neutralization. Cell Reports. 2021:108890.

[18] Xie L, Sun C, Luo C, Zhang Y, Zhang J, Yang J, et al. SARS-CoV-2 and SARS-CoV Spike-RBD Structure and Receptor Binding Comparison and Potential Implications on Neutralizing Antibody and Vaccine Development. bioRxiv. 2020.

[19] Paules CI, Marston HD, Fauci AS. Coronavirus Infections-More Than Just the Common Cold. JAMA. 2020;323(8):707-8.

[20] Sethuraman N, Jeremiah SS, Ryo A. Interpreting Diagnostic Tests for SARS-CoV-2. JAMA. 2020;323(22):2249-51.

[21] Wolfel R, Corman VM, Guggemos W, Seilmaier M, Zange S, Muller MA, et al. Virological assessment of hospitalized patients with COVID-2019. Nature. 2020;581(7809):465-9.

[22] Corman VM, Landt O, Kaiser M, Molenkamp R, Meijer A, Chu DK, et al. Detection of 2019 novel coronavirus (2019-nCoV) by real-time RT-PCR. Euro Surveill. 2020;25(3):2000045.

[23] Chu DKW, Pan Y, Cheng SMS, Hui KPY, Krishnan P, Liu Y, et al. Molecular Diagnosis of a Novel Coronavirus (2019-nCoV) Causing an Outbreak of Pneumonia. Clin Chem. 2020;66(4):549-55.

[24] Chan JF, Yip CC, To KK, Tang TH, Wong SC, Leung KH, et al. Improved Molecular Diagnosis of COVID-19 by the Novel, Highly Sensitive and Specific COVID-19-RdRp/Hel Real-Time Reverse Transcription-PCR Assay Validated In Vitro and with Clinical Specimens. J Clin Microbiol. 2020;58(5).

[25] Xpert® Xpress SARS-CoV-2. https://www.cepheid.com/coronavirus. 2020.

[26] Vivalytic rapid test for COVID-19. https://www.bosch.com/stories/vivalytic-rapid-test-for-covid-19/ 2020 [

[27] ID NOW™ Covid-19. https://www.alere.com/en/home/product-details/id-now-covid-19.html. 2020.

[28] Abbott Launches Molecular Point-of-Care Test to Detect Novel Coronavirus in as Little as Five Minutes. https://abbott.mediaroom.com/2020-03-27-Abbott-Launches-Molecular-Point-of-Care-Test-to-Detect-Novel-Coronavirus-in-as-Little-as-Five-Minutes 2020 [Available from: https://abbott.mediaroom.com/2020-03-27-Abbott-Launches-Molecular-Point-of-Care-Test-to-Detect-Novel-Coronavirus-in-as-Little-as-Five-Minutes.

[29] Perchetti GA, Huang M-L, Mills MG, Jerome KR, Greninger AL. Analytical Sensitivity of the Abbott BinaxNOW COVID-19 Ag CARD. Journal of Clinical Microbiology. 2021;59(3).

[30] Young S, Taylor SN, Cammarata CL, Varnado KG, Roger-Dalbert C, Montano A, et al. Clinical Evaluation of BD Veritor SARS-CoV-2 Point-of-Care Test Performance Compared to PCR-Based Testing and versus the Sofia 2 SARS Antigen Point-of-Care Test. J Clin Microbiol. 2020;59(1).

[31] Shuren J, Stenzel T. The FDA's Experience with Covid-19 Antibody Tests. N Engl J Med. 2021;384(7):592-4.

[32] Choe PG, Kim K-H, Kang CK, Suh HJ, Kang E, Lee SY, et al. Antibody responses 8 months after asymptomatic or mild SARS-CoV-2 infection. Emerging infectious diseases. 2021;27(3):928.

[33] Dan JM, Mateus J, Kato Y, Hastie KM, Yu ED, Faliti CE, et al. Immunological memory to SARS-CoV-2

assessed for up to 8 months after infection. Science. 2021;371(6529).

[34] Merrill AE, Jackson JB, Ehlers A, Voss D, Krasowski MD. Head-to-Head Comparison of Two SARS-CoV-2 Serology Assays. J Appl Lab Med. 2020;5(6):1351-7.

[35] Jaaskelainen AJ, Kuivanen S, Kekalainen E, Ahava MJ, Loginov R, Kallio-Kokko H, et al. Performance of six SARS-CoV-2 immunoassays in comparison with microneutralisation. J Clin Virol. 2020;129:104512.

[36] Charlton CL, Kanji JN, Johal K, Bailey A, Plitt SS, MacDonald C, et al. Evaluation of Six Commercial Mid- to High-Volume Antibody and Six Point-of-Care Lateral Flow Assays for Detection of SARS-CoV-2 Antibodies. J Clin Microbiol. 2020;58(10).

[37] Dou X, Wang E, Hu J, Zong Z, Jiang R, Wang M, et al. Comparison of three automatic chemiluminescent immunoassays for monitoring dynamic profile of SARS-CoV-2 IgG and IgM. J Clin Lab Anal. 2021;35(1):e23681.

[38] Manalac J, Yee J, Calayag K, Nguyen L, Patel PM, Zhou D, et al. Evaluation of Abbott anti-SARS-CoV-2 CMIA IgG and Euroimmun ELISA IgG/IgA assays in a clinical lab. Clin Chim Acta. 2020;510:687-90.

[39] Trabaud MA, Icard V, Milon MP, Bal A, Lina B, Escuret V. Comparison of eight commercial, high-throughput, automated or ELISA assays detecting SARS-CoV-2 IgG or total antibody. J Clin Virol. 2020;132:104613.

[40] Tre-Hardy M, Wilmet A, Beukinga I, Favresse J, Dogne JM, Douxfils J, et al. Analytical and clinical validation of an ELISA for specific SARS-CoV-2 IgG, IgA, and IgM antibodies. J Med Virol. 2021;93(2):803-11.

[41] Catry E, Jacqmin H, Dodemont M, Saad Albichr I, Lardinois B, de Fays B, et al. Analytical and clinical evaluation of four commercial SARS-CoV-2 serological immunoassays in hospitalized patients and ambulatory individuals. J Virol Methods. 2021;289:114060.

[42] iHealth Align. https://ihealthlabs.com/glucometer/ihealth-align/ 2020 [

[43] Nguyen NNT, McCarthy C, Lantigua D, Camci-Unal G. Development of Diagnostic Tests for Detection of SARS-CoV-2. Diagnostics (Basel). 2020;10(11).

[44] Guo J, Chen S, Guo J, Ma X. Nanomaterial Labels in Lateral Flow Immunoassays for Point-of-Care-Testing. Journal of Materials Science & Technology. 2021;60:90-104.

[45] Vashist SK, Luppa PB, Yeo LY, Ozcan A, Luong JHT. Emerging Technologies for Next-Generation Point-of-Care Testing. Trends Biotechnol. 2015;33(11):692-705.

[46] Vashist SK, Mudanyali O, Schneider EM, Zengerle R, Ozcan A. Cellphone-based devices for bioanalytical sciences. Anal Bioanal Chem. 2014;406(14):3263-77.

[47] Roda A, Michelini E, Zangheri M, Di Fusco M, Calabria D, Simoni P. Smartphone-based biosensors: A critical review and perspectives. TrAC Trends in Analytical Chemistry. 2016;79:317-25.

Chapter 9

Molecular Biology of PCR Testing for COVID-19 Diagnostics

Vinita Chittoor-Vinod

Abstract

COVID-19 cases were first reported in December 2019, and since then it has spread quickly to create a global pandemic. This respiratory disease is caused by the SARS-CoV-2 virus. A major contributing factor for the fast spread of this virus is that the infectivity by the asymptomatic carriers is similar to symptomatic patients. Thus, to identify the asymptomatic individuals and to provide the essential treatment and care to COVID-19 patients, we rely heavily on diagnostic assays. Efficient, reproducible and accessible diagnostic tests are crucial in combatting a pandemic. Currently, there are few key detection tests which have been successfully employed to field-use. However, there are constant efforts to enhance their efficacy and accessibility. This chapter aims at explaining the basic principles of the current molecular diagnostic tests, which determine the presence of the virus through the detection of its genetic material. This chapter will aid the readers in understanding the basic workings of these molecular diagnostic tests.

Keywords: molecular diagnostic tests, PCR assays, SARS-CoV-2, COVID-19, RT-PCR, RPA, LAMP, CRISPR-based assays, LFA

1. Introduction

In December 2019 primary cases of COVID-19 were reported in Wuhan (China), which was later declared as a pandemic by WHO in March 2020 [1]. The COVID-19 is caused by the contagious virus SARS-CoV-2 (Severe acute respiratory syndrome coronavirus 2), belonging to the same family as MERS-CoV (Middle East respiratory syndrome coronavirus) and SARS-CoV-1 [2]. Typical symptoms of COVID-19 span a wide range, including fever, dry cough, sore throat and shortness of breath [3]. These symptoms are similar to flu and other respiratory illnesses. In order to provide appropriate care and treatment for COVID-19, it is critical to diagnose SARS-CoV-2 (referred to as CoV-2 hereafter) infections distinctly from other similar diseases. Another complexity to this is that some CoV-2 infected individuals do not exhibit exaggerated symptoms, termed as asymptomatic carriers [4]. It has been shown that the asymptomatic carriers can spread the virus to the same extent as the symptomatic individuals, in the absence of appropriate precautions [4]. Thus, it is imperative to identify all infections efficiently, quarantine and treat appropriately to cease the spread of CoV-2. To achieve this, many diagnostic tests (assays) have been developed and improved by multiple referring (participating) laboratories and CDC (Centers for Disease Control and Prevention). This chapter is focused on simplifying the basic principles of these diagnostic assays. Many scientific review articles which dive deep into the science of CoV-2 diagnostic testing have been published [1, 3, 5–7]. This chapter, however, aims at explaining the same in non-technical terms, intended for a general audience.

2. Biology of SARS-CoV-2

SARS-CoV-2 belongs to the family *Coronaviridae*, similar to SARS-CoV-1. CoV-2 consists of a spherical protein structure of ~80–160 nm diameter [8] (**Figure 1**). This sphere is composed of two lipid layers placed face-to-face close to each other (bilayer). This bilayer is embedded with proteins, collectively referred to as the structural proteins. They include the envelope (E), membrane (M) and spike (S) proteins [2]. The E, M and S-proteins are embedded in the lipid bilayer forming the sphere [9]. The S-proteins stick out of the sphere prominently, giving a spiked crown-like appearance to the virus and thereby conferring the name 'corona' (crown) [2]. They bind to the ACE-2 (human angiotensin-converting enzyme 2) receptors on the host cell membrane to initiate fusion, and therefore are key in the invasion of host cells [10–12]. Encapsulated inside this sphere is the virus genome, which in the case of CoV-2, is a plus (or positive) single-stranded (ss) RNA (ribonucleic acid, ss RNA) [2]. This genetic material is spooled around the nucleocapsid (N) proteins, which are also accounted as structural proteins [2].

The genome of CoV-2 was successfully sequenced by January 2020 [13]. The ss RNA is ~30 kb (kilobases) in length [2], encompassing all the information for protein syntheses and assembly of the new virus particles (virions). There is another group of non-structural proteins (NSPs) which are involved in non-structural functions such as genetic material replication or the assembly of virions [2]. There are 16 such NSPs identified in the CoV-2 genome, which include an RNA-dependent RNA polymerase (RdRP), ExoN (exonuclease) and ORF proteins [2]. RdRP synthesizes new viral genetic material, while ExoN is responsible for genome stability and for removing any errors in the newly synthesized genetic RNA sequence. ORF proteins act as accessory proteins [2].

Viruses have been traditionally categorized in a separate class, from the biotic or living organisms. This is due to their inability to replicate in the absence of a host. In general, the virus invades the host cell, releases its genetic material and hijacks the host machinery for synthesizing its own macromolecules (nucleic acid and proteins) [14]. Upon assembly of virions (new viruses), the host cell is lysed (broken open) to release the new infectious particles [14]. The host cells try to combat the

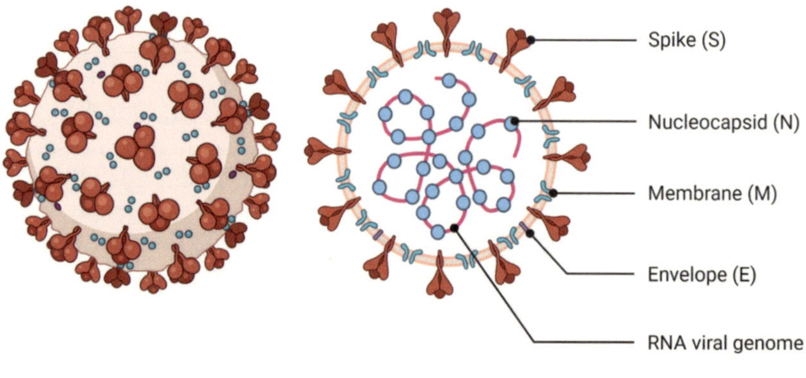

Figure 1.
Cartoon representing the human SARS-CoV-2 virus structure. (Left) Sphere showing the outside of the virus. (Right) A cross-section of the virus sphere depicting the membrane structural proteins (S, M and E), along with the ss RNA genetic material which is wound around the nucleocapsid (N) proteins.

invasion by evoking an immune response specific to the virus (adaptive immunity) [15]. This is attempted through the presentation of fragments of the foreign macromolecules on the host cell surface. These non-indigenous particles, called antigens, are sensed by the immune cells which initiate the production of antibodies against them [15]. Thereafter, any particle resembling the antigen is attacked and cleared by the host immune cells. Antibodies are broadly classified into 5 main immunoglobulin (Ig) classes: G, A, M, E and D. They differ in their structures, capacity to recognize the antigen and occurrence in the course of immune response [15]. These antibodies encompass a structural region which is specific to binding the antigen (called the variable region). The immune response and components are much more complicated than this simple excerpt presented here, and the readers are encouraged to refer to other reviews on the immune system [15].

3. Detection of SARS-CoV-2

The observation that the virus from asymptomatic carriers is equally infectious as those exhibiting clear symptoms of COVID-19 [4, 16], makes it imperative to identify the asymptomatic individuals in order to take appropriate measures for their seclusion and treatment. This is highly dependent on the reliability and accuracy of the diagnostic tests. Further, these assays also permit the recognition of patients with CoV-2 infections at hospitals where it is crucial for their segregation into the COVID-19 specific wards. This is important to prevent further transmission of the virus to admitted and highly vulnerable patient populations. Reliability of a diagnostic test depends on its specificity and sensitivity. Specificity is the ability of the test to correctly detect the negative samples as negative, thus reducing false-positive results [17]. On the other hand, sensitivity is the ability of the test to correctly identify the positive cases as positive, thereby decreasing false-negative results [17]. It is essential that a test is dependable for both these features. False results, either way, will aid in the spread of the virus, and misdirect contact tracing.

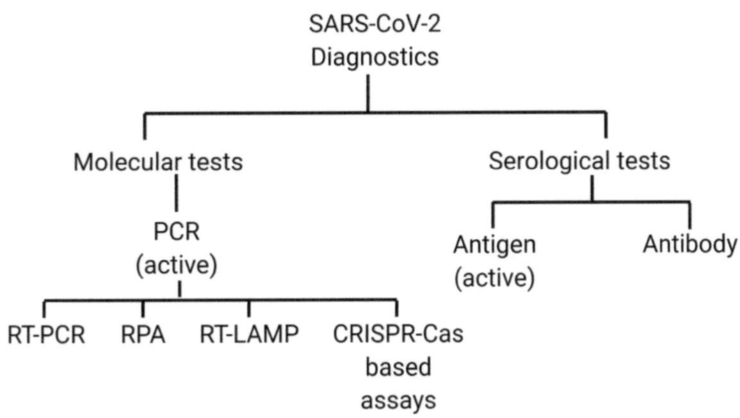

Figure 2.
Categorization of available CoV-2 diagnostic tests. The present diagnostic assays for CoV-2 can be segregated into two broad classes- molecular and serological. Molecular tests determine the presence of the virus by detecting its genome. For molecular assays, specimens can be collected from multiple relevant areas, such as the nasal swab, BAL, etc. Serological tests detect either the presence of the antigen (a protein that is only expressed by the virus) or the antibodies (generated by the host's immune system in response to the infection) in blood samples. While PCR (molecular) and antigen tests detect the presence of the virus at the time of testing, antibody assays mainly determine previous infection. All these tests can identify both, symptomatic and asymptomatic carriers of the virus. The PCR assays include reverse transcription-PCR (RT-PCR), recombinase polymerase amplification (RPA), reverse transcription-loop mediated isothermal amplification (RT-LAMP), and CRISPR-Cas based tests. These PCR assays will be discussed in this chapter.

In the face of a pandemic, such as the one we face currently, a diagnostic assay should have:

- High sensitivity
- High specificity
- Easy read-out method
- Rapid turn-around-time (TAT, time to get the results)
- Low cost
- Easy transport and storage
- High reproducibility

Present diagnostic assays for CoV-2 have been categorized as shown in **Figure 2**.

4. Molecular testing

These diagnostic assays detect the virus through the presence of their genetic material, which is amplified to produce a detectable signal. To fully comprehend the mechanism of these assays, it is essential to first understand the central dogma (**Figure 3**). The common genetic material is DNA (deoxyribonucleic acid), a comparatively more stable nucleic acid than RNA. Generally, DNA is a double-stranded (ds) molecule composed of plus (+) and minus (−) strands [18]. It is made of deoxyribose sugar molecules as backbone and are attached with bases or nucleotides A (adenine), T (thymine), G (guanine) or C (cytosine) [18]. The complementary nature of the bases, i.e. their ability to pair specifically, provides the ds structure. The same feature allows faithful replication of the DNA and syntheses of RNA, thus enabling truthful relaying of the message. The base pairings are A-T and C-G [18]. The deoxyribose (and ribose) sugars provide a directionality to the nuclei acids

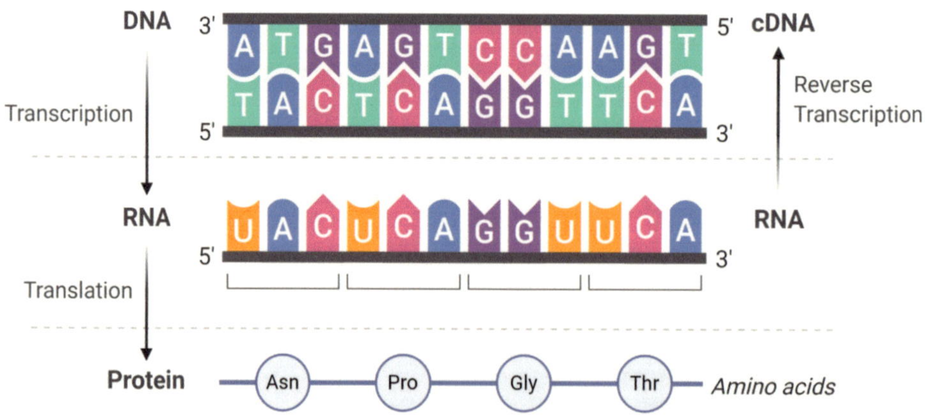

Figure 3.
Central dogma. The message in the double stranded DNA is converted to single stranded RNA by transcription, through complementary base pairing. The code in RNA is converted to proteins by a process called translation (three bases constitute a codon, which represents one amino acid). Amino acids are the building blocks of proteins. RNA can be converted back to double stranded DNA (cDNA) through reverse transcription.

with their chemical groups, 5′ end and 3′ end [19]. All DNA strands are synthesized by DNA polymerases in 5′ - > 3′ direction [19]. The two strands, however, run in opposite directions i.e. the 5′ end of plus strand is closest to the 3′ end of minus strand, while the 3′ end of the plus strand is opposite to the 5′ end of the minus end [19]. Based on the ATGC code (sequence) carried by the plus strand, the minus complementary strand is built [19]. For example, 5′-AGGCTC-3′ sequence on the plus strand will be paired with 5′-GAGCCT-3′.

4.1 DNA to RNA

The information in the genetic material needs to be converted to proteins, which act at the functional level. In this process, a key intermediate is the RNA. The code in the DNA is first converted to RNA through transcription by RNA polymerases [20]. The complementarity of the bases is used to transfer the information faithfully into RNA. Usually, RNA is a ss molecule, with the same complementary base pairings as the DNA. In RNA, T is replaced by U (uracil) which also pairs with A (A-U) [19]. In some viruses, ds RNA serves as the genetic material. However, the rules of complementation and the ss RNA intermediate for protein synthesis remain the same.

4.2 RNA to protein

The code carried by RNA is used for the synthesis of proteins, through translation [20]. Proteins are composed of amino acids building blocks. A codon in the RNA, which is composed of three bases in a specific order, codes for a particular amino acid [20]. So, the sequence of the amino acids in the protein are built according to the sequence of the codons in the respective RNA. Proteins are the macromolecules which acts as support structures, catalyze reactions, relay signaling information, and many other functions.

The dependency of protein synthesis on RNA has been ingeniously employed in the current Pfizer and Moderna vaccines [21]. These vaccines carry an mRNA (messenger RNA) which carries the code for an antigenic fragment of the CoV-2 S-protein [21]. The host cells produce the S-protein fragments which elicit an appropriate immune response. This leads to the production of antibodies that can identify the CoV-2 S-protein upon an actual infection.

5. Polymerase chain reaction (PCR)

PCR is the process of photocopying a specific region (target region) of the DNA, achieved through base complementation. This amplification process is used to produce a detectable signal, which can be correlated to the presence and amount of target DNA present in the reaction (**Figure 4**). In PCR, a specific target region in the DNA sample is demarcated through primers, which are short stretches of DNA ranging from 8–20 nucleotide bases. Short DNA strands are termed as oligonucleotides, where primers are a sub-group which are used in PCR reactions. Primers are complementary to the boundaries of the target region in the DNA sample. In PCR, two primers are required to bind at the 5′ end boundaries, one each for the plus and minus strands. The primers provide a pre-requisite platform for the DNA polymerase to bind and extend the new complementary strands [22], one for each of the two original template strands (**Figure 4B**).

When the starting material for PCR is RNA, as in the case of CoV-2, the RNA template is first reverse transcribed to complementary DNA (cDNA) (**Figure 4A**).

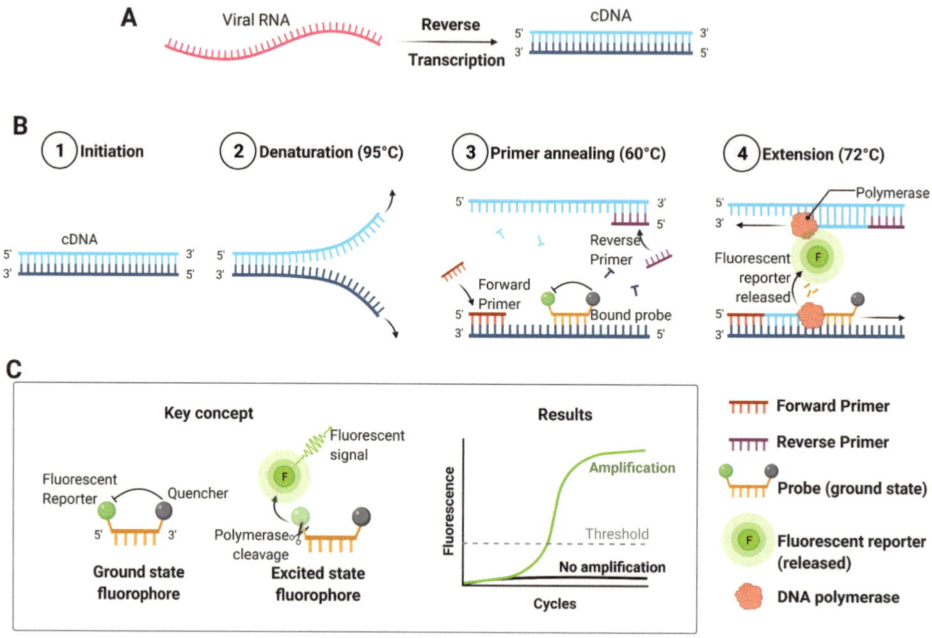

Figure 4.
RT-PCR. (A) Viral ss RNA is converted to ds DNA by the reverse transcriptase enzyme. (B) In PCR, the cDNA acts the template (1). The two strands of the cDNA are separated (denatured) through high heat (2). This allows the annealing of the primers (forward and reverse) and the probe with their complementary regions on the template DNA strands (3). The DNA polymerase extends the primers to synthesize new DNA strands. In this process, the polymerase displaces and separates the fluorescent reporter (F) and the quencher (4). (C) Explanation of the read-out signal generation. At the ground state, the quencher is in close proximity to the reporter, and thus suppresses its emission. Upon cleavage by the polymerase (during extension step), the reporter is released. This relieves its inhibition thereby producing a fluorescent signal. Thus, with an increase in amplification of the template DNA, there is a corresponding increase in the detectable fluorescent signal.

The cDNA then serves as a template for PCR amplification using targeted primers. The conversion of RNA to DNA is achieved through naturally occurring RNA-dependent DNA polymerases, aptly called reverse transcriptase (RT). PCR reactions which depend on the RT enzyme are generally categorized as RT-PCR.

The amplified DNA region was traditionally detected using color or fluorescent agents which bind to ds DNA products [23]. Thus, with an increase in amplification there is an increase in the color/fluorescent signal. PCR read-outs are of two types: quantitative and qualitative. The former, quantitative, yields the amounts of template DNA, either absolute or relative values. On the other hand, qualitative PCR provides information on whether the template DNA is present in a sample. For CoV-2 RNA detection, a simple answer on its presence or absence is essential.

The general types of PCR techniques employed or developed for COVID-19 diagnosis are discussed below.

5.1 Reverse transcriptase-polymerase chain reaction (RT-PCR)

The first diagnostic kit developed to detect the CoV-2 infection was based on RT-PCR. As described above, the viral genomic RNA in the specimen is reverse transcribed to cDNA, followed by PCR amplification of a target gene using primers (**Figure 4**). There are two variants of this reaction: 1-step and 2-steps [3]. In 1-step, reverse transcription and PCR are conducted in the same tube, in tandem. This minimizes the chances of contamination by reducing handling. The 2-steps variation separates the RT reaction which provides cDNA in a separate tube for retention.

This is useful since it is easier to store and handle DNA than RNA, and the cDNA can be used for further testing of other genes, if needed.

Choosing the target gene and region within that gene (usually PCR is directed at amplifying only a small region within a gene) is important, as it needs to be specific to the virus, excluding any overlap with the host genome or any other parasite/virus. For CoV-2 PCR, regions within the N, E, RdRP, S and ORF1ab genes have been successfully used as targets for RT-PCR [3]. It was recommended to use PCRs directed at amplifying at least two target regions for higher specificity. In addition to the viral genes, the human RNase P gene which is present ubiquitously in all cells is also amplified separately [3]. Detection of RNase P ensures that the PCR reaction did receive the specimen. This is important especially in determining negative results for viral gene targets.

During the PCR, the two strands of DNA template (plus and minus strands) are separated using high temperature to break the complementary pairs (reversible). This step is termed as "denaturation" in PCR, which is required to expose the bases for the primers to bind. This is followed by an "annealing" step which is ambient for primer binding to the complementary regions. Entailing this step is "extension" of the primers by DNA polymerase to synthesize complementary product strands. These three key steps are repeated multiple times in the same order to amplify the signal (referred to as PCR cycles). The newly synthesized DNA fragments can then themselves act as templates in the following PCR cycles, thereby giving an exponential amplification pattern. Thus, even a small amount of starting DNA is sufficient to generate a positive signal. Although, the annealing and extension temperatures can be synchronized through appropriate designing of the primers, denaturation requires a higher temperature. This demands the use of thermocyclers for RT-PCR, which can change temperatures of the reaction cyclically. Further, RT-PCR read-out is generally a fluorescent signal which also requires a specific detection instrument. These limit the use of this assay at point-of-care (POC), i.e. use by medical practitioners for instant results to make informed and immediate decisions.

A variation of this conventional assay, TaqMan PCR, was employed as a primary technique for CoV-2 diagnostics [24]. It involves the addition of another oligonucleotide called the probe. This probe, which is complementary to the plus strand is usually positioned towards the center of the target region i.e. between the two opposing primers. Probe is flanked by a fluorescent reporter molecule at its 5′ end and a quencher molecule at the 3′ end (as explained earlier, all oligonucleotides have a direction imparted by the backbone sugar molecules). The fluorescent reporter signal is suppressed by the quencher due to their close proximity. When the probe binds to the plus strand of the template (after denaturation), the DNA polymerase starts synthesizing the new strand from the 3'end of the forward primer (the quencher molecule in the probe 3′ end will not allow the polymerase to start at the probe). In this process, the polymerase cleaves the probe and releases the fluorescent and quencher molecules separately. Due to this irreversible separation, the signal from the fluorescent reporter is uninhibited and detectable. Thus, the level of signal from the reaction is proportional to the amount of new DNA products. TaqMan PCR retains the need for a thermocycler and a fluorescence reader, but provides more specificity than the traditional technique.

During the early stages of the COVID-19 pandemic, samples from multiple individuals were pooled together to reduce the testing times [25]. Upon detecting a positive result, the samples from that pool were individually tested to identify the infected individual/s.

Advantages:

1. RT-PCR is a commonly used assay in most laboratories. Hence, it was easily absorbed as a CoV-2 diagnostic test during the start of this pandemic.

2. It has high specificity, determined by the rigor of the chosen primers/probes.

3. This assay can be easily modified to adapt the mutations of the virus, as reported for CoV-2 S-protein in UK in December 2020 [26].

4. This test has the capability to multiplex. It has been recently modified by the CDC to detect the presence of CoV-2, Influenza strains A and B [3].

5. There is no requirement for a purification step in RT-PCR.

Limitations:

1. This assay depends on a thermocycler and a fluorescence reader, limiting its use at POC.

2. The RT and PCR reactions yield a TAT of ~3–24 hours [27], depending on the number of samples and the handling capacity of the testing center.

5.2 Recombinase polymerase amplification (RPA)

This assay works on the same principle as the RT-PCR but bypasses the need for temperature variations for DNA amplification. It eliminates the denaturation high temperature step, and then combines the annealing and extension steps to a single temperature [28]. The assays which use a single temperature to complete all the reactions are termed as 'isothermal', thus eliminating the need for a thermocycler.

RPA achieves isothermal amplification through the inclusion of a few key components in the reaction mixture (**Figure 5**). The first is the recombinase enzyme, which is incubated with the primers to form a complex, in the presence of a crowding agent (increases viscosity of the solution). The recombinase-primers complex is then added to the reaction with the cDNA derived from viral RNA. Thus, this assay also depends on RNA isolation and RT reaction. The recombinase allows the invasion of the ds cDNA by the primers to bind to their complementary regions. The ss DNA regions (or loops) that are created due to this invasion are stabilized by the binding of ss DNA-binding proteins (SSBPs). This prevents the re-binding of the original template strands (plus and minus). The recombinase enzyme is then displaced from the DNA by a strand-displacing DNA polymerase. This polymerase opens the template DNA structure as it synthesizes new DNA strands emanating from the primer (i.e. strand-displacing). All these components of RPA aim towards the elimination of the denaturation step in the PCR cycle, thus making it isothermal. This assay holds the capacity to be carried out in solid-phase, i.e. on a dry surface with immobilized components [28]. Although the load-of-detection (LOD) and time are compromised in solid-phase RPA [28], this feature can enable the designing of lyophilized kits with minimal storage and transport requirements.

End-point detection of RPA has been vastly calibrated to fit the lateral flow assays (LFA) [28]. This assay yields rapid results in a visual read-out format (**Figure 6**). To adapt RPA to LFA, three different oligonucleotides (2 primers and 1 probe) and a *nfo* nuclease are required. Similar to the TaqMan assay described above, the probe is flanked with a 5′ end antigenic label (usually

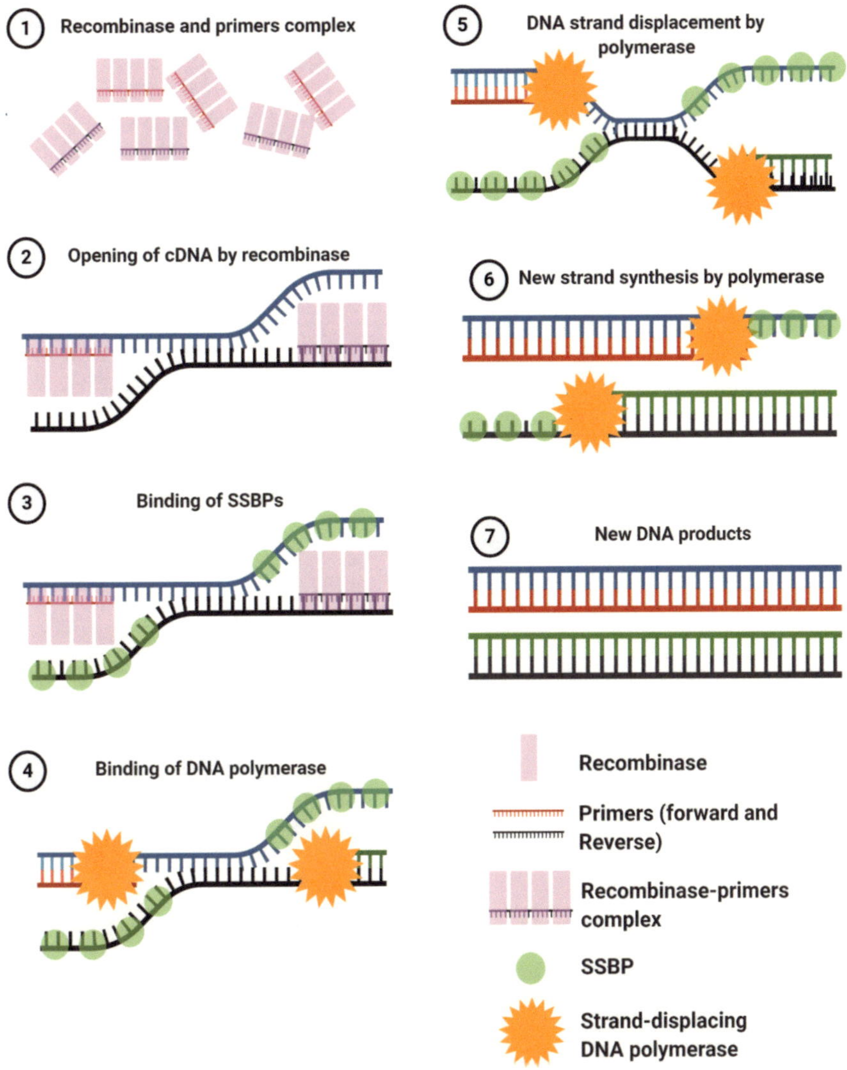

Figure 5.
Recombinase polymerase amplification (RPA). The primers and the recombinase enzyme are allowed to form a complex (1). The recombinase opens up the cDNA template, while the primers bind to their complementary regions (2). The ss DNA regions generated due to the opening of the template structure are stabilized through the binding of the single-strand binding proteins (SSBPs) (3). The DNA polymerase binds to the primers attached to the template DNA, detaching the recombinase (4). The polymerase extends the primers, while opening the ds template on its way. It also moves the SSBPs while synthesizing the new strands (5). New strands are synthesized by the polymerase (6). New ds DNA products which can act as templates for the following amplification cycles (7).

6-Carboxyfluorescein i.e. FAM) and a 3′ end blocking group [28]. The 3′ end group inhibits the DNA polymerase from extending the probe (remember that the polymerase can only add nucleotides at the 3′ end). In addition to these end groups, the probe is also equipped with an abasic nucleotide (tetrahydrofuran) which does not pair with any of the standard bases (A, T, G or C) [28]. This abasic nucleotide creates a fold in the probe that is bound to the complementary template DNA. The *nfo* nuclease recognizes this fold and nicks the probe at this position [28]. The abasic nucleotide is strategically positioned in the probe, such that the nick by the nuclease releases the 3′ end blocking group from the probe/template DNA complex [28]. This opens up the 3′ end for the polymerase to extend the new DNA strand from

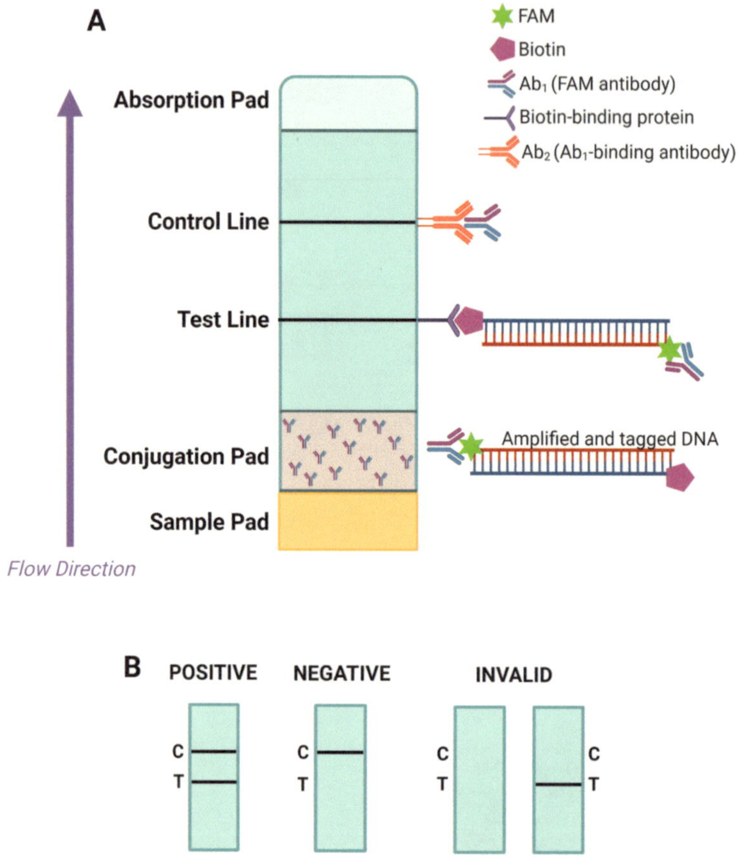

Figure 6.
Lateral flow assay. (A) The strip consists of the regions depicted in the figure. The sample is loaded onto the sample pad. The sample then moves upwards, towards the absorption pad due to capillary action. Sample comprises of the amplified ds DNA products with tags FAM and biotin at two separate ends. From the sample pad, the sample first moves to the conjugation pad which is pre-loaded with Ab_1 (antibodies against FAM). The Ab_1 antibodies bind to the FAM-DNA-biotin products. These complexes move upward and are captured at the test line by the immobilized biotin-binding proteins. This produces a visible test line. The unbound free Ab_1 antibodies (excess) from the conjugation pad also move upwards. These antibodies, however, move past the test line as they do not possess any biotin for interaction at this line. Upon reaching the control line, these antibodies are captured by Ab_2 (antibodies that can bind Ab_1). This interaction produces a visible control line. (B) The appearance of the positive, negative and invalid results. Positive result should show two lines, since it ensures the working of all components of the LFA strip. A conclusive negative result will only produce a control line which is generated by the interaction of immobilized Ab_2 with free unbound Ab_1. All other results are considered invalid.

the probe. The reverse primer (the primer that will bind to the opposite strand) is tagged with a 5'end ligand (usually biotin) [28]. The main feature of these two 5' end tags (FAM and biotin) is the availability of strong binding proteins or antibodies against them. The binding proteins or antibodies are immobilized on LFA strips (dipsticks) at two separate lines, test and control. The test band is coated with biotin-binding proteins (which will capture the 5'end tag of the reverse primer), while the control band is stacked with Ab_2 antibodies (which capture to unbound Ab_1 antibodies, see below). Once the stick is exposed to the sample (either through immersion of the sample pad or loading of the sample) on the sample pad, the sample moves across the conjugation pad which has lyophilized antibodies against FAM (Ab_1). Here the RPA ds DNA products which carry both the tags will be bound by Ab_1. From the conjugation pad, the complex containing Ab_1-RPA products will move further up the strip (due to capillary action) towards the test band. At this juncture, only DNA products which have the biotin tag will be captured by the biotin-binding proteins, showing a positive result. Further movement of these complexes is restricted as the binding proteins are immobilized onto the test line. Along with the complexes, the unbound free Ab_1 antibodies also move up from the conjugation pad. These free antibodies move further up from the test line as they do not carry any biotin. They are captured by the Ab_2 antibodies in the control line. Hence, a positive result should yield two distinct lines in the strip. In case of a negative sample, there is no fruitful conjugation of Ab_1 antibodies on the conjugation pad. However, due to capillary action of the sample, the Ab_1 move up the strip. Although these antibodies will not be captured at the test line, they will be immobilized by Ab_2 on the control line. Thus, a reliable negative result should show one control line on the strip. All other combinations would indicate inconclusive results.

Advantages:

1. Solid-phase RPA can yield kits with minimal needs for transport and storage, thereby significantly improving diagnostics at POC. However, more research is required in improving its LOD and TAT.

2. The LFA compatibility is useful in non-laboratory settings, again increasing its usage at POC.

3. RPA can be easily modified to accommodate the new mutations in target regions.

Limitations:

1. At present, RPA kits are sold by one company. This restricts modifications at the user's end.

2. Prior to LFA, there is a protein purification step to avoid impaired flow of the sample on the strip. This adds to TAT.

3. This assay still requires RNA isolation and reverse transcription steps. These add to the detection times.

5.3 LAMP (loop-mediated isothermal amplification)

LAMP is another isothermal amplification technique which produces long, self-complementary looping DNA strands to generate a detectable signal. This technique employs an engineered DNA polymerase *Bst* 2.0 with strand-displacing feature [29]. This enzyme can separate the two template DNA strands (plus and minus) as it builds the new strand, thus removing the denaturation step from PCR. LAMP is conducted at a single temperature (60–65 °C) [29], conducive to both the annealing and extension steps. Recent modifications include addition of the engineered RT enzyme along with the *Bst* 2.0 polymerase, thus making it a 1-step protocol [29]. Again, this assay still requires RNA isolation from the sample.

Generally, a set of 4 (or 6) specific primers are used in LAMP assay. These primers cover at least six distinct regions, flanking the entirety of the target region. A glimpse of the assay steps is described in **Figure 7**. The self-complementary regions of the primers promote the formation of looped DNA products. This allows LAMP to yield concatemers of various lengths, which are long DNA strands with multiple copies of the target region aligned back to each other [29]. Concatemers multiply the read-out signal at a much faster rate than RT-PCR. The mechanism is explained

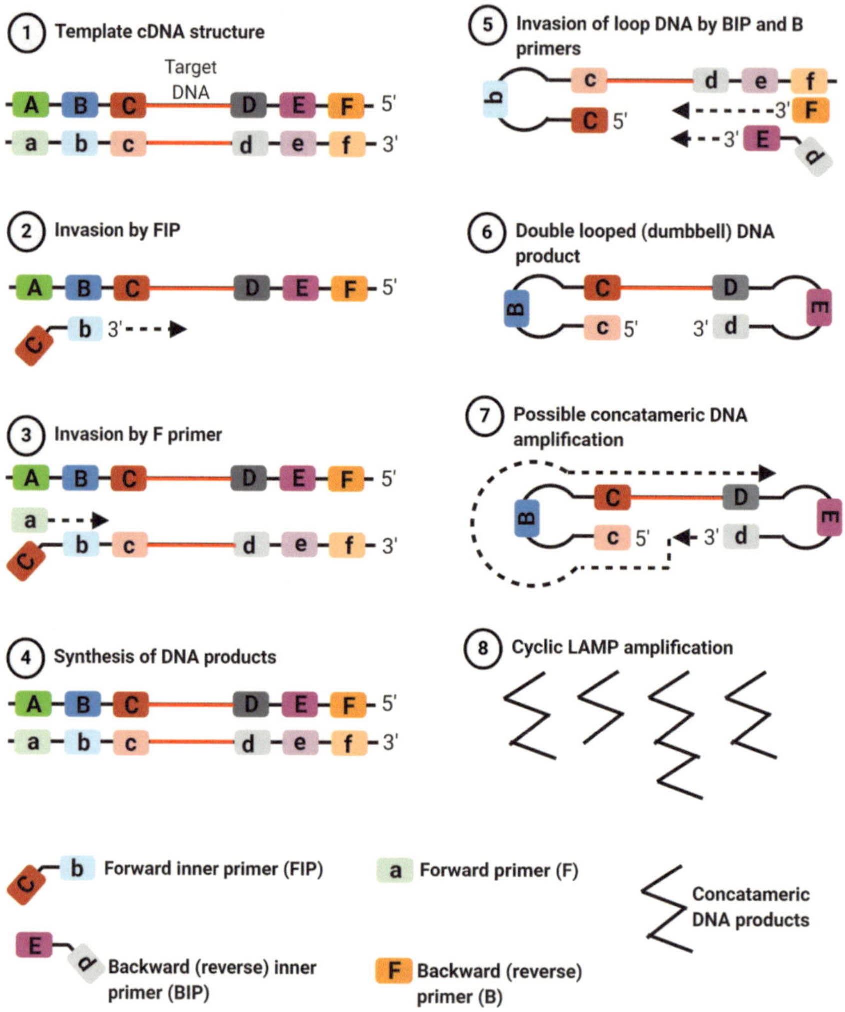

Figure 7.
LAMP. Six specific regions (A, B, C, D, E, F) flanking the target DNA are chosen to design the primers (1). The forwards inner primer (FIP) invades the target DNA. This primer encompasses a self-complementary region (C) on its 5′ end (2). The new strand synthesized with FIP is displaced by the forward primer (3). The DNA products synthesized by the forward primer is similar to the original cDNA template (4). Due to the self-complementarity region on the FIP, it folds on itself forming a loop. This strand is invaded by the backward inner primer (BIP) and backward primer (5). The product formed by BIP on the FIP strand leads to two loops at the ends, forming a dumbbell shaped structure (6). These strands can be extended to form concatemeric DNA products (7). Concatemeric products of variable lengths (8).

in the **Figure** 7. A review article by Thompson and Lei [29] is recommended for further reading on this assay. Here, I would like to highlight the modifications made to RT-LAMP to progress COVID-19 diagnostics.

This detection assay was developed to provide a visible color read-out. A colorimetric detection was incorporated using a simple pH-sensitive dye such as phenol red [29]. The color of this dye is closer to red when the pH is neutral (pH 7.0), and changes towards the yellow spectrum with acidic pH (pH < 7.0). The byproducts of DNA synthesis are acidic, which reduce the pH of the solution. This color change can be easily noted by eye, without any instrument. However, this detection method is limited by the baseline differences in the pH of collected specimens. To circumvent this, fluorescent dyes such as GeneFinder have been employed [29]. This dye produces green color under blue light illuminator to report positive results. Another variation of this assay excluded RNA isolation step to find comparable amplification of the N-protein gene under laboratory conditions [29]. This modification still needs more testing and evaluation with patient samples, prior to field use. After calibration, this assay could significantly reduce the TAT.

Moreover, individual samples can be tagged with specific barcodes in LAMP assay which allow tracing in a pooled sample [29]. A common method of barcoding is the transposase Tn5-adapter system [30]. The original article on this barcoding method is recommended to readers for understanding its mechanism and potential in diagnostics [30]. The barcodes, however, have to be read through NGS (next-generation sequencing), which requires specific lab equipment. This adds time for obtaining the results. It is possible that the bargain between time saved by pooling samples and the time added by NGS could be a deciding factor for the field-use application of this assay.

An important feature of LAMP is its amenability to be paired with other PCR techniques to combine their advantages. So far, the efficacy of LAMP has been tested after merging with RPA, using lab samples [29]. The combined assay is found to have increased sensitivity. RT-LAMP when integrated with CRISPR-Cas12 assay (described below) was shown to reduce detection time considerably [3].

Advantages:

1. This assay is conducted at a single temperature, and thus without a thermocycler.

2. The detection rate is much shorter than other mentioned techniques [3].

3. LAMP offers flexibility to be paired with other assays for improving their detection abilities.

4. This assay can be adapted to lab instrument-free detection methods.

5. Specificity of LAMP is higher than RT-PCR [3].

Limitations:

1. LAMP relies on precisely designed primers. Hence, it is more complicated to accommodate new mutations as compared to RT-PCR [3].

2. Sensitivity of LAMP is lower than the conventional RT-PCR [3].

3. Similar to the previously mentioned techniques, LAMP also requires RNA isolation and reverse transcription.

5.4 CRISPR-based assays

CRISPR (Clustered regularly interspaced short palindromic repeats)-Cas (CRISPR-associated nuclease) technology has been recently tested for its potency in the field of diagnostics. This technique, which was given recognition through the Nobel Prize in Chemistry 2020, is a modified biological process of the bacterial (prokaryotic) adaptive immune system [1]. Here a ss guide RNA (sgRNA or crRNA) leads/guides the CRISPR-Cas complex to the target nucleic acid region [1], owing to its complementarity to this region (**Figure 8**). Upon binding, Cas nuclease cleaves the template nucleic acid [1], along with non-specific cleavage of nearby ss DNA/RNA. This feature is called "collateral cleavage" activity [1], and has been used in

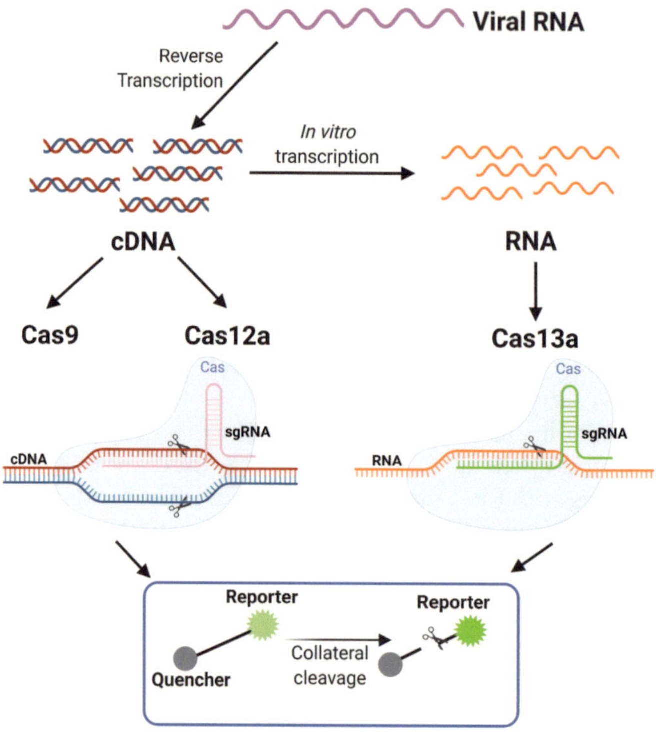

Figure 8.
CRISPR-Cas cleavage system. Viral RNA is reverse transcribed to ds cDNA, which can be further transcribed to amplified RNA through an in vitro system. The cDNA can be processed either through Cas9 or Cas12a, while the ss RNA can be cleaved through Cas13a. The single-guide RNA (sgRNA) or crRNA is complementary to the region of interest, and thus guides the Cas nuclease to the site. After target cleavage, collateral cleavage activity cleave and releases the reporter from quencher inhibition. This produces a detectable fluorescent signal, which is proportional to the amount of target DNA in the reaction.

designing read-out methods for diagnostic tests. This assay is equipped with ss DNA or RNA probes with a fluorescent or traceable reporter molecule, which produces a detectable signal only upon cleavage through collateral activity.

The target for CRISPR-Cas cleavage complex can be modified by changing the crRNA strand sequence, similar to the primers/probes in RT-PCR. Based on the Cas nuclease paired with the crRNA in the assay, the template can vary. For example, Cas13 targets ss RNA, while Cas9 or Cas12 target ds DNA [1]. Thus, in case of CoV-2, the virus ss RNA will need to be reverse transcribed to cDNA which will be either amplified as DNA products or through *in vitro* transcription as RNA products. CRISPR-Cas complexes cannot amplify nucleic acids, and hence rely on other amplification techniques for this (such as previously described methods).

A recently invented SHERLOCK (Specific high-sensitivity enzymatic reporter unlocking) technique includes the crRNA-Cas13a complex to target RNA molecules [1]. This technique uses RPA amplification assay and a non-targeting RNA strand tagged with a fluorescent dye [31]. Patchsung *et al.* [32] used SHERLOCK for CoV-2 diagnostics, targeting the S and ORF1ab genes. This assay has been further modified to suit LFA detection methods, i.e. using paper strips. Another variation of CRISPR-Cas technique is DETECTR, where it is combined with RT-LAMP amplification. This has been tested for CoV-2 E and N genes [33].

Ding *et al.* [34] developed an All-In-One Dual CRISPR-Cas12a (AIOD-CRISPR) assay where all the reactions components are incubated at 37 °C together. This simplifies the diagnostic assay protocol. The AIOD-CRISPR was then modified for a visual color detection in LED blue light illuminator.

Advantages:

1. CRISPR-Cas reactions can be conducted at 37 °C temperature. This is an achievable temperature at POC.

2. This is an isothermal reaction, and thereby does not depend on a thermocycler.

3. The basic CRISPR-Cas technology has the flexibility to be paired with other assays to reap advantages from both techniques.

4. DETECTR assay has a shorter process time as compared to conventional RT-PCR tests [3].

5. The sensitivity of CRISPR-based assays is higher than the other mentioned tests.

6. These assays can be adapted to non-instrumental detection methods like LFA or visible color change under blue light [3, 34].

Limitations:

1. Specificity of CRISPR-based assays is lower than that reported for RT-PCR.

2. These assays also require RNA extraction which adds to TAT.

3. Currently, there is no portable CRISPR-based devices which have been developed for CoV-2. Thus, more research in needed in this field.

4. Calibration of the assays is more complicated than the standard RT-PCR or RPA. Thus, although possible, it will take longer to modify these tests to detect new mutations of the target gene.

6. Conclusion

The current molecular diagnostic tests provide variable degrees of sensitivity and specificity to the detection of SARS-CoV-2. It is clear that at present there is no single assay which fits all the requirements. However, there are constant research efforts aimed at improving the efficiency and accessibility of these assays to meet the growing demand of this pandemic. The improved assays will increase our ability to combat COVID-19 spread, and enhance our preparedness for any future infectious agents by providing a strong platform for building new diagnostic tests.

Acknowledgements

All figures have been created with BioRender.com.

Author details

Vinita Chittoor-Vinod
Stanford University, Palo Alto, California, United States

*Address all correspondence to: chittoor@stanford.edu

'Biotechnology to Combat COVID-19' is a collaborative project with Biotechnology Kiosk

References

[1] Jayamohan H, Lambert CJ, Sant HJ, Jafek A, Patel D, Feng H, Beeman M, Mahmood T, Nze U, Gale BK. SARS-CoV-2 pandemic: a review of molecular diagnostic tools including sample collection and commercial response with associated advantages and limitations. Anal Bioanal Chem. 2020. 10.1007/s00216-020-02958-1

[2] V'Kovski P, Kratzel A, Steiner S, Stalder H, Thiel V. Coronavirus biology and replication: implications for SARS-CoV-2. Nat Rev Microbiol. 2020. 10.1038/s41579-020-00468-6

[3] Nguyen NNT, McCarthy C, Lantigua D, Camci-Unal G. Development of Diagnostic Tests for Detection of SARS-CoV-2. Diagnostics (Basel). 2020;10(11). 10.3390/diagnostics10110905

[4] Gandhi M, Yokoe DS, Havlir DV. Asymptomatic Transmission, the Achilles' Heel of Current Strategies to Control Covid-19. N Engl J Med. 2020;382(22):2158-2160. 10.1056/NEJMe2009758

[5] Pascarella G, Strumia A, Piliego C, Bruno F, Del Buono R, Costa F, Scarlata S, Agro FE. COVID-19 diagnosis and management: a comprehensive review. J Intern Med. 2020;288(2):192-206. 10.1111/joim.13091

[6] Caruana G, Croxatto A, Coste AT, Opota O, Lamoth F, Jaton K, Greub G. Diagnostic strategies for SARS-CoV-2 infection and interpretation of microbiological results. Clin Microbiol Infect. 2020;26(9):1178-1182. 10.1016/j.cmi.2020.06.019

[7] Etievant S, Bal A, Escuret V, Brengel-Pesce K, Bouscambert M, Cheynet V, Generenaz L, Oriol G, Destras G, Billaud G, Josset L, Frobert E, Morfin F, Gaymard A. Performance Assessment of SARS-CoV-2 PCR Assays Developed by WHO Referral Laboratories. J Clin Med. 2020;9(6). 10.3390/jcm9061871

[8] Yang Y, Xiao Z, Ye K, He X, Sun B, Qin Z, Yu J, Yao J, Wu Q, Bao Z, Zhao W. SARS-CoV-2: characteristics and current advances in research. Virol J. 2020;17(1):117. 10.1186/s12985-020-01369-z

[9] Thomas S. The Structure of the Membrane Protein of SARS-CoV-2 Resembles the Sugar Transporter SemiSWEET. Pathog Immun. 2020;5(1):342-63. 10.20411/pai.v5i1.377

[10] Letko M, Marzi A, Munster V. Functional assessment of cell entry and receptor usage for SARS-CoV-2 and other lineage B betacoronaviruses. Nat Microbiol. 2020;5(4):562-569. 10.1038/s41564-020-0688-y

[11] Hoffmann M, Kleine-Weber H, Schroeder S, Kruger N, Herrler T, Erichsen S, Schiergens TS, Herrler G, Wu NH, Nitsche A, Muller MA, Drosten C, Pohlmann S. SARS-CoV-2 Cell Entry Depends on ACE2 and TMPRSS2 and Is Blocked by a Clinically Proven Protease Inhibitor. Cell. 2020;181(2):271-280 e8. 10.1016/j.cell.2020.02.052

[12] Walls AC, Park YJ, Tortorici MA, Wall A, McGuire AT, Veesler D. Structure, Function, and Antigenicity of the SARS-CoV-2 Spike Glycoprotein. Cell. 2020;183(6):1735. 10.1016/j.cell.2020.11.032

[13] Lu R, Zhao X, Li J, Niu P, Yang B, Wu H, Wang W, Song H, Huang B, Zhu N, Bi Y, Ma X, Zhan F, Wang L, Hu T, Zhou H, Hu Z, Zhou W, Zhao L, Chen J, Meng Y, Wang J, Lin Y, Yuan J, Xie Z, Ma J, Liu WJ, Wang D, Xu W, Holmes EC, Gao GF, Wu G, Chen W, Shi W, Tan W. Genomic characterisation and epidemiology of 2019 novel coronavirus: implications for virus

origins and receptor binding. Lancet. 2020;395(10224):565-574. 10.1016/S0140-6736(20)30251-8

[14] Louten J. Virus Replication. Essential Human Virology: Academic Press; 2016. p. 49-70. B9780128009475000041

[15] Dorner T, Radbruch A. Antibodies and B cell memory in viral immunity. Immunity. 2007;27(3):384-392. 10.1016/j.immuni.2007.09.002

[16] Singanayagam A, Patel M, Charlett A, Lopez Bernal J, Saliba V, Ellis J, Ladhani S, Zambon M, Gopal R. Duration of infectiousness and correlation with RT-PCR cycle threshold values in cases of COVID-19, England, January to May 2020. Euro Surveill. 2020;25(32). 10.2807/1560-7917.ES.2020.25.32.2001483

[17] Woloshin S, Patel N, Kesselheim AS. False Negative Tests for SARS-CoV-2 Infection - Challenges and Implications. N Engl J Med. 2020;383(6):e38. 10.1056/NEJMp2015897

[18] Pray L. Discovery of DNA structure and function: Watson and Crick Nature Education2008 [Available from: https://www.nature.com/scitable/topicpage/discovery-of-dna-structure-and-function-watson-397/. https://www.nature.com/scitable/topicpage/discovery-of-dna-structure-and-function-watson-397/

[19] Pray *L. major* molecular events of DNA replication Nature Education2008 [Available from: https://www.nature.com/scitable/topicpage/major-molecular-events-of-dna-replication-413/. https://www.nature.com/scitable/topicpage/major-molecular-events-of-dna-replication-413/

[20] Clancy SB, W. Translation: DNA to mRNA to Protein Nature Education2008 [Available from: https://www.nature.com/scitable/topicpage/translation-dna-to-mrna-to-protein-393/. https://www.nature.com/scitable/topicpage/translation-dna-to-mrna-to-protein-393/

[21] CDC. Understanding mRNA COVID-19 Vaccines [Internet] 2020a [Available from: www.cdc.gov/coronavirus/2019-ncov/vaccines/different-vaccines/mrna.html. www.cdc.gov/coronavirus/2019-ncov/vaccines/different-vaccines/mrna.html

[22] Saiki RK, Gelfand DH, Stoffel S, Scharf SJ, Higuchi R, Horn GT, Mullis KB, Erlich HA. Primer-directed enzymatic amplification of DNA with a thermostable DNA polymerase. Science. 1988;239(4839):487-491. 10.1126/science.2448875

[23] Giglio S, Monis PT, Saint CP. Demonstration of preferential binding of SYBR Green I to specific DNA fragments in real-time multiplex PCR. Nucleic Acids Res. 2003;31(22):e136. 10.1093/nar/gng135

[24] Heid CA, Stevens J, Livak KJ, Williams PM. Real time quantitative PCR. Genome Res. 1996;6(10):986-994. 10.1101/gr.6.10.986

[25] Hirotsu Y, Maejima M, Shibusawa M, Nagakubo Y, Hosaka K, Amemiya K, Sueki H, Hayakawa M, Mochizuki H, Tsutsui T, Kakizaki Y, Miyashita Y, Omata M. Pooling RT-qPCR testing for SARS-CoV-2 in 1000 individuals of healthy and infection-suspected patients. Sci Rep. 2020;10(1):18899. 10.1038/s41598-020-76043-z

[26] CDC. Emerging SARS-CoV-2 variants [Internet] 2020b [Available from: www.cdc.gov/coronavirus/2019-ncov/more/science-and-research/scientific-brief-emerging-variants.html. www.cdc.gov/coronavirus/2019-ncov/more/science-and-research/scientific-brief-emerging-variants.html

[27] Dao Thi VL, Herbst K, Boerner K, Meurer M, Kremer LP, KirrmaierD,FreistaedterA,PapagiannidisD, Galmozzi C, Stanifer ML, Boulant S, Klein S, Chlanda P, Khalid D, Barreto Miranda I, Schnitzler P, Krausslich HG, Knop M, Anders S. A colorimetric RT-LAMP assay and LAMP-sequencing for detecting SARS-CoV-2 RNA in clinical samples. Sci Transl Med. 2020;12(556). 10.1126/scitranslmed.abc7075

[28] Lobato IM, O'Sullivan CK. Recombinase polymerase amplification: Basics, applications and recent advances. Trends Analyt Chem. 2018;98:19-35. 10.1016/j.trac.2017.10.015

[29] Thompson DaL, Y. Recent progress in RT-LAMP enabled COVID-19 detection. Sensors and Actuators Reports. 2020;2(1). https://doi.org/10.1016/j.snr.2020.100017

[30] Schmid-Burgk JL SR, Li D, Hollstein R, Ben-Shmuel A, Israeli O, Weiss S, Paran N, Wilbring G, Liebing J, , Feldman D SM, Lippke B, Sib E, Borrajo J, Strecker J,, Reinhardt J HP, Cleary B, Hölzel M, Nöthen MM, , Exner M LK, Regev A, Zhang F. LAMP-Seq: Population-Scale COVID-19 Diagnostics Using Combinatorial Barcoding. BioRxiv. 2020. https://doi.org/10.1101/2020.04.06.025635

[31] Kellner MJ, Koob JG, Gootenberg JS, Abudayyeh OO, Zhang F. SHERLOCK: nucleic acid detection with CRISPR nucleases. Nat Protoc. 2019;14(10):2986-3012. 10.1038/s41596-019-0210-2

[32] Patchsung M, Jantarug K, PattamaA,AphichoK,SuraritdechachaiS, MeesawatP,SappakhawK,LeelahakornN, RuenkamT,WongsatitT,AthipanyasilpN, Eiamthong B, Lakkanasirorat B, Phoodokmai T, Niljianskul N, PakotiprapheD,ChanaratS,HomchanA, Tinikul R, Kamutira P, Phiwkaow K, SoithongcharoenS,KantiwiriyawanitchC, Pongsupasa V, Trisrivirat D, Jaroensuk J, Wongnate T, Maenpuen S, Chaiyen P, Kamnerdnakta S, Swangsri J, Chuthapisith S, Sirivatanauksorn Y, ChaimayoC,SutthentR,KantakamalakulW, Joung J, Ladha A, Jin X, Gootenberg JS, AbudayyehOO,ZhangF,HorthongkhamN, Uttamapinant C. Clinical validation of a Cas13-based assay for the detection of SARS-CoV-2 RNA. Nat Biomed Eng. 2020;4(12):1140-9. 10.1038/s41551-020-00603-x

[33] Broughton JP, Deng X, Yu G, Fasching CL, Servellita V, Singh J, Miao X, Streithorst JA, Granados A, Sotomayor-Gonzalez A, Zorn K, Gopez A, Hsu E, Gu W, Miller S, Pan CY, Guevara H, Wadford DA, Chen JS, Chiu CY. CRISPR-Cas12-based detection of SARS-CoV-2. Nat Biotechnol. 2020;38(7):870-874. 10.1038/s41587-020-0513-4

[34] Ding X, Yin K, Li Z, Liu C. All-in-One Dual CRISPR-Cas12a (AIOD-CRISPR) Assay: A Case for Rapid, Ultrasensitive and Visual Detection of Novel Coronavirus SARS-CoV-2 and HIV virus. bioRxiv. 2020. 10.1101/2020.03.19.998724

Chapter 10

The Utility of Mechanical Homogenization in COVID-19 Diagnostic Workflows

Zachary P. Morehouse, Rodney J. Nash, Caleb Proctor and Gabriella Ryan

Abstract

The use of mechanical homogenization in patient sample preparation for COVID-19 diagnostics has proven impactful in the face of the global pandemic caused by SARS-CoV-2. Through methods including bead beating and shaker mill homogenization novel approaches to viral detection have been developed and improvements have been made to existing diagnostic workflows for the improvement of throughput and automation capacity. The application of mechanical homogenization techniques has enhanced the sensitivity and methodology for many molecular based approaches to COVID-19 detection and from a variety of sample types ranging from saliva to nasopharyngeal swabs. Additionally, this technology has been used to help increase laboratory safety during sample processing through efficient viral lysis. Herein, the many benefits of mechanical homogenization for COVID-19 detection will be discussed in the context of the many diagnostic workflows currently utilizing the technique.

Keywords: PCR, viral diagnostics, viral detection, antigen diagnostics, antigen detection, molecular diagnostics, COVID-19, homogenization, sample preparation, bead mill, shaker mill, bead beater

1. Introduction

Traditionally the process of mechanical homogenization has been employed in the laboratory setting for the disruption of animal or plant tissues in preparation for downstream molecular applications [1]. However, in the face of a global pandemic this technology has been adapted to increase efficacy and efficiency in viral detection in a variety of COVID-19 diagnostic workflows [2–4].

As the global community began to respond to the spread of SARS-CoV-2, the expansion of public health surveillance programs and community testing protocols became critical objectives [5]. However, the need for rapid expansion in testing capacity caused a tremendous strain on the supply chains providing the equipment and reagents traditionally needed for respiratory virus PCR-based testing [6]. As in most cases, necessity drove innovation. Given the large number of research and academic laboratories equipped to assist in PCR testing, many groups began to offer their assistance in processing patient samples while others began examining novel approaches to viral detection which circumvented the supply chain bottle necks. During the development of these novel testing protocols laboratory safety, diagnostic assay sensitivity and specificity became top priority [5–7]. In an attempt to utilize common laboratory equipment to safely speed up testing efforts, the use of mechanical homogenization was proposed to inactivate the SARS-CoV-2 from nasopharyngeal swabs as a method of increasing safety during processing [2–4, 8].

In brief, mechanical homogenization is the process of using shearing forces applied via mechanical grinding media and rigorous repetitive motion to dissociates a given sample [1]. The parameters at which a sample is processed will impact the degree to which it is dissociated and the quality of the targeted product for downstream applications [1]. In the case of SARS-CoV-2, the goal of mechanical homogenization was to disrupt the viral envelope while still maintaining the integrity of its RNA [2, 3]. This allowed for a reduction in infective potential in the laboratory setting, while preserving the accuracy of polymerase chain reaction (PCR) based diagnostic assays [2, 3].

Following the initial application of mechanical homogenization to COVID-19 swab-based PCR protocols, this technology was adapted to process saliva samples for both antigen and PCR detection workflows [2–4]. Through mechanical homogenization, high viscosity saliva samples were sufficiently processed to allow for automation integration, paving the way for the widespread application of this novel methodology [4, 9].

In this chapter we will further explore the applications of homogenization in response to the COVID-19 pandemic and the multiple diagnostic methodologies this technology has been implemented in and its impact on laboratory safety and overall testing efficiency.

2. Direct-to-PCR testing with shaker mill homogenization of nasopharyngeal swabs

During the late spring of 2020, while SARS-CoV-2 was spreading exponentially and uncontrollably across the globe, testing for this disease was focused entirely on RT-qPCR detection of the virus using US CDC or WHO approved primers [5, 10]. The traditional method for these types of RT-qPCR tests involved two major components. First, the process of virus inactivation and RNA extraction completed through a series of chemical reactions that resulted in purified viral RNA from the provided patient sample [5, 6, 10]. The extracted RNA was then utilized in the second half of this method, amplification and detection [5, 6, 10]. Through RT-qPCR, the purified RNA from the patient sample was combined with the preapproved primers for attempted amplification of the targeted genes, indicating the presence or absence of SARS-CoV-2 depending on the level of amplification seen [5, 6, 10]. The RNA amplification was quantified and reported out as a Cq value, with any Cq less than 40 qualifying as a COVID-19 positive sample per the US CDC and WHO guidelines [10].

The necessity of testing drove up demand for all reagents, machines, and plastics utilized in the RT-qPCR testing method, overstressing the supply chain for these products [5, 8, 9]. Additionally, the need for cold storage of reagents involved in the extraction process and the high price tag on the automated machinery needed to complete both the extraction and detection phases of the traditional testing method, furthered the gap between resource challenged areas and the industrialized regions when it came to COVID-19 testing infrastructure [11, 12]. Areas with the capital needed to create multimillion dollar testing facilities were able to do so, improving their public health response to the pandemic, while those lacking that investment and infrastructure were left with reduced testing capabilities [11]. A critical need arose for a cost efficient, yet safe and effective testing methodology that could be implemented in these resources challenged settings [8, 11].

While the utility of mechanical homogenization in COVID-19 testing was already established as an effective adjunct to the extraction process, improving sensitivity through efficient viral lysis, this process was expanded upon in an attempt to remove the extraction process entirely allowing for direct detection of SARS-CoV-2 from lysed patient samples [2, 3]. The direct-to-PCR approach for COVID-19 testing arose out of necessity to reduce the use of costly reagents in a period where the strain on the supply chain made them difficult to come by [2, 3, 8]. Additionally, this proposed method dramatically reduces cost when compared with the fully automated extraction machinery [2, 3, 8].

In the direct-to-PCR method for viral detection, shaker mill mechanical homogenization was proposed to provide sufficient viral lysis off nasopharyngeal swabs to expose adequate amounts of RNA for RT-qPCR detection [2, 3]. This method was shown to lyse greater than 95% of virus off a nasopharyngeal swab, allowing the resultant lysate to be placed directly into the RT-qPCR reaction as denoted in **Figure 1** [2, 3].

Through proof-of-concept testing with a close relative of SARS-CoV-2, human coronavirus 229E (HCoV-229E), and direct comparison studies between the traditional extraction-based method and the direct-to-PCR method, it was shown that the two methods had above a 94% agreeability in the detection of positive samples [2, 3]. Utilizing the direct-to-PCR method diagrammed in **Figure 1**, shaker mill homogenization was proven to be a viable alternative to the traditional extraction-based method for RT-qPCR detection of SARS-CoV-2 off nasopharyngeal swabs [2, 3].

In addition to the quality of the matched proven efficacy with the traditional, extraction-based methodology, the direct-to-PCR method described utilizing mechanical homogenization also reduces the total cost and time per swab processed [2, 3, 8]. The traditional model for nasopharyngeal swab viral testing cost $10 - $40 USD per swab, when taking into account the extraction kits, automation equipment for extractions, and the RT-qPCR set up [8]. Compared to $3 - $5 USD per swab with the homogenization methodology, given that this workflow does not require additional reagents for viral nucleotide extraction and purification, the only reagent costs are associated with the final RT-qPCR testing [8]. The homogenization equipment utilized in this workflow is sold at a fraction of the cost of the large fully automated extraction machinery.

Along with reducing cost per sample the homogenization workflow reduces the total processing time per sample from approximately 3 hours to 1 hour and 15 minutes [2, 3]. This is accomplished through replacing the extraction and purification steps of the traditional workflow with a 30 sec homogenization step preceding the RT-qPCR [2, 3]. Further supporting the implementation of this workflow into

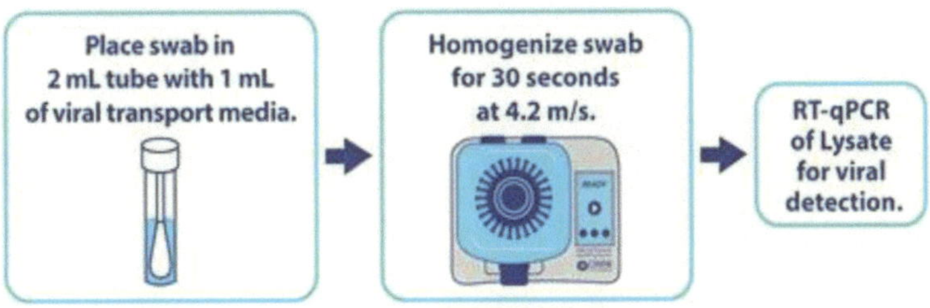

Figure 1.
The direct-to-PCR viral detection methodology using shaker mill homogenization off nasopharyngeal swabs.

the COVID-19 testing repertoire to assist in increasing access to cost effective and timely viral detection methods that maintain sensitivity and specificity when compared to the traditional testing methodologies [8].

3. PCR detection of COVID-19 from saliva utilizing bead beating homogenization

After months of nasopharyngeal swabbing for COVID-19 diagnostic testing, there was a push to look for equally sensitive testing methodologies which provided a more pleasant patient experience during sample collection [4, 6, 9]. By improving the patient experience with testing, the hope was to gain public cooperation with viral surveillance efforts [9, 13]. The high concentration of SARS-CoV-2 particles found throughout the upper respiratory tract led researchers to begin examining the utility of oral swabs or saliva in the current RT-qPCR testing strategies [13, 14].

Saliva samples were shown to have adequate viral loads for reliable RT-qPCR detection, however the high viscosity of the samples made them difficult to pipette preventing the utilization of the fully automated extraction machinery already in place in many large public health testing facilities [9, 13, 14]. Mechanical homogenization in the form of beat beating homogenization was introduced to saliva samples to break up the viscous structure and expose the viral particles [4, 15]. The beat beating strategy utilized ceramic bead media within a 2 mL screw capped sample tube and a mechanical homogenizer to apply rigorous kinetic energy to the saliva sample for 30 seconds to achieve complete dissociation (**Figure 2**) [4, 15]. It was shown that the kinetic energy transferred from the bead beading media homogenized in a sigmoidal pattern was highly effective in dissociating the sample to allow for pipettable lysate that could then be implemented into fully automated extraction-based PCR testing workflows [1, 4, 15]. With the addition of bead beating homogenization to this workflow, the throughput and sensitivity of the assay were dramatically increased [4, 15]. Prior to the implementation of beat beating homogenization, saliva-based testing demonstrated a sensitivity in the mid to low 80% range and throughput was limited to a few hundred samples per day via manual processing [4, 15]. Currently, saliva-based PCR testing utilizing mechanical homogenization prior to extraction procedures demonstrated a 95% sensitivity and 99% specificity, closely matching that of nasopharyngeal swab-based testing for COVID-19 [4, 13–15]. Additionally, with the capability of full automation integration, throughput of sample processing increased from hundreds to thousands of samples per day with the utilization of bead beating homogenization equipment [4, 15].

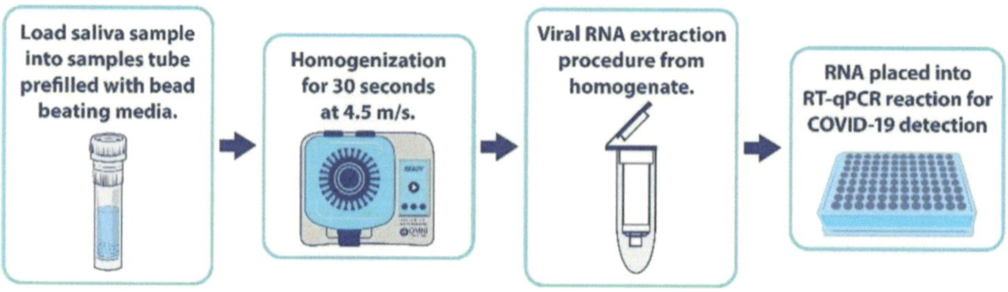

Figure 2.
The methodology for saliva-based testing utilizing bead beating mechanical homogenization for adequate sample dissociation and viral lysis followed by RNA extraction for RT-qPCR viral detection.

Given the similar sensitivity and specificity for SARS-CoV-2 testing, with the improvement in patient experience during sample collection, this method was implemented at universities across the state of Georgia as a community surveillance program [4, 15]. The difference in patient experience from obtaining a nasopharyngeal swab versus a saliva sample for weekly surveillance measures dramatically improved community compliance with testing, validating saliva testing as a viable public health surveillance strategy for COVID-19 propagation in a community [4, 6, 13–15]. Similar entities have now implemented saliva-based testing that utilize front-end mechanical homogenization across the world to improve compliance with public health testing efforts [4, 6, 15].

4. Viral antigen detection from saliva

The United States' Food and Drug Administration (FDA) has approved the use of antigen testing for the detection of SARS-CoV-2 in the summer of 2020 to increase the national testing capacity [6, 16]. Antigen tests are immunoassays that are commonly used in the diagnosis of respiratory pathogens such as influenza [17]. Antigen test are designed to detect the presence of a specific viral antigen, which is defined as a toxin or other foreign substance which induces an immune response [16, 17]. Antigen test are currently approved for nasopharyngeal swab specimens however studies suggest saliva samples may be just as effective in detecting viral antigens [6, 16, 18]. When compared to PCR test, antigen testing is relatively inexpensive, and most test results are available in 15 minutes or less. Antigen test in general are less sensitive than RT-PCR test as well as other nucleic acid amplification test (NAATs) [19]. Alternatively, RT-PCR can amplify and detect minute levels of nucleic acid that cannot be cultured which in this case suggest the presence of viral nucleic acids does not signify contagiousness [20]. Both antigen and nucleic acid tests are optimal when the patient is at their viral load peek [6, 16, 20]. More data is needed to guide the use of antigen tests on asymptomatic individuals and to determine if those who were at one time diagnosed positive for SARS-CoV-2 remain infectious.

The advantage of antigen testing is its convenience and accessibility in the use screening high-risk congregate settings such as primary or secondary educational environments, as well as correctional facilities [16, 21]. Repeat testing could quickly identify infection, therefore allowing implementation of patient quarantine and other preventive measure. However, health care professionals need to understand the limitations of antigen testing [19, 20]. Specifically, the testing factors and analytical performance characteristics, such as sensitivity, specificity, and accurate positive and negative predicted values. The "Holy Grail" for SARS-CoV-2 testing remains to be RT-PCR or some form of nucleic acid amplification testing [21]. Nucleic acid testing should be used to confirm an antigen test to avoid inconsistent and inaccurate results test performance may vary based on specimen choice, quality of specimen, the presence of transport medium, and the amount of time required for transport [20, 21]. Since antigen test are typically less sensitive than NAAT testing, negative results can occur while RT-PCR tests may return a positive result [19]. This may occur is specimen sample is collected early before symptom onset or late in the infection [19, 20]. The specificity of antigen tests is as high as NAAT testing, reducing the likelihood of false positives [16, 21]. False positive will still occur, particularly in communities where prevalence of infection is low [16, 20, 21]. The CDC recommends testing professionals establish infection prevalence for antigen testing based on a rolling average, using the positivity rate of their own SARS-CoV-2 testing over the previous 7–10 days, while considering the clinical and epidemiological context of the person or community being tested [6, 16].

Despite the debated advantages and disadvantages of antigen testing, the concept of saliva-based antigen testing for SARS-CoV-2 detection gained traction due to the ease of use for the patient and potential for rapid turn around time in laboratory processing to support public health efforts. However, as noted in the previous section on saliva-based PCR testing, working with such a viscous material posed difficulty in automation integration prior to the addition of homogenization into the workflow. Antigen testing faced similar difficulties when using saliva for large scale testing, the viscous patient samples required further processing prior to automation integration.

In an attempt to mitigate variations in saliva viscosities and allow for sample integration into high-throughput liquid handler reliant workflows, several protocols were developed to dissociate the saliva samples while maintaining intact antigen for detection [6, 22]. These protocols recommend various combinations of heating and enzyme digestion; heating greater than 60 degrees centigrade for as long as an hour or incubating with Proteinase K as an enzymatic digestion [23]. Reports have found these techniques to be somewhat effective in permitting antigen detection from saliva samples, however inconsistencies have also been scored [18, 20, 23]. Heating can denature the viral proteins and RNA, rendering them undetectable, and enzymes such as Proteinase K is very costly as well as cause degradation of targeted proteins through excessive digestion [20]. Not to mention the suggested incubation periods as great as an hour extends the amount of time required to have a patients' result.

Just as with saliva-based PCR testing, homogenization was proposed as a method for efficient sample disruption [24]. Viscosity in homogenized saliva samples has been shown to be greatly reduced to amounts that are similar to those found in water. Allowing for ease in pipetting and increase throughput using automation and liquid handlers [15]. The various forces found in homogenization are only required for small amounts of processing time, as short as 5 seconds per sample without generating any extra heat during the processing, maintaining the integrity of the antigens targeted. In contrast to other proposed methods for saliva processing in antigen detection, additional enzymes are not required, saving costs and without any needed incubation steps, also saving valuable time during testing.

5. Improving laboratory safety with homogenization

During the COVID-19 global pandemic, safety of all individuals involved in the care of COVID-19 patients as well as laboratory and clinical staff involved in testing for SARS-CoV-2 became a top priority. Given the highly virulent nature of SARS-CoV-2 and the lack of knowledge and treatments we had available, it was essential to neutralize the virus during laboratory testing while preserving the diagnostic capacity of all assays [5]. Employing viral neutralization techniques in the diagnostic workflow was a critical step in increasing the number of facilities available to process COVID-19 patient samples, supporting increased public health testing efforts.

Techniques involving thermal inactivation, chemical neutralization or degradation, enzymatic digestion, and mechanical disruption of samples were all proposed as potential solutions to laboratory safety when handling potential COVID-19 positive patient samples [5, 6]. However, given the global strain on the plastics and chemical reagents needed to complete many of these neutralization steps, the authors felt it was prudent to examine the potential of mechanical sample dissociation in the form of homogenization and its effect on virus neutralization [2, 3, 8]. Ultimately, it was shown that following 30 seconds of homogenization, 98% of the virus in any given sample was inactivated, while still preserving the genetic material for adequate PCR detection [2, 3]. This finding supported expanding the implementation of homogenization in the COVID-19 diagnostic workflow because it could be done both in the laboratory setting, as well as the location of sample collection provided the homogenized sample would be properly refrigerated and transferred for PCR detection within the next 12 hours [2–4, 15].

The mechanical lysis of the SARS-CoV-2 particles in a potentially infectious sample permitted these samples to be processed in a BSL-2 facility, supporting the expansion of laboratory testing facilities equipped to process COVID-19 samples [2, 3, 8]. Without a proven neutralization step, such as mechanical homogenization, all COVID-19 samples would have to be processed in BSL-3 facilities due to the potential risk of exposure to infectious virus. While it is still recommended that the homogenization procedure occur in a biosafety cabinet within a BSL-2 facility, the procedure provides sufficient viral lysis to improve safety when handling potentially infected patient samples and allows additional laboratories to assist with testing in a cost-effective manner [2, 3, 8, 15].

6. Conclusion

Mechanical homogenization has proven its utility in the response to COVID-19 through shaker mill and bead beating technologies implemented in a variety of diagnostic workflows [2–4, 8, 15]. These innovations made possible through effective and efficient viral lysis of SARS-CoV-2 are proving to improve access, speed, and safety while processing patient samples [2–4, 8, 15]. As the global community continues to push innovation to combat COVID-19, mechanical homogenization should be viewed as one of the many repurposed technologies adapted to assist with the response through improving the safety and efficacy of diagnostic testing in a cost-effective manner.

Acknowledgements

The authors would like to acknowledge the laboratory interns and personnel which worked so diligently to support the research efforts of this and all other projects in our laboratory; Mr. Brandon Easparro, Ms. Taylor White, and Ms. Akelachi Okparanta. We would also like to thank Mr. Brent Barton for his contribution to our publications through graphics development, including but not limited to, the graphics used in this manuscript. Additionally, we would like to recognize the following researchers for their assistance in procuring the samples needed to conduct the research studies which allowed us to complete this chapter; Drs. Angel Rivera and Maria Nagy of Quorum X Diagnostics (Tucker, GA, USA), Dr. Michael Shannon of The Georgia Tech Research Institute (Atlanta, GA, USA), Dr. John Roback of Emory University School of Medicine (Atlanta, GA, USA), and Dr. Tonney Nyirenda of the University of Malawi College of Medicine (Blantyre, Malawi).

Conflict of interest

All authors of this chapter are employed by PerkinElmer Inc. in some capacity; however, they have no personal financial incentives in the success or failure of the company, nor was their research referenced in this chapter impacted or influenced by their employment status or any financial incentives. RJ Nash is the owner of

Jeevan BioSciences with personal financial interest in the company; however, none of the research conducted for this chapter directly benefited Jeevan BioSciences, nor did his ownership impact the research.

Thanks

The authors would like to thank Mr. Pete Tortorelli and Mr. Karl Jahn for trusting us enough to support our preliminary research efforts and their continued support of our scholarly activities. Additionally, we would like to acknowledge and thank Ms. Rachel True, Mrs. Rachel Nash, and Mrs. Leah Proctor for their incredible patience, support, and sacrifices made for our research, it does not go unnoticed or unappreciated.

Acronyms and abbreviations

PCR	polymerase chain reaction.
RT-PCR	reverse transcriptase polymerase chain reaction.
RT-qPCR	quantitative reverse transcriptase polymerase chain reaction.
US CDC	US Centers for Disease Control and Prevention.
WHO	World Health Organization.
FDA	Food and Drug Administration.

Author details

Zachary P. Morehouse[1,2,3*], Rodney J. Nash[2,3,4], Caleb Proctor[2] and Gabriella Ryan[2]

1 Michigan State University College of Osteopathic Medicine, East Lansing, MI, USA

2 Omni International Inc, A PerkinElmer Company, Kennesaw, GA, USA

3 Jeevan BioSciences, Tucker, GA, USA

4 Department of Biology, Georgia State University, Atlanta, GA USA

*Address all correspondence to: moreho17@msu.edu

References

[1] Atwood J.A. Systems for Mechanical Sample Lysis and Homogenization for Molecular Biology Applications. In: Micic M. (eds) Sample Preparation Techniques for Soil, Plant, and Animal Samples. Springer Protocols Handbooks. Humana Press, New York, NY: 2016. Pg. 69-84. DOI: 10.1007/978-1-4939-3185-9_6

[2] Morehouse ZP, Proctor CM, Ryan GL, Nash RJ. A novel two-step, direct-to-PCR method for virus detection off swabs using human coronavirus 229E. Virol J. 2020 Aug 25;17(1):129. doi: 10.1186/s12985-020-01405-y. PMID: 32843049; PMCID: PMC7445803.

[3] Morehouse ZP, Proctor CM, Ryan GL, Nash RJ. 693. Shaking Things Up: Direct-to-PCR Viral Detection off Swabs Using Shaker-Mill Homogenization, Open Forum Infectious Diseases, Volume 7, Issue Supplement_1, October 2020, Page S399, https://doi.org/10.1093/ofid/ofaa439.885

[4] Sahajpal NS, Mondal AK, Ananth S, Njau A, Ahluwalia P, Chaubey A, Kota V, Caspary K, Ross TM, Farrell M, Shannon MP, Rojiani AM, Kolhe R. SalivaAll: Clinical validation of a sensitive test for saliva collected in healthcare and community settings with pooling utility for SARS-CoV-2 mass surveillance. medRxiv. 1 September 2020. doi: 10.1101/2020.08.26.20182816

[5] Cheng MP, Papenburg J, Desjardins M, Kanjilal S, Quach C, Libman M, Dittrich S, Yansouni CP. Diagnostic Testing for Severe Acute Respiratory Syndrome-Related Coronavirus 2: A Narrative Review. Ann Intern Med. 2020 Jun 2;172(11):726-734. doi: 10.7326/M20-1301. Epub 2020 Apr 13. PMID: 32282894; PMCID: PMC7170415.

[6] Yüce M, Filiztekin E, Özkaya KG. COVID-19 diagnosis -A review of current methods. Biosens Bioelectron. 2021 Jan 15;172:112752. doi: 10.1016/j.bios.2020.112752. Epub 2020 Oct 24. PMID: 33126180; PMCID: PMC7584564.

[7] Younes N, Al-Sadeq DW, Al-Jighefee H, Younes S, Al-Jamal O, Daas HI, Yassine HM, Nasrallah GK. Challenges in Laboratory Diagnosis of the Novel Coronavirus SARS-CoV-2. Viruses. 2020 May 26;12(6):582. doi: 10.3390/v12060582. PMID: 32466458; PMCID: PMC7354519.

[8] Morehouse ZP, Proctor CM, Ryan GL, Nash RJ. Direct-to-PCR Viral Diagnostic Testing, A Model to Reduce Cost and Increase Access for Underserved Communities. Virology and Mycology. Vol. 9(3):194. 1 December 2020. 9:194.2161-0517.20.09.194

[9] Sahajpal NS, Mondal AK, Njau A, Ananth S, Ghamande S, Hegde M, Chaubey A, M Rojiani A, Kolhe R. COVID-19 screening in a healthcare or community setting: complexity of saliva as a specimen for PCR-based testing. Future Med Chem. 2021 Jan;13(1):9-12. doi: 10.4155/fmc-2020-0255. Epub 2020 Nov 24. PMID: 33228389; PMCID: PMC7684981.

[10] Bustin SA, Nolan T. RT-qPCR Testing of SARS-CoV-2: A Primer. Int J Mol Sci. 2020 Apr 24;21(8):3004. doi: 10.3390/ijms21083004. PMID: 32344568; PMCID: PMC7215906.

[11] Hashmi SK, Murad MH, Theel ES. Screening for SARS-CoV-2: Health Policy Implications in Low- and Middle-Income Countries. Mayo Clin Proc. 2020 Dec;95(12):2606-2608. doi: 10.1016/j.mayocp.2020.10.007. Epub 2020 Oct 15. PMID: 33276834; PMCID: PMC7561345.

[12] Nachega JB, Atteh R, Ihekweazu C, Sam-Agudu NA, Adejumo P, Nsanzimana S, Rwagasore E,

Condo J, Paleker M, Mahomed H, Suleman F, Ario AR, Kiguli-Malwadde E, Omaswa FG, Sewankambo NK, Viboud C, Reid MJA, Zumla A, Kilmarx PH. Contact Tracing and the COVID-19 Response in Africa: Best Practices, Key Challenges, and Lessons Learned from Nigeria, Rwanda, South Africa, and Uganda. Am J Trop Med Hyg. 2021 Feb 11:tpmd210033. doi: 10.4269/ajtmh.21-0033. Epub ahead of print. PMID: 33571138.

[13] Bastos ML, Perlman-Arrow S, Menzies D, Campbell JR. The Sensitivity and Costs of Testing for SARS-CoV-2 Infection With Saliva Versus Nasopharyngeal Swabs : A Systematic Review and Meta-analysis. Ann Intern Med. 2021 Jan 12:M20-6569. doi: 10.7326/M20-6569. Epub ahead of print. PMID: 33428446; PMCID: PMC7822569.

[14] Medeiros da Silva RC, Nogueira Marinho LC, de Araújo Silva DN, Costa de Lima K, Pirih FQ, Luz de Aquino Martins AR. Saliva as a possible tool for the SARS-CoV-2 detection: A review. Travel Med Infect Dis. 2020 Nov-Dec;38:101920. doi: 10.1016/j.tmaid.2020.101920. Epub 2020 Nov 19. PMID: 33220456; PMCID: PMC7674016.

[15] Omni International, A PerkinElmer Company. SARS-CoV-2 Detection in Saliva Using Bead Beating Homogenization and an RT-PCR Test Kit [Internet]. 2021. Available from: https://www.omni-inc.com/index.php/downloads/dl/file/id/122/product/0/202019_sars_cov_2_saliva_app_note_v2.pdf [Accessed: 2021-02-05]

[16] Dinnes J, Deeks JJ, Adriano A, Berhane S, Davenport C, Dittrich S, Emperador D, Takwoingi Y, Cunningham J, Beese S, Dretzke J, Ferrante di Ruffano L, Harris IM, Price MJ, Taylor-Phillips S, Hooft L, Leeflang MM, Spijker R, Van den Bruel A; Cochrane COVID-19 Diagnostic Test Accuracy Group. Rapid, point-of-care antigen and molecular-based tests for diagnosis of SARS-CoV-2 infection. Cochrane Database Syst Rev. 2020 Aug 26;8:CD013705. doi: 10.1002/14651858.CD013705. PMID: 32845525.

[17] Food and Drug Administration, HHS. Microbiology Devices; Reclassification of Influenza Virus Antigen Detection Test Systems Intended for Use Directly With Clinical Specimens. Final order. Fed Regist. 2017 Jan 12;82(8):3609-3619. PMID: 28102980.

[18] Hirotsu Y, Maejima M, Shibusawa M, Nagakubo Y, Hosaka K, Amemiya K, Sueki H, Hayakawa M, Mochizuki H, Tsutsui T, Kakizaki Y, Miyashita Y, Yagi S, Kojima S, Omata M. Comparison of automated SARS-CoV-2 antigen test for COVID-19 infection with quantitative RT-PCR using 313 nasopharyngeal swabs, including from seven serially followed patients. Int J Infect Dis. 2020 Oct;99:397-402. doi: 10.1016/j.ijid.2020.08.029. Epub 2020 Aug 12. PMID: 32800855; PMCID: PMC7422837.

[19] Scohy A, Anantharajah A, Bodéus M, Kabamba-Mukadi B, Verroken A, Rodriguez-Villalobos H. Low performance of rapid antigen detection test as frontline testing for COVID-19 diagnosis. J Clin Virol. 2020 Aug;129:104455. doi: 10.1016/j.jcv.2020.104455. Epub 2020 May 21. PMID: 32485618; PMCID: PMC7240272.

[20] Younes N, Al-Sadeq DW, Al-Jighefee H, Younes S, Al-Jamal O, Daas HI, Yassine HM, Nasrallah GK. Challenges in Laboratory Diagnosis of the Novel Coronavirus SARS-CoV-2. Viruses. 2020 May 26;12(6):582. doi: 10.3390/v12060582. PMID: 32466458; PMCID: PMC7354519.

[21] Yamayoshi S, Sakai-Tagawa Y, Koga M, Akasaka O, Nakachi I, Koh H, Maeda K, Adachi E, Saito M, Nagai H, Ikeuchi K, Ogura T, Baba R,

Fujita K, Fukui T, Ito F, Hattori SI, Yamamoto K, Nakamoto T, Furusawa Y, Yasuhara A, Ujie M, Yamada S, Ito M, Mitsuya H, Omagari N, Yotsuyanagi H, Iwatsuki-Horimoto K, Imai M, Kawaoka Y. Comparison of Rapid Antigen Tests for COVID-19. Viruses. 2020 Dec 10;12(12):1420. doi: 10.3390/v12121420. PMID: 33322035; PMCID: PMC7764512.

[22] Nagura-Ikeda M, Imai K, Tabata S, Miyoshi K, Murahara N, Mizuno T, Horiuchi M, Kato K, Imoto Y, Iwata M, Mimura S, Ito T, Tamura K, Kato Y. Clinical Evaluation of Self-Collected Saliva by Quantitative Reverse Transcription-PCR (RT-qPCR), Direct RT-qPCR, Reverse Transcription-Loop-Mediated Isothermal Amplification, and a Rapid Antigen Test To Diagnose COVID-19. J Clin Microbiol. 2020 Aug 24;58(9):e01438-20. doi: 10.1128/JCM.01438-20. PMID: 32636214; PMCID: PMC7448663.

[23] Azzi L, Maurino V, Baj A, Dani M, d'Aiuto A, Fasano M, Lualdi M, Sessa F, Alberio T. Diagnostic Salivary Tests for SARS-CoV-2. J Dent Res. 2021 Feb;100(2):115-123. doi: 10.1177/0022034520969670. Epub 2020 Oct 31. PMID: 33131360; PMCID: PMC7604673.

[24] Govindaraj S, Daniel M J, Vasudevan SS, Kumaran JV. Changes in salivary flow rate, pH, and viscosity among working men and women. Dent Med Res 2019;7:56-9. doi: 10.4103?dmr.dmr_20_19.

Chapter 11

Development of RT-PCR Based Diagnosis of SARS-CoV-2

Rutuja Sunil Patankar and Vasudeo Pandharinath Zambare

Abstract

In the 2020, COVID-19 pandemic disease created an havoc situation world widely and mainly caused by Severe Acute Respiratory Syndrome Coronavirus-2 (SARS-CoV-2). It has been challenging task for researchers, scientists and medico-pharmaceutical organisations to find out rapid and reliable diagnosis methods. Among the all testing services, a Reverse Transcription Polymerase Chain Reaction (RT-PCR) is the more accurate, rapid and authenticated molecular technique used for most of the diagnosis of major diseases. It has been a global priority to fix the rapid diagnosis method to combat against the pandemic COVID-19. Thus, the present chapter mainly focussing on the progress of RT-PCR method development though various processes of data collection on isolation of whole genome sequence, its primer and method designing. In this scenario, India suddenly become the global leader for vaccine development and hence the challenges and RT-PCR kit development in India and rest of the world has been be discussed. World wide many Government and private agencies and industries have taken an initiative for diagnosis of SARS-CoV-2 hence this chapter also summarised the scope of RT-PCR to combat pandemic situation in future.

Keywords: diagnosis, RT-PCR, COVID-19, SARS-CoV-2, Primers

1. Introduction

Coronavirus outbreak first case found in Wuhan, China in December 2019 [1]. Further, it became a pandemic, affecting the whole world. On February 2020, World Health Organisation (WHO) announced an official name for Coronavirus spread disease as COVID-19 [2]. It primarily targets a respiratory system in humans, as the appearance of symptoms depends on the incubation period, which further relies on the patient's age and the immune system [3].

SARS-CoV-2 as a public health emergency was declared by WHO and thereafter it became essential to find diagnostic tests for early detection and early treatment [4]. Normally the best way to detect any virus from the sample is its isolation and further confirmation by various molecular techniques. But Center for Diseases Control and Prevention (CDC) recommended not to isolate the SARS-CoV-2 as it is a new virus and this practices could be a risky approach and suggested to use patients sample directly for diagnosis [5]. Most of the diagnostic methods are molecular-based hence for diagnosis virus genome study become necessary. On January 2020 the ssRNA - 29870 bp whole sequence of SARS-CoV-2 was reported with GenBank accession number MN908947 [6, 7]. Thus, the basic information of genome sequence helpful for molecular based detection method development specially Polymerase chain reaction (PCR) based methods.

Main focused was on PCR as it is a rapid detection method. Among that Reverse Transcription Polymerase Chain Reaction (RT-PCR) is the most commonly used and still be using the method as it is exactly showing the positive results with great -sensitivity. RT-PCR was said to be a gold-standard for testing coronavirus [8]. RT-PCR can detect the virus from throat, nasopharyngeal swab as well as from stool sample [9]. Early detection using PCR prove to be most sensitive way as negative sample cannot be ruled out. One cohort study found that patients even if not having any symptoms still may be the carrier for viruses thus RT-PCR can detect those at genetic level. Thus, it helps in prevention of nosocomial infection and further spread unknowingly [10].

Sample collection methods also affect the diagnosis results. Thus, WHO and CDC recommended the use of nylon, rayon or any synthetic fibre swabs for sample collection. But shortage of such swabs hammered the testing numbers. Hence, some researchers decided to study the effect of cotton tipped plastic swabs on PCR results and it found that no inhibition effect was seen on PCR [11]. Another method related to heating of sample known as Loop-mediated Isothermal Amplification (LAMP) this works by skipping the RNA extraction process. RNA RT-LAMP sensitivity found to be 97%, while specificity was 99% [12]. Study tried the three viral transmission medium heating treatments named as directly without additives, in a formamide-EDTA buffer and in a RNAsnap™ buffer. Basically, this method skips the RNA extraction process of RT-qPCR by replacing it with heating treatments thus reduces the time for the test and also gives the same result as normal RT-PCR protocol [13]. Similarly, in one study RNA extraction process was skipped and on that place RT-qPCR master mixes were used. Now this helps under such situation where reagent shortage occurs in hospitals. It also expanded the testing capacities [14]. Similar way direct RT-qPCR was used in one of the study found to be an alternative for classical method without RNA extraction [15]. But there are certain limitations in remote areas and portable diagnosis will be preferable using mini PCR based diagnosis kits. One study combined the mini PCR and multi-well plate reader for convenient and portable diagnosis under pandemic situation [16].

As per the available RNA sequences and need of diagnosis method for COVID-19, several RNA extraction kits are available in the market. But due to pandemic situation and rising number of COVID patients, it was under shortage. Thus, magnetic beads base RNA extraction methods were used by various researchers. Silica beads were found to yields RNA and comparable with commercially available QIAcube viral RNA extraction kit which were determined by RT-qPCR and RT-LAMP [17]. Another study due to complexity of protocol was done, in which rather than using transport medium and RNA extraction it was decided to study the use of direct elution of swab and performing RT-qPCR. Elution of dry swabs were done directly in simple TE buffer and tested. Thus, this process simplifies the pre RT-qPCR preparation [18].

Commercial RT-PCR kits are already available in the market and few of them are manufactured by Altona Diagnostics (Hamburg, Germany), BGI (Shenzhen, China), CerTest Biotec (Zaragoza, Spain), KH Medical (Gyeonggi-do, Republic of Korea), Primer Design (Chandler's Ford, UK), R-Biopharm AG (Darmstadt, Germany), and Seegene (Seoul, South Korea). All these kits are the best for detection without any cross-reactivity with another virus and hence can be used for regular diagnosis of SARS-CoV-2 [19]. But the limit of detection (LoD) of kits matters the quality. Earlier China National Medical Products Administration (NMPA) approved 6 PCR kits, but due to time shortage optimisation was not done so LoD might get affected. Thus examination of LoD of this 6 PCR kits with real RNA of the virus was carried. All kits showed different LoD and the poorest LoDs has high chances of giving false negative results. The lab should confirm the performance of the kits and the utilise [20]. Some of the primers and probes for CoV detection has been shown in **Table 1**.

Currently, the RT-PCR test has a 95% specificity and 70% of the sensitivity rate [28, 29]. Self-collected saliva specimens was tested with 6 different molecular diagnostic tests like RTqPCR LDT, SARS-CoV-2 RAT, 3 direct RT-qPCR kits, and RT-LAMP and all tests showed a excellent results. Thus, based on these results, molecular diagnostic method has a great scope ahead [30]. Dr. Aneesh Mehta said that saliva test for coronavirus by PCR is the new type of diagnosis, as it is not invasive method but just spit is required as a sample [31]. This test is said to be a 'SalivaDirect' test developed by a scientist of the Yale School of Public Health, authorised by Food and Drug Administration (FDA) [32].

Most countries have been used Indian Council of Medical Research (ICMR, India) suggested Rapid Antigen Test (RAT) which was available as a kit and direct antigen identification from nasal swab [33]. However several countries found that the negative findings by RAT were shown to be positive by RT-PCR. Thus, according to Dr. Balram Bhargava, Director of ICMR, the RAT was found to offer false-negative outcomes. One of the reports says that around 11% of people found negative by RAT in Delhi, after testing with RT-PCR found to be positive [34]. The Indian Health Ministry and ICMR provided a guideline to re-test the RAT tested negative patients and those who develop symptoms after a few days of the test by RT-PCR [35]. Until now, RT-PCR is the recommended test for all organisations and has been followed. Still, many experts are trying to carry out a number of inventions and studies to make it simpler, more practical and more cost-effective for the whole planet. This book chapter summarised the upto date basics and applied study

Country	Target genes	Sequence	Reference
China	ORF1a	Forward primer: AGAAGATTGGTTAGATGATGATAGT Reverse primer: TTCCATCTCTAATTGAGGTTGAACC Probe:FAM-TCCTCACTGCCGTCTTGTTGACCA-BHQ1	[21]
Hong Kong	N gene	Forward primer: TAATCAGACAAGGAACTGATTA Reverse primer: CGAAGGTGTGACTTCCATG Probe: FAM/ZEN-GCAAATTGTGCAATTTGCGG-IBFQ	[22]
USA	N1 gene	Forward primer: GAC CCC AAA ATCAGCGAA AT Reverse primer: TCTGGTTACTGCCAGTTGAATCTG Probe: FAM-ACCCCGCATTACGTTTGGTGGACC-BHQ1	[23]
USA	N2 gene	Forward primer: TTACAA ACATTGGCCGCA AA Reverse primer: GCGCGACATTCCGAAGAA Probe: FAM-ACA ATTTGCCCCCAGCGTTAG-BHQ1	[24]
USA	N3 gene	Forward primer: GGGAGCCTTGAA TAC ACC AAA A Reverse primer: TGTAGCACG ATTGCAGCATTG Probe: FAM-AYCACATTGGCACCCGCA ATCCTG-BHQ1	[25]
Germany	E gene	Forward primer: ACAGGTACGTTAATAGTTAATAGCGT Reverse primer: ATATTGCAGCAGTACGCACACA Probe: FAM-ACACTAGCCATCCTTACTGCGCTTCG-BBQ	[26]
China	Spike	Forward primer: CCTACTAAATTAAATGATCTCTGCTTTACT Reverse primer: CAAGCTATAACGCAGCCTGTA	[27]

Table 1.
Primers and probes recorded for SARS-CoV-2 real-time reverse transcription PCR assays.

of PCR based diagnosis of SARs CoV-2 including current challenges of diagnosis, protocols and future prospects.

2. Challenges for SARs CoV-2 diagnosis

For treatment of SARs CoV-2, no vaccines is available but it was only the option left out to healthcare sectors that to prevent transmission as soon as possible [26]. So most the countries invested in isolation and detection [26]. The diagnosis of COVID-19 was difficult as it shows symptoms similar to those of flu viruses, thus it was crucial to find the diagnosis as early as possible for management purpose [36]. One of the most important problems in analytical chemistry was highlighted by the COVID-19 pandemic outbreak: the discrepancies between the testing technique (TT) and the testing method (TM) are a common confusion in the clinical field. In addition to the research procedure, TT consists of many steps, such as the collection of specimens, their preservation, storage, transport, labelling and distribution. Pre-test planning procedures for patients are also part of the process. Previously, these procedures, also known as pre-analytical variables, have been identified as the key causes of laboratory testing errors. The most acceptable TT for the TM must be validated during the production of the TM for the identification of the target analyte; otherwise the analysis is performed within a wide range of analytical errors [37]. Successful detection of the virus also depends on time of testing, early or late detection, viral load, sample collection etc. [38].

Further challenge was during the false negative results. It is easy to understand and interpret a perfect test for a disease; the test would only be positive if the disease was present, and it would only be negative if it were absent. However, since all studies have false positives and false negative results, diagnostic tests are not flawless. Test results do not definitively state whether or not there is a disease (or virus). This does not mean that the test is not beneficial; it merely implies that the test results must be probabilistically tested on the basis of test output characteristics, patient data, and disease prevalence [39]. To interpret the results of incomplete tests, two main metrics that characterise the test are needed: diagnostic sensitivity and diagnosis specificity [40]. At present, for commonly used SARS-CoV-2 samples, there is minimal information on these values. To accurately interpret an incomplete test, the approximate probability that the person being evaluated has the disorder must also be considered [39].

The diagnosis was completely relied on two ways Molecular and serological testing as shown in **Figure 1**. Different test among these two categories was tried during a pandemic situation [41].

Currently, RT-PCR is commonly used method by many laboratories due to specificity and fast detection [40]. Some test commonly use for CoV detection has been shown in **Table 2.**

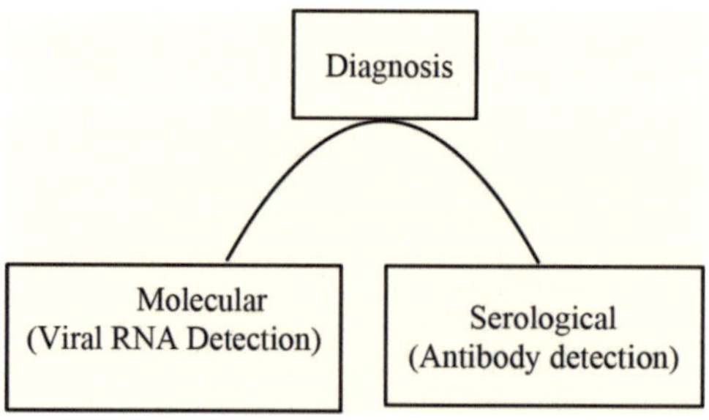

Figure 1.
Two ways of COVID-19 diagnosis.

Tests	Detection	Sample	Advantage	Disadvantage	Reference
Molecular					
RT-PCR	Viral RNA	Nose, throat swab, sputum, stool	Specific Less time	False negative result if viral load is less or if sample is not collected properly.	[24]
Nested RT-PCR	Viral RNA	Nose, throat swab	Highly specific results even in low viral load sample	Cross contamination during protocol	[41]
RT-LAMP	Viral RNA	Nose, throat swab, sputum, stool	Specific Less time	Optimize reaction condition	[42]
CRISPR	Viral RNA	Nose, throat swab, Broncho alveolar lavage fluid	Easy to use Low cost	Can give false result	[8]
Viral sequencing	Viral RNA	Nose, throat swab	Sensitive, convenient	Costly, need trained person, sophisticated instrument	[43]
Serology					
ELISA	Antibody	Blood	Simple and cost effective	Not established for SARS-CoV-2	[44]
Neutralization assay	Antibody	Whole blood, serum, plasma	Quantitative result,	Live virus hence safety required	[37]

Table 2.
Diagnostic testing for SARS-CoV-2.

3. Real-time RT-PCR basics

RT-PCR stands for real-time reverse transcription-polymerase chain reaction. (RT-PCR). It is a technique use to determine the nucleic acid (DNA/RNA) from sample specifically from a virus or bacteria. Currently used for COVID-19 testing. It combines the reverse transcription of RNA into DNA It uses radioactive isotope marker or fluorescent dyes for detection of the targeted gene. It can detect genetic material from nose, throat, stool and sputum sample [45].

4. Real-time RT-PCR protocol

SARS-CoV-2 testing solely depends on patients' health and concern, if the patient is getting some symptoms like cough, fever, headache or related, then the patient can personally take a test by visiting COVID center. If patient is already under medical treatment related to some other health issues, then doctor can recommend a COVID test to that patient for an early treatment. After that the most important part of RT-PCR covid testing is a collection of sample. It is most important as if the sample is not collected properly, it can affect the result as seen in many research [46–48]. CDC has provided the protocol for sample collection and all labs are following this same. Along with that, instruction regarding virus isolation has been given, it is not suppose to be done by an unless it is performed in the BSL-3 laboratory. Sample recommended for collection are nasopharyngeal (NP) and oropharyngeal (OP) swab for RT-PCR [49]. An expert technician can collect the sample from the nose and throat of patient separately by using swab which is individually wrapped. Swab has to be made up of synthetic fiber like plastic or wire shafts. Technician has to follow certain rules while collecting sample like 6 feet of separation, personal protective equipment (PPE) kit, proper gloves and faced covered lid. The sample is to be collected deeply. Once collected it has to be transferred to viral transport medium (VTM). VTM is made up of 2% FBS, 100 μg/mL Gentamicin and 0.5 μg/mL Amphotericin B. Among this 3 ml of media is transferred to sterile screwed capped bottles in which swab is put and stored before further testing [50]. Sample can be stored at 2–8 °C for 72 hours only. If the sample has to be transported for a long distance, then it should be carried in icepack [51].

Once the sample has been collected, then next important and time consuming process is RNA extraction means purification of RNA samples. Most of RNA extraction kits are available in the market shown in **Table 3**, which can be used directly contain lysis buffer and other chemicals which will lyse the virus and RNA will get into solution. First, in order to release the genetic material, the patient's sample is

Kits	Company	Country
Virus RNA Extraction kit		
QIAamp DSP Viral RNA Mini Kit	Qiagen	Hong Kong, Japan, USA
QIAamp Viral RNA Mini Kit		
Chemagic Viral DNA/RNA 300 Kit H96	PerkinElmer chemagen Technologie GmbH	Germany
SARS-CoV-2 Nucleic Acid Kit (RUO)		
MagNA Pure 96 System	Roche	Germany
ANDiS Viral Nucleic RNA Auto Extraction & Purification Kit	3Dmed	China
NucleoMag Dx Pathogen Kit	Macherey-Nagel	France, USA, Switzerland
NucleoSpin RNA Virus		
NucleoMag Virus kit		
Detection kit		
SuperScript III One-Step RT-PCR System with Platinum Taq DNA Polymerase	ThermoFisher	USA
TaqMan Fast Virus 1-Step Master Mix		
SuperScript III Platinum One-Step qRT-PCR Kit		
TaqPath 1-Step RT-qPCR Master Mix, CG		
QuantiTect Probe RT-PCR Kit	Qiagen	Japan
New Coronavirus Nucleic Acid Detection Kit	PerkinElmer chemagen Technologie GmbH	Germany
Respiratory SARS-CoV-2 RT-PCR Panel Assay		
SARS-CoV-2 Real-time RT-PCR Assay		
EURORealTime™ SARS-CoV-2		

Table 3.
Virus extraction and detection kits.

mixed with a solution which lyses the cells. In order to purify RNA, inactivation of RNA activity, denaturation of nucleoprotein complexes and elimination of contaminating DNA and proteins must take place by (phenol which will attract the other protein and break it down, guanidine isothyocynate is also a protein denaturant, RNase inhibitors to inactivate the ribonuclease enzyme) [52]. The resulting cellular debris will then proceed to the RT-PCR stage with the extracted RNA. Further RNA purification is carried by using kit or by centrifugation and solid phase extraction by using column Centrifuge and spin column, which is to be placed in a clean collection tube to collect the supernatant and filtrate is discarded. Again, it has to be washed and centrifuge. Further by using elution buffer RNA is purified.

After purification of viral RNA, the next step is the preparation of the reaction mixture for PCR amplification. In this step master mix has to be used which is premixed concentrated solution that consists of buffer, Reverse transcriptase enzyme nucleotide, forward primer, reverse primer, TaqMan probe, DNA polymerase. Finally, the RNA template to be added and mixed by pulse vortexing. Then load the reaction mixture into a PCR plate which generally contain 96 wells, allowing analysis of several samples at a time. Then place this plate in PCR machine (thermal cycler). Real time RT-PCR is used for detection of new Coronavirus 2019 by amplification of target sequences in Rdrp genes, E gene and N gene. The choice of the target depends on primers and the probe sequences. The first step in RT-PCR is reverse transcription. The first strand complementary DNA synthesis is primed with the PCR reverse primer which hybridizes the complementary part of the virus RNA genome. Reverse transcriptase then add DNA nucleotides onto the 3-prime end of the primer synthesizing DNA complementary of the viral RNA. Then denaturation takes place. Thus PCR consists of a series of cycles consisting of Denaturation, annealing and elongation. In cycle 1, DNA denaturation at 95 °C occurs. The next step at 58 °C allows the annealing of forward primer to complementary part of DNA. In elongation step, DNA polymerase synthesize a new strand complementary to the DNA template by adding nucleotides from the reaction mixture. In 2nd cycle, DNA denaturation form ssDNA, then annealing of primers

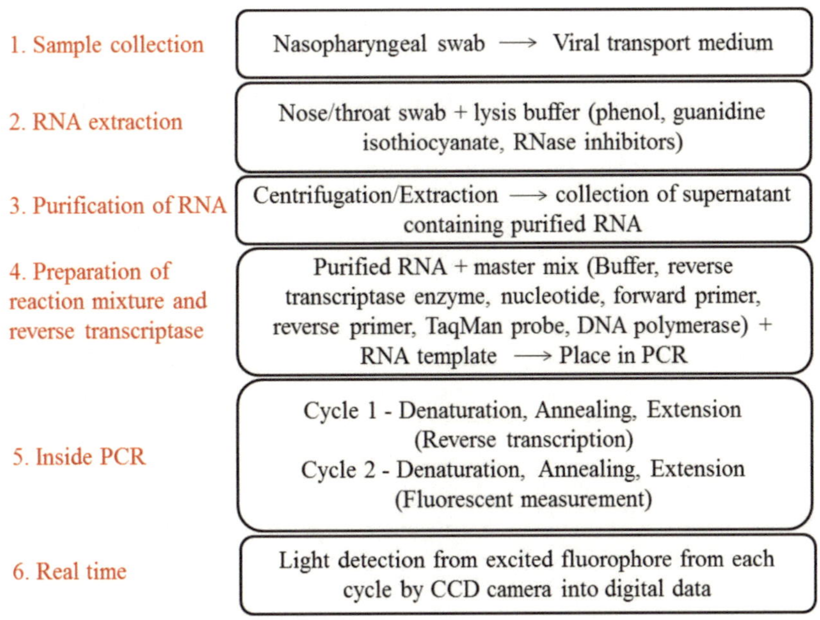

Figure 2.
RT-PCR methodological performance flowchart.

and Taq-man probe to its complementary part of the target DNA. Taq-man probe consist of a fluorophore covalentaly attached to the 5′ end of oligonucleotide probe, the fluorescence is emitted by the fluorophore when is excited by the cyclers light source. Also, this probe consists of quencher at 3′ end. The close proximity of the reporter to the quencher prevents detection of its fluorescence. When polymerase reaches the Taqman probe its endogenous 5′ nuclease activity cleaves the probe, separating the dye from the quencher, with each cycle of PCR more dyes are released, resulting in an increase in fluorescence intensity proportionately to the amount of amplicon synthesized. For the fluorescence signal a tungsten-halogen lamp, an excitation filter, lens, emission filter and charged coupled device (CCD) camera are use which converts light into digital data. A flowchart of the protocol has shown in **Figure 2** [24].

5. Recent development of RT-PCR for SARS-CoV-2 diagnosis

In addition to prevention methods (e.g., hygiene, social distance, isolation of infected individuals, and travel restriction), rigorous community infection testing is essential to track the transmission of the disease as well as educating public policies [53]. Nations that have implemented large research strategies at an early stage like South Korea, Vietnam, and New Zealand have been better able to restrict the spread of the disease. Tests should ideally be simple to sample and evaluate, precise, reliable, scalable and inexpensive. Often, point-of-care tests (POCT) based on antibodies match this definition. However, rapidly emerging epidemics due to novel viruses do not allow antibody-based tests to evolve in a timely manner [54]. Because of the simple adaptability to the nucleotide sequence of the target, viral load tests based on real-time, quantitative RT-PCR (referred to as RTqPCR) are thus an ideal test [55]. This RT-qPCR is currently a reliable test commonly used for the diagnosis of SARS-CoV-2 infected symptomatic and asymptomatic patients [56]. Several scientific and clinical institutions around the world have produced molecular assays to diagnose SARS-CoV-2 and have made RT-qPCR primers and sample sets available to the public [57].

As the genetic code of coronaviruses consists of RNA, its purification of the test samples is a crucial step in RT-qPCR protocols. Officially, institutions in some countries have suggested unique RNA isolation kits for SARSCoV-2 detection [57]. Various virus extraction and detections kits are available in market as shown in **Table 3**. The qRT-PCR has the benefits of high sensitivity, high precision, and a wide variety of sample types that can be use but there are however several factors that influence qRT-PCR outcomes, such as repeated washing, purification and separation of viral nucleic acids, which cause a substantial loss of nucleic acid and increase the risk of fragmentation and hydrolysis of nucleic acid; the number of virus replications below the qRT-PCR detection threshold would also cause false negative effects on the early stage of SARS-CoV-2 infection. So this problem was faced by many laboratories [58]. Some started focusing on RT-LAMP—reverse transcriptase loop-mediated isothermal amplification [59]. Other PCR, which was found to be more potent to detect low viral load was digital droplet PCR (ddPCR) as compared to qRT-PCR but due to limited availability ddPCR instrumentation and lab expertise mostly qRT-PCR is being used [60]. At this point, superior resources are concentrated in all parts of the country to reinforce scientific research. It is assumed that our ability to diagnose and treat patients with new coronavirus pneumonia will develop further with the enhancement and advancement of detection technology.

6. Status in India

Collection of data at one place so that whole country population can refer this data at such a tough situation was a necessity so the Government of India has open an website -https://covid19cc.nic.in/ICMR/login.aspx, which has lots of information regarding testing centers, counting of RT-PCR tests and other antibody–antigen tests, current positive cases, available collection centers with their address contacts etc. Also aligned with ICMR, said to be Covid-19 sample collection management system for rapid antigen, antibody and RT-PCR tests. Lots of RT-PCR kits with variations, are manufactured in India has been shown in **Table 4**.

Kit	Company	Sample required	Website
Fluidigm's Advanta Dx SARS-CoV-2 RT-PCR kit	Fluidigm's Corporation	Saliva	https://www.fluidigm.com/
R-Green kit (SARS COV2-real-time PCR)	Reliance Life Sciences	Throat, nose swab	https://rellife.com/
Dry Swab-Direct RT-PCR test	Centre for Cellular and Molecular Biology (CCMB)	Dry Nasal swab	https://www.ccmb.res.in/
RT-PCR testing kits	iGenetic Diagnostics and BioGenomics	Throat, nose swab	https://www.igenetic.com/
Mylab PathoDetect COVID-19 Qualitative PCR kit	Mylab Discovery Solutions Pvt. Ltd	Throat, nose swab	https://mylabdiscoverysolutions.com/
Real Time PCR kits	Genome Diagnostics Pvt. Ltd.	Nasopharyngeal swab	http://www.genomediagnostics.co.in/about-us.html
GlobalTM diagnostic kit	Equine Biotech	Nasopharyngeal swab	https://covid19.iisc.ac.in/covid-19-rt-pcr-kit/
Corosure Covid-19 diagnostic kit	IIT Delhi	Throat, nose swab	https://home.iitd.ac.in/news-tea-haritaki.php
RT-PCR kit	CSIR-IICT	Throat, nose swab	https://iictindia.org/

Table 4.
RT-PCR kit developed by Indian companies and sample requirement.

7. International status

RT-qPCR assays were already known, but development can lead to better results. Thus, one study was done by targeting two monoplex assays recommended by WHO that was targeted on the envelope gene (E-Sarbeco) and RNA-Dependant RNA Polymerase coding genes (RdRp-IP4). This was combined and test named as 'Duo SARS-CoV-2 RT-qPCR assay'. As already lots of duo assays are commercially available, but this study was done to combine in-house assays. Can be used to reduce the chances of false negative results as it is dual assay [60]. As dual target assays are commercially available, developed specifically to target multiple sites in the viral genome, but mutation rates in virus found to be moderate which can cause problem with respect to results. Some of the tests were done by using 'cobas SARS-CoV-2 E gene qRT-PCR' but some failures were seen due to change in nucleotide at position 26340 of the SARS-CoV-2 gene. So the study was done to identify single nucleotide polymorphism in E gene of the virus. This includes the importance of study regarding mutations in the virus and thus to prevent false negative results [61]. The protocol provided by WHO mention the three assay that is to be performed: First line screening assay - E gene assay, Confirmatory assay - RdRp gene assay, and Additional confirmatory assay - N gene assay [24]. 'Multiplex Real Time PCR' was also use to find its efficacy for SARS-CoV-2 detection. Found to be rapid and accurate method for viral detection [62]. 'Aus Diagnostics respiratory MT-PCR assay' was also found to be reliable and sensitive [63]. Two 'Single-tube nested (STN) real-time RT-PCR assays' specifically targets RdRp/Hel and N genes, found to be 100% specific for detection of SARS-CoV-2 [64]. Even high cost assays were given preference during a pandemic situation like TaqMan-based real-time RT-qPCR which was not even accessible to lots of laboratories. So it was performed by using 2 methods that are SYBR green RT-qPCR and conventional PCR basically standardisation was done of this 2 methods which is cost effective methods and found to give equal results as that of TaqMan-based real-time RT-qPCR [65].

COVID-19 diagnosis now done by one step RT-qPCR by using primers and probes which were developed at different institutes like China CDC, Charite (Germany), The University of Hong Kong, National Institute of Infectious Diseases in Japan (Japan NIID), National Institute of Health in Thailand (Thailand NIH) and US CDC which was announced by WHO [2, 24]. One study performed the analysis of primer-probe sets specifically targeting the N region and RdRp/Orf1 of SARS-CoV-2 by N-assay and RdRp/Orf1 Assays. Primer probe set for N-assay was N (China CDC), HKU-N (HKU), NIID_2019-nCOV_N (Japan NIID), WH-NIC N (Thailand NIH), and 2019-nCoV_N1, -N2, and -N3 (US CDC) and for RdRp/Orf1 Assay RdRp_SARSr (Charite), HKU-ORF1b-nsp14 (HKU), and ORF1ab (China CDC) primer probe set was studied. Results says that NIID_2019-nCOV_N" from the Japan NIID and "ORF1ab" from China CDC gave a good performance for RT-qPCR analysis without any cross-reactivity and non-specific amplifications. This can be used for further diagnosis [66]. Sensitivity of PCR also depends on primer concentration, degeneration and multi target detection. Initial concentration of primer was 300-900 nM but as its concentration rises sensitivity also improves [67]. One study found that concentration upto 400 nM rise the sensitivity [68]. Degenerate primers plays an important role with respect to diversity of SARS-CoV-2. While screening assays with a single target area are more prone to sequence differences than dual or triple-target assays for multi-target identification [67]. Other than this primer length, melting temperature, GC content and annealing temperature also affects the sensitivity of PCR assay [67]. One study attempted to deduce the specific patterns among SARS-CoV-2 isolates and accordingly primers were design targeted to nsp2 gene and further use for diagnosis of probe free real-time RT-PCR. Sensitive and rapid SARS-CoV-2-specific real-time RT-PCR assay COVID-19-nsp2 has therefore been developed [69]. In one research, the efficiency of three novel real-time reverse transcription-PCR (RT-PCR) assays targeting RNA-dependent RNA polymerase (RdRp)/helicase (Hel), spike (S) and nucleocapsid (N) SARS-CoV-2 genes was developed and compared. RNA polymerase (RdRp)/(Hel) assay found to be effective with no cross reactivity with other viruses among samples [27]. Some of the RT-PCR kits manufactured at International level along with sample requirement has been shown in **Table 5**.

Kit Name	Company	Country	Sample required	Website
1copy™ COVID-19 qPCR Multi Kit	1drop Inc.	Korea	Nasal swab	http://www.1drop.co.kr/
ANDiS® SARS-CoV-2 RT-qPCR Detection Kit	3D Medicines	United state	Nasopharyngeal swab	https://www.3dmedcare.com/covid/
CareStart™ COVID-19 MDx RT-PCR	Access Bio, Inc.	United state	Nasopharyngeal swab, Oropharyngeal swab	https://carestart.com/
MOLgen SARSCoV2 Real Time RT PCR	Adaltis S.r.l.	Italy	Nasopharyngeal swabs, oropharyngeal swabs, sputum and bronchoalveolar lavage fluid (BALF).	http://www.adaltis.net/products/molecular-diagnostic-tests/sars-cov2-covid-19/sars-cov2-covid-19/
LyteStar 2019-nCoV RT-PCR Kit 1.0	ADT Biotech	Malaysia	Nasopharyngeal swab, Oropharyngeal swab	http://adt-biotech.com/lytestartm-detection-kits/
AccuPower® SARS-CoV-2 Real-Time RT-PCR kit	BIONEER Corporation	Philippines	Sputum, nasopharyngeal swab, oropharyngeal swab	https://eng.bioneer.com/20-scv-2122.html
VIASURE SARS-CoV-2 S gene Real Time PCR Detection Kit adapted for BD MAX™ System	CerTest Biotec, S.L.	Spain	Respiratory samples	https://www.certest.es/
Simplexa™ COVID-19 Direct RT-PCR Kit	DiaSorin Molecular, LLC	United state	Nasal swab, nasopharyngeal swab, nasal wash/aspirate, and BAL specimens	https://molecular.diasorin.com/us/kit/simplexa-covid-19-direct-kit/
Quick SARS-CoV-2 rRT-PCR Kit	Zymo Research Corp.	United state	Upper respiratory and lower respiratory sample	https://www.zymoresearch.com/
SARS-CoV-2 Nucleic Acid Detection Kit (PCR-Fluorescent Probe Method)	Zybio, Inc.	Philippines	Nasal/throat swab, bronchoalveolar lavage fluids, stool	https://m.zybio.com/en/Product/Molecule/2020-03-24/316.html
Novel Coronavirus (2019-nCoV)/Flu A/Flu B Real-time Multiplex RT-PCR Kit	Zhuhai Haitai Biological Pharmaceutical Co., Ltd	China	Upper respiratory and lower respiratory sample	http://www.zhhaitai.com/
MolecuTech® Real-Time COVID-19	YD Diagnostics Corp.	Korea	Respiratory specimens	http://www.yd-diagnostics.com/2012/eng/channel_02/prt_list.php?selID=37

Kit Name	Company	Country	Sample required	Website
COVID-19 ORF1ab/N Gene PCR Detection Kit	Xi'an Tianlong Science and Technology Co., Ltd	China	Upper respiratory and lower respiratory sample	https://xi-an-tianlong.abraa.com/
Real time RT-PCR Kit for the detection of SARS-CoV-2	Suzhou BTA Biotech Co. Ltd	China	Nasal swab, nasopharyngeal swab, nasal wash/aspirate, and BAL specimens	http://vosunbio.com/
LyoDx® A Freeze-Dried Real-Time RT-PCR Detection Reagent for SARS-CoV-2	SignalDT Biotechnologies (SZ), Inc.	Alameda	Respiratory samples	https://signaldt-biosystems-llc.hub.biz/
SBC SARS-CoV-2 Convective PCR Diagnostic Device/Kit	Schweitzer Biotech Company Ltd	Taiwan	Nasopharyngeal or oropharyngeal swabs	http://covid19.sbc-biotech.com/
RainSure COVID-19 dPCR Detection Kit (lab-based)	RainSure Scientific Co., Ltd	China	Respiratory samples	http://en.rainsurebio.com/
COVID-19 One-Step COVID-19 RT-PCR Kit	Pishtaz Teb Diagnostics	Iran	Nasopharyngeal or oropharyngeal swabs	https://pishtazteb.com/en/pcr/
PerkinElmer® SARS-CoV-2 Realtime RT-PCR Assay	PerkinElmer Inc.	United state	Nasopharyngeal or oropharyngeal swabs	https://www.perkinelmer.com/
SARS-CoV-2 One-Step RT-PCR Kit, RdRp and N Genes, CE-IVD	NZYTech	Portugal	Nasal swab, nasopharyngeal swab, nasal wash/aspirate, and BAL specimens	https://www.nzytech.com/products-services/molecular-diagnostics/sars-cov-2/sars-cov-2-one-step-rt-pcr-kit-rdrp-and-n-genes-ce-ivd/
COVID-19 TaqMan RT-PCR Kit (E/RdRP genes) Dx	Norgen Biotek Corp	Canada	Saliva & Swab Samples	https://norgenbiotek.com/

Table 5.
RT-PCR kits developed by International companies and sample requirement.

8. Future prospects of RT-PCR

PCR method was discovered in 1986 and since then the method is serving medical sectors. In the future, as potential molecular diagnostic methods, PCR will play a significant role. Lots of PCR methods are already used in various research and medical fields, but as we know currently under this pandemic situation RT-PCR has turned out to be a boon in healthcare sectors. Lots of kits have been manufactured throughout the world with some or little variation, thus making it more sensitive, specific and less time consuming. One factor which essential under pandemic situation was a multiple sample analysis in one go [5]. Thus more focus on using portable POC systems, we can imagine the use of micro-fluidics doing concurrent multiple sample analysis. It is possible to analyse immunomagnetic exosomal RNA by using micro-fluidic systems RT-PCR said to be a Chip-based integrated real-time reverse transcription PCR platform [70]. Similar way chip-based RT-PCR digitally can quantify the mRNA in single cell [71].

Scalable, quick, and inexpensive diagnostics of COVID-19 by RT-PCR could help restrict the spread of SARS-CoV-2, saving lives as a result. RNA extraction, however, constitutes an obstacle to the scale-up of experiments. Thus, one research was done directly using the RT-PCR and heat inactivated sample and efficacy was tested. The study proved that is not necessary to carry RNA extraction testing. The study also suggests the use of standard protocols for RT-PCR and transport media by the whole world so the it will become easier to deal with future epidemics. Such RT-PCR said to be an hid RT-PCR (heat-inactivated direct RT-PCR). Sample collection and rather than using transport media, usage of lysis buffer is found to be more efficient as it will directly lys the sample and can be used in RT-PCR without a need of any RNA extraction kit [72].

As *Coronaviridae* family consist many RNA viruses which not only infect the humans but also animals, birds etc. [73]. If we look at the history of this family will see that it has been always serious when it started infecting like in 2002, Severe acute respiratory syndrome coronavirus (SARS-CoV) emerged, in 2012, Middle East respiratory syndrome coronavirus (MERS-CoV), in 2016, swine acute diarrhoea syndrome coronavirus (SADS-CoV) and the latest one which cause pandemic in 2019, severe acute respiratory syndrome coronavirus 2 (SARS-CoV-2) [74]. Among this SADS-CoV infects pigs while other infect humans [75]. This all was controlled well but current 2019 epidemic was beyond control due to lack of diagnosis, medicines and vaccine. For now after all efforts diagnosis for SARS-CoV-2 has been found but as lots of virus under this family can emerge in future and which has already spread in past needed to be studied [76]. So one research was completely done to make a molecular diagnostic kit which can identify almost all CoVs, thus to diagnose easily any virus among this family in future [77]. They designed a semi-nested RT-PCR based upon 38 genome sequences that has been recorded from human and animal CoVs. Thus proved to be a great finding which can diagnose all available CoVs or which can emerge in future too [77].

Lots of research regarding RT-PCR has been done, PCR like nested PCR, ddPCR, two step RT-PCR is an advance and gives more accurate results but labs were not that equipped and it was not possible to set up everything under such pandemic situation. Hence if we think about future this all equipments and facilities have to be adopted by laboratory to deal with emerging epidemics [57].

9. Conclusion

SARs-CoV-2, originated from Wuhan, China and spread all over world, causing a pandemic situation which affected the whole world badly at economic, social, medical level also. Initially it was very difficult to deal with virus as no diagnosis, treatment or vaccine was available, but after lots of efforts of researchers now we have a good diagnosis and control condition in regards spread of infection. Even vaccination has been started in almost all countries. As in the earlier period of pandemic, the diagnosis was the main factor to prevent the spread of the virus. So main focus was on a diagnostic that to on molecular diagnosis as it is more efficient and accurate way of detection. Currently use molecular method is RT-PCR also said to be a gold standard detection method. Lots of RT-PCR kits are now available in most of the countries with little modifications and approvals. The key point to be noticed before the laboratory experiments is the right reliable sampling. Nasopharyngeal and oropharyngeal swabs, which are safer for collection are recommended for screening or early detection. If we talk about a future of RT-PCR advancement in methods like nested PCR, ddPCR, two step RT-PCR have been already done, which is found to be more accurate, but lack of instrumentation and expertise have put it behind, but in future this thing has to be focused and implemented so that the world can deal with any future epidemic.

Author details

Rutuja Sunil Patankar[1] and Vasudeo Pandharinath Zambare[1,2]*

1 School of Science, Sandip University, Nashik, India

2 R&D Department, Om Biotechnologies, Nashik, India

*Address all correspondence to: vasuzambare@gmail.com

References

[1] Christensen, J., Senthilingam, M. (2020) CNN https://edition.cnn.com/2020/01/20/health/whatis-coronavirus explained/index.html.

[2] WHO (2020a) 'Cambodia: WHO strengthens response to COVID-19 with support from the World Bank and UN'https://www.who.int/news-room/feature stories/detail/cambodia-who-strengthens-response-to-covid-19-with-support-from-the-world-bank-and-un.

[3] H. A. Rothan and S. N. Byrareddy, "The epidemiology and pathogenesis of coronavirus disease (COVID-19) outbreak," J. Autoimmun., vol. 109, no. February, p. 102433, 2020, doi: 10.1016/j.jaut.2020.102433.

[4] W. Zhao, J. Zhang, M. E. Meadows, Y. Liu, T. Hua, and B. Fu, "A systematic approach is needed to contain COVID-19 globally," Sci. Bull., vol. 65, no. 11, pp. 876-878, 2020, doi: 10.1016/j.scib.2020.03.024.

[5] H. Zhu, H. Zhang, Y. Xu, S. Laššáková, M. Korabečná, and P. Neužil, "PCR past, present and future," Biotechniques, vol. 69, no. 4, pp. 317-325, 2020, doi: 10.2144/BTN-2020-0057.

[6] W. Zhao, J. Zhang, M. E. Meadows, Y. Liu, T. Hua, and B. Fu, "A systematic approach is needed to contain COVID-19 globally," Sci. Bull., vol. 65, no. 11, pp. 876-878, 2020, doi: 10.1016/j.scib.2020.03.024.

[7] X. Ren et al., "Application and Optimization of RT-PCR in Diagnosis of SARS-CoV-2 Infection," SSRN Electron. J., 2020, doi: 10.2139/ssrn.3546086.

[8] L. J. Carter et al., "Assay Techniques and Test Development for COVID-19 Diagnosis," ACS Cent. Sci., vol. 6, no. 5, pp. 591-605, 2020, doi: 10.1021/acscentsci.0c00501.

[9] D. K. W. Chu et al., "Molecular Diagnosis of a Novel Coronavirus (2019-nCoV) Causing an Outbreak of Pneumonia," Clin. Chem., vol. 7, pp. 1-7, 2020, doi: 10.1093/clinchem/hvaa029.

[10] J. A. Porcel-Vazquez et al., "Usefulness of PCR Screening in the Initial Triage of Trauma Patients During COVID-19 Pandemic," J. Orthop. Trauma, vol. 34, no. 10, pp. e377–e381, 2020, doi: 10.1097/BOT.0000000000001903.

[11] P. Freire, Byron et al. 2020. "Cotton-Tipped Plastic Swabs for SARS-CoV-2 RT-QPCR Diagnosis to Prevent Supply Shortages." Frontiers in Cellular and Infection Microbiology 10(June): 1-4.

[12] A. Sowood et al., "Since January 2020 Elsevier has created a COVID-19 resource centre with free information in English and Mandarin on the novel coronavirus COVID- 19 . The COVID-19 resource centre is hosted on Elsevier Connect , the company ' s public news and information ," no. January, 2020.

[13] J. Alcoba-Florez et al., "Fast SARS-CoV-2 detection by RT-qPCR in preheated nasopharyngeal swab samples," Int. J. Infect. Dis., vol. 97, pp. 66-68, 2020, doi: 10.1016/j.ijid.2020.05.099.

[14] M. R. Hasan et al., "Detection of SARS-CoV-2 RNA by direct RT-qPCR on nasopharyngeal specimens without extraction of viral RNA," PLoS One, vol. 15, no. 7 July, pp. 1-9, 2020, doi: 10.1371/journal.pone.0236564.

[15] N. Lübke et al., "Since January 2020 Elsevier has created a COVID-19 resource centre with free information in English and Mandarin on the novel coronavirus COVID- 19 . The COVID-19 resource centre is hosted on Elsevier Connect , the company ' s public news and information ," no. January, 2020.

[16] E. González-González, G. Trujillo-De Santiago, I. M. Lara-Mayorga, S. O. Martínez-Chapa, and M. M. Alvarez, "Portable and accurate diagnostics for COVID-19: Combined use of the miniPCR thermocycler and a well-plate reader for SARS-CoV-2 virus detection," PLoS One, vol. 15, no. 8 August, pp. 1-13, 2020, doi: 10.1371/journal.pone.0237418.

[17] S. Klein et al., "SARS-CoV-2 RNA extraction using magnetic beads for rapid large-scale testing by RT-qPCR and RT-LAMP," Viruses, vol. 12, no. 8, 2020, doi: 10.3390/v12080863.

[18] S. Srivatsan et al., "Preliminary support for a 'dry swab, extraction free' protocol for SARS-CoV-2 testing via RT-qPCR," bioRxiv Prepr. Serv. Biol., pp. 1-2, 2020, doi: 10.1101/2020.04.22.056283.

[19] P. B. van Kasteren et al., "Comparison of seven commercial RT-PCR diagnostic kits for COVID-19," J. Clin. Virol., vol. 128, no. April, p. 104412, 2020, doi: 10.1016/j.jcv.2020.104412.

[20] X. Wang et al., "Limits of Detection of 6 Approved RT-PCR Kits for the Novel SARS-Coronavirus-2 (SARS-CoV-2)," Clin. Chem., vol. 66, no. 7, pp. 977-979, 2020, doi: 10.1093/clinchem/hvaa099.

[21] K. Ramanathan et al., "Genomic characterisation and epidemiology of 2019 novel coronavirus: implications for virus origins and receptor binding," Lancet, vol. 2020, no. January, pp. 19-21, 2020.

[22] D. K. W. Chu *et al.*, "Molecular Diagnosis of a Novel Coronavirus (2019-nCoV) Causing an Outbreak of Pneumonia," Clin. Chem., vol. 7, pp. 1-7, 2020, doi: 10.1093/clinchem/hvaa029.

[23] Center for Disease Control, "Research Use Only 2019-Novel Coronavirus (2019-nCoV) Real-time RT-PCR Primers and Probes," *CDC's Diagnostic Test COVID-19 Only Supplies*, vol. 19, pp. 2019-2020, 2019, [Online]. Available: https://www.cdc.gov/coronavirus/2019-ncov/lab/virus-requests.html.

[24] V. M. Corman *et al.*, "Detection of 2019 -nCoV by RT-PCR," Euro Surveill, vol. 25, no. 3, pp. 1-8, 2020.

[25] J. F. W. Chan *et al.*, "A familial cluster of pneumonia associated with the 2019 novel coronavirus indicating person-to-person transmission: a study of a family cluster," Lancet, vol. 395, no. 10223, pp. 514-523, 2020, doi: 10.1016/S0140-6736(20)30154-9.

[26] N. Younes et al., "Challenges in Laboratory Diagnosis of the Novel," Mdpi, pp. 1-27, 2020.

[27] S. J. R. Da Silva et al., "Clinical and Laboratory Diagnosis of SARS-CoV-2, the Virus Causing COVID-19," ACS Infect. Dis., vol. 6, no. 9, pp. 2319-2336, 2020, doi: 10.1021/acsinfecdis.0c00274.

[28] Arevalo-Rodriguez et al., "False-Negative Results of Initial Rt-Pcr Assays for Covid-19: a Systematic Review," pp. 1-33, 2020, doi: 10.1101/2020.04.16.20066787.

[29] J. Watson, P. F. Whiting, and J. E. Brush, "Interpreting a covid-19 test result," BMJ, vol. 369, no. May, pp. 1-7, 2020, doi: 10.1136/bmj.m1808.

[30] J. A. Porcel-Vazquez et al., "Usefulness of PCR Screening in the Initial Triage of Trauma Patients During COVID-19 Pandemic," J. Orthop. Trauma, vol. 34, no. 10, pp. e377–e381, 2020, doi: 10.1097/BOT.0000000000001903.

[31] Jamie Ducharme (2020) 'What to Know About COVID-19 Tests, From PCR to Antigen to Antibody'

https://time.com/5880255/covid-19-tests-types/.

[32] Michael Greenwood (2020) 'Quick and affordable saliva-based COVID-19 test developed by Yale scientists receives FDA Emergency Use Authorization' https://news.yale.edu/2020/08/15/yales-rapid-covid-19-saliva-test-receives-fda-emergency- use-authorization.

[33] Kaunain Sheriff M (2020) 'Explained: How rapid antigen tests detect Covid-19, where they will be used in India' https://indianexpress.com/article/explained/how-rapid-antigen-test-detects- coronavirus-where-it-will-be-used-6460735/.

[34] WION (2020) 'Delhi: 11% symptomatic negative tests of RAT found positive via RT-PCR'https://www.wionews.com/india-news/delhi-11-symptomatic-negative-tests-of-rat-found-positive-via-rt-pcr-348153.

[35] Ahmedabad Mirror (2020) 'RAT is out of the bag. Take Covid test again' https://ahmedabadmirror.indiatimes.com/ahmedabad/cover-story/rat-is-out-of-the-bag-take-covid-test-again/articleshow/78048993.cms.

[36] I. A. Mattioli and F. N. Crespilho, "Problems of interpreting diagnostic tests for SARS-CoV-2: Analytical chemistry concerns," An. Acad. Bras. Cienc., vol. 92, no. 4, pp. 1-3, 2020, doi: 10.1590/0001-3765202020201208.

[37] B. C. Behera, R. R. Mishra, and H. Thatoi, "Recent biotechnological tools for diagnosis of corona virus disease: A review," Biotechnol. Prog., no. August, pp. 1-16, 2020, doi: 10.1002/btpr.3078.

[38] E. C. Stites and C. B. Wilen, "The Interpretation of SARS-CoV-2 Diagnostic Tests," Med, vol. 1, no. 1, pp. 78-89, 2020, doi: 10.1016/j.medj.2020.08.001.

[39] Y. Tang, J. E. Schmitz, D. H. Persing, and C. W. Stratton, "crossm Challenges," J. Clin. Microbiol., vol. 58, no. 6, pp. 1-9, 2020.

[40] B. A. Parikh, T. C. Bailey, P. G. Lyons, and N. W. Anderson, "The brief case: 'Not Positive' or 'Not Sure'—COVID-19-negative results in a symptomatic patient," J. Clin. Microbiol., vol. 58, no. 8, pp. 1-6, 2020, doi: 10.1128/JCM.01195-20.

[41] J. Wang et al., "Novel One-Step Single-Tube Nested Quantitative Real-Time PCR Assay for Highly Sensitive Detection of SARS-CoV-2," Anal. Chem., vol. 92, no. 13, pp. 9399-9404, 2020, doi: 10.1021/acs.analchem.0c01884.

[42] M. Crippa, G. B. Bartolucci, F. Toffoletto, and G. Marcer, "Occupational diseases due to allergic and toxic chemicals in health care workers: Fitness for work," Med. del Lav., vol. 103, no. 3, pp. 187-197, 2012.

[43] R. Kumar, S. Nagpal, S. Kaushik, and S. Mendiratta, "COVID-19 diagnostic approaches: different roads to the same destination," VirusDisease, vol. 31, no. 2, pp. 97-105, 2020, doi: 10.1007/s13337-020-00599-7.

[44] W. Zhang et al., "Molecular and serological investigation of 2019-nCoV infected patients: implication of multiple shedding routes," Emerg. Microbes Infect., vol. 9, no. 1, pp. 386-389, 2020, doi: 10.1080/22221751.2020.1729071.

[45] M. Arya, I. S. Shergill, M. Williamson, L. Gommersall, N. Arya, and H. R. H. Patel, "Basic principles of real-time quantitative PCR," Expert Rev. Mol. Diagn., vol. 5, no. 2, pp. 209-219, 2005, doi: 10.1586/14737159.5.2.209.

[46] Y. Li et al., "Stability issues of RT-PCR testing of SARS-CoV-2

for hospitalized patients clinically diagnosed with COVID-19," J. Med. Virol., vol. 92, no. 7, pp. 903-908, 2020, doi: 10.1002/jmv.25786.

[47] A. Piras, D. Rizzo, S. Uzzau, G. De Riu, S. Rubino, and F. Bussu, "Inappropriate Nasopharyngeal Sampling for SARS-CoV-2 Detection Is a Relevant Cause of False-Negative Reports," Otolaryngol. - Head Neck Surg. (United States), vol. 163, no. 3, pp. 459-461, 2020, doi: 10.1177/0194599820931793.

[48] A. Piras et al.,Nasopharyngeal swab collection in the suspicion of Covid-19," no. January, 2020.

[49] A. Nasal et al., "Sheet SARS-CoV-2 (COVID-19) Fact Anterior Nasal (Nares) Specimen Collection for SARS-CoV-2 Diagnostic Testing," no. 6.

[50] CDC, "Preparation of Viral Transport Medium," Centers Dis. Control Prev., vol. 36, no. 4, pp. 268-269, 2004.

[51] U. Jan, "COVID-19 Interim Guidelines for Collecting , Handling, and Testing Clinical Specimens for COVID-19 Summary of Recent Changes Updates as of December 30 , 2020," pp. 1-6, 2021.

[52] G. P. Rédei, "RNA Extraction," Encycl. Genet. Genomics, Proteomics Informatics, pp. 1723-1723, 2008, doi: 10.1007/978-1-4020-6754-9_14747.

[53] P. G. Walker, C. Whittaker, and O. Watson, "Report 12 - The global impact of COVID-19 and strategies for mitigation and suppression | Faculty of Medicine | Imperial College London," vol. 071, no. May, 2020, doi: 10.25561/77735.

[54] S. Report, "COVID 19: Facts and Insights, October 30," pp. 1-142, 2021.

[55] Z. D. Tong *et al.*, "Potential presymptomatic transmission of SARS-CoV-2, Zhejiang Province, China, 2020," Emerg. Infect. Dis., vol. 26, no. 5, pp. 1052-1054, 2020, doi: 10.3201/eid2605.200198.

[56] C. Rothe *et al.*, "Transmission of 2019-nCoV Infection from an Asymptomatic Contact in Germany," N. Engl. J. Med., vol. 382, no. 10, pp. 970-971, 2020, doi: 10.1056/nejmc2001468.

[57] H. G. Barreto, F. A. de Pádua Milagres, G. C. de Araújo, M. M. Daúde, and V. A. Benedito, "Diagnosing the novel SARS-CoV-2 by quantitative RT-PCR: variations and opportunities," J. Mol. Med., vol. 98, no. 12, pp. 1727-1736, 2020, doi: 10.1007/s00109-020-01992-x.

[58] B. Xiao, Q. Zhou, T. Lei, Y. He, and L. Li, "Application of laboratory diagnostic technologies for SARS-CoV-2: current progress and prospect," *Nan Fang Yi Ke Da Xue Xue Bao*, vol. 40, no. 4, pp. 601-605, 2020, doi: 10.12122/j.issn.1673-4254.2020.04.24.

[59] M. F. Österdahl *et al.*, "Detecting SARS-CoV-2 at point of care: preliminary data comparing loop-mediated isothermal amplification (LAMP) to polymerase chain reaction (PCR)," BMC Infect. Dis., vol. 20, no. 1, pp. 1-8, 2020, doi: 10.1186/s12879-020-05484-8.

[60] F. Yu *et al.*, "Quantitative detection and viral load analysis of SARS-CoV-2 in infected patients," Clin. Infect. Dis., vol. 71, no. 15, pp. 793-798, 2020, doi: 10.1093/cid/ciaa345.

[61] Pezzi, Laura et al. 2020. "Development and Evaluation of a Duo SARS-CoV-2 RT-QPCR Assay Combining Two Assays Approved by the World Health Organization Targeting the Envelope and the RNA-Dependant RNA Polymerase (RdRp) Coding Regions." Viruses 12(6): 1-12.

[62] Utilized, Transcription-pcr. 2020. "Crossm A Recurrent Mutation at Position 26340 of SARS-CoV-2 Is

Associated with Failure of the E Gene Quantitative Reverse." 58(10): 1-8.

[63] Hoffmann, Carly A et al. 2020. "Ac Ce Pt e d an Us Cr Ip t Ac Ce Pt e Us Cr." : 1-27.

[64] Attwood, Lucy O et al. 2020. "Since January 2020 Elsevier Has Created a COVID-19 Resource Centre with Free Information in English and Mandarin on the Novel Coronavirus COVID-19 . The COVID-19 Resource Centre Is Hosted on Elsevier Connect , the Company ' sPublic News and Information ." (January).

[65] Dorlass, Erick Gustavo et al. 2020. "Lower Cost Alternatives for Molecular Diagnosis of COVID-19: Conventional RT-PCR and SYBR Green-Based RT-QPCR." Brazilian Journal of Microbiology 51(3): 1117-1123.

[66] Jung et al., "Comparative Analysis of Primer-Probe Sets for RT-qPCR of COVID-19 Causative Virus (SARS-CoV-2)," ACS Infect. Dis., vol. 6, no. 9, pp. 2513-2523, 2020, doi: 10.1021/acsinfecdis.0c00464.

[67] Li, Dandan, Jiawei Zhang, and Jinming Li. 2020. "Primer Design for Quantitative Real-Time PCR for the Emerging Coronavirus SARS-CoV-2." Theranostics 10(16): 7150-7162.

[68] Vijgen, Leen et al. 2008. "A Pancoronavirus RT-PCR Assay for Detection of All Known Coronaviruses." Methods in Molecular Biology 454: 3-12.

[69] Yip, Cyril Chik Yan, Siddharth Sridhar, et al. 2020. "Development and Evaluation of Novel and Highly Sensitive Single-Tube Nested Real-Time Rt-Pcr Assays for Sars-Cov-2 Detection." International Journal of Molecular Sciences 21(16): 1-11.

[70] H. Shao *et al.*, "Chip-based analysis of exosomal mRNA mediating drug resistance in glioblastoma," Nat. Commun., vol. 6, p. 25959588, 2015, doi: 10.1038/ncomms7999.

[71] A. M. Thompson, A. Gansen, A. L. Paguirigan, J. E. Kreutz, J. P. Radich, and D. T. Chiu, "Self-digitization microfluidic chip for absolute quantification of mRNA in single cells," Anal. Chem., vol. 86, no. 24, pp. 12308-12314, 2014, doi: 10.1021/ac5035924.

[72] I. Smyrlaki *et al.*, "Massive and rapid COVID-19 testing is feasible by extraction-free SARS-CoV-2 RT-PCR," Nat. Commun., vol. 11, no. 1, pp. 1-12, 2020, doi: 10.1038/s41467-020-18611-5.

[73] P. Zhou *et al.*, "A pneumonia outbreak associated with a new coronavirus of probable bat origin," Nature, vol. 579, no. 7798, pp. 270-273, 2020, doi: 10.1038/s41586-020-2012-7.

[74] J. Guarner, "Three Emerging Coronaviruses in Two Decades: The Story of SARS, MERS, and Now COVID-19," Am. J. Clin. Pathol., vol. 153, no. 4, pp. 420-421, 2020, doi: 10.1093/ajcp/aqaa029.

[75] P. Zhou *et al.*, "Fatal swine acute diarrhoea syndrome caused by an HKU2-related coronavirus of bat origin," Nature, vol. 556, no. 7700, pp. 255-259, 2018, doi: 10.1038/s41586-018-0010-9.

[76] D. P. Oran and E. J. Topol, "Prevalence of Asymptomatic SARS-CoV2 Infection : A Narrative Review," Ann.Intern. Med., vol. 173, no. 5, pp. 362-367, 2020, doi: 10.7326/M20-3012.

[77] L. Xiu *et al.*, "A RT-PCR assay for the detection of coronaviruses from four genera," J. Clin. Virol., vol. 128, pp. 1-2, 2020, doi: 10.1016/j.jcv.2020.104391.

Chapter 12

Current Status of COVID-19 Diagnostics

Surabhi Dixit and Monal Sharma

Abstract

In December 2019, an unexpected outbreak was caused by novel corona virus, severe acute respiratory syndrome coronavirus 2 (SARS-CoV-2). The lung disease caused by SARS-CoV-2 was given the name of the novel coronavirus disease 2019 (COVID-19) by the World Health Organization (WHO) on February 11, 2020. Since its origin in the Hubei province of Wuhan city in China, now it has spread to 218 countries worldwide. Panic situation created by COVID-19 has compelled researchers and doctors to work collaboratively. To combat with the disease, every control measures are under consideration from drug discovery to vaccine development. In the management of disease, rapid diagnosis is equally important as development of vaccine and drug. At present, various diagnostic kits are available for COVID-19. With the disease progression, global demand for diagnostics is raising. So, this chapter will include the updates on efficient diagnostic assays and future of diagnostic.

Keywords: novel corona virus, COVID-19, SARS-CoV-2, diagnosis, COVID-19 management

1. Introduction

COVID-19 is now a global health emergency as the number of confirmed COVID-19 cases worldwide exceeds 75 million, while the number of global deaths exceeds 1 million. WHO has already declared COVID-19 as a public health emergency of international concern (PHEIC) on January 30, 2020 and a pandemic on March 11, 2020. New COVID-19 cases and deaths are continuously rising. Globally, there have been 106,797,721 confirmed cases and 2,341,145 deaths as per a WHO report on February 11, 2021, since the pandemic started [1, 2]. At the start of pandemic, the regions of the America and Europe were affected badly, contributed 85% of new cases and 86% of new deaths globally. The USA and India are top two countries with more than 10 million confirmed cases and 313,748 and 145,810 deaths, respectively [3]. The infection starts to spread from the seafood wholesale market in Wuhan, China, while the exact origin of the first case remains unclear. Initially, COVID-19 spread, from china to other countries, was due to travelers who got infected in China and then moved outside of the China [4]. Countries who have reported travel-associated spread were Singapore, Japan, Republic of Korea, Malaysia, Vietnam, Australia, the United States of America, Germany, etc. [4, 5]. Current, corona virus outbreak is third after the SARS and MERS corona virus outbreaks. SARS-CoV-2 virus evolved in such a manner that the spread of COVID-19 is more severe than that of the previous severe acute respiratory syndrome (SARS) and the middle east respiratory syndrome (MERS) [6]. Currently, the COVID-19 pandemic has reached to a threatening new phase. New strains from UK with more infectivity are being reported. SARS-CoV-2 belongs to family *Coronaviridae* and order *Nidovirales*. SARS-CoV-2 stands together with two highly pathogenic viruses, SARS-CoV and MERS-CoV as belongs to Betacoronavirus genera [7]. Corona viruses are enveloped, positive-sense, single-stranded RNA viruses. Transmission of SARS-CoV-2 was initiated first from infected animals to humans and then spread rapidly throughout the world via human to human. It spreads via contact to respiratory droplets or aerosols through nosocomial transmission from an infected to uninfected [8]. As COVID-19 causes enormous human casualties and serious economic loss, we are in the urgent need of efficient vaccine and drug development against this dreadful virus. Globally, various serious efforts are being made in this direction. Governments of many countries have taken immediate action and precautionary measures against the virus. Countrywide lockdown were imposed to minimize human contact at public places. Social distancing, hygiene, and self-quarantine limit social interactions and spread of the disease. To control and manage the present pandemic situation the entire world is working and taking necessary steps. To propagate research in this field, governments are providing enough funds for scientists and institutions. To combat with the disease, both preventive and curative approach is considered. We have many potential vaccine candidates that are yet to be approved. Recently in mid November, four groups have reported about the efficacy of their vaccines. Vaccination has been started in many countries like USA, India. Pfizer-BioNTech COVID-19 vaccine and Moderna's COVID-19 vaccine have been approved by FDA recently [9].

To cure the infected patient, several drugs are being tested and used. Drugs that are currently in clinical trials are repurposed drugs, which were designed for other disease including antiviral and antimalarials [10–13]. Other natural product-based formulations are also tested in the management of the disease, for example, Indian giloy (*Tinospora cordifolia*) and ashwagandha [14, 15]. Because of continued spread of COVID-19, accurate diagnosis of people becomes necessary. Rapid screening of an infected person before transmission onto others is essential to curb the disease. Delay and inaccurate diagnosis will give patient a chance to spread the virus. Present pandemic has enforced researchers to work at breakneck speed. As a major contribution toward diagnostic of COVID-19, various detection methods have been developed. Primarily we have molecular-based approaches to confirm suspected cases. Real-time reverse transcription-polymerase chain reaction (RT-PCR)-based testing is the main technique for laboratory diagnosis. Virus antigen- or serological antibody-based assays are also available with the advantage of a short turnaround time for the detection of novel corona virus infection. In this chapter, we will discuss and review the available COVID-19 detection methods and future prospectus of the same.

2. Disease biology

SARS-CoV-2 is a novel corona virus. It is spherical and enveloped. SARS-CoV-2 spans 50–200 nM in diameter. It also contains a typical crown like appearance of coronaviruses due to the presence of 20 nM long spikes like structure on its surface (**Figure 1**). Corona viruses are divided into four genera: alpha-coronavirus (α-CoV), betacoronavirus (β-CoV), gamma-coronavirus (γ-CoV), and delta-coronavirus (δ-CoV). SARS-CoV-2 belongs to β-CoV genera. SARS-CoV-2 is a positive-sense, single-stranded RNA virus with large 29 Kb genome size [16, 17]. Genome wide study demonstrates that SARS-CoV-2 has sequence similarity with the human and bat corona viruses with 82% and 89% sequence homology, respectively [18]. Protein

DOI: http://dx.doi.org/10.5772/intechopen.96955

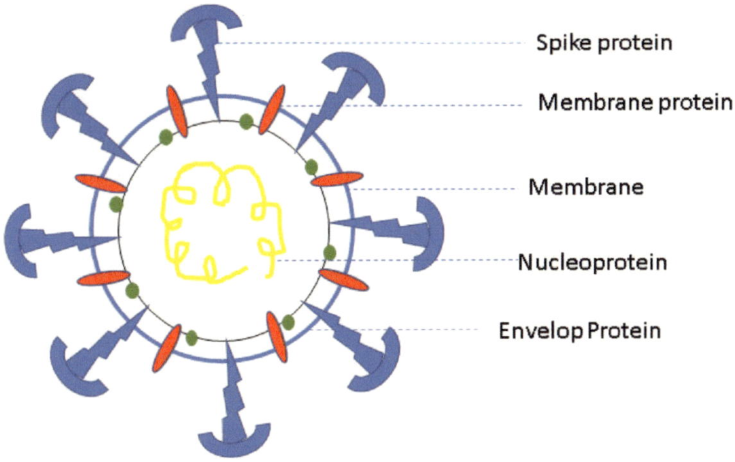

Figure 1.
Schematic diagram showing SARS-CoV-2 structure.

mapping reveals the common protein interaction networks among three CoVs (SARS-CoV-1, MERS-CoV, and SARS-CoV-2) in humans, hence identified molecular mechanisms and potential therapeutic interventions [19]. Genome organization includes sequences for leader region, UTRs, replicase, Spike, Envelope, Membrane, Nucleocapsid protein, 3′UTR, and poly (A) tail sequence [20]. The spike (S), membrane (M), envelope (E), and nucleocapsid (N) are the main four structural proteins of SARS-CoV-2 (**Figure 2**). Spike protein is a club-shaped protein present on the surface of virus and also capable of inducing neutralizing antibodies. It plays a major role in pathogenesis of SARS-CoV-2. M protein is the conserved and abundant protein, which helps virus to maintain its shape. It is also important during budding of viral particles from host cells. Role of E protein is important in viral pathogenesis. Like M protein, E is also a conserved one. Spike, E, and M together form the envelope of SARS-CoV-2. Viral RNA and N protein construct the nucleocapsid of virus [21, 22]. SARS-CoV-2 infects the upper respiratory tract in humans and cause common cold and flu-like infections. Patients suffer from influenza, sore throat, fever, cough, fatigue, and shortness of breath; in few cases, patients also experience gastrointestinal issues, such as diarrhea and vomiting. Severity leads to multiorgan failure and thus causes death [23, 24]. Old age people and individuals suffering from diabetes, hypertension, pulmonary disease, asthma, bronchitis, and cardiovascular disorders are at high risk of severe case of corona disease [24]. It has been reported that bats are the natural reservoir of SARS-CoV-2 like for other human CoVs. SARS-CoV-2 was initially transmitted to humans from infected

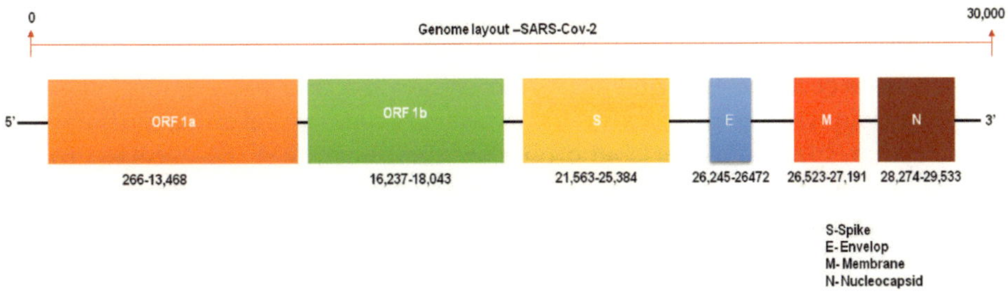

Figure 2.
Genome organization of SARS-CoV-2.

animals in the Wuhan market and then spread globally when human-to-human contact occurs via respiratory droplets or aerosols of infected [16].

At molecular level, when the receptor binding domain of spike protein interacts with human-ACE2 (angiotensin-converting enzyme 2) receptor, it facilitates the binding and subsequent entry of viral particles into host cells. The spike is a heavily glycosylated protein and made up of two subunits, the S1 and the S2. The S1 subunit is again divided into two domains, that is, an N-terminal (S1 NTP) and a C-terminal domain (S1 CTP). RBD is present in C terminal S1 CTP. The RBD shows genomic variability. RBD determines the cellular tropism and host range to be infected by virus [25–27]. Different strains of Corona viruses have variation in binding affinity or human ACE2, thus differ in infection ability, transmission rate, and pathogenicity. In comparison to SARS-CoV (~31 nM) and MERS-CoV (~16.7 nM), SARS-CoV-2 binding affinity (~4.7 nM) is very high [28].

3. Available diagnostic assays

The severity of the disease varies in diagnosed patients ranging from asymptomatic or mild cases to severe cases. The former can be cured by supportive care but the latter depends upon extracorporeal membrane oxygenation. Once patients reached to symptomatic stage, they become contagious and start to shed and spread the virus. Mass screening and accessible diagnostics always play a vital role to constrain the transmission and spread of the virus thus in reduction of mortality rate. Proper infection tracing is needed in the assessment of overall health impacts and statistics. Till now, there are various strategies for diagnosing COVID-19, which are mainly based on viral nucleic acid or antigen detection, and detection of the host's immunological responses. Description about the available test is below:

3.1 Molecular test

Till now, confirmatory diagnosis for COVID-19 is based on molecular approaches only. These are considered to be first-line methods. Nucleic acid testing based on real-time reverse transcription-polymerase chain reaction (RT-PCR) is the main technique for laboratory diagnosis. It involves nucleic acid amplification test to detect unique sequences within SARS-CoV-2 genome. RT-PCR is a two step process. In the first step, viral RNA is converted to cDNA using a reverse transcriptase enzyme, and the second step involves the amplification of only the selected region using gene-specific primers and further quantification is carried out as fluorescently labeled hydrolysis probe produces fluorescent signals [29]. Since the release of entire genome sequence of the virus from scientists of China, many countries, such as England, Germany, South Korea, Turkey, Russia, the USA, India, and China, launched their clinical-grade RT-PCR kits for SARS-CoV-2 detection. For RT-PCR kits, samples are taken from various infected parts of the body, including nasopharyngeal, oropharyngeal, or nasal swabs, upper and lower respiratory tract aspirates, bronchoalveolar lavage, and the sputum [30]. Main components in RT-PCR-based Kits are the reverse transcription and amplification enzymes, specific primers and probes for amplification of the selected viral genome regions, and authorized reagents for negative, positive, and internal controls, target genes, corresponding primer, and probe sequences used in RT-PCR kits so far for SARS-CoV-2 detection. Various research groups have been proposed the use of different set of target genes, corresponding primer, and probe sequences. Generally, the commercial kits based on the RT-PCR are only operated in well-equipped laboratory conditions and require skilled persons [31]. Pixel by

LabCorp COVID-19 Test Home Collection Kit made home collection possible. It contains a specimen biohazard bag, pre-labeled return FedEx envelope, saline tube, insulated specimen pouch, nasal specimen collection, swab gel pack (for sample cooling), shipping box, and the user guideline [32].

Other molecular-based technologies like LAMP, RT-LAMP, and rRT-LAMP amplify nucleic acid isothermally without any use of a thermocycler. DNA polymerase along with multiple primers, six or four as inner and outer primers, is used to amplify the target sequence. In RT-LAMP, analysis of results is done by the change of color, fluorescence, or turbidity in the PCR tubes, which makes it a simple and practical technique. Use of multiple primers gives specificity in results. RT-LAMP is a fast and specific method which completes detection of SARS-CoV-2 in 1–2 h without any need of a trained molecular biologist [33].

Another isothermal nucleic acid amplification based assay is SHERLOCK assay, which also employs the clustered regularly interspaced short palindromic repeats (CRISPR)/CRISPR-associated system (Cas) enzymology for the detection of the target nucleic acid. Upon the binding of CRISPR RNA to the target sequence, the nonspecific endonuclease activity of Cas13 or Cas12 starts, leading to the cleavage of nearby reporter RNAs which generates signal for detection. SHERLOCK is a very specific and sensitive assay for diagnosis as Cas13 does not get activated if two or more mismatches are present in the target RNA, and it can easily discriminate between SARS-CoV-2 and other similar viruses [34].

Advantages:

- RT-PCR is the gold standard for SARS-CoV-2 because it can directly measure the viral genomic parts.
- It is most reliable method for SARS-CoV-2 detection.

Disadvantages:

- It is a tedious, time-consuming protocol.
- When infection of the virus starts to move toward the lower respiratory track, sample collected from throat may give us false negative results.
- It requires laboratories with biosafety level II facility so not suitable for rapid testing.
- Limited number of assay can be performed.
- Sensitivity is low at early stage of infection.
- It can detect the active infection in a patient, not the recovered.

3.2 Antibody test

In an antibody test, existence and concentration of IgG and IgM antibodies is measured in the blood/serum/plasma samples of infected patients. It can determine if the body encounters with a pathogen like SARS-CoV-2 virus. Common antibody tests are based on lateral flow type assays (LFA) and enzyme-linked immunosorbent type assays (ELISA) [35]. An antibody LFA test detects the presence of the specific antibodies in the patient's blood sample. A SARS-CoV-2 antigen(s) is already immobilized on a sample pad. The sample is loaded onto the sample pad at end port where Colloidal gold (CG) or quantum dot (QD)-labeled detection antibodies are present. Sample along with labeled antibodies moves through the strip by capillary action to the test line and control line [36]. If SARS-CoV-2 antibodies are present in the sample, they will be captured by the labeled detection antibody and will bind to the immobilized antigen at test line. Even if the SARS-CoV-2 antibodies are absent in the sample, the gold-labeled antibodies will still be captured at the control line and a band on the strip will appear due to the accumulation of CG or QD.

ELISA tests are performed in multi-well plates coated with the recombinant viral antigen. If antibodies (IgG or IgM) against the SARS-CoV-2 antigen are present in the sample, a binding between coated antigen and SARS-CoV-2 antibodies occurs. Then, secondary anti-human antibodies are added to bind with SARS-CoV-2 Ag-Ab complex. Secondary antibodies are enzyme labeled (usually horseradish peroxidase). Upon addition of an enzyme substrate, a color-changing reaction happens. In the absence of the antibody of interest, no color is generated. In a modified version of ELISA, that is, chemiluminescent immunoassays (CLIA), the binding of the secondary antibody is confirmed by a chemiluminescent substrate [37]. ELISA test is a multistep process that demands a well-equipped lab, but LFA can be used at home without any training [38, 39].

3.3 Antigen test

An antigen is a non-self particle/fragment/molecule that can induce the immune system to produce antibody against pathogens, hence protects the body. The antigen test is also an immunoassay which detects viral components (i.e., S glycoprotein, M protein, or released N protein) or directly virus. Unlike the antibody-based methods, antigen tests detect the active viral infection, not the recovery situation. Because antigens precede antibodies, antigen test could be more reliable than antibody tests. Antigen tests can also be operated on LFA strips for rapid detection or in ELISA plates for increased sensitivity, and high throughput uses [29, 40].

Advantages:

- Antigen tests completes in 15–20 minutes.
- Antigen tests do not require well-equipped labs and highly trained personnel.
- It is cost-effective for both mass screening and application.
- Specificity is higher as it detects direct viral antigen.

Disadvantages:

- Low sensitivity as it requires high level of viral load for testing.

3.4 Other methods

Several other methods for diagnosis have been proposed. Some of them are novel and at research stage and some are based on conventional technology, for example, computed tomography (CT) scans. Aptamers functionalized with quantum dots (Qds), paper-based assays, semiconductor-based binding assays, surface plasmon resonance-based assays, piezoelectric immune sensors, and electrochemical sensors have been developed. A CT scan reveals about the possible abnormalities due to the viral infection in the chest [41]. Other detection

Method	Developer company	References
RT-PCR	Viractor Erofins	[46]
RT-PCR	Bosch	[47]
RT-LAMP	Abbott Laboratories	[48]
SHERLOCK	Howard Hughes Medical Institute	[34]
CMIA	Abbott Laboratories	[49]
Lateral flow assay	Pharmact AG	[50]
Lateral flow assay	ChemBioDiagnostic Systems	[51]
ELISA	Bio-Rad	[52]
Antigen test N protein LFA	Quidel Corporation	[53]

Table 1.
Developed kits for COVID-19 diagnosis.

technologies developed for the identification of SARS-CoV-2 are based on the presence of different biomarkers in bio-fluids. Increased concentrations of C-reactive protein, D-dimer, lymphocytes, leukocytes, and blood platelets and elevated levels of serum urea, creatinine, and cystatin C can be utilized for diagnosis. Biosensors based on plasmonic sensing and field effect transistor (FET) have been developed for mass screening. Localized surface plasmon resonance (LSPR) sensor detects the SARS-CoV-2 nucleic acid with combined use of photo-thermal effect and plasmon sensing [42]. In FET-based biosensors, biological molecules modify the charge distribution of the surface, or they generate a surface potential by binding to the surface, which is further measured as a conductance value [43]. For mass screening of such pandemic, we need a global e-platform to control the spread of the virus which is now possible with emergence of data science and advancement in mobile telecommunications. In this view, mHealth is a useful development, which is an application of mobile devices like smarphones, onboard optics/sensor based patient monitoring devices, and wireless/Bluetooth technology. Such advancements lead to easy collection of large epidemiological data based on contact tracing, automation of inventory mangement, digital, and fast reporting of the new cases. It can also help further in supply chain management of limited resources for affected areas and also help government in policy making [44]. Indian government has also launched "Aarogya setu" app during COVID-19 pandemic [45]. Information about some of the COVID-19 diagnostic kits based on above discussed methods are listed in **Table 1**.

4. Future of diagnostic and conclusion

COVID-19 has emerged as the most severe and terrifying viral infection encountered by us. Considering present pandemic situation, researchers from all around the globe have put strenuous efforts to develop test for COVID-19 diagnosis. They aim to develop a test that shows fast and accurate results, without compromising on the sensitivity and selectivity of the assay. Although present vaccine regime against COVID-19 has lessen the burden on health sector still, we are not aware of the long-term effects of COVID-19. Early medical interventions are only possible if diagnosis of the diseases is done at earlier stages. Many diagnostic tests have been developed which differ from sensitivity to specificity. Every test has disadvantages and advantages over the other methods (**Figure 3**).

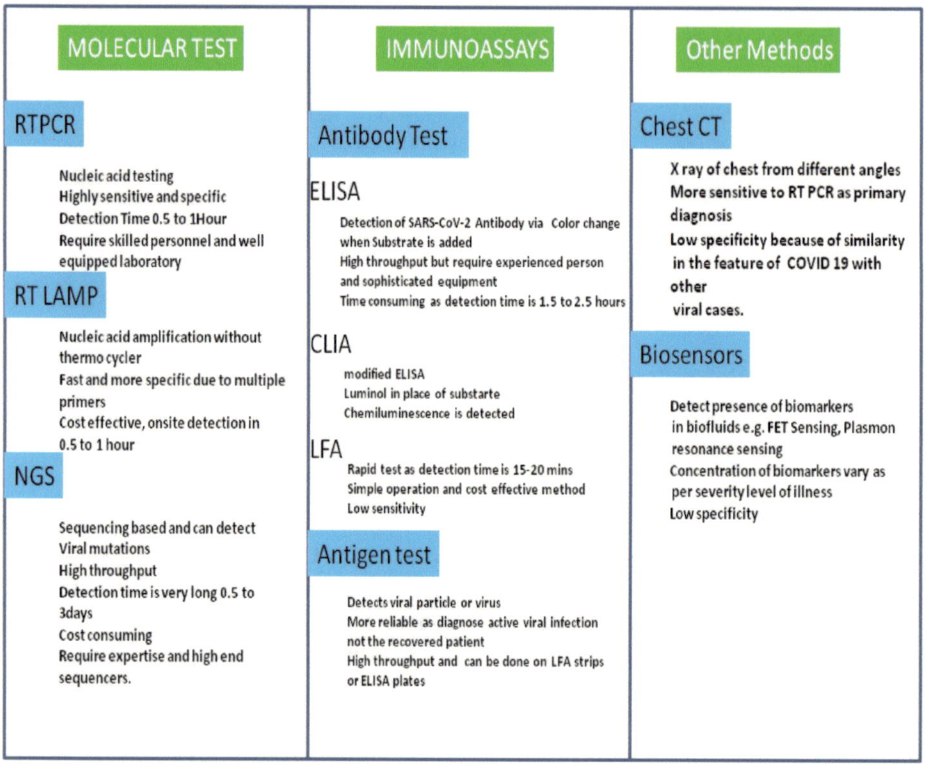

Figure 3.
Comparison of different COVID-19 diagnostic assay.

The genome-based detection of SARS-CoV-2 is solely relied on the RT-PCR method. Existing RT-PCR-based assays are not sensitive enough to detect the COVID-19 in the early stages of infection. Serology tests are rapid and apt for vast screening but they cannot confirm the presence of the active infection. Antigen-based test are also very promising but need development. Despite the excellent effort put by researchers globally, we are still in the need of developing an assay which can detect the SARS-CoV-2 in individuals at the initial stage. For this purpose, early stage biomarkers of COVID-19 should be identified and utilized for development of new assays. In severe conditions, CT scan can be used as complementary diagnostic tool along with RT-PCR [54]. It is reported that physicians took help of CT SCAN to effectively detect COVID-19 infection in RT-PCR false-negative cases. Antigen tests can also be performed along with RT-PCR to support present diagnostics and accelerate the detection speed worldwide. Different manufacturers and laboratories are using various parameters and conditions for testing. We do not have any universal standard for testing. Specimen and collection time needs to be optimized. Such standardization will give consistency in test results [55]. More effort toward research is required for further understanding of the influence of diagnostics. There is still scope in exploring about SARS-CoV-2 virus biology and COVID-19 pathology. Understanding of virus will help in developing more accurate diagnostic and effective treatment. Further research is required in the field of COVID-19 diagnostics to develop a rapid and automated diagnostic test with more sensitivity and specificity. In light of this, the government of India has also announced the call for various research projects for funding. In this direction public, clinicians, industries, and government all should work in coordination to fight against SARS-CoV-2. Global coordination between them is in high demand.

Acknowledgements

DST for funding.

Conflict of interest

The authors declare no conflict of interest.

Author details

Surabhi Dixit[1]* and Monal Sharma[2]

1 School of Environmental Sciences, Jawaharlal Nehru University, New Delhi, India

2 Duke University Medical Center, Durham, North Carolina, USA

*Address all correspondence to: surabhidixit29@gmail.com

References

[1] World Health Organization. Available from: https://www.who.int/emergencies/diseases/novel-coronavirus-2019. 2020. [Accessed: 11 February 2021]

[2] Vashist SK. In vitro diagnostic assays for COVID-19: Recent advances and emerging trends. Diagnostics. 2020;**10**(4):202

[3] COVID-19 coronavirus Pandemic. Available from: https://www.worldometers.info/coronavirus/ [Accessed: 21 December 2020]

[4] Phelan AL, Katz R, Gostin LO. The novel coronavirus originating in Wuhan, China: Challenges for global health governance. Jama. 2020;**323**(8):709-710

[5] Adachi S, Koma T, Nomaguchi M, Adachi A. Commentary: Origin and evolution of pathogenic coronaviruses. Frontiers in Immunology. 2020;**11**:811

[6] Vellingiri B, Jayaramayya K, Iyer M, Narayanasamy A, Govindasamy V, Giridharan B, et al. COVID-19: A promising cure for the global panic. Science of the Total Environment. 2020;**725**:138277

[7] Gorbalenya AE, Baker SC, Baric R, Groot RJ, Drosten C, et al. Severe Acute Respiratory Syndrome-Related Coronavirus: The Species and Its Viruses—A Statement of the Coronavirus Study Group. bioRxiv. 2020:1-20. Available from: https://www.biorxiv.org/content/10.1101/2020.02.07.937862v1

[8] Harapan H, Itoh N, Yufika A, Winardi W, Keam S, Te H, et al. Coronavirus disease 2019 (COVID-19): A literature review. Journal of Infection and Public Health. 2020;**8**:667-673

[9] Available from: https://www.fda.gov/emergency-preparedness-and-response/coronavirus-disease-2019-covid-19/covid-19-vaccines [Accessed: 11 February 2021]

[10] Dong L, Hu S, Gao J. Discovering drugs to treat coronavirus disease 2019 (COVID-19). Drug Discoveries & Therapeutics. 2020;**14**(1):58-60

[11] Gordon DE, Jang GM, Bouhaddou M, Xu J, Obernier K, White KM, et al. A SARS-CoV-2 protein interaction map reveals targets for drug repurposing. Nature. 2020;**583**(7816):459-468

[12] Guy RK, DiPaola RS, Romanelli F, Dutch RE. Rapid repurposing of drugs for COVID-19. Science. 2020;**368**(6493):829-830

[13] Tu YF, Chien CS, Yarmishyn AA, Lin YY, Luo YH, Lin YT, et al. A review of SARS-CoV-2 and the ongoing clinical trials. International Journal of Molecular Sciences. 2020;**21**(7):2657

[14] Kumar V, Dhanjal JK, Kaul SC, Wadhwa R, Sundar D. Withanone and caffeic acid phenethyl ester are predicted to interact with main protease (Mpro) of SARS-CoV-2 and inhibit its activity. Journal of Biomolecular Structure and Dynamics. 2020;**30**:1-3

[15] Balkrishna A, POKHREL S, Singh J, Varshney A. Withanone from *Withania somnifera* May Inhibit Novel Coronavirus (COVID-19) Entry by Disrupting Interactions between Viral S-Protein Receptor Binding Domain and Host ACE2 Receptor. Research Square. 2020:1-26. Available from: https://www.researchsquare.com/article/rs-17806/v1

[16] Wu F, Zhao S, Yu B, Chen YM, Wang W, Song ZG, et al. A new coronavirus associated with human respiratory disease in China. Nature. 2020;**579**(7798):265-269

[17] Wu A, Peng Y, Huang B, Ding X, Wang X, Niu P, et al. Genome composition and divergence of the novel coronavirus (2019-nCoV) originating in China. Cell Host & Microbe. 2020;**27**(3):325-328

[18] Chan JF, Kok KH, Zhu Z, Chu H, To KK, Yuan S, et al. Genomic characterization of the 2019 novel human-pathogenic coronavirus isolated from a patient with atypical pneumonia after visiting Wuhan. Emerging Microbes & Infections. 2020;**9**(1):221-236

[19] Gordon DE, Hiatt J, Bouhaddou M, Rezelj VV, Ulferts S, Braberg H, et al. Comparative host-coronavirus protein interaction networks reveal pan-viral disease mechanisms. Science. 2020;**370**(6521):eabe9403. Available from: https://science.sciencemag.org/content/370/6521/eabe9403/tab-pdf

[20] Lu R, Zhao X, Li J, Niu P, Yang B, Wu H, et al. Genomic characterisation and epidemiology of 2019 novel coronavirus: Implications for virus origins and receptor binding. The Lancet. 2020;**395**(10224):565-574

[21] Bianchi M, Benvenuto D, Giovanetti M, Angeletti S, Ciccozzi M, Pascarella S. Sars-CoV-2 envelope and membrane proteins: Structural differences linked to virus characteristics? BioMed Research International. 2020;**30**:2020

[22] Alsaadi EA, Jones IM. Membrane binding proteins of coronaviruses. Future Virology. 2019;**14**(4):275

[23] Chen N, Zhou M, Dong X, Qu J, Gong F, Han Y, et al. Epidemiological and clinical characteristics of 99 cases of 2019 novel coronavirus pneumonia in Wuhan, China: A descriptive study. The Lancet. 2020;**395**(10223): 507-513

[24] Huang C, Wang Y, Li X, Ren L, Zhao J, Hu Y, et al. Clinical features of patients infected with 2019 novel coronavirus in Wuhan, China. The Lancet. 2020;**395**(10223):497-506

[25] Wu K, Peng G, Wilken M, Geraghty RJ, Li F. Mechanisms of host receptor adaptation by severe acute respiratory syndrome coronavirus. Journal of Biological Chemistry. 2012;**287**(12):8904-8911

[26] Xia S, Zhu Y, Liu M, Lan Q, Xu W, Wu Y, et al. Fusion mechanism of 2019-nCoV and fusion inhibitors targeting HR1 domain in spike protein. Cellular & Molecular Immunology. 2020;**17**:765-767

[27] Yu F, Du L, Ojcius DM, Pan C, Jiang S. Measures for diagnosing and treating infections by a novel coronavirus responsible for a pneumonia outbreak originating in Wuhan, China. Microbes and Infection. 2020;**22**(2):74-79

[28] Wang Q, Zhang Y, Wu L, Niu S, Song C, Zhang Z, et al. Structural and functional basis of SARS-CoV-2 entry by using human ACE2. Cell. 2020;**181**(4):894-904

[29] Green K, Winter A, Dickinson R, Graziadio S, Wolff R, Mallett S, et al. What Tests Could Potentially Be Used for the Screening, Diagnosis and Monitoring of COVID-19 and What Are Their Advantages and Disadvantages. CEBM2020; 2020

[30] Iyer M, Jayaramayya K, Subramaniam MD, Lee SB, Dayem AA, Cho SG, et al. COVID-19: An update on diagnostic and therapeutic approaches. BMB Reports. 2020;**53**(4):191

[31] Corman VM, Landt O, Kaiser M, Molenkamp R, Meijer A, Chu DK, et al. Detection of 2019 novel coronavirus (2019-nCoV) by real-time RT-PCR. Eurosurveillance. 2020;**25**(3):2000045

[32] U.S. Food & Drug Administration. 2020. EUA-LabCorp COVID-19

RT-PCR-Letter of Authorization [WWW Document]. Available from: https://www.fda.gov/media/136148/download

[33] Jiang M, Pan W, Arasthfer A, Fang W, Ling L, Fang H, et al. Development and validation of a rapid, single-step reverse transcriptase loop-mediated isothermal amplification (RT-LAMP) system potentially to be used for reliable and high-throughput screening of COVID-19. Frontiers in Cellular and Infection Microbiology. 2020;**10**:331

[34] Zhang F, Abudayyeh OO, Gootenberg JS. A protocol for detection of COVID-19 using CRISPR diagnostics. A protocol for detection of COVID-19 using CRISPR diagnostics. Cambridge, MA, USA: Broad Institute of MIT and Harvard; 2020;**8**:1-8. Available from: https://www.broadinstitute.org/files/publications/special/COVID-19%20detection%20(updated).pdf

[35] Krammer F, Simon V. Serology assays to manage COVID-19. Science. 2020;**368**(6495):1060-1061

[36] Koczula KM, Gallotta A. Lateral flow assays. Essays in Biochemistry. 2016;**60**(1):111-120

[37] Wan Y, Li Z, Wang K, Li T, Liao P. Performance verification of anti-SARS-CoV-2-specific antibody detection by using four chemiluminescence immunoassay systems. Annals of Clinical Biochemistry. 2020;**57**(6):429-434

[38] Adams E, Ainsworth M, Anand R, Andersson MI, Auckland K, Baillie JK, et al. Evaluation of antibody testing for SARS-Cov-2 using ELISA and lateral flow immunoassays. MedRxiv. 2020

[39] Zhang J, Zhang X, Liu J, Ban Y, Li N, Wu Y, et al. Serological detection of 2019-nCoV respond to the epidemic: A useful complement to nucleic acid testing. International Immunopharmacology. 2020;**88**:106861

[40] Diao B, Wen K, Chen J, Liu Y, Yuan Z, Han C, et al. Diagnosis of acute respiratory syndrome coronavirus 2 infection by detection of nucleocapsid protein. MedRxiv. 2020.

[41] Bernheim A, Mei X, Huang M, Yang Y, Fayad ZA, Zhang N, et al. Chest CT findings in coronavirus disease-19 (COVID-19): Relationship to duration of infection. Radiology. 2020;**295**:200463

[42] Djaileb A, Charron B, Jodaylami MH, Thibault V, Coutu J, Stevenson K, et al. A rapid and quantitative serum test for SARS-CoV-2 antibodies with portable surface plasmon resonance sensing. ChemRvix. 2020;**15**:10-26434

[43] Chen X, Liu Y, Fang X, Li Z, Pu H, Chang J, et al. Ultratrace antibiotic sensing using aptamer/graphene-based field-effect transistors. Biosensors and Bioelectronics. 2019;**126**:664-671

[44] Agrawal M. The Need for next generation diagnostic and surveillance technologies to battle SARS-CoV-2 pandemic. Biotechnology Kiosk. 2020;**2**(4):14-22

[45] Available from: https://www.mygov.in/aarogya-Setu-app/

[46] Viracor Eurofins. 2020. Available from: https://www.viracor-eurofins.com/about-us/newsroom/newsitems/viracor-eurofins-launches-coronavirus-sars-cov-2-rt-pcr-test-with-same-day-results-12-18-hours/ [Accessed: 11 February 2021]

[47] Bosch Global. 2020. Available from: https://www.bosch.com/stories/vivalytic-rapid-test-for-covid-19/ [Accessed: 11 February 2021]

[48] Abbott Laboratories. 2020. Available from: https://www.abbott.com/corpnewsroom/product-andinnovation/detect-covid-19-in-as-little-as-5-minutes.html [Accessed: 11 February 2021]

[49] Abbott Laboratories. 2020. Available from: https://www.abbott.com/corpnewsroom/product-andinnovation/abbott-launches-covid-19-antibody-test.html [Accessed: 11 February 2021]

[50] Pharmact. 2020. Available from: https://www.pharmact.eu/ [Accessed: 11 February 2021]

[51] ChemBio Diagnostic Systems. 2020. Available from: https://chembio.com/dpp-covid-19-igm-igg-system-ous-2/ [Accessed: 11 February 2021]

[52] Bio-Rad. 2020. Available from: https://www.bio-rad.com/featured/en/sars-cov-2-covid-19-testing-solutions.html [Accessed: 11 February 2021]

[53] Quidel. 2020. Available from: https://www.quidel.com/immunoassays/rapid-sars-tests/sofia-sars-antigen-fia [Accessed: 11 February 2021]

[54] Fang Y, Fang Y, Zhang H, Xie J, et al. Sensitivity of chest CT for COVID-19: Comparison to RT-PCR. Radiology. 2020;**200432**

[55] Wang W, Xu Y, Gao R, Lu R, Han K, Wu G, et al. Detection of SARS-CoV-2 in different types of clinical specimens. Jama. 2020;**323**(18):1843-1844

Section 5

Comorbidity and Other Medical Conditions

Chapter 13

COVID-19 and Cancer: Biological Interconnection and Treatment

Nidhi Jyotsana

Abstract

The COVID-19 pandemic has affected more than 125 million lives worldwide and more than 2.5 million people have died so far. Cancer in itself increases the risk of infection especially, cancer patients undergoing cancer-associated treatments are more susceptible to SARS-CoV2 infection. However, many questions related to the biological interconnection between the two diseases remain to be answered. This chapter summarizes some of the biological components that connect cancer to COVID-19 and provide knowledge to not only understand but also, target the co-morbidities.

Keywords: COVID-19, cancer, viral infections, chemotherapy, radiotherapy, immunotherapy, cytokine storm, coagulopathy, ACE2, TMPRSS2

1. Introduction

For past many decades, viral infections have presented a great challenge for cancer patients, on the delivery of cancer care, cancer research, and oncologists. COVID-19 caused by SARS-CoV2 virus continues to spread around the globe and more than 1 million people have been killed due to COVID-19 worldwide (at the time of writing). Though majority of infected people will recover, cancer patients remain at a higher risk to SARS-CoV2 infection and its related severe outcomes. Cancer patients are reported ~3 times more susceptible to SARS-CoV2 infection with possible poor outcomes than individuals without cancer potentially due to their systemic immunosuppressive state caused either by malignancy itself or the anti-cancer treatments. Moreover, the mortality rate of SARS-CoV2 positive cancer patients was reported 6% than 1% for non-cancer patients in China. However, a limited research has been done to understand the biological interconnection between cancer and viral infections. Especially, little is known about the SARS-CoV2 infection biology Therefore, studying whether and how SARS-CoV2 affects cancer and its progression and, vice versa is of utmost importance for (1) the better management of SARS-CoV2 infected cancer patients and, (2) developing novel treatment strategies that can target SARS-CoV2 and/or cancer.

2. Linking viruses and cancer

Viruses are the smallest microorganisms made up of a small number of genes in the form of DNA or RNA surrounded by a protein coating. Viruses enter into a living cell and hijack it's cellular machinery in order to make more copies of itself.

IntechOpen

When a virus enters the body, it triggers the body's immune system. These immune defenses begin with white blood cells which learn to attack and destroy the virus or the virus infected cells. If the body survives the virus attack, the immune system's memory is able to respond more quickly and effectively to subsequent infection by the same virus. This response is called Immunity. Immunity can also be triggered by getting a vaccine. Viruses can be divided into three classes: oncogenic, oncolytic and, non-oncogenic non-oncolytic viruses. The oncogenic viruses (for example, hepatitis C virus, human T-lymphotropic virus, hepatitis B virus) change cells by either integrating their genetic material with the host cell's DNA or enhancing already existing oncogenic genes within the host genome. Thus, the infected cell is regulated by the viral genes and has the ability to undergo abnormal growth. Conflicting results for the relationship between different viruses and various cancer sub-types have been stated in pre-clinical and clinical settings. This is due to the reason that the course and outcome for both, viral infections and cancer and regulated by the type of viral infection, type of cancer and the immune system components involved. For example, a faster growth of melanoma was observed in mice that were challenged with H1N1/influenza A virus due to shunting or diversion of cytotoxic T cells from tumor site to the viral infection site. On the contrary, a slower growth of Lewis lung carcinoma cells was observed in mice following influenza virus infection. Thus, more studies need to be undertaken for clearer context dependent results. Both viruses and cancer invade our normal healthy systems for their growth and proliferation. The inability of our immune system to distinguish between self and non-self, links the severe pathogenesis associated with cancer and viral infections.

3. COVID-19

Coronaviruses are a large family of viruses that can cause mild illnesses, such as the common cold, to more severe diseases such as Severe Acute Respiratory Syndrome (SARS) and Middle East Respiratory Syndrome (MERS). Coronaviruses take their names from the distinctive spikes with rounded tips around their surface, which reminded virologists of the appearance of the sun's atmosphere, known as corona. Coronaviruses are known to primarily target the human respiratory system. COVID-19 represents the seventh member of the coronavirus family that infects humans. Because the novel coronavirus is related to the SARS-associated coronavirus (SARS-CoV), the virus has been named SARS-CoV2. SARS-CoV2 infection may result in mild to severe symptoms that may develop between 2 and 14 days after exposure to the SARS-CoV2 virus. The symptoms of COVID-19 may include shortness of breath, chills, fever, cough, headaches, sore throat, and loss of taste or smell. Additional symptoms including aches, fatigue, nasal congestion and diarrhea may also appear. The illness may cause severe pneumonia and heart problems in some people and may also lead to death. Some people may not develop any symptoms following infection.

SARS-CoV2, by using the spike-like protein on its surface, binds to ACE2 (Angiotensin converting enzyme 2) prior to entry and infection into the host cell. Thus, ACE2 acts as a doorway for the virus that causes COVID-19. ACE2 is a carboxypeptidase enzyme present on the surface of many cell types in tissues like, lungs, heart, blood vessels, kidneys, liver and gastrointestinal tract. The function of ACE2 is to generate small peptides/proteins by cutting up the larger protein angiotensin which then go on to regulate functions in the cells involving wound healing, inflammation and blood pressure regulation, etc.

4. Cancer

Cancer is a broad term for a class of diseases characterized by uncontrolled growth and proliferation of abnormal cells. These normal cells have the ability to infiltrate and destroy normal tissues. The types of treatments that one receives depend on the type of cancer and how advanced it is. Mostly it is a combination of treatments such as chemotherapy, radiotherapy, immunotherapy, hormonal therapy, stem cell transplantation and other targeted therapies. Cancer on its own and its treatment using chemotherapy or radiotherapy weakens one's immune system, reducing the number of infections fighting immune cells and making it harder for one's body to fight infections including the viral infections. And this is why cancer patients who are undergoing or recently underwent chemo/radiotherapy are particularly at higher risk.

5. COVID-19 and cancer

COVID-19 by itself remains biologically novel and not much is known about the role of novel coronavirus SARS-CoV2 in cancer. Some critical questions that need to be answered are (1) Whether SARS-CoV-2 infection cause cancer? (2) Whether SARS-CoV-2 infection increases the risk of cancer? and, (3) Whether SARS-CoV-2 infection affects the survival of cancer patients?

Similar to other severe acute respiratory outbreaks (SARS-CoV, MERS-CoV), comorbidities such as hypertension and malignancy predispose COVID-19 positive patients to adverse clinical outcomes [1–4]. Whether SARS-CoV2 causes or modulates cancer pathobiology, is unknown. However, it is evident that patients undergoing cancer-associated treatments for example, chemo or radiotherapy and CAR-T cell therapy patients are at higher risk of becoming worse following COVID-19 infection [5, 6]. A recent study including 1,590 COVID-19 positive patients in China shows cancer as one of the more serious comorbidities that increase risk with respect to COVID-19 [4, 7]. Therefore, cancer patients receiving anti-tumor therapies should have vigorous screening for COVID-19 infection and their immunosuppressive treatment regimens and dosages potentially decreased in the case of COVID-19 co-infection [8]. For some patients, chemotherapy must be postponed until completion of the antiviral course of therapy, while others cannot be subjected to the viral infection therapy while under treatment for their cancer [9]. The symptoms of COVID-19 in cancer patients are mostly similar to the ones in general population (fever, coughing and shortness of breath) [10, 11]. However, cancer-associated treatments for example, steroids may suppress the fever symptom of COVID-19. The decision on treatment of a COVID-19 positive cancer patient depends on the type of cancer, stage of treatment, and severity of COVID-19. Immune dysregulation and chronic inflammation may be potential drivers of severe outcomes in COVID-19-positive cancer patients. Therefore, a better understanding of the mechanistic link between the two will help to prevent negative effects of infection and also enable the design of novel therapies that target cancer and COVID-19, and co-target both diseases.

6. The biology of interconnection between COVID-19 and cancer

The biological connection between COVID-19 and cancer remains an under-studied area. However, age, ACE2, cytokine storm, and coagulopathy are few strong connecters that link COVID-19 with cancer. A better understanding of these linkers may help us find novel therapy options for the comorbidities.

6.1 Age

Our risk of getting cancer increases with age mostly due to accumulation of mutations with our prolonged exposure to mutagens. In addition, as we grow older, our body's immune system and DNA damage repair system get weaker [12]. In a similar fashion, age has turned out to be a poor prognostic factor for COVID-19 patients. This suggests that age plays a similar role in the progression and pathogenesis of cancer and COVID-19. Further studies should be conducted to identify the molecular interconnection between age, cancer and COVID-19.

6.2 Angiotensin converting enzyme 2 (ACE2)

ACE2 is a carboxypeptidase enzyme that converts angiotensin I to angiotensin 1–9 and angiotensin II to angiotensin 1–7. It is involved in the regulation of heart function and in the protection during acute lung injury [13–15]. SARS-CoV-2 enters human cells through angiotensin 1 converting enzyme 2 (ACE2) [16, 17]. The virus enters via this spike protein, binds to ACE2, and together with ACE2 enters the cell, fuses to the membrane, the virus exists the endosome, and replicates [18]. ACE2 is expressed in multiple organs, including cardiovascular, respiratory, urinary and digestive systems in healthy individuals. The expression levels of ACE2 in cellular subtypes is shown to be viral infection- and interferon-driven [19–21]. Notably, the expression levels of ACE2 are different in cancer cells. According to a recent clinical study, the expression levels of ACE2 gradually increase from healthy control, adenoma, to colorectal cancer patients. This indicates that cancer patients are more likely to be infected with SARS-CoV2. Patients with tumors, expressing higher levels of ACE2, are more susceptible to SARS-CoV2 infection and have poor prognosis [19, 22, 23]. Renal tissue shows higher expression levels of ACE2, and this might explain why most COVID-19 patients have renal dysfunction [18, 24]. Decreased levels of ACE2 were reported in non-small cell lung cancer (NSCLC), and its over-expression had a protective effect in NSCLC and breast cancer via inhibiting cell growth and angiogenesis [25–27]. Due to limited research done in this area, it would be worthwhile to test whether levels of ACE2 increases or decreases in various tissues of cancer patients and COVID-19 patients and how this impacts COVID-19 infection in these patients.

6.3 Cytokine release syndrome

Cytokine release syndrome (CRS) or cytokine storm is a systemic inflammatory response. Cytokine storm can be triggered by pathogenic infections, certain drugs, antibody treatments and, chimeric antigen receptor (CAR)-T cell therapy [28, 29]. Cytokine storm induction is the main cause of inflammation in SARS-CoV-2 infection. Upregulation of cytokines for example, interleukin-6 (IL-6), interleukin-1 beta (IL-1β) in serum, tumor necrosis factor-alpha (TNF-α) are found in COVID-19 patients. Elevated levels of lactate dehydrogenase, and increased levels of circulating monocytes are also common in COVID-19 patients [30, 31]. Such elevated levels of pro-inflammatory cytokines are also observed in cancer patients undergoing immunotherapy and CAR-T cell therapy [32]. The cytokine levels in cancer patients undergoing immunotherapy are higher than the cytokine levels in COVID-19 patients experiencing acute respiratory disease syndrome. The understanding of oncologists in regulating severe inflammatory reaction may prove highly beneficial in these settings. Therefore, anti-inflammatory therapies currently used for cancer patients may be repurposed for the treatment of COVID-19 patients.

6.4 Coagulopathy

Bleeding complications including thrombosis are leading causes of death in cancer patients. Thrombotic events are also commonly associated with the morbidities in COVID-19 patients. Cancer/tumor cells release cytokines, cysteine proteases, tumor micro particles and other pro-coagulants in their microenvironment. Release of such biomolecules can cause an imbalance in hemostasis [33]. Increased levels of D-dimer and prothrombin and decrease in fibrinogen is reported in COVID-19 non-survivor patients at days 10–14 [34–36]. This highlights the significance of regular monitoring and maintenance of these factors in COVID-19 and cancer patients. Therefore, further insights into the molecular interconnections of COVID-19 and cancer disease conditions to coagulopathy may help in reducing the associated mortality in these patients.

6.5 TMPRSS2

Transmembrane Serine Protease 2, TMPRSS2 presents another potential point of connection between cancer and COVID-19. In prostate cancer TMPRSS2 is regulated by the androgen receptor, and the androgen receptor is found not only on prostate cells but on cells of the lung as well. Further investigation is needed to confirm whether the receptor regulates TMPRSS2 in lung tissue, but if it does, androgen-targeted therapies, which are used in the treatment of prostate cancer, could limit SARS-CoV2 infection by downregulating TMPRSS2.

7. Therapeutic options in COVID-19 and cancer patients

Previous studies suggest conflicting results on whether anti-cancer and anti-COVID-19 therapies can be co-administered safely. For example, in over 1000 HCV-positive breast cancer patients, chemotherapy was shown feasible with no significant side effects [37]. However, in another study, ovarian cancer patients undergoing chemotherapy were unable to generate antibody response to the influenza vaccination [38]. Therefore, further efforts are needed to investigate the efficacy and safety of co-administration of anti-cancer and anti-viral drugs and how these outcomes are dependent on the type of cancer, viral infection and therapy.

Vaccination is the most promising approach for preventing a viral infection. Pharmaceutical industries and research organizations across the globe have put great efforts in developing effective and novel vaccine candidates to neutralize SARS-CoV2 virus. Additionally, strategies like repurposing direct preexisting anti-viral drugs as well as convalescent serum from COVID-19 recovered patients have been effectively used. Different monoclonal antibodies (mAbs) that recognize the different epitopes on the viral surface may have improved efficacy in neutralizing the SARS-CoV2 virus. IL-6 inhibitors (for example, tocilizumab and siltuximab mAbs) have been used for the management of cytokine storm in cancer patients receiving CAR-T cell therapy. IL-1, a cytokine upstream of IL-6 which is also upregulated in CRS and IL-1 receptor antagonists such as anakinra have been used to treat arthritis patients. Another class of drugs are nontoxic immune-suppressants known as calcineurin inhibitors that impair T-cell function and thereby reduce cytokine levels. Various viral gene components fundamental for the unchecked proliferation of virus in host cancer cells can serve as therapeutic targets for effective anti-viral therapies. Studying these critical viral components will help the researchers to understand the interconnection between the biology of COVID-19-infected cancer versus normal host cells.

The role of various immune cells for example, T cells, and natural killer (NK) cells in understanding the pathology and therapies of cancer and viral infections is becoming more evident with time. This motivates scientists to enhance their understanding and develop novel immunomodulatory therapeutic strategies for co-targeting these diseases. Functional natural killer (NK) cells can produce antiviral responses against influenza infection and are also reported as potential anti-cancer agents. Additionally, due to their negligible graft vs. host signature, NK cells may provide a safer alternative to co-target cancer and COVID-19. Nanoparticles present excellent vehicles for delivering various disease-associated payloads in vivo. Nanoparticles ornated with recombinant human ACE2 protein on their surface may provide an effective therapeutic option for COVID-19 patients. Following binding to the spike protein of SARS-CoV2 virus, ACE2-conjugated nanoparticles may neutralize the virus and prevent it from binding to the ACE2 receptor present on host cells. Conventional anti-cancer treatment strategies, such as chemo or radiotherapy are unable to distinguish between cancer cells and normal cells. This is a significant drawback and leads to toxicities for patients undergoing treatment. Therapies that directly target viral proteins or generate immune responses against infected cells or cancer cells hold promise for effective and tolerable treatment strategies.

8. Future research perspectives

To understand the pathogenesis of COVID-19 and to connect the link between cancer and COVID-19, we need to develop and study suitable animal models that represent the comorbidity of different cancers and COVID-19 in patients with accuracy. Additionally, the role of specific SARS-CoV2 proteins may be studied by developing chimeric mouse models that express SARS-CoV2 proteins in some tissues. Ziegler et al. demonstrated that ACE2 expressing human cells are the primary targets for SARS-CoV2 infection and that human ACE2 expression in epithelial cells is interferon dependent [20]. Especially, a significantly weaker induction of murine ACE2 was observed in response to interferon or viral infection [20]. Thus, humanized models permissive to SARS-CoV2 infection would closely mimic the human disease condition. Investigating and identifying the relevant immune constituents may lead to new biological strategies to target co-morbidities associated with viral infections and cancer patients. Determining whether active SARS-CoV2 virus leads to cancer in mice would also be an interesting scientific to avenue to better understand the pathology of SARS-CoV2. Clearly, the learnings from cancer biology and cancer therapeutics research will help in establishing clinically effective treatment options for COVID-19 patients (**Figure 1**). It would also be of high relevance to include and study the role of demographic factors in context of cancer and COVID-19 comorbidities.

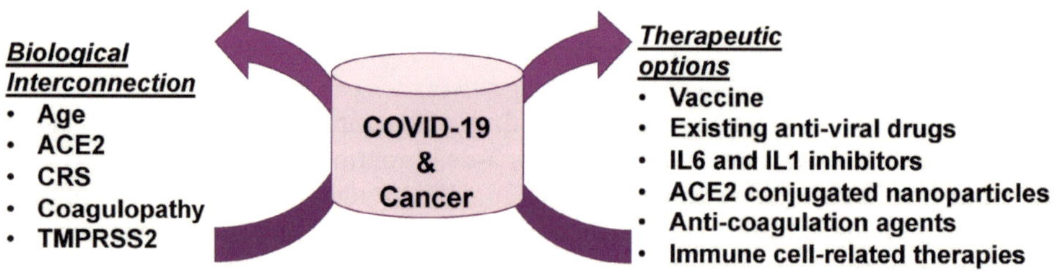

Figure 1.
Interconnection between COVID-19 and cancer.

Author details

Nidhi Jyotsana
Vanderbilt University, Nashville, TN, USA

*Address all correspondence to: nidhi.jyotsana@vanderbilt.edu

References

[1] Mauskopf, J., et al., *The burden of influenza complications in different high-risk groups: a targeted literature review.* J Med Econ, 2013. **16**(2): p. 264-77.

[2] Martinez, A., et al., *Risk factors associated with severe outcomes in adult hospitalized patients according to influenza type and subtype.* PLoS One, 2019. **14**(1): p. e0210353.

[3] Alqahtani, F.Y., et al., *Prevalence of comorbidities in cases of Middle East respiratory syndrome coronavirus: a retrospective study.* Epidemiol Infect, 2018: p. 1-5.

[4] Guan, W.J., et al., *Comorbidity and its impact on 1590 patients with Covid-19 in China: A Nationwide Analysis.* Eur Respir J, 2020.

[5] Liang, W.H., et al., *Clinical characteristics and outcomes of hospitalised patients with COVID-19 treated in Hubei (epicenter) and outside Hubei (non-epicenter): A Nationwide Analysis of China.* Eur Respir J, 2020.

[6] Sahu, K.K., et al., *Facing COVID-19 in the hematopoietic cell transplant setting: A new challenge for transplantation physicians.* Blood Cells Mol Dis, 2020. **83**: p. 102439.

[7] Hanna, T.P., G.A. Evans, and C.M. Booth, *Cancer, COVID-19 and the precautionary principle: prioritizing treatment during a global pandemic.* Nat Rev Clin Oncol, 2020. **17**(5): p. 268-270.

[8] Zhang, L., et al., *Clinical characteristics of COVID-19-infected cancer patients: a retrospective case study in three hospitals within Wuhan, China.* Ann Oncol, 2020.

[9] Borchardt, R.A. and H.A. Torres, *Challenges in managing hepatitis C virus infection in cancer patients.* World J Gastroenterol, 2014. **20**(11): p. 2771-6.

[10] Kalinsky, K., et al., *Characteristics and outcomes of patients with breast cancer diagnosed with SARS-Cov-2 infection at an academic center in New York City.* Breast Cancer Res Treat, 2020.

[11] Leonetti, A., et al., *COVID-19 in lung cancer patients receiving ALK/ROS1 inhibitors.* Eur J Cancer, 2020. **132**: p. 122-124.

[12] White, M.C., et al., *Age and cancer risk: a potentially modifiable relationship.* Am J Prev Med, 2014. **46**(3 Suppl 1): p. S7-15.

[13] Vickers, C., et al., *Hydrolysis of biological peptides by human angiotensin-converting enzyme-related carboxypeptidase.* J Biol Chem, 2002. **277**(17): p. 14838-43.

[14] Tipnis, S.R., et al., *A human homolog of angiotensin-converting enzyme. Cloning and functional expression as a captopril-insensitive carboxypeptidase.* J Biol Chem, 2000. **275**(43): p. 33238-43.

[15] Donoghue, M., et al., *A novel angiotensin-converting enzyme-related carboxypeptidase (ACE2) converts angiotensin I to angiotensin 1-9.* Circ Res, 2000. **87**(5): p. E1-9.

[16] Xu, H., et al., *High expression of ACE2 receptor of 2019-nCoV on the epithelial cells of oral mucosa.* Int J Oral Sci, 2020. **12**(1): p. 8.

[17] Zhou, P., et al., *A pneumonia outbreak associated with a new coronavirus of probable bat origin.* Nature, 2020. **579**(7798): p. 270-273.

[18] Wan, Y., et al., *Receptor Recognition by the Novel Coronavirus from Wuhan: an Analysis Based on Decade-Long Structural Studies of SARS Coronavirus.* J Virol, 2020. **94**(7).

[19] Dai, Y.J., et al., *A profiling analysis on the receptor ACE2 expression reveals the*

potential risk of different type of cancers vulnerable to SARS-CoV-2 infection. Ann Transl Med, 2020. **8**(7): p. 481.

[20] Ziegler, C.G.K., et al., *SARS-CoV-2 Receptor ACE2 Is an Interferon-Stimulated Gene in Human Airway Epithelial Cells and Is Detected in Specific Cell Subsets across Tissues.* Cell, 2020.

[21] Hamming, I., et al., *Tissue distribution of ACE2 protein, the functional receptor for SARS coronavirus. A first step in understanding SARS pathogenesis.* J Pathol, 2004. **203**(2): p. 631-7.

[22] Guan, W.J., et al., *Comorbidity and its impact on 1590 patients with COVID-19 in China: a nationwide analysis.* Eur Respir J, 2020. **55**(5).

[23] Liang, W., et al., *Cancer patients in SARS-CoV-2 infection: a nationwide analysis in China.* Lancet Oncol, 2020. **21**(3): p. 335-337.

[24] Lu, R., et al., *Genomic characterisation and epidemiology of 2019 novel coronavirus: implications for virus origins and receptor binding.* Lancet, 2020. **395**(10224): p. 565-574.

[25] Feng, Y., et al., *The angiotensin-converting enzyme 2 in tumor growth and tumor-associated angiogenesis in non-small cell lung cancer.* Oncol Rep, 2010. **23**(4): p. 941-8.

[26] Feng, Y., et al., *Overexpression of ACE2 produces antitumor effects via inhibition of angiogenesis and tumor cell invasion in vivo and in vitro.* Oncol Rep, 2011. **26**(5): p. 1157-64.

[27] Zhang, Q., et al., *ACE2 inhibits breast cancer angiogenesis via suppressing the VEGFa/VEGFR2/ERK pathway.* J Exp Clin Cancer Res, 2019. **38**(1): p. 173.

[28] Chatenoud, L., et al., *In vivo cell activation following OKT3 administration. Systemic cytokine release and modulation by corticosteroids.* Transplantation, 1990. **49**(4): p. 697-702.

[29] Shimabukuro-Vornhagen, A., et al., *Cytokine release syndrome.* J Immunother Cancer, 2018. **6**(1): p. 56.

[30] Wen, W., et al., *Immune cell profiling of COVID-19 patients in the recovery stage by single-cell sequencing.* Cell Discov, 2020. **6**: p. 31.

[31] Cao, J., et al., *Clinical features and short-term outcomes of 18 patients with corona virus disease 2019 in intensive care unit.* Intensive Care Med, 2020.

[32] Mehta, P., et al., *COVID-19: consider cytokine storm syndromes and immunosuppression.* Lancet, 2020. **395**(10229): p. 1033-1034.

[33] Falanga, A., M. Marchetti, and A. Vignoli, *Coagulation and cancer: biological and clinical aspects.* J Thromb Haemost, 2013. **11**(2): p. 223-33.

[34] Tang, N., et al., *Abnormal coagulation parameters are associated with poor prognosis in patients with novel coronavirus pneumonia.* J Thromb Haemost, 2020. **18**(4): p. 844-847.

[35] Zhou, F., et al., *Clinical course and risk factors for mortality of adult inpatients with COVID-19 in Wuhan, China: a retrospective cohort study.* Lancet, 2020. **395**(10229): p. 1054-1062.

[36] Levi, M., et al., *Coagulation abnormalities and thrombosis in patients with COVID-19.* Lancet Haematol, 2020.

[37] Miura, Y., et al., *The safety of chemotherapy for breast cancer patients with hepatitis C virus infection.* J Cancer, 2013. **4**(6): p. 519-23.

[38] Chu, C.S., et al., *Immunologic consequences of chemotherapy for ovarian cancer: impaired responses to the influenza vaccine.* Vaccine, 2013. **31**(46): p. 5435-42.

Chapter 14

Crosstalk between SARS-CoV-2 and Testicular Hemostasis: Perspective View

R.G. Ahmed

Abstract

The infection of SARS-CoV-2 and its COVID disease caused several economic and social disturbances worldwide. This chapter aimed to determine the severity of SARS-CoV-2 infection on the testicular hemostasis. This overview showed the possible mechanisms of how the SARS-CoV-2 can infect the testes. SARS-CoV-2-induced pneumonia, cytokine storm, and immunosuppressive state may transfer from the respiratory tract to the blood circulation, binding to testicular angiotensin-converting enzyme 2 receptors (ACSE2) and initiate its intracellular replication and action (cytotoxicity), that disrupting the testicular hemostasis. In severe states, COVID-19 disease can increase body/testes temperature, which may destroy the germ cell in the long term. The final mechanism is that SARS-CoV-2 infection causes stress, panic, and anxiety states, causing brain disorders that may perturb the hypothalamic–pituitary-testes-axis (HPTA). This disturbance may then lead to testicular dysfunction. The severity of COVID-19 may be age-dependent and depending on the expression and distribution of testicular ACSE2 receptors. Also, this chapter not only showed the sexual transmission of SARS-CoV-2 but also followed its impact on sexual behavior, pregnancy, and progeny. Thus, maintaining the testicular hemostasis may play a vital role in a healthy life for the offspring. Further research and clinical studies are required to explore this issue.

Keywords: SARS-CoV-2 (COVID-19), Testes, angiotensin-converting enzyme 2 receptor (ACSE2) HPTA, Pregnancy

1. Introduction

The World Health Organization (WHO) confirmed that the infection of SARS-CoV-2 could transfer from human to human via the airway droplet spread, infected surfaces, or fecal route [1–3]. SARS-CoV-2 causes COVID-19 respiratory disease belonging to β-CoV (lineage B) with a duration of 3–6 days [4]. Seah et al. [5] reported that coronaviruses (CoVs) consist of nucleocapsid protein (N) for bounding to RNA genome to make up nucleocapsid, spike protein (S) for binding of host cell receptors to facilitate entry of host cell, an envelope protein (E) for interacting with M to form a viral envelope, and membrane protein (M) for the central organizer of CoV assembly and determining the shape of the viral envelope. SARS-CoV-2 is dissimilar to SARS-CoV in the absence of 8a, longer 8b, and shorter 3b segments and different in the presence of Nsp 2, Nsp3, open reading frame (orf) 2,

Name of virus	Hosts			Classification and incubation period	Transmission of disease/its onset	Epidemiology	Recovery	Complications
	Natural host	Intermediate host	Final host					
SARS-CoV	Bats	Palm civets	Human	β-CoV, lineage B (2–11 days)	Human to human/ sudden	• 2002-2003 in China • Globally thereafter	5–6 weeks	It can damage the testes causing orchitis.
SARS-CoV-2		Malayan pangolins		β-CoV, lineage B (3–6 days)		• 2019-2020 in China • Globally thereafter	2–8 weeks	• It may cause a spermatogenic failure. • It may diminish the sperm concentration and motility.

Table 1.
Overview about the SARS-CoV and testicular complications [10–12].

and orf10 proteins [6–9]. This variance might be the cause of the highly contagious SARS-CoV-2 worldwide. The infection of SARS-CoV-2 can transfer from bats (natural host) to Malayan pangolins (intermediate host) and then to human, as shown in **Table 1** [10–12]. In general, the infection of SARS-CoV-2 can cause a dry cough, diarrhea, fatigue, and disorders in respiratory, circulatory, and renal systems [13–15], and then death [16]. Also, SARS-CoV-2 infection can disrupt the hemostasis of the urinary system [17]. Similar results are recorded in the Middle East respiratory syndrome (MERS-CoV, 2012) and severe acute respiratory syndrome (SARS-CoV, 2002–2003) infected animal models [18].

The current chapter aimed to determine the severity of SARS-CoV-2 infection on the testicular hemostasis and showed the possible mechanisms of how the SARS-CoV-2 can infect the testes. Also, this chapter showed the sexual transmission of SARS-CoV-2 and followed its impact on sexual behavior, pregnancy, and progeny.

2. Observations and discussion

2.1 Possible mechanisms of how the SARS-CoV-2 can infect the testes

As angiotensin-converting enzyme 2 receptors (ACSE2) expression is rich in testes, SARS-CoV-2 may bind these receptors to penetrate cells and initiate its intracellular replication and action (cytotoxicity) that disrupting the testicular hemostasis. Similarly, several studies reported that ACSE2 receptor expression is rich in human male gonads (spermatogonia, Leydig, Sertoli cells, and seminiferous ducts), thus SARS-CoV-2 can bind ACSE2 receptor to disrupt gonadal hemostasis and increase the risk of testicular dysfunction [19–22]. SARS-CoV-2 may cause spermatogenic failure [20]. However, the detection of SARS-CoV-2 in human semen was 1 to 15 patients (6.66%) [23]. More importantly, Li et al. [24] detected the SARS-CoV-2 in the semen of patients with COVID-19 and the semen of recovering cases. However, this study was limited to 50 patients only and a short time. Previously, SARS-CoV and NL63 coronavirus (NL63-CoV) can propagate inside the host cells by binding the cell surface ACE2 [25, 26]. SARS-CoV can disrupt spermatogenesis causing orchitis [27] and infect Leydig cells and testicular epithelial cells [28]. The previous findings could be attributed to SARS-CoV-2-induced pneumonia, neutropenia, lymphopenia, and hypo-albuminemia [29], and immunosuppressive state and cytokine storm [13, 14]. This state could be illustrated by the variation in the levels of several interleukins (IL-1β, IL-10, and IL-4), interferons (interferon-inducible protein 10, and interferon-gamma (IFN-γ)), and monocyte chemoattractant protein 1 (MCP-1) [13, 14]. Alternatively, SARS-CoV can elevate the levels of lipid peroxidation (LPO) and generally reactive oxygen species (ROS), causing oxidative stress (OS) and testicular dysfunction [30].

Another possible mechanism is that in severe states, COVID-19 disease can increase body/testes temperature, which may destroy the germ cell in the long term. Concomitantly, the viral infection-induced fever disrupts the male reproductive homeostasis [22]. In similar, severe fever in SARS-CoV causes congestion and mild fibrosis in the testes, disrupting the testicular hemostasis [27]. There was a reduction in the sperm number and fragmentation in the sperm DNA in males recovering from COVID-19 disease and fever [31, 32]. This variation can deteriorate fertility, delay embryo development, and augment abortion [33]. Importantly, fever alone can damage the spermatogenesis process [34] and destruct the Sertoli and germ cells [27].

The final mechanism is that SARS-CoV-2 infection causes stress, panic, and anxiety states, causing brain disorders that may perturb the hypothalamic–pituitary-testes-axis (HPTA). Also, the disturbance in the hypothalamic–pituitary axis can vary the sex hormones and adrenaline that support sexual activities [35]. SARS-CoV might cause leukocyte infiltration in testes [36], disrupt the functions of Leydig cells and the production of testosterone, destroy the seminiferous epithelium, and damage the blood-testis barrier [27]. Interestingly, the elevation in the level of serum IgG was reported in SARS-CoV patients [37]. This elevation could degenerate the Sertoli and germ cells, causing autoimmune orchitis [27]. Mumps orchitis could be attributed to the reduction in the level of testosterone and an increase in the follicular stimulating hormone (FSH) and luteinizing hormone (LH) levels [38]. In general, the virus can cause orchitis and sterility and increase the risk of the testicular tumor [39–41]. This damage may lead to hypogonadism [42] and decrease the number of Leydig cells [43]. In similar, male infertility might initiate by several viruses such as human papillomavirus (HPV) [44], herpes simplex viruses (HSVs) [45], human immunodeficiency viruses (HIV) [46], hepatitis B virus (HBV) [47], hepatitis C virus (HCV) [48], *Mumps orthorubulavirus* virus (MuV) [49], and Bluetongue virus (BTV) (an arbovirus of ruminants) [50].

2.2 Sexual transmission, sexual behavior, pregnancy, and progeny

The SARS-CoV-2 can transfer via respiratory droplets from human-to-human [51], feces [52], blood [53], or semen [24, 54, 55]. SARS-CoV-2 can form a systemic local infection in the male reproductive system due to the disruption in the barriers between testes, blood, vas deferens, and epididymis barriers [24, 54, 55]. However, the transportation of SARS-CoV-2 through semen was absent during the sexual process [56]. This absence may be due to the defense barrier between the testes and blood [57]. Importantly, real-time polymerase chain reaction (RT-PCR) has failed to designate SARS-CoV-2 sequences in the testicular tissues [43, 58].

The infection of SARS-CoV-2 may transfer during the sexual activity between the couples who have COVID-19 disease [59]. Moreover, saliva contact (physical process) between couples can increase the risk of virus transmission [12, 60]. On the other hand, pregnant women during the last trimester of pregnancy are more vulnerable to SARS-CoV-2 infection [61]. Moreover, cerebral vasculitis [62] and maternofetal T helper 2 (Th2) disorder [63] could damage the placenta. In Iran, 7 from 9 infected pregnant women with SARS-CoV-2 were dead [64]. A few data have supported this route [64]. However, most studies neglected the risk of the vertical route of SARS-CoV-2 between dams and their offspring [65–67]. On the other hand, the infected breast milk with SARS-CoV-2 or the close contact between neonates and infected dams with COVID-19 disease can be other routes for the possibility of SARS-CoV-2 transmission [68].

More importantly, the outbreak of infectious diseases can put the dams and their neonates in a risky state [69]. Likewise, SARS-CoV 2003 might disrupt the maternofetal immune system, causing abortion [70] or intrauterine growth restriction (IUGR) [71]. This disruption may delay neonatal health and cause neurodevelopmental disorders [72]. However, the severity and duration of this disruption on offspring are not identified completely. A healthy dietary supplementation and proper awareness during the perinatal period should be followed during this epidemic period to avoid this disorder. Also, anti-inflammatory treatments will be supportive to treat fertility problems [22].

3. Conclusion

This chapter showed three possible mechanisms of how the SARS-CoV-2 can infect the testes (**Figure 1**): **(1)** SARS-CoV-2 may bind ACSE2, disrupting the

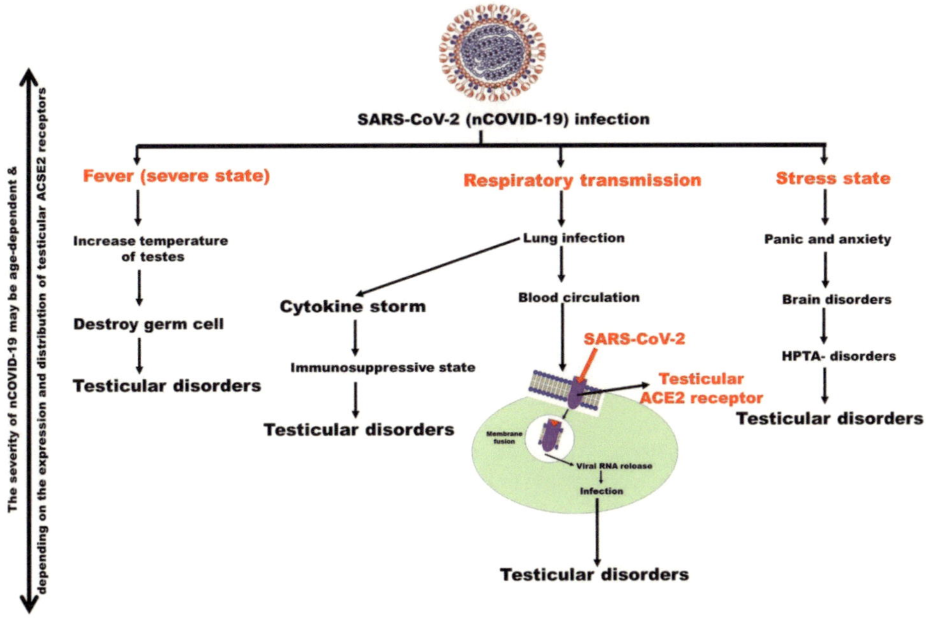

Figure 1.
Summary about the expected mechanisms of SARS-CoV-2 (COVID-19) on testicular hemostasis. Here, ACSE2 is angiotensin-converting enzyme 2, and HPTA is hypothalamic–pituitary-testes-axis.

testicular hemostasis. **(2)** SARS-CoV-2 and its COVID disease can increase the temperature of the testes, destroying the germ cell in the long term. This severity may be age-dependent and depending on the expression and distribution of testicular ACSE2 receptors. **(3)** SARS-CoV-2 and its COVID disease may perturb the HPTA. In the future, SARS-CoV-2 may directly or indirectly change the world's demographics [73]. Thus, preserving the testicular hemostasis may play a dynamic role in a healthy life for the offspring. Additional studies are desired to explore these issues.

4. Recommendations

As there is limited information about the complications of SARS-CoV-2 on reproductive organs, the current findings warrant the risk of the occurrence of orchitis and recommend the following-up and evaluation of the testicular hemostasis (andrological health) in the infected males with SARS-CoV-2. Also, avoid sex activity between the couples who have SARS-CoV-2 infection or symptoms of COVID-19 was recommended. In cases that recovered from COVID-19, the endothelial disorder may cause erectile dysfunction as a pathophysiological condition [74, 75]. Importantly, couples should be avoided the fear of virus transmission during the sexual process because this fear can decrease the sexual desire and quality of sex activity [76]. Moreover, these severe conditions can increase abortion, menstrual disorders, and psychological problems (depression, poor mood, nervousness, or irritability) [77].

On the other hand, recovered dams from symptoms of COVID-19 should use an artificial feeding pump, wash their hands, and wear a mask before and during the breasting feeding process [78]. Evaluation of gonadal function and genital examination for patients recovered from COVID-19 should be warranted. More importantly, the American Society for Reproductive Medicine (ASRM) recommended suspending all types of assisted reproductive techniques (ART), including intrauterine inseminations (IUIs) or in vitro fertilization (IVF) during the COVID-19 pandemic [79], particularly, for patients who have immunocompromised diseases (AIDS, cancer, or malnutrition) or chronic diseases (cardiovascular, hepatic, or renal diseases, hypertension, and diabetes mellitus) [80, 81]. Similarly, the French Biomedicine Agency (ABM) suspended ART during this period [82]. Finally, the social contact between ART professional groups and patients should be online during this period.

Acknowledgements

The author acknowledges all staff in his department for the general assistance.

Funding information

None funding agency found.

Conflict of interest

None stated.

Author details

R.G. Ahmed
Division of Anatomy and Embryology, Zoology Department, Faculty of Science, Beni-Suef University, Beni-Suef, Egypt

*Address all correspondence to: ahmedragab08@gmail.com

References

[1] Yang, H., Wang, C., Poon, L.C., 2020. Novel coronavirus infection and pregnancy. Ultrasound Obstet Gynecol. DOI: 10.1002/uog.22006.

[2] Yeo, C., Kaushal, S., Yeo, D., 2020. Enteric involvement of coronaviruses: is faecal–oral transmission of SARS-CoV-2 possible? Lancet Gastroenterol Hepatol https://doi.org/10.1016/S2468-1253(20)30048-0.

[3] World Health Organization. Novel coronavirus-China [WHO website]. 2020. http://www.who.int/csr/don/12-january-2020-novel-coronavirus-china/en/. Accessed March 18, 2020.

[4] Rasmussen, S.A., Smulian, J.C., Lednicky, J.A., et al., 2020. Coronavirus Disease 2019 (COVID-19) and Pregnancy: What obstetricians need to know. Am J Obstet Gynecol. pii: S0002-9378(20)30197-6. doi:10.1016/j.ajog.2020.02.017.

[5] Seah, I., Su, X., Lingam, G., 2020. Revisiting the dangers of the coronavirus in the ophthalmology practice. Eye ttps://doi.org/10.1038/s41433-020-0790-7.

[6] Angeletti, S., Benvenuto, D., Bianchi, M., et al., 2020. COVID-2019: the role of the nsp2 and nsp3 in its pathogenesis. J. Med. Virol. 2020, 1-5. https://doi.org/10.1002/jmv.25719.

[7] Wu, A., Peng, Y., Huang, B., et al., 2020. Genome composition and divergence of the Novel Coronavirus (2019-nCoV) originating in China. Cell. Host. Microbe. 27, 325-328. https://doi.org/10.1016/j.chom.2020.02.001.

[8] Xu, X., Yu, C., Qu, J., et al., 2020. Imaging and clinical features of patients with 2019 novel coronavirus SARS-CoV-2. Eur. J. Nucl. Med. and Mol. Imaging 1-6. https://doi.org/10.1007/s00259-020-04735-9.

[9] Vellingiri, B., Jayaramayya, K., Iyer, M., et al., 2020. COVID-19: A promising cure for the global panic, Science of the Total Environment (2020), https://doi.org/10.1016/j.scitotenv.2020.138277.

[10] Lam, T., Shum, M., Zhu, H., et al., 2020. Identification of 2019-nCoV related coronaviruses in Malayan pangolins in southern China. BIORXIV. doi: 10.1101/2020.02.13.945485.

[11] Ye, Z-W., Yuan, S., Yuen, K-S., et al., 2020. Zoonotic origins of human coronaviruses. Int. J. Biol. Sci. 16(10), 1686-1697. doi: 10.7150/ijbs.45472.

[12] Zhou, P., Yang, X.L., Wang, X.G., et al., 2020. A pneumonia outbreak associated with a new coronavirus of probable bat origin. Nature https://doi.org/10.1038/s41586-020-2012-7.

[13] Chen, N., Zhou, M., Dong, X., et al., 2020. Epidemiological and clinical characteristics of 99 cases of 2019 novel coronavirus pneumonia in Wuhan, China: A descriptive study. Lancet (London, England). 395, 507-513. https://doi.org/10.1016/S0140-6736(20)30211-7.

[14] Huang, C., Wang, Y., Li, X., et al., 2020. Clinical features of patients infected with 2019 novel coronavirus in Wuhan, China. Lancet 2020; published online Jan 24. https://doi.org/10.1016/S0140-6736(20)30183-5.

[15] Shi, S., Qin, M., Shen, B., et al., 2020. Association of cardiac injury with mortality in hospitalized patients with COVID-19 in Wuhan, China. JAMA Cardiol. doi: 10.1001/jamacardio.2020.0950.

[16] Gates, B., 2020. Responding to Covid-19- A Once-in-a-Century Pandemic? New England Journal of Medicine doi:10.1056/nejmp2003762.

[17] Zou, X., Chen, K., Zou, J., et al., 2020. The single cell RNA seq data analysis on the receptor ACE2 expression reveals the potential risk of different human organs vulnerable to Wuhan 2019 nCoV infection. Frontiers of Medicine. In press.

[18] Channappanavar, R., Perlman, S., 2017. Pathogenic human coronavirus infections: Causes and consequences of cytokine storm and immunopathology, Semin. Immunopathol. 39, 529-539. https://doi.org/10.1007/s00281-017-0629-x.

[19] Fan, C., Li, K., Ding, Y., et al., 2020. ACE2 expression in kidney and testis may cause kidney and testis damage after 2019-nCoV infection. medRxiv preprint doi: https://doi.org/10.1101/2020.02.12.20022418.

[20] Wang, Z., Xu, X., 2020. scRNA-seq profiling of human testes reveals the presence of ACE2 receptor, a target for SARS-CoV-2 infection, in spermatogonia, Leydig and Sertoli cells. Preprints (www.preprints.org) doi:10.20944/preprints202002.0299.v1.

[21] Roychoudhury, S., Das, A., Jha, N.K., et al., 2021. Viral pathogenesis of SARS-CoV-2 infection and male reproductive health. Open Biol. 11, 200347. https://doi.org/10.1098/rsob.20.0347.

[22] Tian, Y., Zhou, L-Q., 2021. Evaluating the impact of COVID-19 on male reproduction. Reproduction 161, R37–R44.

[23] Machado, B., Barcelos Barra, G., Scherzer, N., et al., 2021. Presence of SARS-CoV-2 RNA in semen—cohort study in the United States COVID-19 positive patients. Infect. Dis. Rep. 13, 96-101. https://doi.org/10.3390/idr13010012.

[24] Li, D., Jin, M., Bao, P., et al., 2020. Clinical characteristics and results of semen tests among men with coronavirus disease 2019. JAMA Network Open. 3(5), e208292. doi:10.1001/jamanetworkopen.2020.8292.

[25] Li, W., Sui, J., Huang, I.C., et al., 2007. The S proteins of human coronavirus NL63 and severe acute respiratory syndrome coronavirus bind overlapping regions of ACE2. Virology 367(2), 367-374.

[26] Wu, K., Li, W., Peng, G., et al., 2009. Crystal structure of NL63 respiratory coronavirus receptor-binding domain complexed with its human receptor. Proc Natl Acad Sci U S A, 2009. 106(47), 19970-4.

[27] Xu, J., Qi, L., Chi, X., et al., 2006. Orchitis: a complication of severe acute respiratory syndrome (SARS). Biol Reprod, 74(2), 410-416.

[28] Zhao, J.M., Zhou, G.D., Sun, Y.L., et al., 2003. Clinical pathology and pathogenesis of severe acute respiratory syndrome. Zhonghua Shi Yan he Lin Chang Bing Du Xue Za Zhi 17, 217-221.

[29] Zhang, R., Wang, X., Ni, L., et al., 2020. COVID-19: Melatonin as a potential adjuvant treatment. Life Sciences J. https://doi.org/10.1016/j.lfs.2020.117583.

[30] Dutta, S., Sengupta, P., 2021. SARS-CoV-2 and male infertility: possible multifaceted pathology. Reprod. Sci. In press. (doi:10.1007/s43032-020-00261-z).

[31] Holtmann, N., Edimiris, P., Andree, M., et al., 2020. Assessment of SARS-CoV-2 in human semen-a cohort study. Fertil Steril, S0015-S0282, 30519-7.

[32] Ma, L., Xie, W., Li, D., et al., 2020. Evaluation of sex-related hormones and semen characteristics in reproductive-aged male COVID-19 patients. J Med Virol. In press.

[33] Robinson, L., Gallos, I.D., Conner, S.J., et al., 2012. The effect of sperm DNA fragmentation on miscarriage rates: a systematic review and meta-analysis. Hum Reprod, 27, 2908-2917.

[34] Jung, A.; Schuppe, H.-C., 2007. Influence of genital heat stress on semen quality in humans. Andrologia 39, 203-215.

[35] Bhasin, S., Enzlin, P., Coviello, A., Basson, R. 2007. Sexual dysfunction in men and women with endocrine disorders. Lancet, 369, 597-611.

[36] Hedger, M.P., 1997. Testicular leukocytes: what are they doing? Rev Reprod Fertil 2, 38-47.

[37] National Research Project for SARS Beijing Group, 2003. Dynamic changes of T-lymphocytes and immunoglobulins in patients with SARS. Zhonghua Yi Xue Za Zhi 83, 1014-1017.

[38] Adamopoulos, D.A., Lawrence, D.M., Vassilopoulos, P., et al., 1978. Pituitary-testicular interrelationships in mumps orchitis and other viral infections. Br Med J. 1, 1177-1180.

[39] Tessler, A.N., Catanese, A., 1987. AIDS and germ cell tumors of testis. Urology 30, 203-204.

[40] Pudney, J., Anderson, D., 1991. Orchitis and human immunodeficiency virus type 1 infected cells in reproductive tissues from men with the acquired immune deficiency syndrome. Am J Pathol 139, 149-160.

[41] Oliver, R.T., 1997. Testis cancer. Curr Opin Oncol 9, 287-294.

[42] Ma, L., Xie, W., Li, D., et al., 2020. Effect of SARS-CoV-2 infection upon male gonadal function: A single center-based study. *medRxiv*. Published online March 30, 2020.03.21.20037267. doi:10.1101/2020.03.21.20037267.

[43] Yang, M., Chen, S., Huang, B., et al., 2020. Pathological findings in the testes of COVID 19 patients: Clinical implications. Eur. Urology Focus 6, 1124-1129.

[44] Foresta, C., Pizzol, D., Moretti, A., et al., 2010. Clinical and prognostic significance of human papillomavirus DNA in the sperm or exfoliated cells of infertile patients and subjects with risk factors. Fertility and Sterility, 94(5), 1723-1727. https://doi.org/10.1016/j.fertnstert.2009.11.012.

[45] Amirjannati, N., Yaghmaei, F., Mehdi Akhondi, M., et al., 2014. Molecular and serologic diagnostic approaches; the prevalence of herpes simplex in idiopathic men infertile. Iran Journal of Reproductive Medicine, 12.

[46] Dulioust, E., Le Du, A., Costagliola, D., et al., 2002. Semen alterations in HIV-1 infected men. Human Reproduction, 17(8), 2112-2118. https://doi.org/10.1093/humrep/17.8.2112.

[47] Oger, P., Yazbeck, C., Gervais, A., et al., 2011. Adverse effects of hepatitis B virus on sperm motility and fertilization ability during IVF. Reproductive BioMedicine Online, 23(2), 207-212. https://doi.org/10.1016/j.rbmo.2011.04.008.

[48] Karamolahi, S., Yazdi, R.S., Zangeneh, M., et al., 2019. Impact of hepatitis B virus and hepatitis C virus infection on sperm parameters of infertile men. Int. J. of Reproductive BioMedicine, 17(8), 551-556. https://doi.org/10.18502/ijrm.v17i8.4820.

[49] Otto, W., Mankertz, A., Santibanez, S., et al., 2010. Ongoing outbreak of mumps affecting adolescents and young adults in Bavaria, Germany, Eurosurveillance, 15(50), 3-6. https://doi.org/10.2807/ese.15.50.19748-en.

[50] Puggioni, G., Pintus, D., Melzi, E., et al., 2018. Testicular degeneration and

infertility following Arbovirus infection. J. Virol. 92, 19.

[51] Stadnytskyi, V., Bax, C.E., Bax, A., et al., 2020. The airborne lifetime of small speech droplets and their potential importance in SARS-CoV-2 transmission. Proceedings of the National Academy of Sciences of the United States of America 117, 11875-11877.

[52] Cheung, K.S., Hung, I.F., Chan, P.P., et al., 2020. Gastrointestinal manifestations of SARS-CoV-2 infection and virus load in fecal samples from a Hong Kong cohort: Systematic review and meta-analysis. Gastroenterology S0016-5085: 30448. https://doi.org/10.1053/j.gastr o.2020.03.065.

[53] Yu, F., Yan, L., Wang, N., et al., 2020. Quantitative detection and viral load analysis of SARS-CoV-2 in infected patients. Clinical Infectious Diseases. 71, 793-798. https://doi.org/10.1093/cid/ciaa345.

[54] Li, H., Xiao, X., Zhang, J., et al., 2020. Impaired spermatogenesis in COVID-19 patients. The Lancet 8. https://doi.org/10.1016/j.eclinm.2020.100604 100604.

[55] Li, N., Han, L., Peng, M., et al., 2020. Maternal and neonatal outcomes of pregnant women with COVID-19 pneumonia: a case-control study. Clin Infect Dis https://doi.org/10.1093/cid/ciaa352.

[56] Ibarra, F.P., Mehrad, M., Di Mauro, M.D., et al., 2020. Impact of the COVID-19 pandemic on the sexual behavior of the population. The vision of the east and the west. Int Braz J Urol 46, 104-112.

[57] Wang, S., Zhou, X., Zhang, T., et al., 2020. The need for urogenital tract monitoring in COVID-19. Nat Rev Urol 17, 314-315.

[58] Song, C., Wang, Y., Li, W., et al., 2020. absence of 2019 novel coronavirus in semen and testes of COVID-19 patients. Biol Reprod. 103(1), 4-6.

[59] Cui, P., Chen, Z., Wang, T., et al., 2020. Clinical features and sexual transmission potential of SARS-CoV-2 infected female patients: A descriptive study in Wuhan. China. doi: https://doi.org/10.1101/2020.02.26.20028225.

[60] Zhu, N., Zhang, D., Wang, W., et al., 2020. Novel coronavirus from patients with pneumonia in China, 2019. N Engl J Med 382, 727-733.

[61] Ahmed, R.G., 2021. Novel coronavirus SARS-CoV-2 (COVID-19) and pregnancy: A hypothetical view. Endocrine Metabolic & Immune Disorders - Drug Targets (In Press).

[62] Vivanti, A.J., Vauloup-Fellous, C., Prevot, S., et al., 2020. Transplacental transmission of SARS-CoV-2 infection. Nat Commun 11, 3572. https://doi.org/10.1038/s41467-020-17436-6.

[63] Liu, H., Wang, L-L., Zhao, S-J., et al., 2020. Why are pregnant women susceptible to viral infection: an immunological viewpoint? Journal of Reproductive Immunology doi: https://doi.org/10.1016/j.jri.2020.103122.

[64] Hantoushzadeh, S., Shamshirsaz, A.A., Aleyasin, A., et al., 2020. Maternal death due to COVID-19 disease. American Journal of Obstetrics and Gynecology, 223(1), 109.e1-109.e16. https://doi.org/10.1016/j.ajog.2020.04.030.

[65] Chen, H., Guo, J., Wang, C., et al., 2020. Clinical characteristics and intrauterine vertical transmission potential of COVID-19 infection in nine pregnant women: A retrospective review of medical records. The Lancet, 395(10226), 809-815. https://doi.org/10.1016/S0140-6736(20)30360-3.

[66] Liu, W., Wang, J., Li, W., et al., 2020. Clinical characteristics of 19 neonates born to mothers with COVID-19. Frontiers of Medicine, 14(2), 193-198. https://doi.org/10.1007/s11684-020-0772-y.

[67] Yu, N., Li, W., Kang, Q., et al., 2020. Clinical features and obstetric and neonatal outcomes of pregnant patients with COVID-19 in Wuhan, China: A retrospective, single-centre, descriptive study. The Lancet Infectious Diseases, 20(5), 559-564. https://doi.org/10.1016/S1473-3099(20)30176-6.

[68] Wu, Y., Liu, C., Dong, L., et al., 2020. Coronavirus disease 2019 among pregnant Chinese women: case series data on the safety of vaginal birth and breastfeeding. BJOG: An International Journal of Obstetrics & Gynaecology 127(9), 1109-1115. https://doi.org/10.1111/1471-0528.16276.

[69] Dashraath, P., Jing Lin Jeslyn, W., Mei Xian Karen, L., et al., 2020. Coronavirus disease 2019 (COVID-19) pandemic and pregnancy. Am J Obstet Gynecol. pii: S0002-9378(20)30343-4. doi: 10.1016/j.ajog.2020.03.021.

[70] Al-Haddad, B.J.S., Oler, E., Armistead, B., et al., 2019. The fetal origins of mental illness. Am J Obstet Gynecol. 221(6), 549-562.

[71] Wong, S.F., Chow, K.M., Leung, T.N., et al., 2004. Pregnancy and perinatal outcomes of women with severe acute respiratory syndrome. Am J Obstet Gynecol. 191(1), 292-297. DOI: 10.1016/j.ajog.2003.11.019.

[72] Xu, X., Han, M., Li, T., et al., 2020. Effective treatment of severe COVID-19 patients with tocilizumab. Proc Natl Acad Sci USA, 117(20), 10970-10975. doi: 10.1073/pnas.2005615117.

[73] He, W., Liu, X., Feng, L., et al., 2020. Impact of SARS-CoV-2 on male reproductive health: a review of the literature on male reproductive involvement in COVID-19. Front. Med. 7:594364. doi: 10.3389/fmed.2020.594364.

[74] Sansone, A., Mollaioli, D., Ciocca, G., et al., 2020. Addressing male sexual and reproductive health in the wake of COVID-19 outbreak. J. Endocrinol. Invest. 1-9. http://dx.doi.org/10.1007/s40618-020-01350-1 PMID: 32661947.

[75] Cariani, L., Orena, B.S., Ambrogi, F., et al., 2020. Time length of negativization and cycle threshold values in 182 healthcare workers with Covid-19 in Milan, Italy: An observational cohort study. Int. J. Environ. Res. Public Health 17(15), 5313. http://dx.doi.org/10.3390/ijerph17155313 PMID: 32718008.

[76] Hashem, N.M., Abdelnour, S.A., Alhimaidi, A.R., 2021. Potential impacts of COVID-19 on reproductive health: Scientific findings and social dimension. Saudi Journal of Biological Sciences 28; 1702-1712. DOI: 10.1016/j.sjbs.2020.12.012.

[77] Yuksel, B., Ozgor, F., 2020. Effect of the COVID-19 pandemic on female sexual behavior. Int J Gynaecol Obstet 150, 98-102.

[78] Ferrazzi, E., Frigerio, L., Savasi, V., et al., 2020. Vaginal delivery in SARS-CoV-2-infected pregnant women in Northern Italy: a retrospective analysis. BJOG 127, 1116-1121.

[79] La Marca, A., Niederberger, C., Pellicer, A., et al., 2020. COVID-19: lessons from the Italian reproductive medical experience. INKLINGS, Fertility and Sterility, in press.

[80] Nishi, D., Imamura, K., Watanabe, K., et al., 2020. Internet-based cognitive–behavioural therapy for prevention of depression during pregnancy and in the postpartum (iPDP): a protocol for a large-scale

randomized controlled trial. BMJ Open 10, e036482.

[81] Vaiarelli, A., Bulletti, C., Cimadomo, D., et al., 2020. COVID-19 and ART: the view of the Italian Society of Fertility and Sterility and Reproductive Medicine. Reprod Biomed Online 40, 755-759.

[82] Hamdi, S., Bendayan, M., Huyghe, E., et al., 2020. COVID-19 and andrology: Recommendations of the French-speaking society of andrology (Société d'Andrologie de langue Française SALF). Basic and Clinical Andrology 30, 10.

Chapter 15

COVID-19: A Catalyst for Novel Psychiatric Paradigms - Part 1

Adonis Sfera, Carolina Osorio,
Jose E. Campo Maldonado, Afzaal Jafri, Aaron D. Chokka,
Carlos Manuel Zapata Martín del Campo
and Zisis Kozlakidis

Abstract

Severe acute respiratory syndrome coronavirus-2 (SARS-CoV-2) emerged in the late 2019 and spread rapidly throughout the world, becoming a pandemic in March 2020. It became obvious early that the prognosis of this illness is highly variable, ranging from few mild symptoms to severe complications and death, indicating that aside from the pathogen virulence, host factors contribute significantly to the overall outcome. Like SARS-CoV and Human Coronavirus NL63 (HCoV-NL63-NL63), SARS-CoV-2 enters host cells via several receptors among which angiotensin converting enzyme-2 (ACE-2) are the most studied. As this protein is widely expressed in the lungs, blood vessels, brain, kidney, testes and ovaries, the effects of this virus are widespread, affecting many body tissues and organs. Viral attachment to ACE-2 downregulates this protein, disrupting angiotensin II (ANG II) hydrolysis that in return contributes to the unchecked accumulation of this peptide. ANG II toxicity is the result of excessive activation of ANG II type 1 receptors (AT-1Rs) and N-methyl-D-aspartate NMDA receptors (NMDARs). Overstimulation of these proteins, along with the loss of angiotensin (1–7) (ANG 1–7), upregulates reactive oxygen species (ROS), inflicting end-organ damage (hit 1). However, a preexistent redox impairment may be necessary for the development of SARS-CoV-2 critical illness (hit 2). Here we propose a two-hit paradigm in which COVID-19 critical illness develops primarily in individuals with preexistent antioxidant dysfunction. Several observational studies are in line with the two hit model as they have associated poor COVID-19 prognosis with the hereditary antioxidant defects. Moreover, the SARS-CoV-2 interactome reveals that viral antigen NSP5 directly inhibits the synthesis of glutathione peroxidase (GPX), an antioxidant enzyme that along with glucose-6-phosphate dehydrogenase (G6PD) protect the body from oxidative damage. Indeed, individuals with G6PD deficiency have less favorable COVID-19 outcomes compared to the general population.

Keywords: Sars-CoV-2, antiviral psychotropic drugs, glucose-6-phosphate dehydrogenase, glutathione peroxidase, endocytic pathway, calmodulin

1. Introduction

The COVID-19 pandemic has altered many aspects of daily life, contributing to the higher incidence of psychiatric conditions, including depression, anxiety,

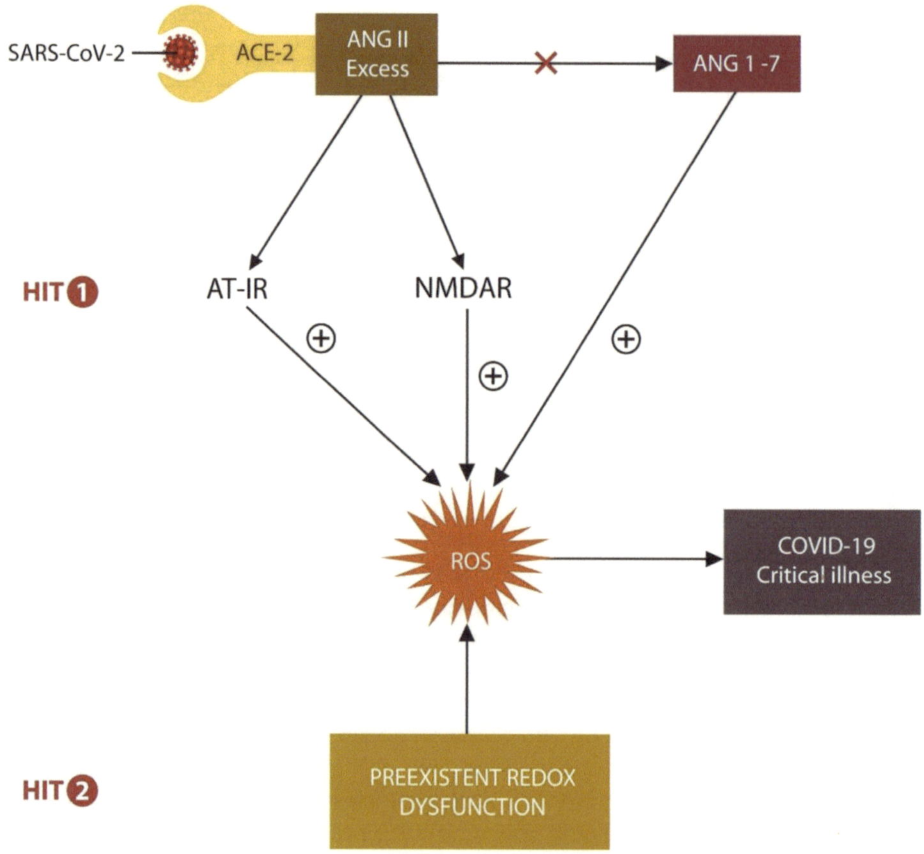

Figure 1.
The two-hit paradigm: Excessive angiotensin II (ANG II) and loss of angiotensin (1–7) (ANG 1–7) generate oxidative stress both directly and indirectly (via ANG II-AT-1R and ANG II-NMDAR axes). COVID-19 critical illness is triggered when a preexistent redox dysfunction (second hit) is present.

posttraumatic stress disorder (PTSD) and substance use [1–8]. In addition, as SARS-CoV-2 is a neurotropic virus, delirium, cognitive impairment and psychosis were demonstrated in up to 40% of infected patients [9–11]. Moreover, like the previous pandemics, COVID-19 may be followed by delayed or even next-generation neuropsychiatric sequelae [12–14]. For example, the offspring of women pregnant during the 1918 influenza pandemic achieved lower education, socioeconomic status, and income as adults, indicating hidden and long-lasting effects [15] (**Figure 1**).

2. COVID-19 and psychotropic drugs

Several psychotropic drugs have been associated with antiviral and antitumor properties, suggesting that they may lower the severity of COVID-19 critical illness [16]. For example, imipramine, clomipramine and the phenothiazine class of drugs have demonstrated efficacy against other viruses, including Ebola, Dengue and West Nile [17–20]. In addition, thioridazine, another phenothiazine, was found to slow the progression of lung cancers, probably by enhancing antitumor immunity [21]. Other antipsychotics evidenced some beneficial effects in patients with glioblastoma and pancreatic cancer, suggesting immuno-oncological properties [22].

The recently published SARS-CoV-2/host protein–protein interaction and phosphorylation studies demonstrated viral interference with several pathways previously implicated in psychiatric disorders and targeted by psychotropic drugs [23, 24]. For example, upon binding to ACE-2, the SARS-CoV-2 virus ingresses host cells via the endocytic pathway (EP), a vesicular system inhibited by chlorpromazine (CPZ) and linked to schizophrenia and neurodegenerative disorders [25, 26]. Indeed, several antipsychotic drugs were found to interact with both the EP and extracellular vesicles (EVs), demonstrating previously unknown mechanisms of action [27, 28]. Other pathways involved in both the SARS-CoV-2 infection and psychiatric illness include autophagy, redox and calmodulin systems, connecting the virus to neuropathology [23, 29–31].

Several studies have associated NMDARs with sigma-1 nonopioid receptor, a protein hijacked by the SARS-CoV-2 to enable viral entry and replication [24, 32]. Indeed, sigma-1 agonists, such as fluvoxamine, sertraline and the antipsychotic drug, haloperidol inhibit exploitation of sigma-1, dampening viral ingress [33–35]. In addition, fluvoxamine was found to decrease ANG II-induced cardiac hypertrophy, indicating protective effects against both the SARS-CoV-2 infection and its complication [36]. Moreover, ifenprodil, an NMDAR antagonist (and sigma-1 receptor agonist), is currently in phase III clinical trials for COVID-19, linking oxidative stress to the severity of SARS-CoV-2 infection [37] (NCT04382924).

In the immune compartment, both COVID-19 and schizophrenia were associated with dysregulated inflammatory processes and lower levels of regulatory T cells (Tregs), suggesting possible autoimmune pathology [38–40]. In contrast, antipsychotic drugs were found to upregulate Tregs, lowering autoimmune inflammation [39]. Indeed, NMDARs are abundantly expressed not only in the central nervous system (CNS) but also in the immune compartment where they regulate T-cell proliferation in response to antigens. Along these lines, NMDAR antagonists, including antipsychotic drugs upregulate Tregs, enhancing immunological tolerance that in return decreases neuroinflammation [41].

In the following sections, we take a closer look at the SARS-CoV-2 interactome, looking for pathways altered by viral infection, psychiatric disorders and the action mechanism of psychotropic drugs. In other words, learning from the virus to design better psychiatric treatments (**Table 1**).

SARS-CoV-2	Phenothiazines	References
Internalization via EP endocytosis	Inhibit EP endocytosis	[42]
Lowers autophagy	Augment autophagy	[43]
Augments calmodulin	Lower calmodulin	[44]
Augments sigma-1 receptor signaling	Lower sigma-1 receptor signaling	[45]
Lower regulatory T cells (Tregs) number	Upregulate the number of regulatory T cells (Tregs)	[39]

Table 1.
Phenothiazine class of antipsychotic drugs oppose several SARS-CoV-2 actions.

3. The SARS-CoV-2 interactome and viral infection

SARS-CoV-2 is an enveloped, positive-sense, single-stranded, RNA virus with a genome of 30 kb, encoding for 29 viral proteins. These proteins target about 332 human molecules, some of which are also involved in psychiatric disorders and the action mechanism of psychotropic drugs [24]. The virus accesses host cells via its spike (S) glycoprotein that attaches to the cell surface receptor ACE-2 [46]. Viral binding is mediated by TMPRSS2, a human protease, that cleaves S antigen into the S1 subunit, the receptor binding site, and S2, the mediator of viral fusion with host cell membranes [47]. Upon fusion the virus is internalized through the EP pits that join the early and late endosomes, reaching the lysosomes. The later, link the EP to autophagy via autolysosomes (autophagosomes fused with lysosomes) (**Figure 2**).

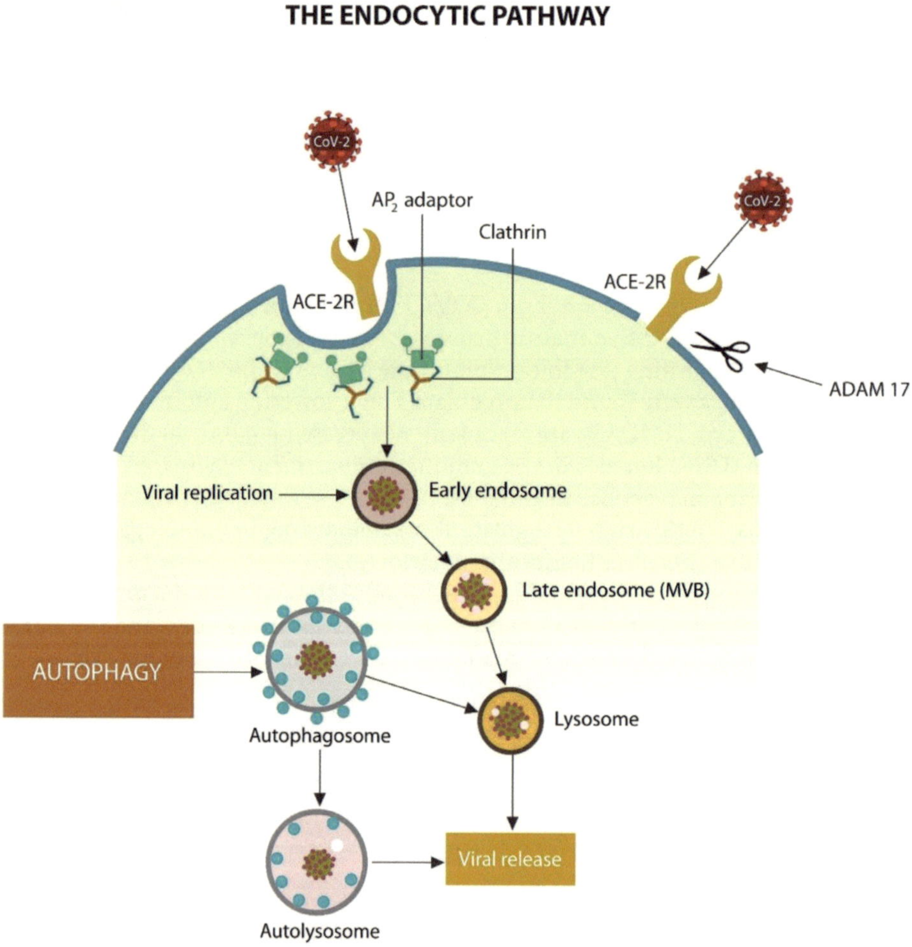

Figure 2.
Upon receptor binding and fusion, SARS-CoV-2/ACE-2 complexes enter human cells through the endocytic pathway (EP) pits early and late endosomes that subsequently join the lysosomes. Lysosomes link the EP to autophagy as authophagosomes (that can also carry the virus) fuse with the lysosomes, engendering the autolysosomes. Viruses are released from the endoplasmic reticulum - Golgi intermediate compartment (ERGIC) (not shown) to the cell surface, either individually or packed in extracellular vesicles (EVs). Viruses connected to ACE-2 receptors that are not endocytosed are shed by ADAM17. Both endocytosis and shedding contribute to ACE-2 downregulation, a marker of COVID-19 critical illness.

The SARS-CoV-2 protein–protein interaction studies have reported that 40% of viral proteins interact with human EP, indicating that vesicular trafficking plays a crucial role in COVID-19 pathogenesis [24]. In addition, several viral proteins usurp mitochondria and autophagy, cellular systems associated with host antiviral defenses [48]. Indeed, the SARS-CoV-2 interactome revealed that the virus hijacks both the mammalian target of rapamycin complex 1 (mTORC1), the master regulator of autophagy, and the E3 ubiquitin ligases in the outer mitochondrial membrane [24].

Upon release from EP into the cytosol, the SARS-CoV-2 virus replicates and assembles in the endoplasmic reticulum - Golgi intermediate compartment (ERGIC) from which the viral progeny is released at the cell surface [49].

4. The SARS-CoV-2/ACE-2 attachment

Novel studies have reported that the S antigen of SARS-CoV-2 virus attaches with high affinity to ACE-2 receptors, promoting oxidative stress by several mechanisms, including ANG 1–7 downregulation, ANG II accumulation and NMDRs or AT-1Rs overstimulation (**Figure 1**) [49–54].

Aside from the S antigen, several other SARS-CoV-2 proteins interact directly with the human molecules, disrupting numerous pathways, including EP, epigenome, mitochondria and autophagy (**Table 2**).

SARS-CoV-2 proteins	Human proteins	References psychiatric pathology
NSP4, NSP8, ORF9C	Mitochondrial dysfunction/oxidative stress	[55]
NSP2, NSP6, NSP7, NSP10, NSP13, NSP15, ORF3A, E, M, ORF8	Endocytic pathway (EP)	[56]
NSP6, ORF9C	Sigma receptors, Autophagy	[57]
NSP5, NSP8, NSP13, E	Epigenome	[58, 59]

Table 2.
The SARS-CoV-2 non-S antigen interactions with human proteins.

Both the S antigen and non-S-induced molecular changes affect molecular pathways previously associated with schizophrenia and autism. For example, excessive NMDAR activation and externalization of phosphatidylserine (PS) on the outer leaflet of plasma membrane was documented in both COVID-19 critical illness and schizophrenia [60]. This is relevant because PS exposure has been linked to dysregulated immunosuppression and the activation of coagulation cascade, changes associated with severe COVID-19 and some psychiatric disorders [61, 62]. With the same token, NMDAR/PS exposure facilitates SARS-CoV-2 endocytosis via the EP [63–65]. Interestingly, PS externalization was associated with schizophrenia as it inhibits monoamine oxidase B (MAO-B), a dopamine (DA) metabolizing enzyme [66]. Loss of MAO-B with subsequent DA upregulation is believed to trigger psychosis, linking PS exposure to severe psychiatric conditions. Furthermore, other studies have associated normal aging with EP upregulation, likely explaining the increased risk of COVID-19 complications in elderly [67].

5. ACE-2 downregulation

The SARS-CoV-2 fusion with host cellular membrane occurs at the level of EP pits, structures comprised of the clathrin heavy chains and adaptor protein 2 (AP2), molecules altered by both schizophrenia and the psychotropic drugs [25, 68–70] (**Figure 2**).

The SARS-CoV-2/ACE-2 complexes that are not endocytosed, are shed by ADAM17, contributing to ACE-2 downregulation and increased COVID-19 severity. The exacerbation of SARS-CoV-2 infection is likely the result of virus/ACE-2 complexes dissemination throughout the body via the circulatory system, increasing infectivity (**Figure 3**) [71].

Novel studies have shown that oxidative stress can directly activate ADAM17, triggering ACE-2 downregulation [72, 73]. This takes place as NMDARs interacts with dopamine 1 receptors (D1Rs) activating ADAM17 to excessively cleave ACE-2 from the cell membranes [74–76]. Moreover, ADAM17 can be activated directly by viral proteins NSP6 and ORF9C interaction with sigma-1 receptors [24, 77] (**Table 2**). Furthermore, PS exposure at the cell surface facilitates ACE-2 downregulation, suggesting that the virus may utilize multiple mechanisms to lower this protein and enable infectivity [78].

Another novel study found that ACE-2 contains a calmodulin-binding site, implicating calcium in ADAM17 activation and COVID-19 critical illness [79, 80].

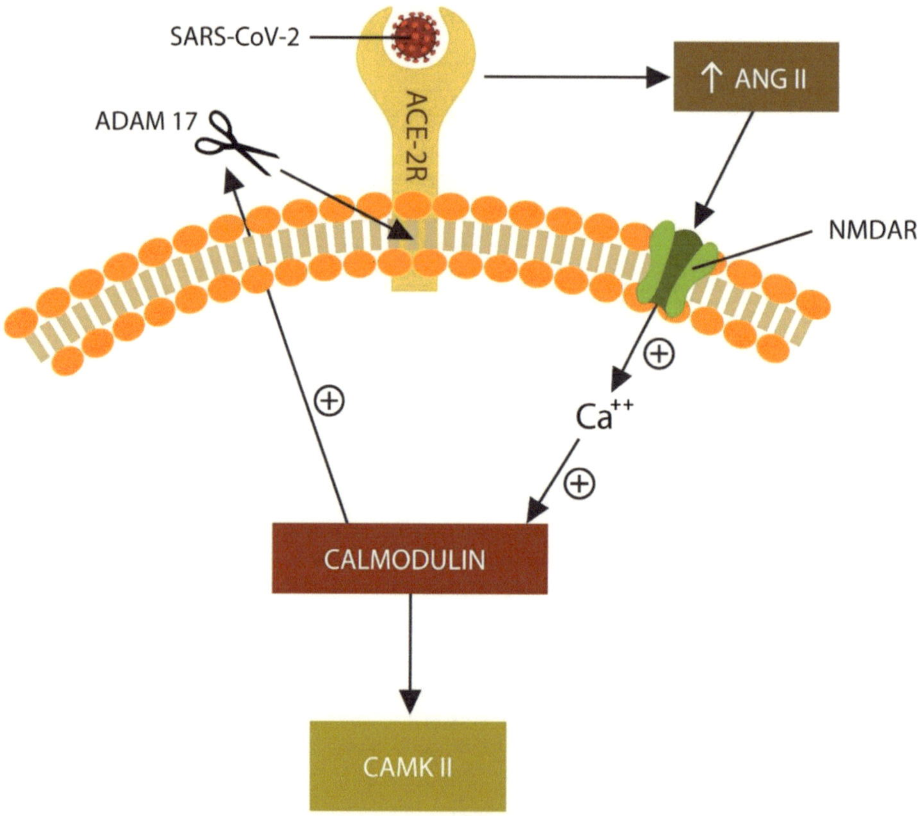

Figure 3.
Activation of ANG II-NMDAR axis results in intracellular calcium influx and calmodulin upregulation. Calmodulin-activated ADAM17 orchestrates the shedding of ACE-2/SARS-CoV-2 complexes, leading to ACE-2 downregulation and high infectivity by ACE-2/SARS-CoV-2 circulatory dissemination.

Indeed, it was established that intracellular calcium influx via NMDARs upregulates calmodulin, activating ADAM17 (**Figure 3**) [81, 82]. On the other hand, calmodulin antagonists, including psychotropic drugs amitriptyline, phenothiazines and melatonin, inhibit ACE-2 downregulation and the odds of COVID-19 complications [83]. In addition, recent studies found that SARS-CoV-2 could activate calcium/calmodulin-dependent protein kinase II (CAMK II), linking the virus further to excitotoxicity (excessive intracellular calcium) [23].

Taken together, ADAM17 promotes ACE-2 downregulation via oxidative stress mediated by NMDARs-upregulated intracellular calcium, mechanisms involved in schizophrenia, drug addictions and COVID-19 critical illness [83–86].

6. COVID-19: a catalyst for novel psychiatric paradigms - part 2

6.1 The virus and madness

The connection between viruses, and psychiatric disorders has been around for many centuries. In the ancient world, Thucydides reported "total and immediate loss of memory" in the survivors of "plague of Athens", a disease suggestive of viral encephalitis [87, 88]. In our time, MRI studies have associated herpes simplex encephalitis, a condition marked by amnesia, with specific neuroimaging markers, linking viruses to cognition [89]. In addition, novel genetic studies have demonstrated that the HK2 retrovirus, frequently detected in the genome of drug addicts, was an ancestral pathogen incorporated into human DNA [90]. Over the past century, numerous studies linked in utero or early postnatal viral infections with the development of schizophrenia and autism later in life [91]. For example, women pregnant during the 1964 rubella epidemic in the United States gave birth to offspring that frequently developed autism or schizophrenia, suggesting that other viruses, probably including COVID-19, may have similar outcomes [92, 93]. In addition, obsessive–compulsive disorder (OCD), schizophrenia, attention deficit hyperactivity disorder (ADHD) and Tourette syndrome were traced to prenatal viral infections [94]. Neurodegenerative disorders, especially Parkinson's disease (PD), were documented to surge after prior pandemics, including the 1918 influenza, suggesting that COVID-19 may promote neurodegeneration [95]. On the positive side, the SARS-CoV-2 virus may prompt the development of novel PD therapies, including angiotensin receptor blockers (ARBs) and angiotensin-converting enzyme inhibitors (ACEi) that have demonstrated efficacy in animal models [96].

Aside from linking prenatal viral exposure to severe psychiatric illness, several new studies reported that dormant CNS viruses could also engender this pathology [97]. For example, a recent report found that compared to controls, patients with schizophrenia demonstrated higher titers of Borna disease virus (BDV) immune complexes [98]. Others have connected influenza A, varicella-zoster, herpes simplex, hepatitis C and human immunodeficiency virus with the development of serious psychiatric disorders [99].

Autoantibodies against NMDARs, demonstrated in some schizophrenia patients, were recently found to be the result of molecular mimicry between the M2 protein of influenza A virus and NMDARs [100, 101]. Indeed, several large epidemiological studies found increased prevalence of autoimmune diseases in patients with schizophrenia, indicating that autoantibodies may be the result of either molecular mimicry or virus-induced modifications in human proteins [102]. For example, the molecular resemblance between an H1N1 influenza antigen and human hypocretin molecule triggers narcolepsy as virus-induced hypocretin modification may elicit autoantibodies [103]. Along these lines, the NMDAR partial antagonist, memantine, utilized in Alzheimer's disease (AD), was found to possess immunosuppressant properties [39, 103, 104]. Indeed, prior studies have demonstrated memantine efficacy against Trypanosoma cruzi, a disease with established autoimmune pathogenesis [105].

Untreated patients with schizophrenia were reported to be at high risk of COVID-19 complications, probably due to SARS-CoV-2-associated neuroinflammation, an established risk factor of many psychiatric disorders. On the other hand, psychotropic drugs with anti-inflammatory properties may lower the SARS-CoV-2-mediated neuroinflammation, explaining the protective effects of these agents [24, 106].

6.2 COVID-19 and acquired antioxidant defects

According to the two-hit paradigm presented here, the COVID-19 prognosis is likely determined by the status of premorbid redox reserves, especially those comprised of the antioxidant enzymes G6PD and GPX. These proteins maintain homeostasis by neutralizing ANG II-activated NADPH oxidase (NOX) [107]. NOX upregulation was documented in patients with neurodegenerative disorders, schizophrenia, and suicidal behaviors, linking CNS pathology to redox system failure [108–110].

G6PD is a potent antioxidant enzyme that lowers NOX by upregulating the synthesis of NADPH and glutathione (GSH) [111]. Conversely, G6PD deficiency was associated with hemolysis and endothelial dysfunction caused by lower GSH and increased oxidative stress [111].

We surmise that the SARS-CoV-2 virus engenders acquired deficits of G6PD and GPX via ANG II-aldosterone upregulated NOX [112] (**Figure 4**). When COVID-19-induced deficiency of antioxidant enzymes occurs on the background of a hereditary G6PD deficit (observed in some populations with ancestral exposure to malaria), the resultant redox failure trigger COVID-19 critical illness [113] (**Figure 4**).

Several recent studies have supported this model as they established that G6PD deficient individuals, including many African Americans, are more likely to develop COVID-19 critical illness [6, 7, 114–116]. Moreover, G6PD deficiency was associated with cardiovascular disease, hypertension, liver fibrosis and iron dyshomeostasis, indicating the importance of redox balance in this pathology [117–121].

6.2.1 Malaria and COVID-19 prognosis

Malaria is an old enemy of mankind that throughout the past centuries exacted a heavy toll on the population of Africa and the surrounding regions. Residents of these areas have gradually developed phenotypes of plasmodium-resistant erythrocytes, including G6PD deficiency, thalassemia, and hemoglobin C, to protect against malaria [122]. Although these modified red blood cells may block plasmodial ingress, individuals with these changes are more susceptible to hemolysis and iron-mediated oxidative stress that in turn promote infections, hypertension, cancer and neuropsychiatric disorders [123–126]. Indeed, both *Plasmodium falciparum* and the SARS-CoV-2 virus induce redox dysfunctions conducive to these pathologies.

Neuropsychiatric manifestations of malaria have been known since the ancient era however, they were more thoroughly studied only in World War I when French Army physicians encountered malaria during the campaign in Northern Greece [127–129]. More recent studies demonstrated that ROS play a major role in the pathogenesis of malaria and the CNS manifestations of this infection. For example, excessive ROS were shown to directly activate nucleotide-binding oligomerization domain-like receptor family, pyrin domain-containing-3 (NLRP3) inflammasomes, molecular

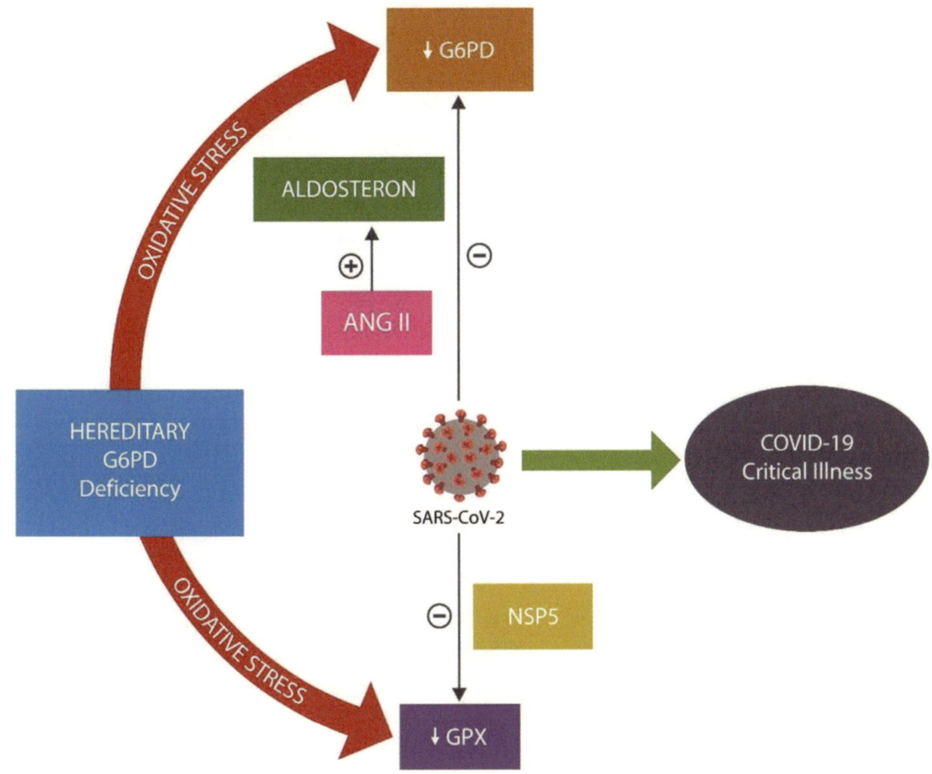

Figure 4.
The SARS-CoV-2 virus causes oxidative stress by inhibiting both GPX (directly) and G6PD (indirectly via ANG II and aldosterone-upregulated NOX). Individuals with hereditary G6PD deficiency are at higher risk for developing COVID-19 critical illness as the loss of antioxidant enzymes is more profound and oxidative stress higher.

structures involved in numerous pathological processes, including t psychiatric disorders [130, 131]. Interestingly, some antipsychotic drugs, including clozapine, function as NLRP3 inhibitors, indicating anti-neuroinflammatory properties [132]. The SARS-CoV-2 interactome established that viral protein OPR3a can activate NLRP3 directly, suggesting a pathway for virus-induced neuroinflammation [133, 134].

Several studies reported that *Plasmodium falciparum*-infected red blood cells externalize PS, a phenomenon observed in severe COVID-19 illness [135]. On the other hand, CPZ was demonstrated to bind PS, promoting eryptosis (elimination of infected red blood cells) with improvement of malaria symptoms [136, 137]. Interestingly antimalarial drugs, chloroquine and hydroxychloroquine operate by inhibiting the EP, a common mechanism of action with some antipsychotic drugs, including CPZ [138]. Since erythrocytes with externalized PS were also documented hypertension, further studies are needed to clarify the role of PS in illness and eryptosis as a possible therapeutic intervention [138, 139]. Indeed, CPZ has been utilized routinely in the emergency treatment of uncontrolled hypertension, indicating a possible role of eryptosis in addition to the well-established CPZ effects on alpha-adrenergic receptors [140].

6.2.2 Malaria exposure and the risk of COVID-19

Population groups throughout the world with exposure to malaria during the previous centuries were found to be at higher risk of hereditary G6PD deficiency and antioxidant failure. This background increases the odds not only of viral infections but also of other redox disorders, including hypertension, cancer and cardiac disease. For example, 12.2% of African American males and 4.1% of females are G6PD deficient, indicating a potentially higher risk of COVID-19 complications [141]. Indeed, novel studies found a 2.4 percent higher COVID-19 mortality in African Americans compared to Whites, Asians or Latinos [142].

Moreover, the lower GSH and nitric oxide (NO) levels in African Americans compared to other groups, places this population at higher risk of both hypertension and prostate cancer, suggesting that the SARS-CoV-2 infection may precipitate these complications [143–149]. In this regard, African Americans with COVID-19 should be routinely assessed for G6PD deficiency and supplemented with the widely available antioxidant, N-acetylcysteine [150].

Oxidative stress was demonstrated to directly trigger hypertension by resetting the CNS baroreflex, therefore the G6PD-deficient individuals could be more prone to COVID-19-related cardiovascular complications [151]. On the other hand, ARBs and ACEi lower ANG II-mediated ROS, likely averting these complications [152–157]. Indeed, the lower utilization of ARBs and ACEi in the treatment of hypertensive African Americans may place this population at higher risk of COVID-19 critical illness [158]. Although numerous clinical trials supported the efficacy of ARBs and ACEi in African Americans, these drugs are rarely utilized in this population as an initial therapeutic options [158, 159]. This is significant as both ARBs and ACEi appear to lower COVID-19 mortality rate, probably by dampening oxidative stress-ACE-2 downregulation. For example, a novel study found that COVID-19 patients treated with ACEi or ARBs at the time of initial infection had fewer unfavorable outcomes and lower mortality rate compared to individuals unexposed to these drugs [160].

Taken together, the SARS-CoV-2-upregulated ANG II, triggers hypertension and cardiovascular disease by augmenting oxidative stress and altering the baroreceptor setting. Individuals with G6PD deficiency are at increased risk of both hypertension and COVID-19 critical illness, indicating alignment with the two-hit paradigm presented here.

7. Conclusion

The COVID-19 pandemic has exacerbated the disease course in many psychiatric patients as mandatory social isolation and decreased frequency of therapeutic meetings promoted fear and uncertainty in this fragile population. The restrictive measures associated with the pandemic have often led to decreased medication adherence, increased depression, anxiety and substance use disorders, often contributing to unfavorable outcomes.

On a positive note, the SARS-CoV-2 virus may be a catalyst for a better understanding of the role of viruses in the pathogenesis of psychiatric illness. As SARS-CoV-2 (and probably other viruses) utilize the molecular machinery involved in severe psychiatric disorders, the clarification of these mechanisms may help with the development of better therapies. Indeed, the EP and antioxidant enzymes may become the new psychiatric paradigms, expanding the current dopamine and serotonin models to include viruses and microbes in psychopathology.

Author details

Adonis Sfera[1*], Carolina Osorio[2], Jose E. Campo Maldonado[3], Afzaal Jafri[1], Aaron D. Chokka[1], Carlos Manuel Zapata Martín del Campo[5] and Zisis Kozlakidis[4†]

1 Patton State Hospital, San Bernardino, CA, United States

2 Department of Psychiatry, Loma Linda University, Loma Linda, CA, United States

3 Department of Medicine, The University of Texas Rio Grande Valley, Edinburg, TX, United States

4 International Agency for Research on Cancer, World Health Organization, Lyon, France

5 National Institute of Cardiology "Ignacio Chávez", Mexico City, Mexico

*Address all correspondence to: dr.sfera@gmail.com

† Where authors are identified as personnel of the International Agency for Research on Cancer/WHO, the authors alone are responsible for the views expressed in this article and they do not necessarily represent the decisions, policy or views of the International Agency for Research on Cancer/WHO.

References

[1] Mathewson AC, Bishop A, Yao Y, Kemp F, Ren J, Chen H, Xu X, Berkhout B, van der Hoek L, Jones IM. Interaction of severe acute respiratory syndrome-coronavirus and NL63 coronavirus spike proteins with angiotensin converting enzyme-2. J Gen Virol. 2008 Nov;89(Pt 11):2741-2745. doi: 10.1099/vir.0.2008/003962-0. PMID: 18931070; PMCID: PMC2886958.

[2] Verdecchia P, Cavallini C, Spanevello A, Angeli F. The pivotal link between ACE2 deficiency and SARS-CoV-2 infection. Eur J Intern Med. 2020;76:14-20. doi:10.1016/j.ejim.2020.04.037

[3] Sfera A, Osorio C, Jafri N, Diaz EL, Campo Maldonado JE. Intoxication With Endogenous Angiotensin II: A COVID-19 Hypothesis. Front Immunol. 2020;11:1472. Published 2020 Jun 19. doi:10.3389/fimmu.2020.01472

[4] Sasi, Sreethish, et al. "A case of COVID-19 in a patient with asymptomatic hemoglobin D thalassemia and glucose-6-phosphate dehydrogenase deficiency." The American Journal of Case Reports 21 (2020): e925788-e925781.

[5] Al-Aamri, Maryam Ali, et al. "A saudi G6PD deficient girl died with pediatric multisystem inflammatory syndrome-COVID-19." MedRxiv (2020).

[6] Vick, Dan J. "Glucose-6-phosphate dehydrogenase deficiency and COVID-19 infection." Mayo Clinic Proceedings. Vol. 95. No. 8. Elsevier, 2020.

[7] Taylor EW, Radding W. Understanding Selenium and Glutathione as Antiviral Factors in COVID-19: Does the Viral Mpro Protease Target Host Selenoproteins and Glutathione Synthesis?. Front Nutr. 2020;7:143. Published 2020 Sep 2. doi:10.3389/fnut.2020.00143

[8] Simon NM, Saxe GN, Marmar CR. Mental Health Disorders Related to COVID-19-Related Deaths. JAMA. 2020 Oct 20;324(15):1493-1494. doi: 10.1001/jama.2020.19632. PMID: 33044510.

[9] Parra A, Juanes A, Losada CP, et al. Psychotic symptoms in COVID-19 patients. A retrospective descriptive study. Psychiatry Res. 2020;291:113254. doi:10.1016/j.psychres.2020.113254

[10] Rogers JP, Chesney E, Oliver D, et al. Psychiatric and neuropsychiatric presentations associated with severe coronavirus infections: a systematic review and meta-analysis with comparison to the COVID-19 pandemic. Lancet Psychiatry. 2020;7(7):611-627. doi:10.1016/S2215-0366(20)30203-0

[11] Banerjee D, Viswanath B. Neuropsychiatric manifestations of COVID-19 and possible pathogenic mechanisms: Insights from other coronaviruses. Asian J Psychiatr. 2020;54:102350. doi:10.1016/j.ajp.2020.102350

[12] Saunders-Hastings PR, Krewski D. Reviewing the History of Pandemic Influenza: Understanding Patterns of Emergence and Transmission. Pathogens. 2016 Dec 6;5(4):66. doi: 10.3390/pathogens5040066. PMID: 27929449; PMCID: PMC5198166.

[13] Manjunatha N, Math SB, Kulkarni GB, Chaturvedi SK. The neuropsychiatric aspects of influenza/swine flu: A selective review. Ind Psychiatry J. 2011;20(2):83-90. doi:10.4103/0972-6748.102479

[14] Steinman G. COVID-19 and autism. Med Hypotheses. 2020;142:109797. doi:10.1016/j.mehy.2020.109797

[15] Fletcher JM. The effects of in utero exposure to the 1918 influenza pandemic on family formation. Econ

Hum Biol. 2018;30:59-68. doi:10.1016/j.ehb.2018.06.004

[16] Plaze M, Attali D, Petit AC, et al. Repurposing chlorpromazine to treat COVID-19: The reCoVery study. Encephale. 2020;46(3):169-172. doi:10.1016/j.encep.2020.05.006

[17] Zhao Y, Ren J, Fry EE, Xiao J, Townsend AR, Stuart DI. Structures of Ebola Virus Glycoprotein Complexes with Tricyclic Antidepressant and Antipsychotic Drugs. J Med Chem. 2018 Jun 14;61(11):4938-4945. doi: 10.1021/acs.jmedchem.8b00350. Epub 2018 May 21. PMID: 29741894.

[18] Bocci G, Bradfute SB, Ye C, Garcia MJ, Parvathareddy J, Reichard W, et al. Virtual and In Vitro Antiviral Screening Revive Therapeutic Drugs for COVID-19. ACS Pharmacology & Translational Science(2020). DOI: 10.1021/acsptsci.0c00131

[19] Otręba, Michał, Leon Kośmider, and Anna Rzepecka-Stojko. "Antiviral activity of chlorpromazine, fluphenazine, perphenazine, prochlorperazine, and thioridazine towards RNA-viruses. A review." European journal of pharmacology 887 (2020): 173553.

[20] Wang, Yancui, et al. "Inactivation of Zika virus in plasma and derivatives by four different methods." Journal of medical virology 91.12 (2019): 2059-2065.

[21] Shen J, Ma B, Zhang X, et al. Thioridazine has potent antitumor effects on lung cancer stem-like cells. Oncol Lett. 2017;13(3):1563-1568. doi:10.3892/ol.2017.5651

[22] Tuan NM, Lee CH. Penfluridol as a Candidate of Drug Repurposing for Anticancer Agent. Molecules. 2019;24(20):3659. Published 2019 Oct 11. doi:10.3390/molecules24203659

[23] Bouhaddou M, Memon D, Meyer B, et al. The Global Phosphorylation Landscape of SARS-CoV-2 Infection. Cell. 2020;182(3):685-712.e19. doi:10.1016/j.cell.2020.06.034

[24] Gordon DE, Jang GM, Bouhaddou M, Xu J, Obernier K, White KM, O'Meara MJ, Rezelj VV, et al. SARS-CoV-2 protein interaction map reveals targets for drug repurposing. Nature. 2020 Jul;583(7816):459-468. doi: 10.1038/s41586-020-2286-9. Epub 2020 Apr 30. PMID: 32353859; PMCID: PMC7431030.

[25] Schubert KO, Föcking M, Prehn JH, Cotter DR. Hypothesis review: are clathrin-mediated endocytosis and clathrin-dependent membrane and protein trafficking core pathophysiological processes in schizophrenia and bipolar disorder? Mol Psychiatry. 2012 Jul;17(7):669-681. doi: 10.1038/mp.2011.123. Epub 2011 Oct 11. PMID: 21986877.

[26] Wu F, Yao PJ. Clathrin-mediated endocytosis and Alzheimer's disease: an update. Ageing Res Rev. 2009 Jul;8(3):147-149. doi: 10.1016/j.arr.2009.03.002. Epub 2009 Mar 21. PMID: 19491039.

[27] Kano SI, Dohi E, Rose IVL. Extracellular Vesicles for Research on Psychiatric Disorders. Schizophr Bull. 2019;45(1):7-16. doi:10.1093/schbul/sby127

[28] Daniel JA, Chau N, Abdel-Hamid MK, Hu L, von Kleist L, Whiting A, Krishnan S, Maamary P, Joseph SR, Simpson F, Haucke V, McCluskey A, Robinson PJ. Phenothiazine-derived antipsychotic drugs inhibit dynamin and clathrin-mediated endocytosis. Traffic. 2015 Jun;16(6):635-654. doi: 10.1111/tra.12272. Epub 2015 Apr 9. PMID: 25693808.

[29] Vucicevic L, Misirkic-Marjanovic M, Harhaji-Trajkovic L, Maric N,

Trajkovic V. Mechanisms and therapeutic significance of autophagy modulation by antipsychotic drugs. Cell Stress. 2018;2(11):282-291. Published 2018 Oct 25. doi:10.15698/cst2018.11.161

[30] Novak G, Seeman P, Tallerico T. Increased expression of calcium/calmodulin-dependent protein kinase IIbeta in frontal cortex in schizophrenia and depression. Synapse. 2006 Jan;59(1):61-68. doi: 10.1002/syn.20211. PMID: 16247765.

[31] Yao JK, Keshavan MS. Antioxidants, redox signaling, and pathophysiology in schizophrenia: an integrative view. Antioxid Redox Signal. 2011;15(7):2011-2035. doi:10.1089/ars.2010.3603

[32] Pabba M, Sibille E. Sigma-1 and N-Methyl-d-Aspartate Receptors: A Partnership with Beneficial Outcomes. Mol Neuropsychiatry. 2015;1(1):47-51. doi:10.1159/000376549

[33] Friesland M, Mingorance L, Chung J, Chisari FV, Gastaminza P. Sigma-1 receptor regulates early steps of viral RNA replication at the onset of hepatitis C virus infection. J Virol. 2013;87(11):6377-6390. doi:10.1128/JVI.03557-12

[34] Cobos EJ, Entrena JM, Nieto FR, Cendán CM, Del Pozo E. Pharmacology and therapeutic potential of sigma(1) receptor ligands. Curr Neuropharmacol. 2008;6(4):344-366. doi:10.2174/157015908787386113

[35] Lee IT, Chen S, Schetz JA. An unambiguous assay for the cloned human sigma1 receptor reveals high affinity interactions with dopamine D4 receptor selective compounds and a distinct structure-affinity relationship for butyrophenones. Eur J Pharmacol. 2008;578(2-3):123-136. doi:10.1016/j.ejphar.2007.09.020

[36] Tagashira H, Bhuiyan S, Shioda N, Hasegawa H, Kanai H, Fukunaga K. σ1-receptor stimulation with fluvoxamine ameliorates transverse aortic constriction-induced myocardial hypertrophy and dysfunction in mice, Am J Physiol, 2010, vol. 299 (pg. H1535-H1545)

[37] Hashimoto K. Activation of sigma-1 receptor chaperone in the treatment of neuropsychiatric diseases and its clinical implication. J Pharmacol Sci. 2015 Jan;127(1):6-9. doi: 10.1016/j.jphs.2014.11.010. Epub 2014 Dec 4. PMID: 25704012.

[38] Gladstone DE, Kim BS, Mooney K, Karaba AH, D'Alessio FR. Regulatory T Cells for Treating Patients With COVID-19 and Acute Respiratory Distress Syndrome: Two Case Reports. Ann Intern Med. 2020 Jul 6:L20-0681. doi: 10.7326/L20-0681. Epub ahead of print. PMID: 32628535; PMCID: PMC7370819.

[39] Kelly DL, Li X, Kilday C, Feldman S, Clark S, Liu F, Buchanan RW, Tonelli LH. Increased circulating regulatory T cells in medicated people with schizophrenia. Psychiatry Res. 2018 Nov;269:517-523. doi: 10.1016/j.psychres.2018.09.006. Epub 2018 Sep 5. PMID: 30195746; PMCID: PMC6207456.

[40] May M, Beauchemin M, Vary C, Barlow D, Houseknecht KL. The antipsychotic medication, risperidone, causes global immunosuppression in healthy mice. PLoS One. 2019;14(6):e0218937. Published 2019 Jun 26. doi:10.1371/journal.pone.0218937

[41] Kahlfuß S, Simma N, Mankiewicz J, et al. Immunosuppression by N-methyl-D-aspartate receptor antagonists is mediated through inhibition of Kv1.3 and KCa3.1 channels in T cells. Mol Cell Biol. 2014;34(5):820-831. doi:10.1128/MCB.01273-13

[42] Negreira-Caamaño M, Piqueras-Flores J, Martínez-DelRio J, et al. Impact of Treatment with

Renin-Angiotensin System Inhibitors on Clinical Outcomes in Hypertensive Patients Hospitalized with COVID-19 [published online ahead of print, 2020 Sep 19]. High Blood Press Cardiovasc Prev. 2020;1-8. doi:10.1007/s40292-020-00409

[43] Dutta D, Donaldson JG. Search for inhibitors of endocytosis:Intended specificity and unintended consequences. Cell Logist. 2012;2 (4):203-208. doi:10.4161/cl.23967

[44] Vucicevic L, Misirkic-Marjanovic M, Harhaji-Trajkovic L, Maric N, Trajkovic V. Mechanisms and therapeutic significance of autophagy modulation by antipsychotic drugs. Cell Stress. 2018;2(11):282-291. Published 2018 Oct 25. doi:10.15698/cst2018.11.161

[45] Prozialeck WC, Weiss B. Inhibition of calmodulin by phenothiazines and related drugs: structure–activity relationships. J Pharmacol Exp Ther. 1982 Sep;222 (3):509-516. PMID: 6286920.

[46] Zhou, P., Yang, XL., Wang, XG. et al. A pneumonia outbreak associated with a new coronavirus of probable bat origin. Nature 579, 270-273 (2020). https://doi.org/10.1038/s41586-020-2012-7

[47] Mahendran ASK, Lim YS, Fang CM, Loh HS, Le CF. The Potential of Antiviral Peptides as COVID-19 Therapeutics. Front Pharmacol. 2020;11:575444. Published 2020 Sep 15. doi:10.3389/fphar.2020.575444

[48] Carmona-Gutierrez D, Bauer MA, Zimmermann A, et al. Digesting the crisis: autophagy and coronaviruses. Microb Cell. 2020;7(5):119-128. Published 2020 May 4. doi:10.15698/mic2020.05.715

[49] Hassanpour M, Rezaie J, Nouri M, Panahi Y. The role of extracellular vesicles in COVID-19 virus infection [published online ahead of print, 2020 Jun 13]. Infect Genet Evol. 2020;85:104422. doi:10.1016/j.meegid.2020.104422

[50] Xu J, Sriramula S, Lazartigues E. Excessive Glutamate Stimulation Impairs ACE2 Activity Through ADAM17-Mediated Shedding in Cultured Cortical Neurons. Cellular and Molecular Neurobiology. 2018 Aug;38(6):1235-1243. DOI: 10.1007/s10571-018-0591-8.

[51] Zhang F, Liu C, Wang L, Cao X, Wang YY, Yang JK. Antioxidant effect of angiotensin (1-7) in the protection of pancreatic β cell function. Mol Med Rep. 2016 Sep;14(3):1963-9. doi: 10.3892/mmr.2016.5514. Epub 2016 Jul 13. PMID: 27430410; PMCID: PMC4991744.

[52] Sommer A, Kordowski F, Büch J, Maretzky T, Evers A, Andrä J, Düsterhöft S, Michalek M, Lorenzen I, Somasundaram P, Tholey A, Sönnichsen FD, Kunzelmann K, Heinbockel L, Nehls C, Gutsmann T, Grötzinger J, Bhakdi S, Reiss K. Phosphatidylserine exposure is required for ADAM17 sheddase function. Nat Commun. 2016 May 10;7:11523. doi: 10.1038/ncomms11523. PMID: 27161080; PMCID: PMC4866515.

[53] Doumas M, Patoulias D, Katsimardou A, Stavropoulos K, Imprialos K, Karagiannis A. COVID19 and increased mortality in African Americans: socioeconomic differences or does the renin angiotensin system also contribute? [published online ahead of print, 2020 Jul 15]. J Hum Hypertens. 2020;1-4. doi:10.1038/s41371-020-0380-y

[54] Welch WJ. Angiotensin II-dependent superoxide: effects on hypertension and vascular dysfunction. Hypertension. 2008;52(1):51-56. doi:10.1161/HYPERTENSIONAHA.107.090472

[55] Krutetskaya ZI, Melnitskaya AV, Antonov VG, Nozdrachev AD. Sigma-1 Receptor Antagonists Haloperidol and Chlorpromazine Modulate the Effect of Glutoxim on Na + Transport in Frog Skin. Dokl Biochem Biophys. 2019 May;484(1):63-65. doi: 10.1134/S1607672919010186. Epub 2019 Apr

[56] Shao L, Martin MV, Watson SJ, et al. Mitochondrial involvement in psychiatric disorders [published correction appears in Ann Med. 2011 Jun;43 (4):329]. Ann Med. 2008;40 (4):281-295. doi:10.1080/07853890801923753

[57] Ryder PV, Faundez V. Schizophrenia: the "BLOC" may be in the endosomes. Sci Signal. 2009;2(93):pe66. Published 2009 Oct 20. doi:10.1126/scisignal.293pe66

[58] Tsai SY, Pokrass MJ, Klauer NR, De Credico NE, Su TP. sigma-1 receptor chaperones in neurodegenerative and psychiatric disorders. Expert Opin Ther Targets. 2014;18(12):1461-1476. doi:10.1517/14728222.2014.97

[59] Pishva E, Creese B, Smith AR, Viechtbauer W, Proitsi P, van den Hove DLA, Ballard C, Mill J, Lunnon K. Psychosisassociated DNA methylomic variation in Alzheimer's disease cortex. Neurobiol Aging. 2020 May;89:83-88. doi: 10.1016/j.neurobiolaging.2020.01.001. Epub 2020 Jan 8. PMID: 32007278.

[60] Gasull T, Sarri E, DeGregorio-Rocasolanó N, Trullas R. NMDA receptor overactivation inhibits phospholipid synthesis by decreasing choline-ethanolamine phosphotransferase activity. J Neurosci. 2003 May 15;23(10):4100-7. doi: 10.1523/JNEUROSCI.23-10-04100.2003. PMID: 12764097; PMCID: PMC6741076.

[61] Hoirisch-Clapauch S, Amaral OB, Mezzasalma MA, Panizzutti R, Nardi AE. Dysfunction in the coagulation system and schizophrenia. Transl Psychiatry. 2016;6(1):e704. Published 2016 Jan 5. doi:10.1038/tp.2015.204

[62] Jayarangaiah A, Kariyanna PT, Chen X, Jayarangaiah A, Kumar A. COVID-19-Associated Coagulopathy: An Exacerbated Immunothrombosis Response. Clin Appl Thromb Hemost. 2020;26:1076029620943293. doi:10.1177/1076029620943293

[63] Glebov, O.O. Tonic NMDA receptor signalling shapes endosomal organisation in mammalian cells. Sci Rep 10, 9315 (2020). https://doi.org/10.1038/s41598-020-66071-0

[64] Sicari D, Chatziioannou A, Koutsandreas T, Sitia R, Chevet E. Role of the early secretory pathway in SARS-CoV-2 infection [published correction appears in J Cell Biol. 2020 Sep 7;219(9):]. J Cell Biol. 2020;219(9):e202006005. doi:10.1083/jcb.202006005

[65] Hasanagic S, Serdarevic F. Potential role of memantine in the prevention and treatment of COVID-19: its antagonism of nicotinic acetylcholine receptors and beyond. Eur Respir J. 2020;56(2):2001610. Published 2020 Aug 13. doi:10.1183/13993003.01610-2020

[66] Tachiki KH, Buckman TD, Eiduson S, Kling AS, Hullett J. Phosphatidylserine inhibition of monoamine oxidase in platelets of schizophrenics. Biol Psychiatry. 1986 Jan;21(1):59-68. doi: 10.1016/0006-3223(86)90008-9. PMID: 3942801.

[67] Alsaqati M, Thomas RS, Kidd EJ. Proteins Involved in Endocytosis Are Upregulated by Ageing in the Normal Human Brain: Implications for the Development of Alzheimer's Disease. J Gerontol A Biol Sci Med Sci. 2018 Mar 2;73(3):289-298. doi: 10.1093/gerona/glx135. PMID: 28655199.

[68] Bayati A, Kumar R, Francis V, McPherson PS. SARS-CoV-2 uses clathrin-mediated endocytosis to gain access into cells. BioRxIv (2020) doi: https://doi.org/10.1101/2020.07.13.201509

[69] Garcia MD, Formoso K, Aparicio GI, Frasch ACC, Scorticati C. The Membrane Glycoprotein M6a Endocytic/Recycling Pathway Involves Clathrin-Mediated Endocytosis and Affects Neuronal Synapses. Front Mol Neurosci. 2017;10:296. Published 2017 Sep 20. doi:10.3389/fnmol.2017.00296

[70] Sharp SI, Hu Y, Weymer JF, et al. The effect of clozapine on mRNA expression for genes encoding G protein-coupled receptors and the protein components of clathrin-mediated endocytosis. Psychiatr Genet. 2013;23(4):153-162. doi:10.1097/YPG.0b013e32835fe51d

[71] Heurich A, Hofmann-Winkler H, Gierer S, Liepold T, Jahn O, Pöhlmann S. TMPRSS2 and ADAM17 cleave ACE2 differentially and only proteolysis by TMPRSS2 augments entry driven by the severe acute respiratory syndrome coronavirus spike protein. J Virol. 2014 Jan;88(2):1293-307. doi: 10.1128/JVI.02202-13. Epub 2013 Nov 13. PMID: 24227843; PMCID: PMC3911672.

[72] Pagliaro P, Penna C. ACE/ACE2 Ratio: A Key Also in 2019 Coronavirus Disease (Covid-19)?. Front Med (Lausanne). 2020;7:335. Published 2020 Jun 18. doi:10.3389/fmed.2020.00335

[73] Brill A, Chauhan AK, Canault M, Walsh MT, Bergmeier W, Wagner DD. Oxidative stress activates ADAM17/TACE and induces its target receptor shedding in platelets in a p38-dependent fashion. Cardiovasc Res. 2009;84(1):137-144. doi:10.1093/cvr/cvp176

[74] Chen G, Greengard P, Yan Z. Potentiation of NMDA receptor currents by dopamine D1 receptors in prefrontal cortex. Proc Natl Acad Sci U S A. 2004;101(8):2596-2600. doi:10.1073/pnas.0308618100

[75] Ladepeche L, Dupuis JP, Bouchet D, et al. Single-molecule imaging of the functional crosstalk between surface NMDA and dopamine D1 receptors. Proc Natl Acad Sci U S A. 2013;110(44):18005-18010. doi:10.1073/pnas.1310145110

[76] Pei L, Lee FJ, Moszczynska A, Vukusic B, Liu F. Regulation of dopamine D1 receptor function by physical interaction with the NMDA receptors. J Neurosci. 2004;24(5):1149-1158. doi:10.1523/JNEUROSCI.3922-03.2004

[77] Li J, Liu B, Gao X, et al. Overexpression of sigma-1 receptor inhibits ADAM10 and ADAM17 mediated shedding in vitro [published correction appears in Protein Cell. 2012 May;3(5):400]. Protein Cell. 2012;3(2):153-159. doi:10.1007/s13238-012-2006-9

[78] Wang G, Coleman CG, Chan J, et al. Angiotensin II slow-pressor hypertension enhances NMDA currents and NOX2-dependent superoxide production in hypothalamic paraventricular neurons. Am J Physiol Regul Integr Comp Physiol. 2013;304(12):R1096-R1106. doi:10.1152/ajpregu.00367.2012

[79] Lai ZW, Lew RA, Yarski MA, Mu FT, Andrews RK, Smith AI. The identification of a calmodulin-binding domain within the cytoplasmic tail of angiotensin-converting enzyme-2. Endocrinology. 2009;150(5):2376-2381. doi:10.1210/en.2008-1274

[80] Lambert DW, Clarke NE, Hooper NM, Turner AJ. Calmodulin interacts with angiotensin-converting enzyme-2 (ACE2) and inhibits shedding of its ectodomain. FEBS Lett.

2008;582(2):385-390. doi:10.1016/j.febslet.2007.11.085

[81] Ermak G, Davies KJ. Calcium and oxidative stress: from cell signaling to cell death. Mol Immunol. 2002 Feb;38(10):713-721. doi: 10.1016/s0161-5890(01)00108-0. PMID: 11841831.

[82] Ataman ZA, Gakhar L, Sorensen BR, Hell JW, Shea MA. The NMDA receptor NR1 C1 region bound to calmodulin: structural insights into functional differences between homologous domains. Structure. 2007;15(12):1603-1617. doi:10.1016/j.str.2007.10.012

[83] Ragia G, Manolopoulos VG. Inhibition of SARS-CoV-2 entry through the ACE2/TMPRSS2 pathway: a promising approach for uncovering early COVID-19 drug therapies [published online ahead of print, 2020 Jul 21]. Eur J Clin Pharmacol. 2020;1-8. doi:10.1007/s00228-020-02963-4

[84] Novak G, Seeman P, Tallerico T. Schizophrenia: elevated mRNA for calcium-calmodulin-dependent protein kinase IIbeta in frontal cortex. Brain research. Molecular Brain Research. 2000 Oct;82(1-2):95-100. DOI: 10.1016/s0169-328x(00)00188-1.

[85] Soto-Vega E, Meza I, Ramírez-Rodríguez G, Benitez-King G. Melatonin stimulates calmodulin phosphorylation by protein kinase C. J Pineal Res. 2004 Sep;37(2):98-106. doi: 10.1111/j.1600-079X.2004.00141.x. PMID: 15298668.

[86] Wei Y, Wang R, Teng J. Inhibition of Calcium/Calmodulin-Dependent Protein Kinase IIα Suppresses Oxidative Stress in Cerebral Ischemic Rats Through Targeting Glucose 6-Phosphate Dehydrogenase. Neurochem Res. 2019 Jul;44(7):1613-1620. doi: 10.1007/s11064-019-02785-6. Epub 2019 Mar 27. PMID: 30919283.

[87] Mujtaba S, He Y, Zeng L, Yan S, Plotnikova O, Sachchidanand, Sanchez R, Zeleznik-Le NJ, Ronai Z, Zhou MM. Structural mechanism of the bromodomain of the coactivator CBP in p53 transcriptional activation. Mol Cell. 2004 Jan 30;13(2):251-263. doi: 10.1016/s1097-2765(03)00528-8. PMID: 14759370.

[88] Cunha BA. The cause of the plague of Athens: plague, typhoid, typhus, smallpox, or measles? Infectious Disease Clinics of North America. 2004 Mar;18(1):29-43. DOI: 10.1016/s0891-5520(03)00100-4.

[89] Kapur N, Barker S, Burrows EH, Ellison D, Brice J, Illis LS, Scholey K, Colbourn C, Wilson B, Loates M. Herpes simplex encephalitis: long term magnetic resonance imaging and neuropsychological profile. J Neurol Neurosurg Psychiatry. 1994 Nov;57(11):1334-1342. doi: 10.1136/jnnp.57.11.1334. PMID:

[90] Karamitros T, Hurst T, Marchi E, Karamichali E, Georgopoulou U, Mentis A, Riepsaame J, Lin A, Paraskevis D, Hatzakis A, McLauchlan J, Katzourakis A, Magiorkinis G. Human Endogenous Retrovirus-K HML-2 integration within RASGRF2 is associated with intravenous drug abuse and modulates transcription in a cell-line model. Proc Natl Acad Sci U S A. 2018 Oct 9;115(41):10434-10439. doi: 10.1073/pnas.1811940115. Epub 2018 Sep 24. PMID: 30249655; PMCID: PMC6187174.

[91] McGrath JJ, Pemberton MR, Welham JL, Murray RM. Schizophrenia and the influenza epidemics of 1954, 1957 and 1959: a southern hemisphere study. Schizophr Res. 1994 Dec;14(1):1-8. doi: 10.1016/0920-9964(94)90002-7. PMID: 7893616.

[92] Hutton J. Does Rubella Cause Autism: A 2015 Reappraisal?. Front Hum Neurosci. 2016;10:25. Published

2016 Feb 1. doi:10.3389/fnhum.2016.00025

[93] Brown AS, Begg MD, Gravenstein S, Schaefer CA, Wyatt RJ, Bresnahan M, Babulas VP, Susser ES. Serologic evidence of prenatal influenza in the etiology of schizophrenia. Arch Gen Psychiatry. 2004 Aug;61(8):774-780. doi: 10.1001/archpsyc.61.8.774. PMID: 15289276.

[94] Khandaker GM, Zimbron J, Dalman C, Lewis G, Jones PB. Childhood infection and adult schizophrenia: a meta-analysis of population-based studies. Schizophr Res. 2012;139(1-3):161-168. doi:10.1016/j.schres.2012.05.023

[95] Henry J, Smeyne RJ, Jang H, Miller B, Okun MS. Parkinsonism and neurological manifestations of influenza throughout the 20th and 21st centuries. Parkinsonism Relat Disord. 2010;16(9):566-571. doi:10.1016/j.parkreldis.2010.06.012

[96] Perez-Lloret S, Otero-Losada M, Toblli JE, Capani F. Renin-angiotensin system as a potential target for new therapeutic approaches in Parkinson's disease. Expert Opin Investig Drugs. 2017 Oct;26(10):1163-1173. doi: 10.1080/13543784.2017.1371133. Epub 2017 Aug 29. PMID: 28836869.

[97] Breier A. 39. VIRUSES AND SCHIZOPHRENIA: IMPLICATIONS FOR PATHOPHYSIOLOGY AND TREATMENT. Schizophr Bull. 2018;44(Suppl 1):S61-S62. doi:10.1093/schbul/sby014.158

[98] Zaliunaite V, Steibliene V, Bode L, Podlipskyte A, Bunevicius R, Ludwig H. Primary psychosis and Borna disease virus infection in Lithuania: a case control study. BMC Psychiatry. 2016;16(1):369. Published 2016 Nov 3. doi:10.1186/s12888-016-1087-z

[99] Coughlin SS. Anxiety and Depression: Linkages with Viral Diseases. Public Health Rev. 2012;34(2):7. doi:10.1007/BF03391675

[100] Kępińska AP, Iyegbe CO, Vernon AC, Yolken R, Murray RM, Pollak TA. Schizophrenia and Influenza at the Centenary of the 1918-1919 Spanish Influenza Pandemic: Mechanisms of Psychosis Risk. Front Psychiatry. 2020;11:72. Published 2020 Feb 26. doi:10.3389/fpsyt.2020.00072

[101] Blanpied TA, Clarke RJ, Johnson JW. Amantadine inhibits NMDA receptors by accelerating channel closure during channel block. J Neurosci. 2005 Mar 30;25(13):3312-22. doi: 10.1523/JNEUROSCI.4262-04.2005. PMID: 15800186; PMCID: PMC6724906.

[102] Eaton WW, Byrne M, Ewald H, Mors O, Chen CY, Agerbo E, Mortensen PB. Association of schizophrenia and autoimmune diseases: linkage of Danish national registers. Am J Psychiatry. 2006 Mar;163(3):521-528. doi: 10.1176/appi.ajp.163.3.521. PMID: 16513876.

[103] Luo G, Ambati A, Lin L, Bonvalet M, Partinen M, Ji X, Maecker HT, Mignot EJ. Autoimmunity to hypocretin and molecular mimicry to flu in type 1 narcolepsy. Proc Natl Acad Sci U S A. 2018 Dec 26;115(52):E12323-E12332. doi: 10.1073/pnas.1818150116. Epub 2018 Dec 12. PMID: 30541895; PMCID: PMC6310865.

[104] Rejdak K, Grieb P. Adamantanes might be protective from COVID-19 in patients with neurological diseases: multiple sclerosis, parkinsonism and cognitive impairment. Multiple Sclerosis and Related Disorders. 2020;42:102163 10.1016/j.msard.2020.102163

[105] Damasceno FS, Barisón MJ, Pral EM, Paes LS, Silber AM. Memantine, an antagonist of the NMDA glutamate receptor, affects cell proliferation, differentiation and the

intracellular cycle and induces apoptosis in Trypanosoma cruzi. PLoS Negl Trop Dis. 2014;8(2):e2717. Published 2014 Feb 27. doi:10.1371/journal.pntd.0002717

[106] Kozloff N, Mulsant BH, Stergiopoulos V, Voineskos AN. The COVID-19 Global Pandemic: Implications for People With Schizophrenia and Related Disorders. Schizophr Bull. 2020 Jul 8;46(4):752-757. doi: 10.1093/schbul/sbaa051. PMID: 32343342; PMCID: PMC7197583.

[107] Wen H, Gwathmey JK, Xie LH. Oxidative stress-mediated effects of angiotensin II in the cardiovascular system. World J Hypertens. 2012;2(4):34-44. doi:10.5494/wjh.v2.i4.34

[108] Tarafdar A, Pula G. The Role of NADPH Oxidases and Oxidative Stress in Neurodegenerative Disorders. Int J Mol Sci. 2018;19(12):3824. Published 2018 Nov 30. doi:10.3390/ijms19123824

[109] Schiavone, S., Neri, M., Mhillaj, E. et al. The NADPH oxidase NOX2 as a novel biomarker for suicidality: evidence from human post mortem brain samples. Transl Psychiatry 6, e813 (2016). https://doi.org/10.1038/tp.2016.76

[110] Wang X, Pinto-Duarte A, Sejnowski TJ, Behrens MM. How Nox2-containing NADPH oxidase affects cortical circuits in the NMDA receptor antagonist model of schizophrenia. Antioxid Redox Signal. 2013 Apr 20;18(12):1444-62. doi: 10.1089/ars.2012.4907. Epub 2012 Oct 18. PMID: 22938164; PMCID: PMC3603498.

[111] Stanton RC. Glucose-6-phosphate dehydrogenase, NADPH, and cell survival. IUBMB Life. 2012;64(5):362-369. doi:10.1002/iub.1017

[112] Rajamohan SB, Raghuraman G, Prabhakar NR, Kumar GK. NADPH oxidase-derived H(2)O(2) contributes to angiotensin II-induced aldosterone synthesis in human and rat adrenal cortical cells. Antioxid Redox Signal. 2012;17(3):445-459. doi:10.1089/ars.2011.4176

[113] Buinitskaya Y, Gurinovich R, Clifford G. Wlodaver CG, Kastsiuchenka S. Centrality of G6PD in COVID-19: The Biochemical Rationale and Clinical Implications. Front. Med., 22 October 2020 | https://doi.org/10.3389/fmed.2020.584112

[114] Jain SK, Parsanathan R, Levine SN, Bocchini JA, Holick MF, Vanchiere JA. The potential link between inherited G6PD deficiency, oxidative stress, and vitamin D deficiency and the racial inequities in mortality associated with COVID-19. Free Radic Biol Med. 2020;161:84-91. doi:10.1016/j.freeradbiomed.2020.10.002

[115] Youssef JG, Zahiruddin F, Youssef G, et al. G6PD deficiency and severity of COVID19 pneumonia and acute respiratory distress syndrome: tip of the iceberg?. Ann Hematol. 2021;100(3):667-673. doi:10.1007/s00277-021-04395-1

[116] Guillin OM, Vindry C, Ohlmann T, Chavatte L. Selenium, Selenoproteins and Viral Infection. Nutrients. 2019;11(9):2101. Published 2019 Sep 4. doi:10.3390/nu11092101

[117] Moossavi S, Besharat S, Sharafkhah M, et al. Inverse Association of Plasma Level of Glutathione Peroxidase with Liver Fibrosis in Chronic Hepatitis B: Potential Role of Iron. Middle East Journal of Digestive Diseases. 2016 Apr;8(2):122-130. DOI: 10.15171/mejdd.2016.17.

[118] Rodrigo, R., González, J. & Paoletto, F. The role of oxidative stress in the pathophysiology of hypertension. Hypertens Res 34, 431-440 (2011). https://doi.org/10.1038/hr.2010.264

[119] Hecker PA, Leopold JA, Gupte SA, Recchia FA, Stanley WC. Impact of glucose-6-phosphate dehydrogenase deficiency on the pathophysiology of cardiovascular disease. Am J Physiol Heart Circ Physiol. 2013;304(4): H491-H500. doi:10.1152/ajpheart. 00721.2012

[120] Conrad M, Kagan VE, Bayir H, et al. Regulation of lipid peroxidation and ferroptosis in diverse species. Genes Dev. 2018;32(9-10):602-619. doi:10.1101/gad.314674.118

[121] Li, J., Cao, F., Yin, Hl. et al. Ferroptosis: past, present and future. Cell Death Dis 11, 88 (2020). https://doi.org/10.1038/s41419-020-2298-2

[122] Kwiatkowski DP. How malaria has affected the human genome and what human genetics can teach us about malaria. Am J Hum Genet. 2005;77(2):171-192. doi:10.1086/432519

[123] Bocchetta A. Psychotic mania in glucose-6-phosphate-dehydrogenase-deficient subjects. Ann Gen Hosp Psychiatry. 2003;2(1):6. Published 2003 Jun 13. doi:10.1186/1475-2832-2-6

[124] Manjurano A, Sepulveda N, Nadjm B, et al. African glucose-6-phosphate dehydrogenase alleles associated with protection from severe malaria in heterozygous females in Tanzania. PLoS Genet. 2015;11(2):e1004960. Published 2015 Feb 11. doi:10.1371/journal.pgen.1004960

[125] Fibach E, Dana M. Oxidative Stress in β-Thalassemia. Mol Diagn Ther. 2019 Apr;23(2):245-261. doi: 10.1007/s40291-018-0373-5. PMID: 30484264.

[126] Chirico EN, Pialoux V. Role of oxidative stress in the pathogenesis of sickle cell disease. IUBMB Life. 2012 Jan;64(1):72-80. doi: 10.1002/iub.584. Epub 2011 Nov 30. PMID: 22131167.

[127] Weiss MG. The interrelationship of tropical disease and mental disorder: conceptual framework and literature review (Part I--Malaria). Cult Med Psychiatry. 1985 Jun;9(2):121-200. doi: 10.1007/BF00117368. PMID: 4017618.

[128] Paisseau G. Malaria during the War. Lancet (1919) pp.749-751 pp.

[129] Singh VB, Kumar H, Meena BL, Chandra S, Agrawal J, Kanogiya N. Neuropsychiatric Profile in Malaria: An Overview. J Clin Diagn Res. 2016;10(7):OC24-OC28. doi:10.7860/JCDR/2016/19035.8169

[130] Kim HK, Andreazza AC, Elmi N, Chen W, Young LT. Nod-like receptor pyrin containing 3 (NLRP3) in the post-mortem frontal cortex from patients with bipolar disorder: A potential mediator between mitochondria and immune-activation. J Psychiatr Res. 2016 Jan;72:43-50. doi: 10.1016/j.jpsychires.2015.10.015. Epub 2015 Oct 26. PMID: 26540403.

[131] Wang X, Pinto-Duarte A, Sejnowski TJ, Behrens MM. How Nox2-containing NADPH oxidase affects cortical circuits in the NMDA receptor antagonist model of schizophrenia. Antioxid Redox Signal. 2013 Apr 20;18(12):1444-62. doi: 10.1089/ars.2012.4907. Epub 2012 Oct 18. PMID: 22938164; PMCID: PMC3603498.

[132] Giridharan VV, Scaini G, Colpo GD, et al. Clozapine Prevents Poly (I:C) Induced Inflammation by Modulating NLRP3 Pathway in Microglial Cells. Cells. 2020;9(3):577. Published 2020 Feb 28. doi:10.3390/cells9030577

[133] Siu KL, Yuen KS, Castaño-Rodriguez C, Ye ZW, Yeung ML, Fung SY, Yuan S, Chan CP, Yuen KY, Enjuanes L, Jin DY. Severe acute respiratory syndrome coronavirus ORF3a protein activates the NLRP3

inflammasome by promoting TRAF3-dependent ubiquitination of ASC. FASEB J. 2019 Aug;33(8):8865-8877. doi: 10.1096/fj.201802418R. Epub 2019 Apr 29. PMID: 31034780; PMCID: PMC6662968.

[134] Shah A. Novel Coronavirus-Induced NLRP3 Inflammasome Activation: A Potential Drug Target in the Treatment of COVID-19. Front Immunol. 2020;11:1021. Published 2020 May 19. doi:10.3389/fimmu.2020.01021

[135] Argañaraz GA, Palmeira JDF, Argañaraz ER. Phosphatidylserine inside out: a possible underlying mechanism in the inflammation and coagulation abnormalities of COVID-19. Cell Commun Signal. 2020 Dec 27;18(1):190. doi: 10.1186/s12964-020-00687-7. PMID: 33357215; PMCID: PMC7765775.

[136] Hylén U, Eklund D, Humble M, Bartoszek J, Särndahl E, Bejerot S. Increased inflammasome activity in markedly ill psychiatric patients: An explorative study. J Neuroimmunol. 2020 Feb 15;339:577119. doi: 10.1016/j.jneuroim.2019.577119. Epub 2019 Nov 26. PMID: 31786499.

[137] Eda S, Sherman IW. Cytoadherence of malaria-infected red blood cells involves exposure of phosphatidylserine. Cell Physiol Biochem. 2002;12(5-6):373-384. doi: 10.1159/000067908. PMID: 12438774.

[138] Koka S, Lang C, Boini KM, Bobbala D, Huber SM, Lang F. Influence of chlorpromazine on eryptosis, parasitemia and survival of Plasmodium berghe infected mice. Cell Physiol Biochem. 2008;22(1-4):261-268. doi: 10.1159/000149804. Epub 2008 Jul 25. PMID: 18769053.

[139] Delvecchio R, Higa LM, Pezzuto P, et al. Chloroquine, an Endocytosis Blocking Agent, Inhibits Zika Virus Infection in Different Cell Models. Viruses. 2016;8(12):322. Published 2016 Nov 29. doi:10.3390/v8120322

[140] Wang J, Chen S, Bihl J. Exosome-Mediated Transfer of ACE2 (Angiotensin-Converting Enzyme 2) from Endothelial Progenitor Cells Promotes Survival and Function of Endothelial Cell. Oxid Med Cell Longev. 2020 Jan 18;2020:4213541. doi: 10.1155/2020/4213541. PMID: 32051731; PMCID: PMC6995312.

[141] Viskin S, Berger M, Ish-Shalom M, Malov N, Tamari M, Golovner M, Kehati M, Zeltser D, Roth A. Intravenous chlorpromazine for the emergency treatment of uncontrolled symptomatic hypertension in the pre-hospital setting: data from 500 consecutive cases. Isr Med Assoc J. 2005 Dec;7(12):812-815. PMID: 16382707.

[142] Chinevere TD, Murray CK, Grant E Jr, Johnson GA, Duelm F, Hospenthal DR. Prevalence of glucose-6-phosphate dehydrogenase deficiency in U.S. Army personnel. Mil Med. 2006 Sep;171(9):905-907. doi: 10.7205/milmed.171.9.905. PMID: 17036616.

[143] Doumas M, Patoulias D, Katsimardou A, Stavropoulos K, Imprialos K, Karagiannis A. COVID19 and increased mortality in African Americans: socioeconomic differences or does the renin angiotensin system also contribute? [published online ahead of print, 2020 Jul 15]. J Hum Hypertens. 2020;1-4. doi:10.1038/s41371-020-0380-y

[144] Mata-Greenwood E, Chen DB. Racial differences in nitric oxide-dependent vasorelaxation. Reprod Sci. 2008;15(1):9-25. doi:10.1177/1933719107312160

[145] Lavender, N.A., Benford, M.L., VanCleave, T.T. et al. Examination of polymorphic glutathione S-transferase (GST) genes, tobacco smoking and prostate cancer risk among Men of

African Descent: A case-control study. BMC Cancer 9, 397 (2009). https://doi.org/10.1186/1471-2407-9-397

[146] Hutchings A, Purcell WM, Benfield MR. Peripheral blood antigen-presenting cells from African-Americans exhibit increased CD80 and CD86 expression. Clin Exp Immunol. 1999;118(2):247-252. doi:10.1046/j.1365-2249.1999.01051.x

[147] Akaberi D, Krambrich J, Ling J, et al. Mitigation of the replication of SARS-CoV-2 by nitric oxide in vitro [published online ahead of print, 2020 Sep 21]. Redox Biol. 2020;37:101734. doi:10.1016/j.redox.2020.101734

[148] Xiao J, Cohen P, Stern MC, Odedina F, Carpten J, Reams R. Mitochondrial biology and prostate cancer ethnic disparity. Carcinogenesis. 2018 Dec 13;39(11):1311-1319. doi: 10.1093/carcin/bgy133. PMID: 30304372; PMCID: PMC6292412.

[149] Feairheller DL, Park JY, Sturgeon KM, et al. Racial differences in oxidative stress and inflammation: in vitro and in vivo. Clin Transl Sci. 2011;4(1):32-37. doi:10.1111/j.1752-8062.2011.00264.x

[150] Miripour ZS, Sarrami-Forooshani R, Sanati H, et al. Real-time diagnosis of reactive oxygen species (ROS) in fresh sputum by electrochemical tracing; correlation between COVID-19 and viral-induced ROS in lung/respiratory epithelium during this pandemic. Biosens Bioelectron. 2020;165:112435. doi:10.1016/j.bios.2020.112435

[151] Ibrahim H, Perl A, Smith D, et al. Therapeutic blockade of inflammation in severe COVID-19 infection with intravenous N-acetylcysteine. Clin Immunol. 2020;219:108544. doi:10.1016/j.clim.2020.108544

[152] de Queiroz TM, Monteiro MM, Braga VA. Angiotensin-II-derived reactive oxygen species on baroreflex sensitivity during hypertension: new perspectives. Front Physiol. 2013;4:105. Published 2013 May 13. doi:10.3389/fphys.2013.00105

[153] Guimarães, D. D., Carvalho, C. C., and Braga, V. A. (2012). Scavenging of NADPH oxidase-derived superoxide anions improves depressed baroreflex sensitivity in spontaneously hypertensive rats. Clin. Exp. Pharmacol. Physiol. 39, 373-378.

[154] Braga, V. A. (2010). Dietary salt enhances angiotensin-II-induced superoxide formation in the rostral ventrolateral medulla. Auton. Neurosci. 155, 14-18

[155] Inukai T, Yoshida N, Wakabayashi S, Inukai Y, Matsutomo R, Takanashi K, Nakamachi T, Takebayashi K, Aso Y, Takahashi K. Angiotensin-converting enzyme inhibitors and angiotensin II receptor blockers effectively and directly potentiate superoxide scavenging by polymorphonuclear leukocytes from patients with type 2 diabetes mellitus. Am J Med Sci. 2005 May;329

[156] Cianchetti S, Del Fiorentino A, Colognato R, Di Stefano R, Franzoni F, Pedrinelli R. Anti-inflammatory and anti-oxidant properties of telmisartan in cultured human umbilical vein endothelial cells. Atherosclerosis. 2008 May;198(1):22-28. doi: 10.1016/j.atherosclerosis.2007.09.013. Epub 2007 Oct 22. PMID: 17950296.

[157] Heringer-Walther S, Batista EN, Walther T, Khosla MC, Santos RA, Campagnole-Santos MJ. Baroreflex improvement in shr after ace inhibition involves angiotensin-(1-7). Hypertension. 2001 May;37(5):1309-1314. doi: 10.1161/01.hyp.37.5.1309. PMID: 11358946

[158] Eguchi K, Shimizu M, Hoshide S, Shimada K, Kario K. A bedtime dose of

ARB was better than a morning dose in improving baroreflex sensitivity and urinary albumin excretion--the J-TOP study. Clin Exp Hypertens. 2012;34(7):488-492. doi: 10.3109/10641963.2012.666604. Epub 2012 Apr 25. PMID: 22533496.

[159] Williams SF, Nicholas SB, Vaziri ND, Norris KC. African Americans, hypertension and the renin angiotensin system. World J Cardiol. 2014;6(9):878-889. doi:10.4330/wjc.v6.i9.878

[160] Flack JM, Mensah GA, Ferrario CM. Using angiotensin converting enzyme inhibitors in African-American hypertensives: a new approach to treating hypertension and preventing target-organ damage. Curr Med Res Opin. 2000;16(2):66-79. PMID: 10893650.

Chapter 16

Frequency of Hyperglycemia in Patients with Covid-19 Infection and Pneumonia

Valeriy Ivanovich Vechorko, Evgeny Mikhailovich Evsikov, Oksana Alekseevna Baykova, Natalya Vadimovna Teplova and Dmitriy Aleksandrovich Doroshenko

Abstract

Diabetes mellitus can increase the risk of death in COVID-19 by 12 times, according to the portal of the us Centers for disease control and prevention. Coronavirus-infected diabetics are six times more likely to need inpatient treatment, and diabetes is the second most severe complication in COVID-19 after cardiovascular diseases. The state of carbohydrate metabolism in patients with COVID-19 has not been sufficiently studied in clinical studies. Isolated studies indicate that viral infection may be accompanied by an increase in the concentration of glycated hemoglobin in patients with viral pneumonia. To assess the frequency of hyperglycemia and diagnosis of newly diagnosed diabetes mellitus in patients with COVID-19 and acute lung damage aged 41–80 years, who were hospitalized in a repurposed infectious diseases hospital in Moscow with a diagnosis of pneumonia. In the observational study analyzed laboratory and clinical diagnostic data of 278 patients who had, according to the anamnesis and the medical conclusions of impaired glucose tolerance and manifested forms of diabetes, including 163 men and 115 women, aged 41–80 years, admitted to the hospital for diagnosis and treatment in the period from 12.04.2020 on 10.11.2020 of diagnoses according to ICD-10: U07.1 Coronavirus infection. In the selected groups of patients, the initial and subsequent fasting blood glucose levels were analyzed after 8 hours without food intake on a stationary automatic analyzer and using portable glucose, meters using diagnostic test strips. The concentration of glucose and ketones in the urine was determined by a semi-quantitative method. We evaluated the dynamics of indicators when detecting pathological values of glucose concentration. Glucose levels above 6.4 mmol/l were taken as pathological. In patients aged 41–80 years who were hospitalized with covid-19 infection and pneumonia, fasting hyperglycemia was diagnosed in 31–47%, glucosuria in 1.9–6.1%, ketonuria – 20.4-46.2% of cases, in different age groups. In 16.6–31.3% of cases in patients with covid-19,after treatment and regression of changes in the lungs, normalization of glucose levels was observed, but in 14.8–16.7% of the changes persisted, and in 9–13% of them, after an additional study, newly diagnosed diabetes mellitus was diagnosed. Hyperglycemia was significantly more often detected in patients with arterial hypertension of 2–3 degrees of severity and with a tendency to reliability, in patients with obesity of 2–3 degrees. Lipid metabolism disorders (hypertriglyceridemia and hypercholesterolemia), which are characteristic of changes in carbohydrate metabolism in patients with impaired glucose tolerance and diabetes, were significantly more often diagnosed in patients with covid-19 than in the group of patients with acute and chronic lung pathology without proven infection with this virus, but only in the group of patients aged 41–60 years. Covid-19 infection complicated by pneumonia occurs in individuals aged 41–80 years with a high incidence of hyperglycemia and ketonuria. The incidence of newly diagnosed diabetes mellitus in such patients is 9–13%.

Keywords: Covid-19 infection, pneumonia, hyperglycemia, diabetes mellitus

1. Introduction

The available data so far indicatethat in SARS-CoV-2, the nature of the pathology goes beyond acute respiratory infection [1–4]. Researchers identify 2 more disease periods associated with SARS-coronavirus-2 infection, including a rare hyperinflammatory syndrome after an acute period and late inflammatory andvirological complications [1, 2]. These 3 disease periods not only determine the time course of SARS-CoV-2 infection at the population level, but also reflect the possible multiple organ involvement [1, 2, 5]. Patients may have pronounced cardiovascular and gastrointestinal lesions, and dermatological and cutaneous-mucous manifestations, such as giperosmolarna with Kawasaki disease [1, 2]. Laboratory studies can reveal elevated inflammatory markers (e.g., levels of C-reactive protein and ferritin), a coagulopathy (e.g. D-dimer) and elevated cardiac markers (troponin level), [6, 7]. According to the available data and according to some experts, the COVID-19 developing trebovatelna process or COVID-19-associated coagulopathy [5, 8, 9].

To the development of the disease most often predispose:

- cardiovascular diseases, especially arterial hypertension;
- diabetes mellitus;
- chronic lung disease;
- cancer (in particular, hematological malignancies, lung cancer, and metastasis);
- chronic kidney disease;
- obesity;
- smoking;
- immunodeficiency states;
- chronic liver diseases [10, 11].

According to sources from the Chinese center for disease control and prevention (February 2020) and who information materials [12, 13], the death rate from COVID-19 largely depends on the age of patients and the presence of chronic diseases, including diabetes mellitus (**Figure 1**). Based on the study of 72,314 cases of COVID-19, the researchers obtained the following statistics: patients suffering from cardiovascular diseases had a mortality rate of 13.2%, with verified diabetes mellitus 9.2%, with arterial hypertension 8.4%, with chronic forms of diseases respiratory tract 8%, with oncological pathology 7.6% [12, 13].

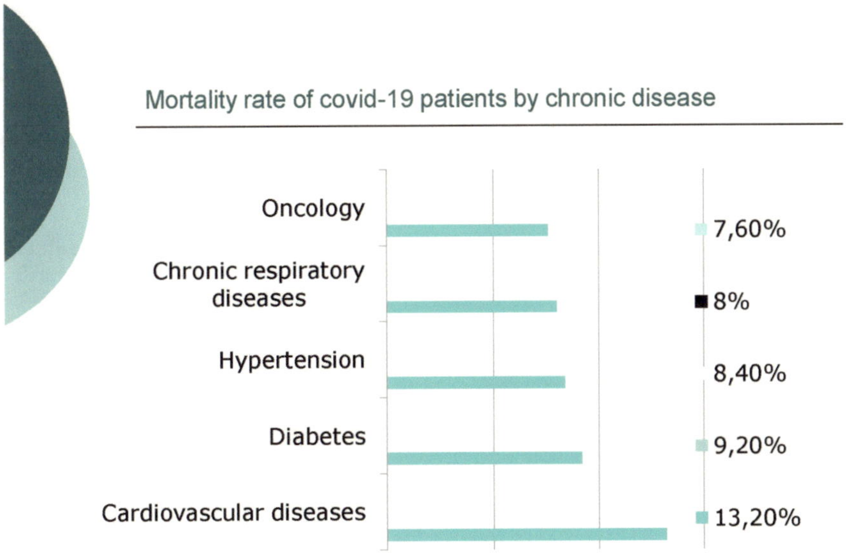

Figure 1.
Mortality rate of covid-19 patients by chronic disease (sources: WHO, Chinese authorities as of February 2020), [12, 13].

Diabetes can increase the risk of death in COVID-19 by 12 times, according to the portal of the US Centers for disease control and prevention [14]. Coronavirus-infected diabetics are six times more likely to need hospital admission and inpatient treatment, and diabetes is the second most severe complication in COVID-19 after cardiovascular disease [15].

The state of carbohydrate metabolism in patients with COVID-19 has not been sufficiently studied in clinical studies. Isolated studies indicate that viral infection may be accompanied by an increase in the concentration of glycated hemoglobin in patients with viral pneumonia [16–18].

2. Purpose and objectives of the study

To assess the frequency of fasting hyperglycemia and the frequency of diagnosis of newly diagnosed diabetes mellitus in patients with COVID-19 and acute lung damage aged 41–80 years, who were hospitalized in a repurposed infectious diseases hospital in Moscow with a diagnosis of pneumonia.

3. Material and methods

We have analyzed laboratory and clinical diagnostic data of 278 patients who had, according to the anamnesis and the medical conclusions of impaired glucose tolerance and manifested forms of diabetes, including 163 men and 115 women, aged 41–80 years, admitted to the hospital for diagnosis and treatment in the period from 12.04.2020 on 10.11.2020 of diagnoses according to international classification of diseases and causes of death revision 10 (ICD-10): U07.1 Coronavirus infection caused by a virus COVID-19, virus identified (confirmed by laboratory testing regardless of the severity of clinical signs or symptoms); J12.9 community acquired pneumonia. Patients 'data were archived in the city computer system of DZM KIS EMIAS (unified medical information and analytical system Department of health of the city of Moscow). All patients were admitted to the hospital with fever symptoms, cough complaints, and shortness of breath. After inpatient treatment, all patients showed regression of inflammatory changes in the lungs and improvement of their condition. Patients were divided into groups depending on their age and the results of biochemical (PCR diagnostics and enzyme immunoassay for determining the concentration of M and G-immunoglobulins) and clinical-radiological studies

Namber. Disease, degree of respiratory failure	Group 2 (41–60 years old) (n = 57)	Group 4 (61–80 years old) (n = 59)	The difference in percentages
1. Segmental pneumonia of one lung	1 (1.7%)	0	1.7%
2. Focal pneumonia of one lung	2(3,5%)	0	3,5%
3. Lobar pneumonia of one lung	11(19,3%)	15(25,4%)	6,1%
4. Polysegmental pneumonia of 2 lungs	8(14%)	14(23,7%)	9,7%
5. Acute bronchitis	0	2(3,4%)	3,4%
6. Chronic bronchitis, exacerbation	4(7%)	5 (8.5%)	1.5%
7. Chronic obstructive bronchitis (COBD), exacerbation	6(10,5%)	9(15,2%)	4,7%
8. COBD out of exacerbation	9(15,8%)	4((6,8%)	9%
9. Bronchial asthma	9(15,8%)	4((6,8%)	9%
10. Bronchiectasis	0	2(3,4%)	3,4%
11. Benign formation of the bronchus	0	1(1,7%)	1,7%
12. Pneumosclerosis	3(5,3%)	9(15,2%)	9,9%
13. Emphysema of the lungs	1(1,7%)	4(6,8%)	5,1%
14. Bullous emphysema	0	2(3,4%)	3,4%
15. 1-sided hydrothorax	3(5,3%)	4(6,8%)	1,5%
16. 2-sided hydrothorax	8(15,8%)	5(8,5%)	7,3%
17. Exudative pleurisy	2(3,5%)	3(5,1%)	1,6%
18. Pneumothorax	0	2(3,4%)	3,4%
19. Atelectasis lungs	0	2(3,4%)	3,4%
20. Pulmonary embolism (PE) of the 1st lung	8(14%)	1(1.7%)	12.3%
21. PE of 2 lungs	1(1,7%)	0	1,7%
22. Stagnation in the pulmonary circulation (stagnation in the MCC)	2(3,5%)	2(3,4%)	0,1%
23. Acute respiratory viral infections	1(1,7%)	0	1,7%
24. Sleep apnea syndrome	1(1,7%)	0	1,7%
25. Respiratory failure 0	. 1(1,7%)	1(1,7%)	0
26. Respiratory failure 1 degree	. 2(3,4%)	4(6,8%)	3,4%
27. Respiratory failure 2 degree	2(3,4%)	0	3,4%

Table 1.
The nature of the respiratory system pathology and the frequency of respiratory failure in two groups of patients without clinical, radiological and biochemical signs of COVID-19.

MSCT (multispiral computed tomography of the chest and lung radiography) performed in all 278 patients. Diagnosis COVID-19 was verified from 162 patients, including 86 men and 76 women who were divided into two groups according to age: 1st - 86 patients at the age from 41 to 60 years, an average of 50.7 ± 1.8 years, men 50(58.1 per cent), women 36(41.9 percent) and 3-group, 76 patients aged 61 to 80 years, an average of 70.3 ± 2.6 years, men 36,women 40. The comparison group consisted of 116 patients, including 77 men and 39 women with pathology of respiratory system coming to the hospital on an emergency basis with referral physician diagnosis of SMP J12.9 community acquired pneumonia, in which the results of the study in the hospital signs of infection COVID-19 have been identified. By age, these patients were divided into two groups: group 2–57 patients aged 41–60 years, average 50.2 ± 2.4, men 36, women 21 and group 4–59 patients, including 41 men and 18 women, age from 61 to 80 years, average age 66.3 ± 1.5 years. The nature of the pathology of the lungs and respiratory system in patients without signs of covid-19 infection is shown in **Table 1**.

The nature of lung damage according to the chest MSCT method and the severity of respiratory failure in patients with COVID-19 and pneumonia are shown in **Table 2**.

In the selected groups of patients, theinitial and subsequent fasting blood glucose levels were analyzed after 8 hours without food intake on a stationary automatic analyzer and using portable glucose, meters using diagnostic test strips. The concentration of glucose and ketones in the urine was determined by a semi-quantitative method. We evaluated the dynamics of indicators when detecting pathological values of glucose concentration. Glucose levels above 6.4 mmol/l were taken as pathological.

Number Disease	Group 1 (41–60 years old) (n = 86)	Group 3 (61–80 years old) (n = 76)	The difference in percentages
1. Pneumonia of the 1st lung	6(7%)	5(6,6%)	0,4%
2. Pneumonia of 2 lungs	69(80,2%)	63(82,9%)	2,7%
3. No pneumonia	11(12,8%)	8(10,5%)	2,3%
4. MSCT scan 1(the degree of lung damage according to the results of multispiral computed tomography)	31(41,3%)	21(27,6%)	13,7%
5. MSCT scan 2	36(48%)	47(61,9%)	13,9%
6. MSCT scan 3	8(10,7%)	7(9,2%)	1,5%
7. MSCT scan 4	0	1(1,3%)	1,3%
8. Respiratory failure 0	4(4,6%)	3(3,9%)	0,7%
9. Respiratory failure 1 degree	4(4,6%)	2(2,6%)	2%
10. Respiratory failure 2 degree	0	3(3,9%)	3,9%

Note: MSCT scan 0 Lungs are clean, there are no lesions. CT1 Focal inflammatory processes filling no more than 25% of alveoli. CT2 Half of the lung tissue is affected. CT3 Up to 75% of lungs are involved in the pathological process. CT4 Bilateral interstitial pneumonia, complete filling of the lung tissue with exudate. The condition is designated by the term respiratory distress syndrome, requires connection to a ventilator. From the site: https://tyubik.net/lecheniye-preparatami/991-kt-1-2-3-4-chto-jeto-znachit-pri-koronaviruse .html.

Table 2.
The frequency of detection of pneumonia in one and two lungs, the severity of pneumonia according to the criteria of multispiral computed tomography of the lungs, and the severity of respiratory failure in two groups of patients of different ages with COVID-19 (number of cases, frequency in %).

To assess hyperglycemia and diabetes, the "criteria for newly diagnosed diabetes mellitus" were used [World Health Organization, WHO, 9 June 2012]:

- Diabetes symptoms + increased venous blood plasma glucose concentration of 11.1 mmol/l when measured randomly. A measurement is considered random at any time of the day, without taking into account the time since the last meal. The classic symptoms of diabetes are polyuria, polydipsia, and weight loss in the absence of obvious causes.

- Fasting glucose concentration in blood plasma is 7.0 mmol/l or in whole blood 6.1 mmol/l. Measurement of glucose concentration is considered to be performed on an empty stomach, if at least 8 hours have passed after a meal.

- The concentration of glucose in blood plasma is 11.1 mmol/l 2 hours after taking 75 g of glucose (glucose tolerance test).

If there are no symptoms of diabetes, a second test should be performed on a different day to confirm the diagnosis. If the diagnosis cannot be confirmed by the level of fasting glycemia or by random measurement, a glucose tolerance test is performed.

Note: The normal concentration of fasting plasma glucose is considered to be 6.1 mmol/l. Impaired glucose tolerance is diagnosed when the fasting plasma glucose concentration is 6.1–7.0 mmol/l. A preliminary diagnosis of diabetes mellitus is established at an fasting plasma glucose concentration of 7.0 mmol/l. The diagnosis of diabetes must be confirmed.

At values above 7.0 mmol/l, according to WHO recommendations, 2012, a glucose tolerance test was performed and the level of glycosylated hemoglobin in the patient's peripheral blood was determined. The level of triglycerides and cholesterol in the blood serum was determined using a Getpremier spectrophotometer (USA). The level of pathologically elevated triglyceride concentrations was considered to be values above 2.8 mmol/l, cholesterol concentrations above 5.2 mmol/l.

Exclusion criteria. The sample did not include patients with worsening of pneumonia, transfer to the intensive care unit, death due to complications of covid infection, cirrhosis of the liver, oncopathology and hemoblastosis, chronic kidney disease of stages 4 and 5, purulent lung lesions, heart failure above stage 2A, with previously diagnosed diabetes and glucose tolerance disorders.

Methods of statistical processing of the obtained data. All the results of the study were processed statistically using the Exsel and Statgraphics software packages (version 2.6). The student's "t-test" was used to compare continuous variables. The Chi – square test or Fisher's exact test were used to evaluate a feature that characterizes the frequency of the phenomenon. The values were compared with the non-Gaussian distribution using the Mann–Whitney U-test. The average intergroup differences of the same type of indicators were compared with the assessment of the reliability of the detected differences.Were considered to be reliable values at $p < 0{,}05$.

4. Results and discussion

The detection rate of hyperglycemia exceeded 30% in group 1 of patients aged 41–60 years with COVID-19 and pneumonia, hyperglycemia persisted during the hospital follow - up period – in 14%, and the frequency of newly diagnosed diabetes mellitus exceeded 9% (**Table 3**). For all these parameters, we did not find any

Number	Indicator	Group 1 (n = 86, men 50, women 36) Patients with COVID-19 and pneumonia	Group 2 (n = 57, men 36, women 21) Patients with lung pathology	Difference in %	The significance of differen-ces, p
1.	Increased blood glucose concentration	27(31,4%)	27(47,4%)	16%	>0,05
2.	Normal concentration of glucose in the blood	59(68,6%)	30(52,6%)	16%	>0,05
3.	The frequency achieved of normoglycemia at higher rate	17 of 27 (63%)	21 of 27 (77.8%)	14.8%	>0,1
4.	Frequency of preservation of hyperglycemia during the period of inpatient treatment	4 of 27 (14.8%)	4 of 27 (14.8%)	0	>0,5
5.	Frequency identified the glycosuria	4 of 65 (6.1%)	1 of 47 (2.1%)	4%	>0.3
6.	Average values of glucose concentration in urine (mmol/l)	17,6 ± 3,86 (2,8–56)	1,7	—	—
7.	Without glucosuria	61 of 65 (93.9%)	46 of 47(97,9%)	4%	>0,3
8.	Ketonuria rate	30 of 65 (46.2%)	6 of 47 (12,8%)	33,4%	<0,01
9.	The average values of the concentration of ketones in the urine (mmol/l)	1,99 ± 0,26 (0,1-7,8)	3,52 ± 0,56 (0,1–10)	43,4%	<0,001
10.	No detected ketonuria	35 of 65 (53.8%)	41 of 47(87,2%)	33,4%	<0,01
11.	Newly diagnosed diabetes (DM)	8 of 86 (9.3%)	5 of 57 (8,8%)	0,5%	> > 0,5

Table 3.
Frequency of diagnosis of hyperglycemia, glucosuria, ketonuria and newly diagnosed diabetes mellitus in groups of patients aged 41–60 years with COVID-19 and pneumonia (group 1) and in patients with respiratory system damage without COVID-19 infection (group 2).

significant differences from the average values in the 2nd comparison group.The frequency of diagnosis of ketonuria in urine was 3.6 times higher in group 1 (the difference was statistically significant, p).

In the study of lipid metabolism in groups of patients it was found that pukazatel the frequency of hypertriglyceridemia was 25% in the 1st group of patients and was significantly higher than the values of the comparison group - 2-group, in which cases the improvement in the levels of TG in peripheral blood have been identified (**Table 4**). The average values of the concentrations of this lipid was also significantly higher in patients with COVID-19 and pneumonia (group 1), by 43.4% ($p < 0,001$). The frequency of hypercholesterolemia was higher in the 1st group of patients – in 22.2% of patients and exceeded by 18.4% (significantly, p).

The frequency of hyperglycemia detection exceeded 45% in group 3 patients aged 61–80 years with COVID-19 and pneumonia, hyperglycemia persisted during the hospital follow - up period – in 16.7%, and the frequency of newly diagnosed diabetes mellitus exceeded 13% (**Table 5**). In these parameters, except for the frequency of hyperglycemia preservation, we did not detect significant differences from the average values in group 4 comparison.

This indicator was 20.4% higher in the 1st group of patients, the difference was significant ($p < 0.05$). The frequency of diagnosis of ketonuria in urine was 2.0 times higher in group 1 (the difference is statistically unreliable, $p > 0.2$), but the average concentration of ketone bodies was 47.9% lower (significantly, $p < 0,001$).

We did not detect any cases of pathological elevation of TG levels in peripheral blood in groups 3 and 4 of patients (**Table 6**). The Mean values of the concentration of this lipid also did not differ significantly and significantly in patients with COVID-19 and pneumonia (group 3), and in patients of the comparison group (group 4). The frequency of hypercholesterolemia was also higher in the 4th group of patients – in 23.6% of patients and exceeded by 14.7% (unreliable, $p > 0,05$).

To clarify the nature of the association of hyperglycemia with comorbidity and the nature of therapy in patients with COVID-19 and pneumonia, we compared the

Number	Indicator	Group 1 (n = 86) Patients with COVID-19 and pneumonia	Group 2 (n = 57) Patients with lung pathology	Difference in %	Significance of differen-ces, p
1.	Frequency of hypertriglyceridemia	25%	0	25%	<0.03
2.	Without hypertriglyceridemia	75%	100%	25%	<0,03
3.	The average values of triglycerides concentration in blood (mmol/l)	2,43 ± 0,49 (0,76-6,81)	1,39 ± 0,08 (1,14-1,80)	42,8%	<0,001
4.	Frequency of hypercholesterolemia	22,2%	4%	18,4%	<0,05
5.	Frequency of normocholesterolemia	77,8%	96%	18,4%	<0,05
6.	Average values of concentration of cholesterol in blood (mmol/l)	3,86 ± 1,07 (0,62-7,75)	3,95 ± 0,98 (1,83-5,31)	2,3%	>0,3

Table 4.
The nature of changes in the concentration of triglycerides and cholesterol in peripheral blood in patients aged 41–60 years with COVID-19 and pneumonia (group 1) and in patients with respiratory system damage without COVID-19 infection (group 2), M ± m, the frequency of the sign in % and the significance of differences.

Number	Indicator	Group 3 (n = 76, male 36, female 40) Patients with COVID-19 and pneumonia	Group 4 (n = 59, men 41, women18) Patients with lung pathology	Difference in %	The significance of differences
1.	Elevated blood glucose	36 of 76 (47.3%)	35 of 59 (59,3%)	12%	> > 0,1
2.	The normal concentration of glucose in blood	40 of 76(52.7%)	24 of 59(40.7%)	12%	>0,1
3.	Frequency achieved normoglycemia at higher rate	28 of 36 (77.8%)	20 of 35 (57.1%)	20.7%	<0,05
4.	Frequency of preservation of hyperglycemia during the period of inpatient treatment	6 of 36 (16,7%)	5 of 35 (14.3%)	2.4%	>0,3
5.	The identified frequency of glycosuria	1 of 54 (1.9%)	8 of 48 (16.7%)	14,8%	>0,1
6.	Average values of glucose concentration in urine (mmol/l)	5.5	2,35 ± 0,74 (0,1–5,6)	—	
7.	Without glucosuria	53 of 54 (98.1%)	40 of 48 (83,3%)	14,8%	>0,1
8.	Ketonuria rate	11 of 54 (20.4%)	5 of 48 (10,4%)	10%	>0,2
9.	The average values of the concentration of ketones in the urine (mmol/l)	1,27 ± 0,21 (0,1-6,0)	2,44 ± 0,37 (0,1–8)	47,9%	<0,001
10.	No detected ketonuria	43 of 54 (79.6%)	43 of 48 (89,6%)	10%	>0,2
11.	Newly diagnosed DM	10 of 76 (13.1%)	5 of 59(8,5%)	4,6%	>0,3

Table 5.
Frequency of diagnosis of hyperglycemia, glucosuria, ketonuria and newly diagnosed diabetes mellitus in groups of patients aged 61–80 years with COVID-19 and pneumonia (group 3) and in patients with respiratory system damage without COVID-19 infection (group 4).

frequency of diseases recorded in medical records in 162 patients aged 41–80 years, including 63 with hyperglycemia and 99 with normoglycemia (**Table 7**). A statistically significant association with hyperglycemia was confirmed only for the diagnosis of grade 2–3 hypertension (arterial hypertension) – the difference between the groups was 22.8% ($p < 0,03$). The sign of grade 2–3 obesity was 16.8% more common in patients with hyperglycemia, the difference is on the verge of statistical significance ($p > 0.05$).

The study conducted in patients aged 41–80 years admitted to the hospital with suspected covid-19 infection revealed fasting hyperglycemia in 31–47% of different age groups, and newly diagnosed DM in 9–13% of patients. Comparison with groups of patients with acute and chronic lung pathology did not allow us to note significant and significant differences in these indicators. These data suggest that the development of covid infection with the addition of pneumonia is a significant factor in both the development of transient hyperglycemia and the manifestation of diabetes mellitus.

n/a number	Indicator	Group 3 (n = 76, male 36, female 40) Patients with COVID-19 and pneumonia	Group 4 (n = 59, men 41, women 18) Patients with lung pathology	Difference in %	Significance of differences
1.	Frequency of hypertriglyceridemia	0	0	0	—
2.	Without hypertriglyceridemia	100%	100%	0	0
.	The average values of triglycerides concentration in blood (mmol/l)	1,31 ± 0,08 (0,80-1,73)	1,45 ± 0,15 (0,62-2,25)	9,6%	>0,2
4.	Frequency of hypercholesterolemia	2,7%	> > 0,3	14,7%	>0,1
5.	Without hypercholesterolemia	91,1%	76,4%	14,7%	>0,1
6.	Average values of concentration of cholesterol in blood (mmol/l)	3,93 ± 0,83 (1,44-5,74)	4,04 ± 1,48 (3,19-7,43)	2,7%	>0,5

Table 6.
The nature of changes in the concentration of triglycerides (TG) and cholesterol (CH) in peripheral blood in patients aged 61–80 years with COVID-19 and pneumonia (group 3) and in patients with respiratory system damage without COVID-19 infection (group 4), M ± m, the frequency of the sign in % and the significance of differences.

Number	Indicator, type of pathology, treatment method	The frequency difference between	The accuracy of the indicator R
1.	Hypertension of 2–3 degrees of severity	22.8%	<0.03
2.	Grade 2–3 obesity	16.8%	>0.05
3.	Uterine fibroids (women)	11,1%	>0,2
4.	Paroxysmal and permanent-functional form of atrial fibrillation	10%	>0.2
5.	Chronic alcoholic disease	7.4%	>0.3
6.	Intracoronary transluminal angioplasty (TLAP) procedures, stenting	6.3%	>0.3
7.	Viral hepatitis B, C	6%	>0.3

Table 7.
The degree of difference in the frequency of certain forms of pathology and treatment measures in patients with COVID-19 and pneumonia aged 41–80 years, which prevailed in patients with hyperglycemia (n = 63), compared with patients with normal blood glucose concentration (n = 99).

Our data are confirmed by the results obtained in previous studies on the clinical assessment of the course of covid-19 in patients at a hospital in Wuhan (China). Thus, the authors reported that of 99 infected individuals, it was shown that 52% had elevated glucose levels, and in some patients with viral pneumonia, virus infection was accompanied by an increase in the concentration of glycated hemoglobin [19].

According to our data, in 16.6–31.3% of patients after treatment and regression of changes in the lungs, normalization of glucose levels was also observed, but in 14.8–16.7% the changes persisted, and in 9–13% of them, after an additional study, newly diagnosed diabetes mellitus was diagnosed. From these data, it can be assumed that the effect of covid-viral infection on carbohydrate metabolism in patients with pneumonia is observed mainly in the acute period of the disease, but in some patients, the disease in subsequent periods may manifest previously existing prerequisites for the development of chronic pathology (diabetes mellitus).

A feature of carbohydrate metabolism disorders in patients with COVID-19 and pneumonia in our study was a high frequency of ketonuria – more than 45% of patients aged 41–60 years studied in group 1. In the 3rd group of older patients, this pattern was less pronounced, the frequency of ketonuria exceeded 20%. We tried to link this feature of changes in the metabolism of ketone bodies with the vastness of the lung lesion and impaired gas exchange. However, a comparison of the rates of respiratory failure of varying severity in groups 1–3 of patients with COVID-19, as well as indicators of the severity of lung damage according to the diagnostic criteria of the chest MSCT method (multispiral computed tomography of the chest), did not reveal significant and significant differences between the groups. Based on the obtained data, we suggested that viral antigens can change the parameters of tissue membrane permeability for glucose in patients, with an increase in under-oxidized ketone bodies in the bloodstream and an increase in their urinary excretion. The rate of elimination of ketone bodies in the urine was apparently, higher in patients with COVID-19 in group 1 aged 41–60 years than in group 3, 61–80 years, which can be explained by a more preserved filtration function of the kidneys in the younger part of patients with this infection.

To date, apparently, only a few studies have estimated the prevalence of acidosis and ketoacidosis in a large number (n = 658) hospitalized patients with confirmed COVID-19 [20]. Of this sample, 42 (6.4%) patients had positive urine or serum ketones, with only three of 42 (7%) meeting the American Diabetes Association criteria for decompensated ketoacidosis (DKA). People with ketosis were about twice as likely to develop diabetes in this study, and three people who developed DKA were diagnosed with diabetes [20]. In a review and analytical article by employees from the Italian University and the Nephrological Center of Naples (Campania University, "Luigi Vanvitelli", and Nefrocenter Research & Nyx Start-UP, Naples, Italy), the nature of keto-acidotic conditions in patients with COVID-19 is analyzed The authors believe that at the onset of diabetes such conditions may include the so-called pre-diabetic state (impaired fasting glucose and impaired glucose tolerance), which occur with persistently normal levels of glycated hemoglobin, in addition, with a temporary hyperglycemic effect, usually observed in any acute or severe inflammatory disease, or symptoms and signs of ketoacidosis in patients, causes decompensated diabetes [21]. In actual clinical practice, clinicians may classify any event that occurs in people with high blood sugar levels as decompensated ketoacidosis (DKA), regardless of whether it was a real case of DKA or the accumulation of ketones was a consequence of respiratory acidosis potentiated by malnutrition (ion-controlled ketosis). A factor of keto-acidosis can also be a high concentration of inflammatory markers in the blood of patients with COVID-19, which is also typical for DKA, regardless of the concomitant disease [22, 23].

This assumption is confirmed by the results of studies in groups of patients with COVID-19 indicators of lipid metabolism. Since the natural type of lipid changes in diabetes mellitus, according to the literature, hypercholesterolemia are the most common types of lipid changes in diabetes mellitus, we analyzed these lipid parameters. The frequency of both hypertriglyceridemia and hypercholesterolemia in the group of patients aged 41–60 years with COVID-19 and pneumonia exceeded 22% and was significantly higher than in the comparison group of patients of similar age without this viral infection. However, we did not find such differences in the groups of older patients. These data allowed us to assume that COVID-19 infection to a greater extent can affect glucose-dependent mechanisms of lipid exchange of triglycerides and cholesterol in patients with pneumonia at the age of 61 years than in older patients in whom lipid changes often cause not acute, and chronic factors associated with age-related changes of liver function and central hemodynamics. To clarify this issue, we analyzed the frequency of diagnosis of various forms of pathology, including cardiovascular, in patients with COVID-19 and pneumonia with hyperglycemia and normoglycemia in the general group of patients aged 41–80 years. The comparison allowed us to establish that hyperglycemia was significantly more often detected in patients with arterial hypertension of 2–3 degrees of severity and-with a tendency to reliability-more often in patients with obesity of 2–3 degrees. Neither coronary atherosclerosis (confirmed by coronary angiography and coronary stenosis plastic surgery), nor the frequency of previously developed cardiosclerosis with damage to the cardiac conduction system and the development of atrial fibrillation, nor liver damage in viral hepatitis and chronic alcoholism in the groups of patients with COVID-19 and pneumonia had a significant direct relationship with the frequency of detected cases of hyperglycemia.

5. Conclusions

1. In patients aged 41–80 years who were hospitalized with covid-19 infection and pneumonia, fasting hyperglycemia was diagnosed in 31–47%, glucosuria in 1.9–6.1%, ketonuria – 20.4-46.2% of cases, in different age groups.

2. In 16.6–31.3% of cases in patients with covid-19, after treatment and regression of changes in the lungs, normalization of glucose levels was observed, but in 14.8–16.7% of the changes persisted, and in 9–13% of them, after an additional study, newly diagnosed diabetes mellitus was diagnosed.

3. Hyperglycemia was significantly more often detected in patients with arterial hypertension of 2–3 degrees of severity and with a tendency to reliability, in patients with obesity of 2–3 degrees. Lipid metabolism disorders (hypertriglyceridemia and hypercholesterolemia), which are characteristic of changes in carbohydrate metabolism in patients with impaired glucose tolerance and diabetes, were significantly more often diagnosed in patients with covid-19 than in the group of patients with acute and chronic lung pathology without proven inyion with this virus, but only in the group of patients aged 41–60 years.

Conflict of interest

Didn't show up.

Authors' contribution

Vechorko V. I.-the idea of research. Writing sections "research Results", "discussion of results", "Conclusions". Doroshenko D. A.-description of research methods.

Evsikov E. M.-a set of materials, statistical processing, design of the article text. Baykova O. A.-writing the section "Introduction", design of the article text. Teplova N.V. - writing the chapter "Discussion of results".

Annotation

History of the issue

Already in the initial period of studying the prognostic significance and danger to human health and life of the state of infection with the COVID-19 virus in January–April 2020, mainly thanks to research from Chinese medical centers, it was clarified that factors contributing to lung damage are highly likely the course of the disease in severe form, include: advanced age [6]; diabetes [6, 7, 24]; obesity [25]; chronic lung diseases [14], including asthma [12]; heart disease [12, 16]; hypertension [14]; chronic kidney disease [14].

In one of the first clinical observations of 41 COVID-19-infected people in Wuhan, China, it was shown that in 32% of cases, COVID-19 was combined with other diseases, including diabetes (20%), hypertension (15%) and cardio-vascular diseases (15%), [16]. Another report of patients who were discharged or died at clinics in Wuhan between January 1, 2020 and March 8, 2020 reported that patients with COVID-19 with diabetes had worse outcomes compared to patients of the same sex and age without diabetes. Advanced age and concomitant arterial hypertension independently contributed to the hospital death of patients with diabetes [6]. The results obtained at the Wuhan Jin Yin Tang Hospital showed that in intensive care units, 17% of patients suffered from chronic diseases, including diabetes (17%), cerebrovascular diseases (13.5%), chronic heart disease (10%) and T. D. During treatment in 35% of critically ill patients, hyperglycemia was a concomitant pathology, and mortality among patients with diabetes was 77.7% [16, 26].

In a retrospective study of 138 patients with COVID-19, from a clinic in this city in China, published on February 7, 2020, it was shown that 46.4% of patients had one or more comorbidities, of which 10% had diabetes, while in wards Intensive care (ICU) 22.2% of patients had diabetes, that is, 2 times more often [26]. The study of the relationship between diabetes and mortality and severity of COVID-19, as well as in determining the prevalence of diabetes in patients with COVID-19, has also been conducted in several meta-analyzes. Employees from the Institute of Gastroenterology, Delhi, India (Institute of Liver, Gastroenterology, & Pancreatico-Biliary Sciences, Sir Ganga Ram Hospital, New Delhi, India). searched PubMed for case–control studies in English published between January 1 and April 22, 2020 that had data on diabetes in patients with COVID-19. The incidence of diabetes was compared between patients with and without a combined mortality or severity endpoint. Included 33 studies (16,003 patients).. The authors found that diabetes was significantly associated with mortality from COVID-19 with a pooled odds ratio of 1.90 [24]. Another meta-analysis conducted by researchers at the Faculty of Medicine, Universitas Pelita Harapan, Tangerang, Indonesia analyzed data from 6452 patients from 30 studies. A meta-analysis showed that diabetes was associated with an incidence of combined adverse outcomes (relative risk, RR 2.38) and its subgroup, which included mortality (RR 2.12), severe COVID-19 (RR 2.45), acute respiratory distress syndrome (ARDS) (RR 4.64) and disease progression (RR 3.31). It was concluded that diabetes was associated with mortality, severe COVID-19, ARDS and disease progression in patients with COVID-19 [7].

From the statistics of the 2020 epidemic in the North American continent, it follows that diabetes mellitus can increase the risk of death from COVID-19 by 12 times, according to the portal of the US Centers for Disease Control and Prevention. Patients infected with coronavirus with diabetes are six times more likely to need hospitalization for inpatient treatment, and diabetes is in second place in terms of severity of complications in COVID-19 after cardiovascular disease [10]. According to the China Cardiometabolic and Cancer Cohort (4C) nationwide study, compared with patients with normal glucose tolerance, people with impaired glucose tolerance or diabetes had a high risk of lung infection with a multifactorial adjusted odds ratio (OR; 95% CI) 1.56 (1.02–2.37) and 1.63 (1.01–2.61), respectively [27]. Epidemiological evidence from the United States suggests that diabetes is associated with a high risk of infectious disease. People with diabetes are at increased risk of bacteremic pneumococcal infection and are reported to have a high risk of nosocomial bacteremia with mortality rates up to 50% [28]. At the same time, the state of carbohydrate metabolism in patients with COVID-19 who have not previously suffered from diabetes has not been sufficiently studied in clinical studies. Hyperglycemia, even in people with no previous diabetes, has often been observed in complicated coronavirus disease 2019 (COVID-19), [17, 18]. Hyperglycemia in COVID - 19 is a strong predictor of a worse prognosis and an increased likelihood of death [18]. In the above-cited study of patients with COVID-19, conducted at the Wuhan Jin Yin Tang Hospital, with the participation of 99 infected people, it was shown that 52% of those infected had elevated glucose levels, and in some patients with viral pneumonia, infection with the virus was accompanied by an increase in the concentration glycated hemoglobin [16].

Goal and tasks

To assess the incidence of hyperglycemia and diagnosis of newly diagnosed diabetes mellitus in patients with COVID-19 and acute lung damage at the age of 41–80 years, hospitalized in a repurposed infectious diseases hospital in Moscow with a diagnosis of pneumonia.

Material and methods

The observational study analyzed laboratory and clinical diagnostic data of 278 patients who did not have, according to the anamnesis and the presented medical reports, signs of impaired glucose tolerance and manifest forms of diabetes mellitus, including 163 men and 115 women aged 41–80 years admitted to hospital for diagnosis and treatment in the period from 12.04.2020 to 10.11.2020 with diagnoses according to ICD-10: U07.1 Coronavirus infection. In the selected groups of patients, the initial and subsequent levels of fasting blood glucose were analyzed, after 8 hours without food, on a stationary automatic analyzer and using portable glucometers using diagnostic test strips. The concentration of glucose and ketones in urine was determined by a semi-quantitative method. The dynamics of indicators was assessed when pathological values of glucose concentration were detected. Glucose levels above 6.4 mmol/L were considered pathological.

Results

In patients aged 41–80 years hospitalized with covid-19 infection and pneumonia, fasting hyperglycemia was diagnosed in 31–47%, glucosuria in 1.9–6.1%, ketonuria - 20.4-46.2% of cases, in different age groups. In 16.6–31.3% of cases in patients with covid-19, after treatment and regression of changes in the lungs, there was a normalization of glucose levels, but in 14.8–16.7% of cases persisted, and in 9–13% of them, after an additional study, newly diagnosed diabetes mellitus was diagnosed. Hyperglycemia was significantly more often detected in patients with arterial hypertension of 2–3 degrees of severity and with a tendency to reliability, in patients with obesity 2–3 degree. Lipid metabolism disorders (hypertriglyceridemia and hypercholesterolemia), characteristic of changes in carbohydrate metabolism with impaired glucose tolerance and diabetes, were significantly more often diagnosed in patients with covid-19 than in the group of patients with acute and chronic lung pathology without proven infection with this virus, but only in the group of patients age period 41–60 years.

Conclusion

Covid-19 infection complicated by pneumonia occurs in persons aged 41–80 years with a high incidence of hyperglycemia and ketonuria. The incidence of newly diagnosed diabetes mellitus in such patients is 9–13%.

Author details

Valeriy Ivanovich Vechorko[1], Evgeny Mikhailovich Evsikov[1,2*], Oksana Alekseevna Baykova[1,2], Natalya Vadimovna Teplova[2] and Dmitriy Aleksandrovich Doroshenko[1]

1 City Clinical Hospital No. 15 named after O.M. Filatov of the Moscow Department of Health, Russia, Moscow

2 Russian National Research Medical Institute named after N.I. Pirogov, Russia, Moscow

*Address all correspondence to: dr.evsikov@gmail.com

References

[1] Abrams JY, Godfred-Cato SE, Oster ME и др. Multisystem inflammatory syndrome in children associated with severe acute respiratory syndrome coronavirus 2: a systematic review. J Pediatr. Опубликовано онлайн 5 августа 2020 г. doi: 10.1016/j.jpeds.2020.08.003

[2] Morris S.B; Schwartz N.G; Patel P.P; Abbo L., и др. Case Series of Multisystem Inflammatory Syndrome in Adults Associated with SARS-CoV-2 Infection — United Kingdom and United States, March–August 2020. MMиBP Morb Wkly Rep. 2020; 69 (40): 1450-1456. DOI: 10.15585/mmwr.mm6940e1

[3] Carfì A.; Bernabei R.; Landi F. et al. Persistent Symptoms in Patients After Acute COVID-19. Gemelli Against COVID-19 Post-Acute Care Study Group. JAMA. 2020;324(6):603-605. doi:10.1001/jama.2020.12603

[4] Del C. R., Collins L. F. C, Malani P. Long-term Health Consequences of COVID-19. JAMA. 2020; 324 (17): 1723-1724.

[5] COVID-19 и полиорганная патология. Возможности успешного лечения вирусной инфекции и её осложнений. Общество специалистов по сердечной недостаточности. Мареев В. Ю. Лекция. 13 июня 2020 https://youtu.be/jhVp9vJiwB4. РФ.Москва

[6] Qiao Shi [1 2], Xiaoyi Zhang [3], Fang Jiang [4], Xuanzhe Zhang [2], Ning Hu [2], Chibu Bimu [2], Jiarui Feng [5], Su Yan [2], Yongjun Guan [2], Dongxue Xu [3], Guangzhen He [6], Chen Chen [2], Xingcheng Xiong [1], Lei Liu [1], Hanjun Li [1], Jing Tao [1], Zhiyong Peng [7], Weixing Wang [8]. Clinical Characteristics and Risk Factors for Mortality of COVID-19 Patients With Diabetes in Wuhan, China: A Two-Center, Retrospective Study. Diabetes Care. 2020 Jul;43(7):1382-1391. doi: 10.2337/dc20-0598. Epub 2020 May 14.

[7] Ian Huang [1], Michael Anthonius Lim [2], Raymond Pranata [3]. Diabetes mellitus is associated with increased mortality and severity of disease in COVID-19 pneumonia - A systematic review, meta-analysis, and meta-regression. Diabetes Metab Syndr.. Jul-Aug 2020;14(4):395-403. doi: 10.1016/j.dsx.2020.04.018. Epub 2020 Apr 17.

[8] Cuker A., Peyvandi F. Coronavirus disease 2019 (COVID-19): Hypercoagulability. Literature review, 2020. BMJ Best Practice.

[9] Connors J.M., Levy J.H. Thromboinflammation and the hypercoagulability of COVID-19 // J. Thromb. Haemost. 2020 // www.hematology.org/covid-19/covid-19-and-coagulopathy. J Thromb Haemost 2020 Jul;18(7):1559-1561. doi: 10.1111/jth.14849. Epub 2020 May 26.

[10] Centers for Disease Control and Prevention. People who are at higher risk for severe illness // www.cdc.gov/coronavirus/ 2019-ncov/need-extra-precautions/ people-at-higher-risk.html.

[11] Zhang C., Shi L., Wang F.-S. Liver injury in COVID-19: management and challenges // Lancet Gastroenterol. Hepatol. 2020. Vol. 5. № 5. P. 428-430.

[12] Рекомендации ВОЗ для населения в связи с распространением нового коронавируса (2019-nCoV): мифы и ложные представления. Дата обращения: 08.02.2020.

[13] “Solidarity” clinical trial for COVID-19 treatments (англ.). World Health Organization (16 October 2020). Дата обращения: 17 октября 2020.

[14] CDC. Interim Clinical Guidance for Management of Patients with

Confirmed Coronavirus Disease (COVID-19) (англ.). U. S. Centers for Disease Control and Prevention (11 February 2020). Дата обращения: 25 апреля 2020. Архивировано 25 апреля 2020 года.

[15] Диабет может увеличивать риск смерти при COVID-19. https://ria.ru/20200727/1574954095.html. МОСКВА, 27 июля 2020 г. — РИА Новости.

[16] Huang C, Wang Y, Li X, et al. Clinical features of patients infected with 2019 novel coronavirus in Wuhan, China. Lancet. 2020; 395(10223): 497-506.

[17] Zhang Y, Li H, Zhang J, et al. The clinical characteristics and outcomes of diabetes mellitus and secondary hyperglycaemia patients with coronavirus disease 2019: A single-centre, retrospective, observational study in Wuhan. Diabetes Obes Metab. 2020. https://doi.org/10.1111/dom.14086.

[18] Li H, Tian S, Chen T, et al. Newly diagnosed diabetes is associated with a higher risk of mortality than known diabetes in hospitalized patients with COVID-19. Diabetes Obes Metab. 2020; 22(10): 1897-1906.

[19] Chen N, Zhou M, Dong X, et al. Epidemiological and clinical characteristics of 99 cases of 2019 novel coronavirus pneumonia in Wuhan, China: a descriptive study. Lancet. 2020; 395(10223): 507-513.

[20] Li J, Wang X, Chen J, Zuo X, Zhang H, Deng A. COVID-19 infection may cause ketosis and ketoacidosis. Diabetes Obes Metab. 2020; 1-7. https://doi.org/10.1111/dom.14057.

[21] Gentile S ,Strolo F ,Andrea Mambro MD ,Antonio Ceriello MD COVID-19, ketoacidosis and new-onset diabetes: Are there possible cause and effect relationships among them? Diabetes, Obesity and Metabolism.Volume 22, Issue 12 First published: 13 August 2020 ,https://doi.org/10.1111/dom.14170

[22] Ceriello A, De Nigris V, Prattichizzo F. Why is hyperglycaemia worsening COVID-19 and its prognosis? Diabetes Obes Metab. 2020; 1-2. https://doi.org/10.1111/dom.14098.

[23] Stentz FB, Umpierrez GE, Cuervo R, Kitabchi AE. Proinflammatory cytokines, markers of cardiovascular risks, oxidative stress, and lipid peroxidation in patients with hyperglycemic crises. Diabetes. 2004; 53: 2079-2086.

[24] Yongli Yan [1], Yan Yang [1], Fen Wang [1], Huihui Ren [1], Shujun Zhang [1], Xiaoli Shi [1], Xuefeng Yu [1], Kun Dong [2]. Clinical characteristics and outcomes of patients with severe covid-19 with diabetes. BMJ Open Diabetes Res Care. 2020 Apr;8(1):e001343. doi: 10.1136/bmjdrc-2020-001343.

[25] Глыбочко П.В., Фомин В.В., Авдеев С.Н. и др. Клиническая характеристика 1007 больных тяжелой SARS-CoV-2 пневмонией, нуждавшихся в респираторной поддержке (рус.) Клиническая фармакология и терапия: журн. — 2020. — 17 мая (т. 29, № 2). — С. 21—29. — ISSN 0869-5490.

[26] Wang D, Hu B, Hu C, et al. Clinical characteristics of 138 hospitalized patients with 2019 novel coronavirus-infected pneumonia in Wuhan, China. JAMA. 2020. doi: 10.1001/jama.2020.1585.

[27] Li M, et al. Diabetes Care. 2020. PMID: 32540923 Mian Li [1], Yu Xu [1], Qin Wan [2], Feixia Shen [3], Min Xu [1], Zhiyun Zhao [1], Jieli Lu [1], Zhengnan Gao [4], Gang Chen [5], Tiange Wang [1], Yiping Xu [1], Jiajun Zhao [6], Lulu Chen [7], Lixin Shi [8], Ruying Hu [9], Zhen Ye [9], Xulei Tang [10], Qing Su [11], Guijun Qin [12], Guixia Wang [13],

Zuojie Luo [14], Yingfen Qin [14], Yanan Huo [15], Qiang Li [16], Yinfei Zhang [17], Yuhong Chen [1], Chao Liu [18], Yiming Mu [19], Youmin Wang [20], Shengli Wu [21], Tao Yang [22], Li Chen [23], Xuefeng Yu [24], Li Yan [25], Huacong Deng [26], Guang Ning [1], Yufang Bi [27], Weiqing Wang [27]. Individual and Combined Associations of Modifiable Lifestyle and Metabolic Health Status With New-Onset Diabetes and Major Cardiovascular Events: The China Cardiometabolic Disease and Cancer Cohort (4C) Study. Diabetes Care. 2020 Aug;43(8):1929-1936. doi: 10.2337/dc20-0256. Epub 2020 Jun 15.PMID: 32540923

[28] American Diabetes A. 4. Comprehensive medical evaluation and assessment of comorbidities: standards of medical care in diabetes-2020. Diabetes Care. 2020; 43(Suppl 1): S37- S47.

Chapter 17

Refocusing Functional Anatomy and Immunology of the Respiratory Mucosa in the Advent of Covid-19

Humphrey Simukoko

Abstract

Atmospheric oxygen is an indispensable element required in order for mammalian cells to function normally. The mammalian respiratory system, through pulmonary ventilation and gas diffusion, provides the physical mechanisms by which oxygen gains access to all body cells and through which carbon dioxide is eliminated from the body. The network of tissues and organs of the respiratory system helps the mammalian body cells to absorb oxygen from the air to enable the tissues and organs to function optimally. The advent of the coronavirus disease 2019 (Covid-19) Pandemic caused by the severe acute respiratory syndrome coronavirus 2 (SARS-CoV-2) has stimulated heightened and refocused interest in the study of various aspects of the respiratory system. The SARS-CoV-2 targets the respiratory system mucosal cells and in a cascade of biological processes curtails the ability of the respiratory system to absorb and deliver oxygen to the pulmonary blood and body cells often resulting in severe disease and/or death. The mucosa and submucosa of the respiratory tract are adapted to provide both innate and adaptive immune defense mechanisms against pathogens including the SARS-CoV-2. The entire respiratory tract is covered by a mucosa that transitions in its structural and functional characteristics from the upper respiratory tract to the lower respiratory tract. This chapter provides an overview of the functional anatomy and immunology of the respiratory tract covering the mucosa from the upper respiratory tract all the way up to the alveolar epithelium. In the advent of the covid-19 pandemic, a broader perspective and understanding of the anatomy and immunology of the respiratory tract will enable general readers and researchers to fully appreciate the discourse in covid-19 research as it affects the respiratory tract.

Keywords: Covid-19, SARS-CoV-2, Respiratory tract, Pandemic, Coronavirus, immunology

1. Introduction

The novel Coronavirus disease of 2019 (covid-19) caused by the Severe Acute Respiratory Syndrome (SARS) Coronavirus (CoV)-2 was first reported in Wuhan, China in December 2019 and had continued to ravage the world, causing widespread respiratory health problems and mortalities. The virus targets mainly the respiratory tract. It enters the lungs through the upper respiratory tract and attacks alveoli epithelial type2 (AT2) cells [1]. Many patients succumb to pneumonia in severe SARS-CoV-2 infections.

In the advent of the covid-19 pandemic, there had been a renewed focus on the mammalian respiratory anatomy and physiology. In this regard, this calls for a broader perspective and understanding of the anatomy and physiology of the respiratory system. This chapter therefore provides an overview of the functional anatomy and immunology of the respiratory tract in the context of the covid-19 pandemic.

2. Anatomical organization of the respiratory tract

The mammalian respiratory system consists of tissues and organs whose main function is to ensure exchange of oxygen and carbon dioxide between the organism and the external environment. From the functional perspective, the respiratory system is viewed as consisting of a conducting part and a gaseous exchange part while from a purely anatomical perspective the respiratory system is viewed as being composed of an upper respiratory component and a lower respiratory component.

The conducting part of the respiratory system, also known as the conducting airways, is that part of the respiratory system that merely transports gases from the external environment to the lungs and from the lungs to the external environment, while the gaseous exchange part is that part of the respiratory system that is responsible for the diffusion of gases (particularly oxygen and carbon dioxide) into and out of the blood capillaries of the lungs. Structures from the nasal cavity up to the terminal bronchioles constitute the conducting part of the respiratory tract. The conducting part also serves a protective function by conditioning the air that has been inhaled [2]. Conditioning of the inspired air by the conducting airways includes heating the air to body temperature, filtering out harmful gases and particles such as dust and bacteria as well as saturating the air to 100% relative humidity [2]. In trapping and filtering out harmful gases and particles, the respiratory tract uses a mucociliary escalator or mucociliary blanket. The mucociliary escalator is composed of cilia, mucus and a layer of fluid known as the periciliary layer. The fluid on the surface of the airways is constantly propelled by cilia from near the lungs to regions far away from the lungs towards the nasal cavity to be expelled.

The conducting part terminates at the terminal bronchioles before transforming into the gaseous exchange zone. The gaseous exchange zone is located within the lung parenchyma. The components of the gaseous exchange zone consist of the respiratory bronchioles, alveolar ducts and alveolar sacs together with their alveoli [2]. The gaseous exchange zone is a thin membrane that exists between the alveoli space and the pulmonary capillary blood. The pulmonary capillary blood network thoroughly covers the alveoli walls and receives the major cardiac output of the right ventricle via the pulmonary trunk [2–3].

The entire mammalian respiratory tract from the nasal cavity to the bronchi tree is lined by a mucus membrane known as the respiratory mucosa. The respiratory mucosa consists of epithelial cells that sit on top of a layer of loose connective tissue. The main function of the respiratory mucosa is to prevent pathogens and noxious particles from reaching the lungs. In most parts of the respiratory tract, the respiratory mucosa secretes a thick protective mucus layer. Generally, the respiratory mucosa consists of a pseudostratified columnar epithelium and an underlying loose connective tissue known as the lamina propria. The epithelium normally transitions in structure from the nasal cavity towards the lungs starting with a pseudostratified columnar epithelium in the nasal cavity and ending with a simple squamous or cuboidal epithelium in the alveoli. The respiratory mucosa contains different types of epithelial cells that range from ciliated columnar to simple squamous. Within the respiratory tract epithelial cells are found mucus-secreting cells such as goblet cells and some specialized glands containing both mucus and serous cells [4].

Throughout the respiratory tract from the nasal cavity to the alveoli, sheets of cells cover the internal surface. The sheets of cells, known as epithelium, differ in structure and function depending on the location within the respiratory tract. The major part of the respiratory tract, from the nasal cavity to the bronchi, is lined by a pseudostratified columnar epithelium. From the bronchi downwards to the bronchioles, the epithelium changes into a simple columnar to cuboidal epithelium. The epithelium then changes in the alveoli to become a thin squamous epithelium that allows for gaseous exchange to take place. The epithelial cells sit on top of a basement membrane below which lies a layer of loose connective tissue known as the lamina propria [4].

Anatomically, the respiratory tract is viewed as consisting of the upper and lower parts. The upper respiratory tract consists of the nasal cavity and adjoining paranasal sinuses, pharynx and the portion of larynx above the vocal folds. The lower respiratory tract comprises of the lower parts of the larynx, the trachea, bronchi, bronchioles and the alveoli [5].

3. The upper respiratory tract

The upper respiratory tract is composed of the nose and nasal cavity, the pharynx and the larynx. It is the first entry point for air and other potentially harmful substances including bacteria and viruses. The upper respiratory tract functions in the filtration, warming and humidification of the inspired air. In addition, the upper respiratory tract contains nerve endings of the first cranial nerve known as the olfactory nerve which is responsible for detecting odors in the inspired air. This section provides an account of the functional anatomy of the major components of the upper respiratory tract particularly the nasal cavity and pharynx.

3.1 The nasal cavity

Up to 90% or more of inspiration occurs through the nose and therefore the nasal cavity is an important site for initial infection by most microorganisms including SARS-CoV-2. Moreover, SARS-CoV-2 infection via the ocular route is hypothesized to occur via drainage of virus-laden tears into the nasal cavity through the nasal lacrimal duct [6–8].

The air entering the respiratory tract is usually dry, cold and containing potentially harmful particulate matter. Therefore, the major function of the nasal cavity is to humidify and warm the inspired air. As the air passes through the nasal cavity, airborne particles are filtered off including microorganisms before the air reaches the lower respiratory tract. In addition, the nasal cavity is an olfactory (smell) organ and also helps in draining and clearing the paranasal sinuses and lacrimal ducts [7].

Entrance into the nasal cavity is provided by the nostrils, which are two external openings into the nasal cavity. The nasal cavity consists of the nasal skeleton which is made up of a combination of parts of bones such as the maxilla, the ethmoid, the perpendicular part of the palatine bone and the medial pterygoid plate. The nasal cavity is divided into two separate cavities by a cartilaginous nasal septum. Each half of the nasal cavity consists of a roof, floor, medial wall and lateral wall. The nasal septum is made up of cartilage and bone. In contrast to the lateral walls, the floor and the roof of the nasal cavity which are covered by a pseudostratified columnar epithelium, the nasal septum is covered by squamous epithelium [9]. The posterior boundary of the nasal cavity is provided by the choanae also known as posterior nasal apertures. The choanae open into the nasopharynx [10–12].

Four paranasal sinuses surround the nasal cavity in humans. These are the frontal sinuses (superior anterior), ethmoid sinuses (superior), paired maxillary sinuses (lateral), and sphenoid sinuses (posterior). The paranasal sinuses communicate with the nasal cavity through ducts that drain through ostia, which empty into spaces located on the lateral wall. Only the sphenoid paranasal sinus empties into the posterior roof of the nasal cavity [13].

There are three recognizable regions within each half of the nasal cavity: the nasal vestibule, respiratory region and olfactory region.

3.1.1 Nasal vestibule

The first part of the nasal cavity immediately posterior to the nostrils is the nasal vestibule. The initial half of the nasal vestibule is covered by a keratinized stratified squamous epithelium that contains hairs known as vibrissae. The function of the vibrissae is to filter inhaled particles. The second half of the nasal vestibule is covered by a pseudostratified ciliated columnar epithelium [14, 15].

3.1.2 Respiratory region

The respiratory region is the main part of the nasal cavity and is that part which houses the nasal conchae (or turbinate bones) and meatuses. Nasal conchae are curved shelves of bone that protrude from the lateral walls of the nasal cavity. The spaces between the nasal conchae are referred to as meatuses. The main functions of the respiratory region are to humidify and warm the inspired air and to trap and eliminate particulate matter. The respiratory region is covered in respiratory epithelium (pseudostratified ciliated columnar epithelium) and mucous cells.

As the air passes through the nasal cavity, it is warmed to body temperature and is humidified to near 100%. The warming and humidification of the inspired air is aided by the neuromuscular network within this region. The neuromuscular network of the respiratory region regulates airflow within the nasal cavity by controlling the blood volume in the erectile tissue on the turbinate bones. Under normal physiological conditions, the erectile tissue is continuously stimulated by the sympathetic nervous system to prevent nasal congestion [13].

Airborne particles that escape trapping in the nasal vestibule become trapped in the mucous produced by the respiratory nasal mucosa. The trapped particles are then eliminated by the ciliated cells of the mucociliary system which sweep mucous and trapped particles at a rate of 1 cm per minute into the naso-pharynx for further expulsion [16].

3.1.3 Olfactory region

One of the most commonly reported neurological indicators of SARS-CoV-2 infection is the temporary loss of smell (anosmia). Studies suggest that anosmia better predicts SARS-CoV-2 infection than other well-known symptoms such as fever and cough. Furthermore, studies suggest that the novel coronavirus changes the sense of smell in patients not by directly affecting neurons but by affecting the function of sustentacular or supporting cells [17, 18].

The olfactory region is a small area located at the superior apex of the nasal cavity and the ethmoturbinates and is lined with olfactory receptor cells. The olfactory region is responsible for sensing odors in inspired air. It is lined by an olfactory epithelium which is made up of a pseudostratified epithelium that contains olfactory sensory receptor cells, supporting cells and mucus secreting glands. The olfactory receptor neuron is a bipolar cell that gives rise to a small-diameter, unmyelinated axon at its basal surface that transmits olfactory information centrally. At its apical surface, the receptor neuron gives rise to a single process that expands into a knob-like protrusion from which several microvilli, called olfactory cilia, extend into a thick layer of mucus [19]. The fibers of the olfactory sensory receptor cells have their axonal projections onto the olfactory bulb of the brain [20, 21]. For efficient detection of odors in the inspired air, afferent (in-coming) airflow needs to be directed orthonasally (straight) and retronasally (backwards) in order for the nasal olfactory epithelium to pick up the odor [13]. The odor particles become trapped in the mucous and bind to odorant-binding proteins that concentrate and help to solubilize the odor particles. The odor particles then get attached to olfactory receptors located on the cilia of olfactory cells. Upon stimulation of the odor receptors, the odor signals are transmitted up through the cribriform plate to synapse with neurons of the olfactory bulb which then send the signals through the olfactory nerve (CNI) into the secondary neurons for higher processing. A unique feature of the olfactory receptors is that a single receptor cell can detect only one odorant type [13, 20, 22, 23].

3.1.4 Nasal conchae (turbinate bones) and meatuses

Nasal conchae, also known as turbinate bones, are any of several thin, scroll-shaped bony elements originating from the lateral walls of the nasal cavity. Each half of the nasal cavity has three turbinate bones named superior, middle and inferior turbinates. The superior and middle turbinates extend from the ethmoid bone. The inferior turbinate bone is independent of the superior and middle turbinates. The inferior turbinate is the most anteriorly located and therefore the first of the turbinate bones to come into contact with inspired air. The turbinate bones, particularly the anteriorly located inferior turbinate, are involved in innate and adaptive immune reactions of the nasal cavity [14].

Nasal meatuses are spaces found between the turbinate bones and the nasal cavity walls. There are four meatuses in the nasal cavity: the superior meatus, the middle meatus and the inferior meatus.

Superior meatus. The superior meatus is located inferior to the superior turbinate and superior to the middle turbinate bones; this is the drainage site of the posterior ethmoid sinus.

Middle meatus. The middle meatus is located inferior to the middle turbinate and superior to the inferior turbinate. This is the drainage site of the frontal, anterior ethmoid, and maxillary sinuses.

Inferior meatus. The inferior meatus is located inferior to the inferior turbinate and superior to the floor of the nasal cavity. The nasolacrimal duct drains tears from the lacrimal sac at the medial canthus of the eye into the anterior portion of this meatus via Hasner's valve [13].

3.1.5 Blood supply and lymphatics of the nasal cavity

The nasal cavity has a rich vascular supply which allows it to effectively regulate humidity and temperature of the inhaled air. The nasal cavity is also supplied by a network of lymphatic vessels which drain into various lymph nodes located in the pharyngeal region and the neck.

3.1.5.1. Blood supply

The function of warming and humidifying the inspired air in the nasal cavity is achieved by an elaborate network of blood vessels. The mucosa of the nasal cavity enlarges and shrinks due to sympathetic innervation of the nasal vasculature.

The main sources of arterial blood to the nasal cavity are the internal and external carotid arteries [24]. The internal carotid artery gives off the ophthalmic artery which in turn gives off two main branches to the nasal septum: the anterior and posterior ethmoidal arteries and the dorsal nasal artery. The anterior ethmoid artery supplies the lateral nasal wall and the nasal septum. The posterior ethmoid artery supplies the superior turbinate and the nasal septum [9, 14].

The external carotid artery gives off the maxillary artery and facial artery. The maxillary artery gives off a smaller artery known as the descending palatine artery which then passes through the pterygopalatine fossa through the palatine canal before it branches into the greater and lesser palatine arteries. The greater palatine artery enters the greater palatine foramen on the posterior aspect of the palate before traversing the palate anteriorly to enter the nasal cavity via the incisive canal. The greater palatine artery supplies the septum and the floor of the nasal cavity. The sphenopalatine artery, a branch of the maxillary artery, supplies the middle and inferior turbinate bones as well as the posterior part of the nasal septum [25].

The facial artery, a branch of the external carotid artery, gives rise to three arteries namely, the superior labial artery, the lateral nasal artery and the angular artery. The three arteries supply the nasal septum, nasal vestibule and dorsal nasal cavity respectively [25].

A common site of epistaxis (nose bleeding) in the nasal cavity commonly occurs at Kiesselbach's plexus (Little's area) located in the anterior nasal septum. This plexus is a vascular anastomosis between the anterior ethmoid artery, superior labial artery, greater palatine artery and the terminal branch of the posterior septal branch of the sphenopalatine artery [26]. The names of the veins that drain the nasal cavity follow those of the arteries with which they pair.

3.1.5.2. Lymphatic drainage of the nasal cavity

In general, the main functions of the lymphatic system in the nasal cavity include transportation of old leukocytes from the lymph nodes in the vicinity of the nasal cavity to the blood and transportation of antigen-presenting cells (APCs) to the lymph nodes in order to trigger an immune response.

Lymph from the vestibule of the nasal cavity is drained into the submandibular lymph nodes. The anterior one third of the nasal cavity is drained by lymphatic vessels that deposit their lymph fluid in the submaxillary lymph nodes. The posterior two thirds of the nasal cavity including the ethmoid sinuses is drained by lymphatic vessels that deposit lymph partly into the retropharyngeal lymph nodes and partly into the superior deep cervical lymph nodes [27].

3.1.6 Nerves of the nasal cavity

The first cranial nerve (olfactory-CNI) transmits signals from the nasal cavity to the brain to provide the sense of smell. The olfactory epithelium is in the superior portion of the nasal cavity. Within this epithelium are sensory cilia that project up through the cribriform plate to the olfactory bulb. From the olfactory bulb, signals are sent through the olfactory nerve proper to a network of secondary neurons for processing before ending up in the brain [28].

Sensory innervation to the external and internal parts of the nasal cavity is provided by the trigeminal nerve through its two branches the ophthalmic nerve and maxillary nerve [29].

3.1.7 Paranasal sinuses

The nasal cavity is extended by the paranasal sinuses. These are air-filled cavities found in some bones surrounding the nasal cavity. In the human, there are four pairs of paranasal sinuses which are named based on the bones in which they are found. The four sinuses are: the maxillary, frontal, sphenoid, and the ethmoid. The inner surfaces of the four paranasal sinuses are lined by a ciliated pseudostratified epithelium containing mucus-secreting goblet cells. Paranasal sinuses may serve in lightening the weight of the head, humidifying and warming of inspired air, increasing the resonance of speech, providing mechanical rigidity and increasing olfactory surface area [10].

4. The lower respiratory tract

All the structures from the trachea down to the alveoli constitute components of the lower respiratory tract. The components of the lower respiratory tract with support from the rib cage and diaphragm pull in the inspired air from the upper respiratory tract and transport it to the alveoli where oxygen is absorbed into the blood stream and carbon dioxide is released in exchange.

5. Functional anatomy of the lower respiratory tract mucosa

The mucosa of the respiratory tract is lined by a pseudostratified columnar epithelium which consists of a variety of cells (**Figure 1**). It has been estimated

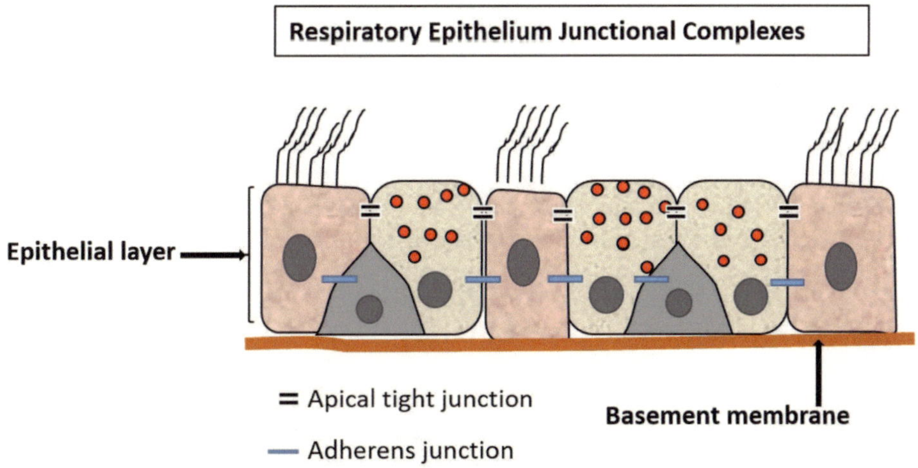

Figure 1.
Schematic diagram showing apical junctional complexes found in the respiratory airway epithelium. Shown in this diagram are tight junctions (black) and adherens (blue). Apical junctional complexes are a key component of the innate immune system in the respiratory tract that form between two neighboring cells. Apical junctional complexes consist of mainly tight junctions and adherens junctions. Tight junctions control intercellular movements of ions and other molecules while adherens junctions are responsible for the initiation and maintenance of cell-cell adhesion.

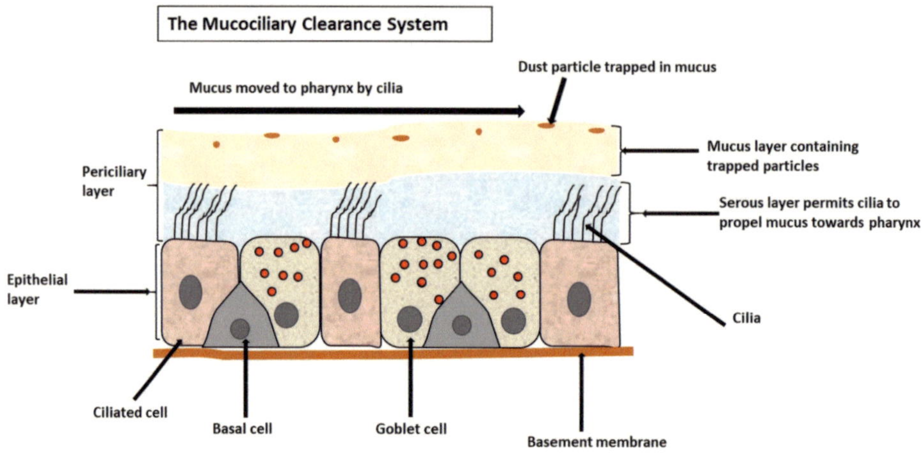

Figure 2.
Schematic diagram showing the components of the mucociliary clearance system. The mucus layer traps particles suspended in the inhaled air. The trapped particles are then propelled by cilia with the aid of the serous layer towards pharynx.

that the total number of cells covering the lower human respiratory tract is 10^{10} cells that covers a surface area of 2,500cm^3 [30]. The pseudostratified columnar epithelium consists of four major cell types which lie on a continuous basement membrane. The four major cell types of the pseudostratified columnar epithelium are the ciliated, secretory, undifferentiated intermediate and basal cells (**Figure 1**). The function of the basal and the undifferentiated intermediate cells is to act as the progenitors of the other respiratory epithelium cells. The ciliated columnar cell type is the most predominant cell of the respiratory epithelium. It rests on a basement membrane and tapers towards the surface. On its luminal surface, the ciliated cells bear numerous cilia which distinguish them from other cell types. Cilia are hair-like cellular organelles that project from the surface of the cell [31, 32]. The luminal surface of each ciliated cell contains about 200–300 cilia. Each of the cilia on the luminal surface of the upper airways is estimated to be about 0.25 μm in diameter with a height of about 6.5 μm. The dimensions are smaller in the lower respiratory tract. In addition, there are numerous microvilli on the apical surface of the ciliated cells. The role of the microvilli is to ensure trans-epithelial movement of fluids and electrolytes. Ciliated cells are interconnected by tight junctions (**Figure 2**). These tight junctions are specialized protein structures that are responsible for regulating the passage of solutes and ions across the epithelial barrier [30, 33]. Thus, the tight junctions act as sieves that only allow the passage of selected substances.

6. Immune mechanisms of the respiratory tract

Respiratory infections are among the top 5 causes of high morbidity and mortality globally. Respiratory infections pose a continuous threat to humans due to their easy dissemination via aerial transmission as evidenced recently by the covid-19 pandemic [34].

A number of factors play different roles in the defense mechanism of the respiratory tract. The defense mechanism of the respiratory tract exists within two broad categories i.e. the humoral immunity and cell-mediated immunity components. In addition, the physical or innate immune defense mechanism plays a critical role as the first line defense mechanism within the respiratory tract. The innate defense mechanism of the respiratory tract consists of non-specific physical barriers that can prevent noxious substances from accessing the delicate part of the respiratory system such as the alveoli thereby averting injury to those components.

The respiratory immune response consists of multiple tiers of cellular responses that are engaged in a sequential manner in order to control infections. In addition, specific mechanisms are in place to promote disease tolerance in response to respiratory infections. Various physical barriers, cell types and chemicals are involved in the respiratory system immune response and coordinate pathogen clearance and tissue repair within the respiratory tract [35]. The immune response within the respiratory tract follows an ordered, stepwise program of engagement of distinct tiers of defense [36].

Local sensor cells first detect the invading microorganism. This detection event can trigger cell-intrinsic defense responses that contain the pathogen, lead to secretion of chemo-attractants to recruit rapid responder cells such as neutrophils, and alert lung-resident lymphoid cells through the secretion of first order cytokines. The complex interplay between resident and infiltrating immune cells and secreted innate immune proteins shapes the outcome of host-pathogen, host-allergen, and host-particle interaction within the mucosal airway compartment [37].

6.1 Airway barrier defenses

The first line of defense against infection in the respiratory tract is the mucosal epithelium. The pulmonary epithelium initially acts as a physical barrier between the airway lumen and the vasculature. The epithelium provides the physical barrier by the formation of tight junctions that include claudins, occludins, and adherens.

The physical and chemical barrier to the airways is provided by four major cell types. These cells include ciliated cells, mucus-secreting goblet cells, and club cells, which produce antimicrobial compounds. Basal cells, along with club cells serve as regional progenitor cells to replenish the other cell types [38]. The proportion of each cell type, and the associated defense mechanisms, are compatible with the airway diameter. In the human respiratory tree, ciliated cells and mucus-secreting cells create the barrier defense in larger airways, whereas mucus-secreting cells become less frequent and secretory cells become more predominant in smaller airways. Within the alveoli, alveolar type 1 cells facilitate gas exchange whereas alveolar type 2 cells secrete pulmonary surfactant [35].

6.2 The mucociliary system as a respiratory tract defense barrier

Arguably, the most important component of the innate immune mechanism of the respiratory tract is the mucociliary systems. The mucociliary system is one of the primary mechanisms for protecting the respiratory tract tissues. It operates through the coordinated functions of mucus and cilia that trap and eliminate inhaled materials. Mucociliary action also ensures elimination of dead endogenous cells and debris [39].

The mucociliary clearance system (**Figure 2**) refers to the composite structures within the respiratory tract that are responsible for eliminating mucus and potentially harmful foreign materials from the respiratory tract. It is a self-cleansing mechanism of the respiratory tract and forms the major first line defense mechanism of the lungs [16]. The main components of the mucociliary clearance apparatus are the cilia found on columnar ciliated cells and the mucus produced by mucus secretory cells known as goblet cells. A layer of fluid and mucus known as the airway surface or periciliary layer covers the airways and this layer of fluid and mucus is constantly propelled by cilia from the distal to the proximal lungs [16].

The mucociliary clearance is a component of the innate immune defense mechanism [40]. In order for the lungs to perform normally, a properly functioning mucociliary escalator is cardinal. Problems with components of the mucociliary escalator, either the mucus or cilia, may cause airway blockage which may result in accumulation of harmful germs and particulate matter, thereby causing damage to the lungs [36]. High morbidity and mortality in many respiratory diseases have been attributed to dysfunctions in components of the mucociliary escalator including abnormal biophysical properties of mucus and ciliopathy [41]. Furthermore, some studies had shown that the majority of the pre-existing conditions that increased the risk of death from COVID-19 are the same diseases that were affected by long-term exposure to air pollution particularly exposure to fine particulate matter [42]. This may indicate that damage to the mucociliary escalator may be responsible for the high risk to covid-19 infection and other respiratory infections among people chronically exposed to air pollution. Treatment to reduce abnormalities of components of the mucociliary escalator have been shown to improve outcomes in respiratory diseases indicating the importance of the mucociliary escalator in pulmonary defense.

6.2.1 Role of cilia in mucociliary clearance

It has been estimated that cilia beat about 12 to 15 HZ in waves that are well coordinated. This ciliary motion has been observed to be metachronal i.e. back-to-front and is directed towards the pharynx [43]. With this motion, particulate matter trapped in mucus including bacteria and viral particles is moved towards the pharynx by being propelled through the vocal cords and glottis. As a result of this constant ciliary movement, an estimated 30 ml of respiratory mucus is discharged into the oral or nasal cavity or swallowed [43].

6.2.2 The role of basal cells in mucociliary clearance

Basal cells of the respiratory epithelium have the capability to differentiate into ciliated and secretory cells and hence can restore the normal structure of the respiratory epithelium after injury. The stimulus for differentiation into ciliated or secretory cells is by exposure to the luminal air [44]. The differentiation of basal cells into ciliated and secretory cells has been attributed to the activation of the transcription factor forkhead boxJ1 (FOXJ1) and the regulatory factor X [45]. Thus, the basal and intermediate cells impart regeneration capacity to various regions of the airway. In the human respiratory tract, the highest epithelial regeneration capacity is found in the large airways (trachea and bronchi) whose regeneration capacity is estimated to be about 8 times higher than in the smaller airways [36].

6.3 Adaptive immune response of the lower respiratory tract

The respiratory tract is constantly exposed to the external environment which contains numerous particles and molecules that can potentially trigger an inflammatory reaction. An important anatomical feature of the respiratory system in general and the lungs in particular is that it has a large surface area of epithelium that is constantly exposed to the external environment and, at the same time, is highly vascularized. This anatomical feature makes the respiratory tract and the lungs to be the major portal of entry for many pathogens including a wide array of respiratory viruses [46].

The respiratory immune system must discriminate between potentially harmful pathogens and those that are innocuous. Most diseases of the respiratory tract involve contributions from both the innate and adaptive immune systems. Complex interactions occur during most respiratory tract infections. A number of systems are involved in the overall immune responses within the respiratory tract and include epithelium-immune system interactions, early effector mechanisms, the influence of the microbiome and immunomodulatory and regulatory pathways [47].

As opposed to the innate immune system, the adaptive immune system (or acquired immune system) is highly specific to a particular pathogen. The adaptive immunity is also able to provide long-term immune protection. The cells responsible for carrying out the acquired immune response are the lymphocytes.

Many respiratory tract viral infections result in mild, self-limited disease. However, other viruses like the SARS-CoV-2 and certain type A influenza virus strains such as the highly pathogenic avian H5N1 viruses can produce severe and frequently fatal infections and can also target epithelial cells of the conducting airways [5].

Many types of immune cells such as dendritic cells, macrophages, neutrophils, eosinophils, and B and T lymphocytes, contribute to lung immunity. Cell-mediated

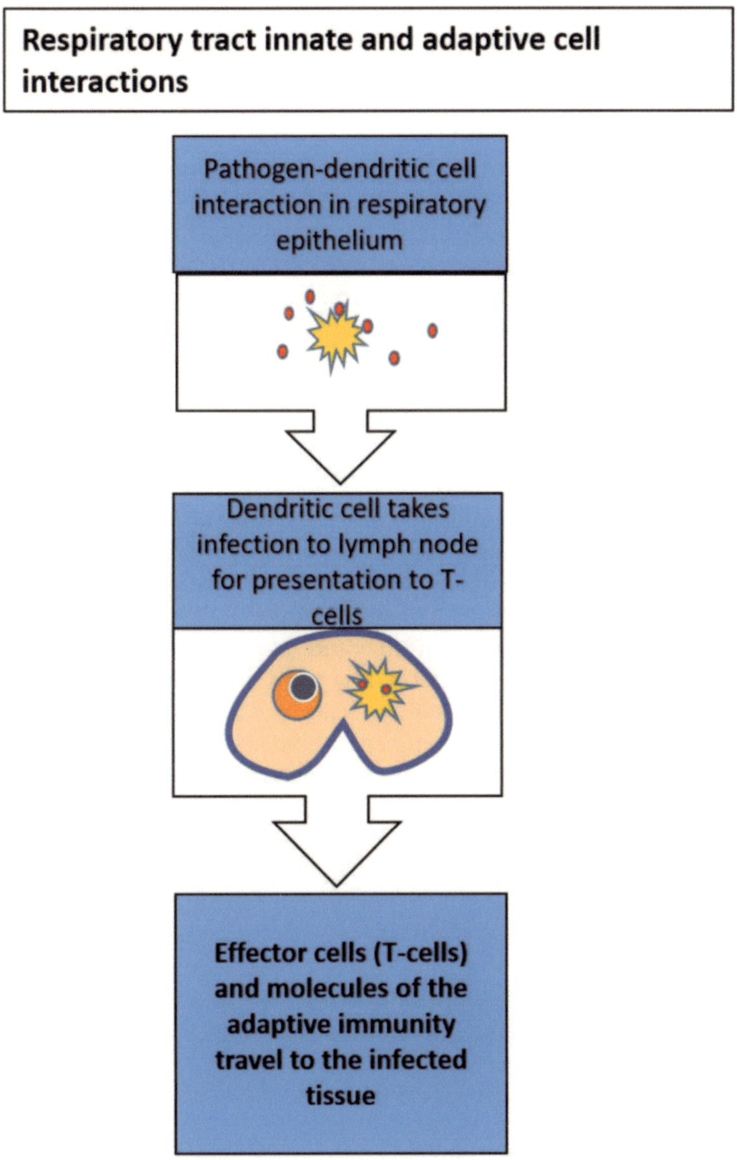

Figure 3.
Adaptive immune responses build and shape innate immune responses.

adaptive immune responses are key against all classes of pulmonary pathogens including viruses, various bacteria and fungi. Adaptive immune responses build upon and shape innate immune responses (**Figure 3**). They depend on sequential pairwise interactions between three cell types: T-cells, Natural Killer (NK) cells, and Dendritic Cells (DCs).

Dendritic cells (DCs) are also known as accessory cells whose function is to ingest and process antigen material and then present it on their surfaces to the T cells. DCs migrate to local lymph nodes once activated by antigens and within the lymph nodes they interact with T cells and B cells to initiate and orchestrate the adaptive immune response. Thus, dendritic cells act as messengers between the innate and the adaptive immune systems [48].

Upon virus exposure, dendritic cells in the lungs mature and traffic to the local draining lymph nodes (cervical and mediastinal lymph nodes), where they display peptide antigen to naïve CD4 T cells. After being exposed to antigen, the antigen-specific T cells then become activated and initiate a program of proliferation and differentiation, resulting in the production of effector cells that have the capacity to migrate to the lung and terminate the infection [46]. T cells mediate viral clearance via cytokine production or direct cytolytic mechanisms which may be either perforin or Fas mediated pathways [49].

During the course of a respiratory virus infection, pools of memory T cells are established that persist for the life of the individual. These CD4 T cells differ significantly from their naive precursors in that they persist at a high frequency, generate rapid effector functions in response to antigen exposure, have distinct cytokine production profiles, have low requirements for co-stimulation, and have reduced susceptibility to apoptosis. Many memory cells can be found in secondary lymphoid organs, such as the draining lymph nodes and the spleen [46, 50, 51].

7. Conclusion

The respiratory system will continue to attract attention in terms of research particularly during and in the post covid-19 era. Thus, understanding the functional anatomy and immunology of the respiratory tract will be cardinal. Respiratory diseases will undoubtedly continue to be major public health problems worldwide, with unpredictable morbidities and mortalities. To date, although considerable progress had been in understanding the functional anatomy and immunology of the respiratory tract, there was need to put the subject in the context of the covid-19 pandemic in order to complement the prevailing research efforts in combating covid-19. Much remains to be done in terms of predicting respiratory disease prior to symptoms and also in the development of novel and new treatments in a more personalized manner [52, 53].

Acknowledgements

The author is grateful to the University of Zambia for providing unlimited internet access and library facilities and to Biotechnology Kiosk and Intech for publishing the work.

Conflict of interest

The author declares no conflict of interest.

Author details

Humphrey Simukoko
Department of Biomedical Science, School of Veterinary Medicine, Africa Centre of Excellence for Infectious Diseases of Humans and Animals (ACEIDHA), University of Zambia, Lusaka, Zambia

*Address all correspondence to: h.simukoko@unza.zm

'Biotechnology to Combat COVID-19' is a collaborative project with Biotechnology Kiosk

References

[1] Vallamkondu, J., John, A., Wani, W. Y., Ramadevi, S. P., Jella, K. K., Reddy, P. H., & Kandimalla, R. SARS-CoV-2 pathophysiology and assessment of coronaviruses in CNS diseases with a focus on therapeutic targets. *Biochimica et biophysica acta. Molecular basis of disease*, 2020. *1866*(10), 165889. https://doi.org/10.1016/j.bbadis.2020.165889

[2] Kia'i N, Bajaj T. Histology, Respiratory Epithelium. [Updated 2020 Jul 3]. In: StatPearls [Internet]. Treasure Island (FL): StatPearls Publishing; 2020 Jan-. Available from: https://www.ncbi.nlm.nih.gov/books/NBK541061/

[3] Haddad M, Sharma S. Physiology, Lung. [Updated 2020 Jul 22]. In: StatPearls [Internet]. Treasure Island (FL): StatPearls Publishing; 2020 Jan-. Available from: https://www.ncbi.nlm.nih.gov/books/NBK545177/

[4] Guyton, Arthur C.; Hall, John E. *Textbook of medical physiology* (11th ed.). 2005. Philadelphia: W.B. Saunders. ISBN 0-7216-0240-1.

[5] Braciale, T. J., Sun, J., & Kim, T. S. Regulating the adaptive immune response to respiratory virus infection. *Nature reviews. Immunology*, 2012. *12*(4), 295-305. https://doi.org/10.1038/nri3166

[6] Camner P, Bakke B. Nose or mouth breathing? Environ Res. 1980; 21:394-398.

[7] Sun C.B, Wang Y.Y, Liu G.H, Liu Z. Role of the Eye in Transmitting Human Coronavirus: What We Know and What We Do Not Know. https://www.scilit.net/article/3498497ae4fd4d7954701bba57684bda. Accessed December, 2, 2020.

[8] Gengler, I., Wang, J. C., Speth, M. M., & Sedaghat, A. R. Sinonasal pathophysiology of SARS-CoV-2 and COVID-19: A systematic review of the current evidence. *Laryngoscope investigative otolaryngology*, 2020. *5*(3), 354-359. https://doi.org/10.1002/lio2.384

[9] Oneal RM, Beil Jr RJ, Schlesinger J. Surgical anatomy of the nose. Otolaryngol Clin North Am. 1999 Feb;32(1):145-81.

[10] Cappello ZJ, Minutello K, Dublin AB. Anatomy, Head and Neck, Nose Paranasal Sinuses. [Updated 2020 Sep 20]. In: StatPearls [Internet]. Treasure Island (FL): StatPearls Publishing; 2020 Jan-. Available from: https://www.ncbi.nlm.nih.gov/books/NBK499826/

[11] AlJulaih GH, Sharma P, Lasrado S. StatPearls [Internet]. StatPearls Publishing; Treasure Island (FL): Sep 3, 2020. Anatomy, Head and Neck, Nose Bones.

[12] Galarza-Paez L, Marston G, Downs BW. StatPearls [Internet]. StatPearls Publishing; Treasure Island (FL): Aug 21, 2020. Anatomy, Head and Neck, Nose.

[13] Sobiesk J. L and Munakomi S. Anatomy, Head and Neck, Nasal Cavity. [Updated 2020 Jul 27]. In: StatPearls [Internet]. Treasure Island (FL): StatPearls Publishing; 2020 Jan-. Available from: https://www.ncbi.nlm.nih.gov/books/NBK544232/

[14] Patel R.G. Nasal Anatomy and Function. Facial Plast Surg. 2017 Feb;33(1):3-8.

[15] Lafci Fahrioglu S, VanKampen N, Andaloro C. StatPearls [Internet]. StatPearls Publishing; Treasure Island (FL): Aug 11, 2020. Anatomy, Head and Neck, Sinus Function and Development.

[16] Londino, J. D.; Collawn, J. F.; Matalon, S. Regulation of Airway

Lining Fluid in Health and Disease. In *Comparative Biology of the Normal Lung*, 2nd ed.; Richard, A. P., Ed.; Academic Press, **2015**; pp 467-477

[17] Brann, D.H., Tsukahara, T., Weinreb, C., Lipovsek, M., Van den Berge, K., Gong, B., Chance, R., Macaulay, I.C., Chou, H.-J., Fletcher, R.B., et al. (2020). Non-neuronal expression of SARS-CoV-2 entry genes in the olfactory system suggests mechanisms underlying COVID-19-associated anosmia. Science Advances **6**, eabc5801.

[18] Bryche, B., St Albin, A., Murri, S., Lacote, S., Pulido, C., Ar Gouilh, M., Lesellier, S., Servat, A., Wasniewski, M., Picard-Meyer, E., (2020). Massive transient damage of the olfactory epithelium associated with infection of sustentacular cells by SARS-CoV-2 in golden Syrian hamsters. Brain, behavior, and immunity. 2020. 10.1016/j.bbi.2020.06.032

[19] Purves D, Augustine GJ, Fitzpatrick D. Editors. Neuroscience. 2nd edition. Sunderland (MA): Sinauer Associates; 2001. The Olfactory Epithelium and Olfactory Receptor Neurons. Available from: https://www.ncbi.nlm.nih.gov/books/NBK10896/

[20] Salazar I. The nasal cavity and its olfactory sensory territories. *Frontiers in neuroanatomy*, 2015. *9*, 31. https://doi.org/10.3389/fnana.2015.00031

[21] Munger SD, Leinders-Zufall T, Zufall F. Subsystem organization of the mammalian sense of smell. *Annu Rev Physiol. 2009; 71():115-40.*

[22] Tcatchoff L Claude N, Jean-Claude P, Loïc B. A single lysyl residue defines the binding specificity of a human odorant-binding protein for aldehydes, FEBS Letters, 2006. Volume 580, Issue 8, (2102-2108) ISSN 0014-5793, https://doi.org/10.1016/j.febslet.2006.03.01

[23] Briand L., Eliot C., Nespoulous C., Bezirard V., Huet J-C., Henry C., Blon F., Trotier D., Pernollet J-C. Evidence of an Odorant-Binding Protein in the Human Olfactory Mucus: Location, Structural Characterization, and Odorant-Binding Properties *Biochemistry*, 2002. 41, 23, 7241-7252

[24] Widdicombe J. Microvascular anatomy of the nose. Allergy. 1997;52(40 Suppl):7-11.

[25] MacArthur F.J and McGarry G.W. The arterial supply of the nasal cavity. Eur Arch Otorhinolaryngol. 2017 Feb;274(2):809-815.

[26] Krulewitz NA and Fix ML. Epistaxis. Emerg Med Clin North Am. 2019 Feb;37(1):29-39.

[27] Koroulakis A and Agarwal M. Anatomy, Head and Neck, Lymph Nodes. [Updated 2020 Jul 27]. In: StatPearls [Internet]. Treasure Island (FL): StatPearls Publishing; 2020 Jan-. Available from: https://www.ncbi.nlm.nih.gov/books/NBK513317/

[28] Gomez Galarce M, Yanez-Siller JC, Carrau RL, Montaser A, Lima LR, Servian D, Otto BA, Prevedello DM, Naudy CA. Endonasal anatomy of the olfactory neural network: Surgical implications. Laryngoscope. 2018 Nov;128(11):2473-2477.

[29] Huff T, Daly DT. StatPearls [Internet]. StatPearls Publishing; Treasure Island (FL): Jul 31, 2020. Neuroanatomy, Cranial Nerve 5 (Trigeminal)

[30] Tilley, A. E., Walters, M. S., Shaykhiev, R., & Crystal, R. G. Cilia dysfunction in lung disease. *Annual review of physiology*, 2015. *77*, 379-406. https://doi.org/10.1146/annurev-physiol-021014-071931

[31] Carvalho-Santos Z, Azimzadeh J, Pereira-Leal JB, Bettencourt-Dias M.

Evolution: tracing the origins of centrioles, cilia, and flagella. J. Cell Biol. 2011. 194: 165-75

[32] Satir P, Christensen ST. Structure and function of mammalian cilia. Histochem. Cell Biol. 2008. 129: 687-93

[33] Knight DA, Holgate. The airway epithelium: structural and functional properties in health and disease. *ST Respirology. 2003 Dec; 8(4):432-46.*

[34] Garmendia J, Gonzalo-Asensio J Editorial: Update on the Immune Mechanisms Against Respiratory Pathogens. Front. Immunol. http://doi.org/10.3389/fimmu.2019.01730.

[35] Iwasaki, A., Foxman, E. F., Molony, R. D. Early local immune defences in the respiratory tract. *Nature reviews. Immunology*, 2017. *17*(1), 7-20. https://doi.org/10.1038/nri.2016.117

[36] Iwasaki A, Medzhitov *R*. Control of adaptive immunity by the innate immune system. *Nat Immunol. 2015 Apr; 16(4):343-53.*

[37] Hartl D, Tirouvanziam R, Laval J, Greene C.M, Habiel D, Sharma L, Yildirim A.O, Dela Cruz C.S, Hogaboam C.M. Innate Immunity of the Lung: From Basic Mechanism to Translational Medicine. J Innate Immun. 2018. 10: 487-501

[38] Galeas-Pena, M., McLaughlin, N., & Pociask, D. The role of the innate immune system on pulmonary infections, *Biological Chemistry*, 2019. *400*(4), 443-456. doi: https://doi.org/10.1515/hsz-2018-0304

[39] Benam, K. H., Vladar, E. K., Janssen, W. J. & Evans, C. M. Mucociliary defense: emerging cellular, molecular, and animal models. *Ann. Am. Thorac. Soc*. 2018. **15**, S210–S215.

[40] Rutland J, Morgan L and de Iongh R. Respiratory Ciliary Dysfunction. In *Pediatric Respiratory Medicine (Second Edition)*; Lynn M. Taussig and Louis I. Landau., Ed., Academic Press. **2008**; pp 979-98. https://doi.org/10.1016/B978-032304048-8.50071-2

[41] Boucher RC. 2007. Airway surface dehydration in cystic fibrosis: pathogenesis and therapy. Annu. Rev. Med. 58: 157-70

[42] Sanderson MJ, Sleigh MA. Ciliary activity of cultured rabbit tracheal epithelium: beat pattern and metachrony. J Cell Sci. 1981;47:331-47. pmid:7263784

[43] Bottier M, Blanchon S, Pelle G, Bequignon E, Isabey D. A new index for characterizing micro-bead motion in a flow induced by ciliary beating: Part I, experimental analysis. PLOS Computational Biology 2017. 13(7): e1005605. https://doi.org/10.1371/journal.pcbi.1005605

[44] Gerovac BJ, Valencia M, Baumlin N, Salathe M, Conner GE, Fregien NL. 2014. Submersion and hypoxia inhibit ciliated cell differentiation in a Notch dependent manner. Am. J. Respir. Cell Mol. Biol. 2014. 51: 516-25

[45] Didon L, Zwick RK, Chao IW, Walters MS, Wang R, et al. 2013. RFX3 modulation of FOXJ1 regulation of cilia genes in the human airway epithelium. Respir. Res. 2013. 14: 70 16.

[46] Woodland, D. L., and Scott, I. T cell memory in the lung airways. *Proceedings of the American Thoracic Society*, 2005. *2*(2), 126-131. https://doi.org/10.1513/pats.200501-003AW

[47] Lloyd C. M. Chair's Summary: Innate and Adaptive Immune Responses in Airway Disease. 2014. https://doi.org/10.1513/AnnalsATS.201405-210AW

[48] Curtis J. L. Cell-mediated adaptive immune defense of the lungs. *Proceedings of the American Thoracic*

Society, 2005. *2*(5), 412-416. https://doi.org/10.1513/pats.200507-070JS

[49] Eichelberger M, Allan W, Zijlstra M, Jaenisch R, Doherty PC. Clearance of influenza virus respiratory infection in mice lacking class I major histocompatibility complex-restricted CD8+ T cells. *J Exp Med.* 1991 *Oct 1; 174(4):875-80.*

[50] Woodland DL, Hogan RJ, Zhong W. Cellular immunity and memory to respiratory virus infections. *Immunol Res.* 2001*; 24(1):53-67.*

[51] Dutton R. W, Swain S. L, Bradley L. M. The generation and maintenance of memory T and B cells. *Immunol Today.* 1999 *Jul; 20(7):291-3.*

[52] Kiley JP. Advancing respiratory research. *Chest*. 2011;140(2):497-501. doi:10.1378/chest.11-0774

[53] Simukoko H. and Mujuni, B.; Options for covid-19 therapeutics: aerosolized inhalation antibody conjugated nanoparticles, Biotechnology Kiosk, Vol 2, Issue 8, PP: 4-16 (2020); DOI: https://doi.org/10.37756/bk.20.2.8.1

Section 6

Drugs Therapeutics Treatments

Chapter 18

Cellular Therapy as Promising Choice of Treatment for COVID-19

Duygu Koyuncu Irmak and Erdal Karaoz

Abstract

In the pandemic of COVID-19, while living normals have been changing, there have been a huge effort globally to find out effective and safe treatment agents and vaccines. As of now, the advances show the progress in vaccine development, however the treatment of the COVID-19 is yet not fully specified. The drugs, i.e. antibiotics, antivirals, antimalarians, even anti-HIV agents which have been known already were taken out of the shelves and brought into use in different combinations. On the other hand, the cellular treatment, more specifically the mesenchymal stem cell therapy has been encouraged, resulting in various evidence published all over the world. This chapter aims to compile the published information, in means of methods, disease manifestations, results and limitations, about the stem cell treatment of the COVID-19 and to provide a source of harmonized reference for scientific society.

Keywords: mesenchymal stem cell, cellular therapy, regenerative, restorative, personalised medicine

1. Introduction

Since the global living routine have been dramatically changed by a novel virus called SARS-CoV-2, scientific community has been working hard on the understanding of the pathophysiology of the COVID-19 infection caused by this virus, and the methods of preventing and treating the disease. The spectrum of clinical manifestations of COVID-19 varies from asymptomatic or somewhat mild-disease (81%) to severe clinical conditions characterized by respiratory failure requiring mechanical ventilation (14%) and to critical systemic presentations with multiple organ dysfunction syndromes or failures (5%) [1, 2].

There is a huge effort to develop vaccines, some are developed and received the accelerated access at the moment, however, there is no specific antiviral treatment recommended or appreved for COVID-19, yet. Current therapeutic strategies are only supportive and oxygen therapy represents the primary treatment intervention for patients with severe pneumonia. The medications that have already been known such as anti-viral, anti-malarial, and anti-inflammatory agents have been taken from the shelves and began to be used as the emergency state action to improve the recovery of the patients and increase the survival. Whilst these treatments can improve patient's recovery and survival to some extend, these therapeutic strategies do not lead to unequivocal restoration of the lung damage inflicted by this disease [3]. The outcome so far shows that the antibiotics are ineffective; although systemic corticosteroids seem be effective, they also reduce the immune system activity and thus its ability to fight against the infection. It is of crucial importance to save the patients with severe COVID-19 pneumonia, to prevent and even reverse the cytokine storm along with inhibiting the viral replication [4].

The cellular therapies with mesenchymal stem cells (MSCs) are attracting attention as they could offer a new therapeutic approach in this context. These stem cells have broad pharmacological effects, including anti-inflammatory, immunomodulatory, regenerative, pro-angiogenic and even anti-fibrotic properties [5].

Stem cells, in particular MSCs, exert their immunomodulatory, anti-oxidant, and reparative therapeutic effects likely through secreted extracellular vesicles (EVs), and therefore, could be beneficial, alone or in combination with other therapeutic agents, in patients diagnosed with COVID-19 [3, 6]. They are are emerging as new promising treatments, since they could not only attenuate the inflammation but also regenerate the lung damage caused by COVID-19 [7, 8].

In this chapter, we outline the information about this novel virus, and the pathophysiology of the COVID-19 infection, the mechanisms of cytokine storm and lung damage caused by SARS-CoV-2 virus and how mesenchymal stem cells (MSCs) can be utilized to hamper this damage by harnessing their regenerative properties. The potential of these ancestor cells in the enhanced clinical utility in treating the COVID-19 patients along with the opportunuties major roadblocks to progressing these promising curative therapies toward mainstream treatment for COVID-19 have also been evaluated.

2. SARS-CoV-2 infection: what to focus

2.1 SARS-CoV-2 virus

Belonging to the β Coronavirus family, SARS-CoV2 is a single-stranded RNA, enveloped virus of 50-200 nm diameter [9]. Spike Glycoprotein (S) is the vital protein consisting of three S1-S2 heterodimers that bind to angiotensin-converting enzyme 2 (ACE2) receptor on type II pneumocyte in the lung tissue [3, 9, 10]. Besides S protein, enetically SARS-CoV-2 is constructed on structural proteins of membrane (M), envelope (E), and nucleocapsid (N) proteins. Spread of the virus is managed by the high affinity of S proteins to ACE2 receptors that are expressed in human organs, principally in lung alveolar epithelial cells and enterocytes of the small intestine [11, 12].

Once the SARS-CoV-2 virus enters into the type II pneumocyte and capillary endothelium by endocytosis, it increases in the cytoplasm. Apoptosis is induced by yhe stress in the pneumocytes. Besides, the viral RNA acts as a pathogen-associated molecular pattern and is recognized by the pattern recognition receptor or toll-like receptors. Subsequent chemokine attraction causes neutrophil migration and activation. Then the destruction of the alveolar-capillary walls occur. This leads to the lost interface between the intra-alveolar space and the stroma. Therefore, fluid leaks through and fills into the alveolar spaces [13, 14].

One of the prominent features of SARS-CoV-2 is its being more inclinable to infect the human lung and higher, 3.20-fold faster, duplication time than SARS-CoV [15].

2.2 The development of the SARS-CoV-2 infection

2.2.1 In the society

Modes of transmission occurs through droplet transmission, fecal-oral route, conjunctiva and fomites [13, 14]. Also, the local transmission can be traced back to the patient's body fluids such as respiratory droplets, saliva, feces, and urine [15]. The virion is stabilized at lower temperatures, i.e., 4 °C has higher survival than 22 °C [16, 17].

Before the clinical symptoms presentation, during the symptomatic stage and even during the recovery period, the patients with COVID-19 can spread the infection, because SARS-CoV-2 virions are shed throughout the clinical course.

When it comes to the residence time of the SARS-CoV-2 virion on surfaces, it has been known that the viable residence time of SARS-CoV-1 in aerosols, copper, cardboard, stainless steel, and plastic are 3 h, 4 h, 24 h, 48 h, and 72 h, respectively [18].

2.2.2 In the clinics

2.2.2.1 Clinical presentation of COVID-19

The symptoms and relevant clinical presentations of COVID-19 was deeply elaborated in WHO-China joint report [19]. Cases of 85%, present with pyrexia in but only 45% are febrile on early presentation [20]. Cough is seen in 67.7% of patients and sputum is seen in 33.4%. Cases show respiratory symptoms such as dyspnea (18.6%), sore throat (13.9%), and nasal congestion (4.8%) [20]. General symptoms such as muscle or bone aches (14.8%), chills (11.4%), and headache (13.6%) are also seen [20]. Gastrointestinal symptoms including nausea/vomiting and diarrhea are observed in 5% and 3.7% of the cases, respectively. These clinical presentations of COVID-19 were consistent in similar studies on COVID-19 cases in China [21–24].

In SARSCoV- 2 infected severe cases, fatal acute respiratory distress syndrome (ARDS), associated with monocyte and macrophage infiltration, diffuse alveolar damage, and cellular fibromyxoid exudates have been confirmed [25, 26] with mortality reported as high as 52.4% [27]. At the 7th–10th days of the manifestations of immune dysregulation, including cytokine release syndrome with elevated cytokine levels (IL-6, IL-8, IL-1, IL2R, IL-10, and TNF-α), lymphopenia (in CD4+ and CD8+ T cells), and decreases in IFN-γ expression in $CD4^+$ T cells [26–28]. It is suggested that the cytokine storm or response may weaken the adaptive immunity against COVID-19 infection, [29] which is associated with atrophy of the secondary lymphoid tissues [25]. The risk of the success of the anti-inflammatory treatment comes from the secondary infections [30].

In severely damaged the lung tissue the ARDS develops which can further turns to septic shock. These two complications are the major issues in intensive care unit (ICU) care. The mortality from COVID-19 in patients older than 60 years, with smoking history, and comorbid medical conditions including but not limited to hypertension, cardiovascular and cerebrovascular disease, and diabetes also occurs from these complications. Notably, smoking and older age group patients tend to have a higher density of ACE2 receptors [13].

Asymptomatic or presymptomatic infection takes its naming from the patients which are the most majority of the all cases have no symptoms although they test positive for SARS-Cov-2 by reverse-transcriptase polymerase chain reaction (RT-PCR). The rest of the cases demonstrate the symptoms of fever (98%), cough (76%), dyspnoea (55%) and myalgia or fatigue (44%). Other signs, such as sputum production (28%), headache (8%), haemoptysis (5%) and diarrhoea (3%), may also be present [31]. On the other hand, the severe cases are seen in the clinics and are typically characterised by pneumonia and usually accompanied by the complications of ARDS [31, 32], acute cardiac injury [33], and secondary infections [34].

ARDS is the most significant complication in severe cases of COVID-19, and it affects 20–41% of hospitalized patients [31, 35] besides, heart failure, renal failure, liver damage, shock and multi-organ failure have also been observed as complications.

Clinical manifestation severity has been seen in a stratification which depends on symptomatology [36] (**Figure 1**). Adult COVID-19 cases may be grouped as follows [37, 38]:

1. Mild: The cases with any of the various signs and symptoms of COVID-19 (e.g. muscle pain, fever, malaise, headache, cough, sore throat) but the absence of breath shortness, dyspnoea or abnormal chest imaging.

2. Moderate: The cases with showing signs of lower respiratory illness by clinical assessment or imaging and peripheral oxygen saturation (SpO^2) ≥ 94% (room air at sea level).

3. Severe: The cases characterized by breathing rates ≥30 breaths/min, SpO^2 < 94% (room air at sea level); a ratio of arterial partial pressure of oxygen to fraction of inspired oxygen (PaO^2/FiO^2) less than 300 mmHg, or lung infiltrates greater than 50%.

4. Critical: The patients presenting with respiratory failure requiring mechanical ventilation, septic shock and/or multiple organ dysfunctions [36].

As the RNA expression is detectable across a wide range of human tissues [39], it is thought that the multi-organ dysfunction is probably linked to the expression pattern of ACE2 gene. The cells, tissues and organs most affected are those with high ACE2 expression, the entry receptor or opening doors for SARS-Cov-2. The research has shown that ACE2 is abundantly expressed in the epithelia of the lung and small intestine in humans, for possible routes of the SARS-Cov-2 [40]. Since the recent data suggest that cell-surface expression on the lungs is below the detection limit [41], it has been proposed that the COVID-19 disease pathology would not be directly correlate with ACE2 cell-surface protein expression [41]. As reported for the heart and kidneys, the said disparity may be linked to the selective, transient expression of ACE2 [42, 43].

Health condition of the patients suddenly detoriates in the later stages of diseases progression. Death comes right after the fast multiple organs' failure and ARDS. Cytokine storm has been indicated as the causal factor for ARDS and multiple organ failure [44, 45]. WHO has announced the case fatality rate of

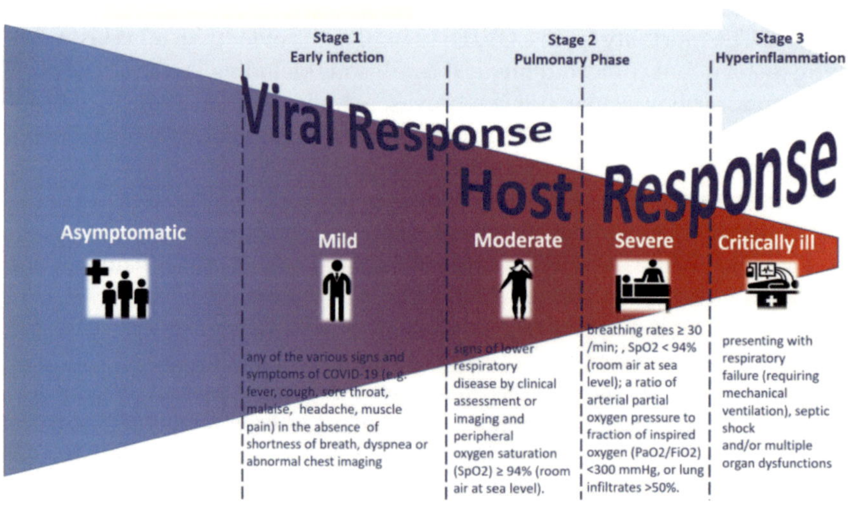

Figure 1.
Clinical stages and the manifestations of COVID-19 disease.

COVID-19 as ranging from 0.3 to 1%, higher than that of influenza A which is 0.1%. The epidemiological studies reported from the countries implementing COVID-19 mitigation strategies revealed that almost 80% of patients of COVID-19 had no symptoms or mild disease, whereas 14% of the patients had severe symptoms, and 6% of them were in critical condition [46].

2.2.2.2 COVID-19 disease management

The management of viral pneumonia is supportive in absence of specific treatment. The most dominating symptoms are fever and dry cough, therefore the first-line antipyretic agent antitussive medications [47]. Oxygen supplementation at 5 L/min must be administered for patients requiring ARDS treatment and the oxygen saturation target must be ≥92–95% in pregnant cases, ≥90% in other cases [48].

Conventionally, the complications of septic shock and acute kidney injury should be managed with relevant sepsis and renal replacement therapies [49]. In the middle to later course of COVID-19, some of the cases may develop overlapping bacterial and/or fungal infection. In these cases, the empiric antimicrobial treatment should be provided.

The WHO has been recommending the usage of extracorporeal membrane oxygenation in the patients who sustain hypoxia refractory to supplementary oxygen [49]. Or else, the convalescent plasma and IgG are used as rescue therapy in critical cases, without any solid evidence for the benefit of this practice. Most of the cases demonstrate vital health measures to control COVID-19 spreading. If the public health measures are not taken properly, there will be a patient burden that exceeding the volume of ICU beds and mechanical ventilation, as seen in the crisis in Italy. Hence, the objective of the COVID-19 management lies on the maintenance of social distancing to suppress the rapid emergence inflow of new cases. This epidemiological approach is called as flattening of the curve. The public health interest should be for identifying and isolating the infective cases, attain and maintain contact tracing and isolation [50].

3. The pathophysiology of the SARS-CoV-2 infection: what we know

3.1 Cytokine storm

The story of the cytokine 'breeze' transformation to the 'storm' starts with the infection of the cell through receptor–ligand interactions which activates massive numbers of leucocytes, particularly B cells, T cells, natural killer cells, monocytes, dendritic cells and macrophages. The release of inflammatory cytokines from these cells attract and activate more white blood cells. Cytokine breeze starts locally post-primary infection with appearing classical signs of inflammation including, calour (heat), dolour (pain), rubor (redness), tumour (swelling or oedema) and loss of function. At the beginning, the localized response works for eliminating the trigger. The host response involving the increase in blood flow, facilitation of leucocyte extravasation and delivery of plasma proteins to the site of injury, increase in body temperature and pain triggering spreads throughout the body via systemic circulation. These responses along with the host repair processes results in either gradually restored organ function or recovery happening by fibrosis which may lead organ dysfunction [51, 52].

Fibroblasts proliferate and invade the intra-alveolar zone constructing fibroblast foci. This seems as the beginning of the pulmonary fibrosis pathogenesis [53]. Lung sections from two patients with early-phase COVID-19 pneumonia demonstrated the characteristics similar to this initiation step of fibrosis [54]. Fibroblast foci were observed in the airways, besides the edema, type II pneumocyte hyperplasia with infiltration of inflammatory cellular and multinucleated cells. Some reactive epithelial hyperplasia areas are also abundant alveolar macrophages [54]. The SARS-CoV-2 caused progressing injury of the alveolar zone, apears to establish a pro-inflammatory microenvironment triggering this aberrant response with partial replacement of normal tissue by fibrous tissue. Since the severe and critical COVID-19 presentations show strong involvement of inflammatory components and possibly loss of resident stem cell stocks, the research is focused in investigating the role of cellular therapy using immune response-suppressing MSCs for COVID-19 therapy [55].

In COVID-19, the extend of the cytokine release can be the ground for the diversity of the clinical manifestations. The term 'cytokine breeze' meaning a mild/nonlethal cytokine release response to infection includes the symptoms of increased local temperature (heat), myalgia, arthralgia, nausea, rash, depression, and other mild flu-like symptoms. The compensatory repair process in the body is launched for the reparation of the organs and tissues affected. The term 'cytokine strom' is used to describe the similar sudden and uncontrolled cytokine releases observed in autoimmune, hemophagocytic lymphohistiocytosis, sepsis, cancers, acute immunotherapy responses, and infectious diseases [56, 57].

All these cytokine strom ailments were not only observed in SARS-Cov-2, but also previously reported in SARS-Cov-1 and MERS-Cov cohorts [58, 59]. Hyperinflammation, though, is characteristic for SARS-Cov-2 which is a unique immunological feature of COVID-19. The data reported from recovered and seriously ill patients suggests that there is a significant relationship between severe inflammation and mortality. The main components of the cytokine strom are the critical pro-inflammatory immune elements in the inflammation site [51]. Once the immune system is activated by infection, drug or any stimulus, the cytokines (IFN, IL, chemokines, CSF, TNF, etc.) are released in high levels into the circulation leading to deleterious and diffuse impact on multiple organs.

At the moment, the factors responsible for triggering the inflammatory sequence resulting in cytokine strom are still ambiguous. It is attributed to an imbalance in immune-system regulation resulting from increasing immune cell activation via TLR or other mechanism and decreasing in anti-inflammatory response.

Altough the local and systemic cytokine responses of host to theinfection are essential parts of the host's initial response to infection, a cytokine strom, due to the harmful effects on the host, almost always is a pathological process [31]. Normally, to keep the pathogen under control, the cytokines released from natural killer (NK) cells and macrophages, activated T cells, and humoral immunity work to resolve the inflammation, along with the antibody-dependent cell-mediated cytotoxicity [60]. When looked in some more detail, epithelial cells produce local cytokines like IFN-α/β and IL-1β which can protect neighbouring cells by stimulating IFN-stimulated gene expression. This also activates the immune competent cells such as NK cells. In turn, the lytic potential of NK cells increased and IFN-γ secretion is potentiated [61]. IFN-γ actives the resident macrophages which amplifies TLR-mediated stimulation, specifically induce the high NK cells release [62]. On one side, the IL-12 acts to increase NK IFN-γ secretion, on the other side, increased levels of IL-6 also may limit the immune response by its effects on the cytotoxic activity of NK cells via the down-regulation of intracellular perforin and granzyme B levels [63]. The disease does not regress but progress further, the activities of the T cells and humoral responses causes additional cytokine responses. This process, like pouring petrol on fire, results in greater or sustained antigen release and added TLR ligands from viral-induced cytotoxicity [64]. Concurrently, an insufficient negative feedback mechanism by IL-10 and IL-4 would be expected to increase the severity of cytokine responses toward a cytokine storm. The exacerbated fire of the lethal cytokine storm reveals widespread alveolar damage characterized by hyaline membrane formation and infiltration of interstitial lymphocytes [65, 66]. In COVID-19 disease, a cytokine storm is demonstrated frequently in patients with severe-to-critical symptoms; concurrently the lymphocytes and NK cell counts are sharply reduced with elevations in levels of D-dimer, C-reactive protein (CRP), ferritin, and procalcitonin which are the inflammation biomarkers [67].

As the reported evidence regarding the immunological response to SARS-CoV-2 is quite limited, we are able to compile and interpret the relevant information from the published information. After the host is invaded by the virus, host innate immune system through pattern recognition receptors (PRRs) including C-type lectin-like receptors, Toll-like receptor (TLR), NOD-like receptor (NLR), and RIG-I like receptor (RLR), is the first to pick out [68]. The inflammatory factors' expression, dendritic cells' maturation, and type I interferons (IFNs) synthesis are promoted by the virus for basically two main purposes: limiting the spread of the virus, and phagocytosis of the viral antigens [68]. Whilst the escape of the virus from the immune responses is facilitated by the N protein of the virus [69], a strong troop of the adaptive immune response joins the combat against the virus, with its elements of T lymphocytes including CD4+ and CD8+ T cells. CD4+ T cells stimulate B cells to produce virus-specific antibodies, and CD8+ T cells directly kill virus-infected cells. T helper cells produce proinflammatory cytokines to enhance the antiinflammatory process. Paradoxically, SARS-CoV-2 induces the apoptosis of the T cells, hence inhibit their function. The major role of humoral immunity over its complements such as C3a and C5a and antibodies cannot be overlooked in the fight against the virus [70, 71]. Here comes another paradox where the immune system overreaction of the generates a large amount of free radicals locally causing severe damages to the lungs and other organs, even multi-organ failure and even death [62, 72].

In severe cases, it has been reported that SARS-CoV-2 affects heart, kidney, liver, GI-system, resulting in multiple organ dysfunction and in some cases even death [73]. One study supports that the novel virus also could potentially infect the enterocytes through a ACE2 enzyme; as ACE2 is highly expressed on enterocytes may help to explain why diarrhea occurs with acute infection as well as the fecal shedding observed [74]. Since the ACE-2 receptors are also expressed on other tissues like kidney, liver, heart and digestive system organs; thus, explaining the rapid progression towards systemic inflammatory conditions as observed in critically ill patients [75]. Hence, it is worth to consider that the infection spreading in broader scale would have impact the inflammatory cascade sources in a number of tissues in several organs, besides the lung.

4. The treatment options in SARS-CoV-2: what to use

Based on evidence from laboratory, animal, and clinical studies, the WHO recommends the drugs for treatment of COVID-19 includes Remdesivir, Lopinavir/Ritonavir, Lopinavir/Ritonavir with interferon beta-1a, chloroquine, and hydroxychloroquine [76].

Remdesivir is a monophosphoramide prodrug that causes premature termination of viral RNA replication. It was developed against Ebola, MERS-CoV, and SARS-CoV, before the COVID-19 pandemic shook the globe. Potent interference of remdesivir with the NSP12 polymeras3e of SARS-CoV-2 was shown in vitro despite intact ExoN proofreading activity [73, 77]. It is suggested that when the baricitinib which is an inflammatory drug used in combination with anti-viral drugs like Remidesivir, increases the potential of the drug to reduce viral infection [78, 79].

The Lopinavir/Ritonavir drugis a protease inhibitors combination. It is usually used to treat HIV infection; from the laboratory experiments, it is evident that these drugs could be used to treat the COVID-19 infections [80]. The lopinavir and ritonavir are used as a regimen single-agent or combination with either ribavirin or interferon-α [81]. It is also reported that the interferon beta-1a, which is used to treat multiple sclerosis, can also be used as a remedial approach for COVID-19 disease [73].

A randomised controlled trial (ChiCTR 2000029308) aimed to evaluate the efficiency and safety of lopinavir and ritonavir in severe COVID-19 patients, comparing lopinavir-ritonavir (n: 99) to standard care (n: 100). There was a significant difference in the time to clinical improvement between the two groups on day 14, whereas this difference was not statistically significant on day 28. The decrease of 5.8% in mortality at 28 days and the length of stay in the ICU reduced as five days in the lopinavir-ritonavir treatment [82].

Spike protein from virus binds to ACE2 or CD147 on the host cell, mediating viral invasion and dissemination of virus among other cells [55, 83]. In addition to ACE2, it has recently been demonstrated that S protein of novel virus also binds to CD147. Meplazumab which is an anti-CD147 humanized antibody, co-immunoprecipitation, ELISA, and immuno-electron microscope were handled to demonstrate the new CD147 path of viral invasion. This importanty evidence has been providing a key target for the development and administration of specific anti-SARS-CoV-2 medicines [84].

ACE Inhibitor and Angiotensin Receptor-1 Blocker are also medications used for the curative purposes of COVID-19. As already mentioned, SARS-CoV-2 enters the type II pneumocytes via the ACE2 receptor. Functionally ACE2 receptor has a mutual physiological action to ACE1, it converts the angiotensin II back into angiotensin I. Thus, patients taking receptor blocker will have an increased plasma angiotensin II. On the contrary, patients taking inhibitor will have low angiotensin II levels [85, 86]. Its effect in the alveolar tissue is still unknown. Discontinuation of ACEi or ARBs is not recommended yet as hypertension is an acute risk of discontinuation and can exacerbate the clinical course and increase mortality of COVID-19 if infected by SARS-CoV-2. Although chloroquine is an anti-malarial medication, it can inhibit pH-dependent stages of replication in viruses, as well as having immunomodulation which is dependent on the suppression of cytokines (IL-6 and TNF-α) production and dissemination. Secondary COVID-19 rates can be minimized with pre- and post-exposure prophylaxis in an individual with document exposure to SARS-CoV-2. Therefore, hydroxychloroquine has been hypothesized to be an adequate chemoprophylaxis candidate to reduce secondary COVID-19 [87].

WHO recommends to continue the use of ibuprofen as antipyretic agent, yet the first-line antipyretic remains to be acetaminophen.

The use of systemic corticosteroids in the management of ARDS secondary to viral pneumonia is debatable. The rationale behind this that the corticosteroids prolong the viral shedding time and maintain a systemic anti-inflammatory condition. This will minimize the precipitation of ARDS, dyspnea, and severe pneumonia.

The systemic corticosteroid usage in the management of ARDS developed due to viral pneumonia is still under discussion. The aim of this medication use is that corticosteroids prolong the viral shedding time and maintain a systemic anti-inflammatory state that will minimize the precipitation of ARDS, dyspnea, and severe pneumonia [76].

Considerable amount of protection is provided by the convalescent plasma collected from donors who have survived an infectious disease by developing antibodies is considered to provide a great degree of protection for recipients affected by the emerging virus [88]. Convalescent plasma is an old tool that has been successfully used to treat numerous infectious diseases, including the 2003 SARS-CoV-1 epidemic, 2009–2010 H1N1 influenza virus pandemic, and 2012 MERS-CoV epidemic [88–91] for which there is no effective treatment.

Based on the clinical effectiveness of convalescent plasma, such as signs of improvement approximately 1 week after convalescent plasma transfusion, effectively neutralizing SARS-CoV-2, leading to impeded inflammatory responses and improved symptom conditions without severe adverse events the FDA has granted clinical permission for applying convalescent plasma to the treatment of critically ill COVID-19 patients [92]. Antibiotics with immunomodulatory actions are used in therapy with antiviral drugs and to avoid secondary infections, such as bacterial and fungal infections in patients. Besides their antimicrobial function, antibiotics such as Azithromycin show immunomodulatory properties, which can reduce inflammatory macrophage polarization and inhibit NF-κB signaling pathways, minimizing the hyperinflammation damage. Since the beginning, antibiotics have been used with good results in mortality reduction and shortening of intubation time in COVID-19 disease [93, 94].

The expressive number of deaths and confirmed cases of SARS-CoV-2 call for an urgent demand of effective and available drugs for COVID-19 treatment. Currently, multiple avenues for therapies are being explored.

5. The mesenchymal stem cells or medicinal signalling cells

Human mesenchymal stromal cells are also recognised as mesenchymal stem cells and medicinal signaling cells (MSCs). The reason of why the MSCs are named as 'mesenchymal' is their residence in the mesodermal niche, and their multipotency. They are also termed as mesenchymal stromal cells, if they fulfill the minimum criteria of adherence, expression of CD105, CD73, and CD90, absence of CD45, CD34, CD14 or CD11b, CD79a or CD19, and HLA-DR cell surface markers as well as gives rise to descendant lineages including myocytes, adipocytes, chondrocytes, and osteocytes [95, 96] as characterized by International Society of Stromal Therapy (ISCT) in 2005 [97].

Since initial isolation from the bone marrow (BM), MSCs have been found in numerous adult and fetal-derived organs/tissues such as adipose tissue, dental pulp, umbilical cord, and placenta [98]. For translational research, MSCs are categorized into different generations according to their preparation strategy as minimally manipulated, culture-expanded, lineage induced, or genetically modified [99].

Another recommendation of naming is "medicinal signaling cells", as inspired by the fact that these cells possess the properties of homing and secrete bioactive factors that possess the immunomodulatory and regenerative potential. These features give these cells the ability to act as drugs in situ and they have shown site-specific therapeutic outcomes. The infused exogenous MSCs were shown to signal resident stem cells of the patient to repair the damage via their bioactive factors instead of undergoing their differentiation [100]. For both research and clinical purposes, large amounts of MSCs can be isolated from the embryo, fetus as well as adult stem cell sources, including bone marrow, umbilical cord blood, adipose tissue, menstrual blood, Wharton's jelly, amniotic fluid and human deciduous teeth [101, 102].

Our age is the time of MSCs, thanks to the self-renewal and differentiation properties, have already demonstrated a promising role in treating numerous life-threatening diseases as part of the modern research and regenerative medicine [103]. Depending on their origin, stem cells can be divided into three categories of embryonic, fetal and adult stem cells [104]. Indeed, fetal and embryonic stem cells have a higher potential than adult stem cells. The adults stem cells are more used in the research and development because they have the availability and less ethical issues. Bone marrow, fat tissue, human dental pulp and umbilical cord blood are amongs the numerous sources of adult stem cells, which are of crucial importance in regenerative medicine. The technology, moreover, allow these stem cells to be isolated and protected in stem cell banks under low temperature for many years without losing their potential. Particularly, the umbilical cord blood and bone marrow are the reservoirs of both hematopoietic stem cells and MSCs. It has been known that the MSCs are the most explored and exploited categories of stem cells in treating various disorders [102].

MSCs have the differentiation capacity toward trilineage paraxial mesodermal derivates such as bone, cartilage, and fat. Besides, immunomodulatory properties of MSCs allow for expansion of therapeutic use of them in regenerative medicine in inflammatory diseases, in addition to the allogeneic allogeneic use [105–108]. Interestingly, the first published evidence in the allogeneic MSCs use in inflammatory disease is a pediatric case with acute refractory graft-vs-host-disease (GVHD) in 2004 in which MSCs derived form bone marrow were given. In this study, the patient transplanted MSCs survived in well condition 1 year after MSC treatment, while other 24 patients having severe GVHD showed the median survival rate as 2 months [109]. After this pioneering evidence, MSC immunomodulation has shown to be broad-based, best detailed for CD4 lymphocytes but also for dendritic cells and natural killer cells [110, 111]. As evident by the increasing MSC trials focusing on immune/inflammatory diseases in recent years which are accounted for almost one-third of the trials, the clinical importance of the immunomodulatory properties is compromised [112–114]. General charateristics of the MSCs is their being fibroblast shaped cells which are plastic adherent; fulfilling the criteria of stem cells and MSC as well as stromal cell types [109, 115]. The immunomodulatory activities are suggested to include:

a. inhibition of the proliferation and function of dendritic cells, T and B cells, as well as NK cells.

b. polarization of monocyte to anti-inflammatory macrophages called M2 cells.

c. production of IL-10 and decreased production of TNF-α and IL-12 [116, 117].

In addition, MSCs have powerful antifibrotic effects which may alleviate lung fibrosis [118, 119].

Lately, there have been increasing reports revealing that the MSCs induce therapeutic characteristics by releasing bioactive substances known as secretomes in a paracrine path [120]. The soluable proteins such as chemokines, growth factors, cytokines, and extracellular vesicles (EVs) including microvesicles and exosomes present in the MSC-secretomes [121]. MSCs, like all other stem cells, when the culture medium or secretome are injected into the patients, show paracrine signalling to take in these molecules to the cells in vicinity [122]. The exosomes contain bioactive molecules, including microRNAs (miRNA), transfer RNAs (tRNA), long noncoding RNAs (lncRNA), growth factors, proteins, and lipids. Of note, the lipid content of the exosomes is an added value by facilitating the infusion of the exosomes attracted to the plasma membrane of the neighboring cells [123]. Once the molecules content of the secretome is internalized, the neighboring cells modulate various downstream pathways, including immunomodulation, suppression of apoptosis, prevention of fibrosis, and remodelling or repair of the damaged tissues [120, 124].

Several studies with drugs targeting GM-CSF, IL-6, IL-1, IL-2 and TNF-α is already in the pipeline which aims to calm down the inflammatory response in COVID-19 patients. MSCs are well-known for their immuno-modulatory properties including the anti-inflammatory cytokines/chemokines secretion, anti-apoptotic effect and their reparative ability for the damaged epithelial cells. Their inherent nature to migrate towards injured lungs and secretion of paracrine factors which protects and repair alveolar cells; make MSCs a potential therapeutic option for COVID-19 treatment. Recently, MSCs have been widely studied from basic research to clinical trials particularly for immune-mediated inflammatory diseases such as systemic lypus erythematous (SLE) and GVHD [125–127].

6. The mesenchymal stem cell treatment in COVID-19: what to prove

The therapy using MSCs usually covers the processes of isolation, culture, subculture, proliferation, and differentiation of exogenously obtained stem cells, which are then transplanted into patients for immune regulation and microenvironment repair. The therapy success determinants are the safety and efficacy for any treatment. Hence the safety and effectiveness of MSCs are important as shown in a number of clinical trials besides fundamental studies.

MSCs have been widely used in the treatment of inflammatory diseases, such as in graft vs. host disease [128] and lupus erythematosus [129]. Some studies have shown that MSCs have definite efficacy in improvement in cardiovascular, kidney, liver, and other diseases [130, 131].

MSCs are able to regulate the immune response by controlling the function and proliferation of various immune cells. They alsocan inhibit monocyte differentiation into dendritic cells (DCs) which results in upregulation of regulatory cytokines and downregulation of inflammatory cytokines [132]. It was suggested that systemic administration of MSC resulted in reduction of H5N1 influenza virus-induced mortality in older patients with severe pulmonary illness [133]. Also, in patients with H7N9 induced ARDS, a significant improvement in survival rate was observed [134]. So far, MSC transplantation in human subjects with diverse disease conditions has not showed any severe adverse events [135]. Therefore, it is plausible that MSC-therapy can be used to treat COVID-19 patients.

MSCs are evaluated as one of the most promising candidates for SARS-CoV-2 infection treatment. Since the key target for the treatment of SARS-CoV-2 infection resides in the cytokine storm management in lungs, MSCs are well-suited considering their main mechanism of action is through their immunomodulatory and anti-inflammatory properties [129].

MSCs have immunomodulatory effects and they:

1. prevent uncontrolled cytokine or inflammatory factors production,

2. inhibit excessive immune responses, and.

3. reduce immune damage to tissues and organs.

Having the immunemodulatory properties, MSCs not only take part in suppressing immune injury, but also replace and repair damaged tissue and inhibit lung fibrosis. Treating COVID-19 with MSCs has presented considerably good results [136]. Stem cell therapy can suppress the storm of cytokine release, promote endogenous repair by improving the microenvironment, slow the progression of acute lung inflammation down and relieve the symptoms of respiratory distress [137]. The reports suggested that the potentially COVID-19 can be successfully treated with MSCs therapy by the MSC regulation mechanism of the immune system. Studies revealed that when the MSCs are exposed to an inflammatory microenvironment, they can regulate immune cells and inflammatory factors, such as cytokines, leading the alterations in the specific or nonspecific immune responses in vivo. The said modulation is shown to be related to exosomes or the cytokines secreted by MSCs, such as transforming growth factor (TGF)-b, prostaglandin (PG)E-2, and interleukin (IL)-10 [138, 139].

The regulation of the T and B lymphocytes' functions is of special interest as it has been done in several ways. One of these is the T cell proliferation, which is controlled by inflammatory stimulation. A study on cell cycle analysis revealed that T cell subsets can be blocked at the G0/G1 phase. Another way of modulation is that the MSCs can control T cell function via cytokines, by releasing TGF-β, inhibiting the immune activity of Th17 cells, inducing their altering to form T regulatory cell Treg cells, or secreting hepatocyte growth factor to regulate the Th17/Treg cell balance [140]. The modulation of the B cells' proliferation, differentiation, and antibody secretion by the MSCs is also important, since MSCs can affect the G0/G1 phase transition of B cells and regulate the antibody secretion ability of B cells through various transcription pathways [141]. MSCs help to regulatory B cells to multiply; these B cells express IL-10. MSCs activate T cells to release interferons, as well. Suppression of activated B cells regulates the immune function of B cells, and MSCs can also affect innate immune cells, including macrophages and dendritic cells, to realize immune regulation. Under inflammatory conditions, MSCs regulate macrophage function, as well [142]. Once the proinflammatory macrophages (M1) secrete the inflammatory agents, activated MSCs can up-regulate the cyclooxygenase (COX)-2 signal and increase PGE2 secretion. This thereby promotes the transformation of macrophages from activated proinflammatory type to selectively activated anti-inflammatory type (M2).

The MSCs releasing the anti-inflammatory factor TSG-6 and the CD44 macrophages act collectively to destroy the interaction between CD44 and toll-like receptor-2, inhibit the nuclear factor-jB signal downstream, and reduce the inflammatory response [143]. On the other hand, the MSCs can secrete HGF under endotoxin stimulation to induce differentiation into regulatory dendritic cells and alleviate acute lung injury [144].

As explored by research, COVID-19 patients' blood have large numbers of inflammatory factors including interferon-c, interferon-inducible protein-10, and monocyte chemoattractantprotein-1. Additionally, when the patients staying in ICU is compared with the patients in the inpatient clinics, the concentration of granulocyte colony-stimulating factor (G-CSF), MCP-1, tumor necrosis factor (TNF)-a, and other inflammatory factors were shown to be dramaticaly higher in the ICU patients, hence there is a positive correlation between the severity of the cytokine storm and the clinical manifestations of COVID-19 [145]. As discussed previously (see section 2.2.2) COVID-19 have a variety of clinical manifestations changing from a mild disease to a severe disease. This change in severity results both from complications of the viral infection and the cytokine storm. The cytokine storm damaging effects are well-known. Cytokine storm in patients with severe COVID-19 can lead to the release of nitricoxide, which affects the normal systolic and diastolic function of blood vessels, thereby causing hypotension and multi-organ hypoxia [146]. Severe patients have IL-6 levels ten-times higher than those in non-severe patients. In addition, the IL-6 levesl are closely related to the serum SARS-CoV-2 virus load and vital signs of patients. Some study reports have now shown that tozumab (anti-IL-6 receptor) use can prevent worsening of the disease [147]. The MSCs of umblical cord origin, can also inhibit monocyte activation and IL-6 production to inhibit the development of cytokine storm, these result in the improved patient's prognosis. It has been reported that the microenvironment having high IL-6 levels, lead the MSCs to produce cytokines and exosomes enriched with mirR-455-3p, thus calming cytokine storm down and treating acute inflammatory injury. However, the effect of MSCs on cytokine storm in patients with COVID-19 still needs further confirmation [148].

MSCs may suppress ARDS exacerbation and pulmonary fibrosis. Studies have revealed that, once infused or transplanted intravenously, MSCs can reside in the lungs and help improving the microenvironment of the lungs, protecting alveolar epithelial cells, promoting neovascularization, and preventing pulmonary fibrosis

[149, 150]. So it seems that one of the most important outcome of the MSC treatment is its reparative action. The reperative function of the MSCs is managed over a variety of the cytokines, particularly keratinocyte growth factor (KGF) [151]. KGF functions through promoting alveolar fluid clearance and alleviating the acute lung injury induced by endotoxin by up-regulating ACE-2 [152]. Another up-regulation managed by KGF is that the activity of sodium potassium ATP enzyme in alveolar cells, resulting in the improvement in alveolar fluid transport, and this play a therapeutic role in ARDS and lung injury [153].

MSCs may have bacteriostatic role. There was a controversy in whether the virus could cause MSCs to lose their function when the MSCs are invaded by bacteria. Although conducted in limited number of patient size, the clinical trial reported from Beijing, showed that the COVID-19 virus could not infect umbilical cord MSCs that were infused intravenously [136]. MSCs can exert their anti-COVID-19 virus effect through direct and indirect mechanisms, according to the recent research. Direct function of the MSCs can be lined up as the direct anti-viral effect by secreting antibacterial peptides and proteins, indoleamine 2,3-dioxygenase, IL-17, and other molecules. MSCs can activate a large number of anti-virus genes independent of interferon, such as the IFITM gene, which can encode protein structures that prevent viruses from invading cells [154]. When it comes to the indirect function of the MSCs combating against COVID-19, they also exhibit an indirect antiviral effect through regulating the coordination of pro-inflammatory and anti-inflammatory actors of the patient's immune system and inducing the macrophages' functions [155–157].

The in vitro sepsis model, ARDS model, and alveolar epithelial fibrosis model use in the research activities demonstrated the immunoregulation and antibacterial and antiviral values of MSCs [156, 157]. Studies show that MSCs secrete at least four AMPs including, antibacterial peptide LL-37, human defensin 2, hepcidin, and lipocalin-2. The function of these AMPs includes killing cells, inhibiting the synthesis of essential proteins, DNA, and RNA of infected cells, interacting with certain targets in infected cells, and playing an active regulatory role in the infection and inflammatory progress of COVID-19 patients [158].

The therapeutic properties of the MSCs against SARS-CoV-2 infection include:

1. Apoptosis induction via activated T-cells alleviating excessive immune responses.

2. Regeneration and maintenance of the homeostasis in specific lung injuries.

3. Release of cytokines to inhibit neutrophil intravasation and enhance macrophage differentiation which helps attenuate inflammation and also promotes the release of extracellular vesicles which deliver microRNA, mRNA proteins and metabolites into host cells post lung injury which promotes repair regeneration and lung function restoration. Therefore MSCs should be considered as a potential treatment for critically ill patients with SARS-CoV-2 infection [159, 160].

6.1 MSC clinical studies

It has been observed that most of the clinical trials for COVID-19 treatment have used allogeneic stem cell source. The curative effect of MSCs in the treatment of COVID-19 has been shown by the two recent clinical trials. In one of them, human umbilical cord derived MSCs were used in three consecutive intravenous infusions administered to patients with COVID-19; it was reported from this trial that subject demonstrated the neutrophil levels decreased significantly, lymphocytes increased, $CD4^+$ T and $CD8^+$ T cells returned to normal level, and vital signs were improved, after the second intravenous infusion [161]. The other trial recruited seven patients with COVID-19 (two mild cases, four severe cases, and one critical case) to receive one intravenous MSC transplantation each. According to the published results, The patient's regulatory dendritic cell population increased, the level of the pro-inflammatory factor TNFa decreased, and the level of antiinflammatory factor IL-10 increased, after 2–4 days after MSC transplantation [136]. This was a pilot study Clinical grade MSCs were injected intravenously (1×10^6 cells/kg body weight) and the patients were followed-up for 14 days. From clinical point of view, a significant reduction in clinical symptoms and pneumonia infiltration was observed in chest CT of critically ill COVID-19 patient within 2–4 days of MSC-therapy. An increase in peripheral lymphocyte levels, decrease in C-reactive protein (CRP), drastic disappearance of activated cytokine-secreting immune cells ($CXCR3^+CD4^+$T-cells, $CXCR3^+CD^8$ + T-cells and $CXCR^3$ + NK-cells) and restoration of regulatory DC cell population to normal levels was observed after day 6 of MSC transplantation. From cytokines point of view, the level of anti-inflammatory cytokine IL-10 was increased and the levels of serum pro-inflammatory cytokine TNF-α was significantly decreased. These were considered as the indicators of the efficient regulation of cytokine storm in COVID-19 patients on MSC transplantation. On the other hand, the absence of ACE-2 receptor and TMPRSS2 on the transfused MSCs affirmed that they cannot get infected with SARS-Cov-2, suggesting the beneficial effects of the MSC-therapy in COVID-19 infection. The authors suggested that this clinical trial showed that transplantation of MSCs can improve the prognosis of patients with COVID-19 [145]. In a case report of one critically all COVI-19 case who is 65-year-old woman with underlying with type-II diabetes and hypertension, it was reported that after receiving MSC-based treatments her health improved and she left the ICU. The authors of this case report proposed that the possible effects of hUCMSCs might be anti-inflammation and tissue repair to COVID-19 patient. They also suggested that MSCs could down regulate proinflammatory cytokines and chemokines and increase IL-10 and VEGF which could promote the lung repair [161]. The patient didn't respond to any anti-viral drug and the disease progressed to multiple organ injury. During this critical stage when the patient is ventilated, hUC-MSC was infused in 3 consecutive administrations in 50 × 106 cells/dose. After second MSC administration, ventilator was removed as the vital signs had improved with gradual decrease in serum albumin and CRP levels. CT images showed no infiltration patches of pneumonia by the end of MSC infusions. These results suggest that hUC-MSC can be beneficial for patient who showed resistantance to anti-viral drugs. The therapeutic potential of MSCs in viral infections and immunomodulation capabilities to alleviate the cytokine storm, are being tested in clinical studies that have been initiated to further evaluate their efficiency for COVID-19 treatment.

The evidence pf the published results of the clinical trials in which the MSC transplantation is used for curative purposes, shows the beneficial effect of MSCs on the treatment of severe patients. However, more clinical data are still needed to confirm its effectiveness [162].

Several anti-viral drugs such as remdesivir, favipiravir, ribavirin functioning as RNA dependent RNA polymerase inhibitors, lopinavir, ritonavir which are protease inhibitors and drugs suc as hydroxychloroquine targeting endocytic pathway are being evaluated for COVID-19 but standard therapeutics yet not available. To fight against the cytokine storm, immune-therapy targeting TNFα, IL-1, IL-2, and IL-6 and are evaluated. One of the promising immune-modulators is the MSCs administered as add-on therapy can surmount the severity of COVID-19 infections. Recent studies have shown that MSC-therapy significantly dampens the cytokine storm in critically ill COVID-19 patients [163].

The published results of MSC add-on therapy for ARDS, with focused clinical outcome measures' analysis on safety, efficacy, and related immunologic and pulmonary responses [164]. The clinical studies have demonstrated that MSC therapy is safe and has the potential to mitigate inflammatory and physiologic damage for a variety of conditions involving the central nervous, [165] cardiac, [166] renal, [167] gastrointestinal, [168] and respiratory [169, 170] systems. The data in the literature suggests similar results for MSC therapy for treating ARDS in COVID-19.

As expected, safety is the most important matter for all new therapies, especially in patients at high risk for death from the condition being treated and was carefully evaluated for MSC-treated patients in the clinical trials published. According to the literature review, out of the 200 ARDS patients were treated with intravenously or intratracheally administered MSCs or placebo, 30patients died in the active treatment group. None of these 30 deaths were found to be related to MSC therapy. Also, no other SAEs attributed to the MSC therapy. Some transient adverse effects reported, but all of them resolved on its own in short term. This safety profile is consistent with the experience of other human clinical trials involving MSC therapy [165, 171].

The clinical trials of cell-based therapy using MSCs and their safety has been reported in several clinical trials related to GVHD and SLE [127, 172–174]. The approach of MSC transplantation has been used to treat H7N9-induced ARDS patients and the outcome showed significant reduction in mortality rates [134]. Similarly, the study of MSC-based treatment for SARS-CoV-2 suggested that MSCs lack SARS-CoV-2 infection-vital receptors (ACE2- and TMPRSS2-); so MSCs are SARS-CoV-2 infection-free. Also, the these cells' infusion in SARSCoV- 2-infected patients improved the outcomes because of their extraordinary immunosuppressant potential [136].

The potential efficacy of MSC therapy for ARDS in COVID- 19-infected patients is reported from a phase 1 trial. There were 9 patients enrolled. In-hospital mortality was reported as 33.3% (3/9), including two with septic shock and one with ventilator-induced severe pneumomediastinum and subcutaneous emphysema. No serious prespecified cell infusion-associated or treatment-related adverse events was identified in any patient. The circulating inflammatory (CD14CD33/CD11b+CD16+/CD16+MPO+/CD11b+MPO+/CD14CD33+) and MSC markers (CD26+CD45-/CD29+CD45-/CD34+CD45-/CD44+CD45-/CD73+CD45−/CD90+CD45-/CD105+CD45-/CD26+CD45-) were reported as progressively reduced and the immune cell markers such as Helper-T-cell/Cytotoxity-T-cell/Regulatory-T-cell were notably increased after cell infusion. As a result, this phase I clinical trial showed that a single-dose intravenous infusion of hUC-MSCs was safe with favourable outcome in nine ARDS patients [175]. According to the available evidence, SARS-CoV-2 affects not only the lung, but also the heart and kidney with reported cardiomyopathy and kidney injury [171, 176]. It has been reported that the improved resolution of multiple organ failure or increased organ failure-free days with MSC treatment, which further supports their consideration for clinical use.

The safety and efficacy profile of MSCs is well-constituted based on the results from several completed clinical studies conducted on the therapeutic potential of these therapies in lung diseases such as ARDS [134, 177] as well as broncho-pulmonary dysplasia cardiovascular diseases), diabetes [178, 179] and also spine injuries [180]. Although it has been still in experimental phase, the stem cell types investigated for possible cure of SARS-CoV-2 infections include human induced pluripotent stem cells. Recently, it has been reported that when iPSCs were exposed to SARS-CoV-2, it was presented a deleterious effect on the cells in vitro where the pluripotency of iPSCs was lost leading to fibroblast-like phenotype [181, 182]. Therefore, evidence-based selection of stem cell type for the treatment of COVID-19 is critical for safety and efficacy.

Wraping up, it seems the MSC-therapy, when applied as add-on treatment, suppresses the over activated immune system through its immuno-modulatory properties and promotes the tissue repair of alveolar cells in lung microenvironment of SARS-CoV-2 infected patients. Clearly, the data of the recent studies are encouraging, however they have major limitations such as the small-sized patient recruitment. Hence, the need for larger randomized control trials to establish the effectiveness and safety of MSC-therapy in SARS-Cov-2 infection is obvious.

The immense knowledge available with reference to the mechanism of action of MSCs and their effective potencies at a specific disease stage makes MSCs as an promising and effective therapeutic candidate.

6.2 Mesenchymal stem cell treatment action of mechanism

It has been demonstrated that MSCs have broad immunomodulatory, anti-inflammatory capacity [183, 184], as well as regenerative properties [185]. MSCs can induce the repair of damaged tissue, and eventually prevent long-term lung damage resulting from COVID- 19. The stabilization of the endothelial fluid leakage and maintenance of the alveolar-capillary barrier function are also characteristics demonstrated by MSCs; obviously, these features are irrevocable to decrease lung permeability and attenuating the development of interstitial lung oedema [186]. These are the main grounds for the MSC based cellular therapy as potentially effective treatment for COVID-19 infection.

Severe cases of COVID-19 infection is characteristic with high levels of cytokines in the plasma, particularly IL-6 which is a biomarker of inflammation and immune response. From this perspective, clinical trials using the medications such as Sarilumab and Tocilizumab, the antibodies anti-IL6 receptors, has been testing such therapeutic strategy in hospitalized COVID-19 infected patients.

Azithromycin is an antibiotic with immunomodulatory effects and invasion inhibitory activity. That is why this drug has been also administrated for the therapy of chronic inflammatory conditions, such as bronchiolitis and rosacea. Although the exact mechanisms of this anti-inflammatory effect are still not fully known, some studies presented a reduction of IL-6 levels after azithromycin treatment [187, 188]. What is more, another study has demonstrated that azithromycin increases rhinovirus-induced interferons and interferon-stimulated mRNA and protein expression as well as decreases rhinovirus replication and release, resulting in induced anti-viral responses in epithelial cells of the human brochiols [189].

After administered systemically, the majority of MSCs reside in the vascular bed of lungs through the interactions with the capillary endothelial cells. When labelled MSCs are traced, it was seen that most are cleared within 24–48 h, and there can be persistence in injured or inflamed lungs for a longer period [190]. It has been suggested that the apoptosis and subsequent efferocytosis and phagocytosis by resident inflammatory and immune cells could be amongst the clearance process [191]. MSCs can secrete various soluble mediators including anti-inflammatory cytokines [192], antimicrobial peptides [193], angiogenic growth factors, as well as extracellular vesicles [194] in their vicinity.

There are evidence for cell–cell transmission of mitochondria from MSCs to respiratory epithelial and immune cells [195]. This reveals the release of anti-inflammatory mediators is specific for the inflammatory lung environment and is mediated through differential activation of damage- and pathogen-associated molecular pathogen receptors expressed on MSC surfaces [196, 197]. Amongst these receptors, Toll-like receptors are crucial; since these are activated by viral RNA in COVID-19 and viral unmethylated CpG-DNA (e.g. TLR9). This leads to modulate the pathways of cell signalling resulting in MSC activation [198]. MSCs derived angiopoietin-1 and keratinocyte growth factor (KGF) contribute to the reparation or restoration of alveolar–capillary barriers disrupted as part of ARDS pathogenesis [199]. On the other hand, the specific inhibitory microRNAs in extracellular vesicles are also described as mediating the protective effects of MSCs in pre-clinical models of infectious or non-infectious acute lung injuries [200].

6.3 Developing the stem cells as advanced medical products for COVID-19

Currently, there are 82 clinical trials investigating the therapeutic potential of mesenchymal stem cells in COVID-19 patients that are registered on clinicaltrials.gov website; out of all these, 70 trials have (83%) the MSCs as therapeutic agent being tested. The allogeneic bone-marrow or umbilical cord-derived MSCs transplanted intravenously on three different occasions is involved in 21 studies (63%). Most of these trials are either recruiting patients or have not yet started the enrolment. MSCs have been investigated and reported in ARDS both in pre-clinical [201] and clinical settings [127]. Now that, a number of promising trials are currently underway, which could revolutionize the regenerative or MSC-based cellular treatment prospects for severe COVID- 19 patients.

Regardless of how urgent the development of MSC-based therapies for COVID-19 is, it is critically important that the manufacturing of MSCs is in compliance with good manufacturing practices (GMP) and follows strict regulations prior to being approved for the use in humans.

The current findings clearly show that there is a huge unmet need for globally coordinated approach to support to conduct multicentre clinical trials aiming to demonstrate safety and effectiveness of various types of stem cells to treat health complications of novel virus. Also, there is a need in biomedical research and development to establish the most effective stem cell types that are ideally suited for the treatment of the complications.

The development of the stem cell advanced medicinal products will also require: (a) GMP compliant technologies to enable massive stem cell production, and (b) testing platforms that mimic human pathophysiology as much as possible, such as 3D bio-printed organoids, organon- chip, to allow targeted screening and rapid testing of stem cells safety and efficacy. EVs appears as an attractive alternative to cell–based therapy, recently. EVs have several advantages compared to the whole cell therapy including lower risk of oncogenic effects, lower susceptibility to harm by hostile disease tissues and for longer-term storage. The long-term storage is fundamental to make the treatment accessible globally and it surrounds the requirement to have expensive GMP cell manufacturing facilities. The production of EVs must follow the same strict guidelines that apply to stem cells and any EV-based therapy needs to be approved by the health authorities after being tested in clinical trials to demonstrate and confirm the safety and efficacy.

6.4 Stem cells route of delivery

In most clinical trials investigating the MSC treatments of SARS-CoV-2 infection so far, MSCs are delivered via the intravenous route by infusion. The direct target of the intravenous route is not the lungs, that is why the inhalation route delivering the cells directly to lungs could be theoretically more effective. However, the inhalation route has the risk of not able to manage the uniform delivery of cells to lungs [202]. The evidence is being more and more visible to suggest that the curative potential of MSCs is attributed mostly to their secreted EVs via paracrine effects [203].

As evident from several clinically available inhaled medications for chronic lung disease, the inhalation route of delivering therapeutics to the lungs is a more direct route with lower the number of adverse effects, compared to the intravenous route. However, it must be appropriately managed for inhaled administration of a treatment in COVID-19 patients in the hospital setting. Many studies have showed the feasibility of delivering stem cells via spray for direct pulmonary delivery with high viability [204]. Inhalation route of stem cell administration is an opportunity for efficient delivery of stem cells directly to the lungs, yet it needs further research and proof of concept.

7. Conclusion

Once the globe has suddenly got into the pandemic of COVID-19, all the scientific community has been making every effort to understand the etiology, pathophysiology, societal and clinical aspects of the SARS-CoV-2 viral infection all over the world. As of time this chapter is compiled, there are several vaccines developed in several countries. However, despite all the efforts, there is yet no specific and validated treatment for the infection. Instead, the medicinal products already available are being used in all clinical presentations, including antivirals, antibiotics, antimallarians, ans the agents aiming to take the disease under control. Here, taking the available published evidence in place, we elaborated the structure and pathophysiological aspects which are treatment targets to fight against the pandemic of our age. In this context the mesenchymal stem cells apear as advanced medicinal product of the cellular treatment option. Having the available knowledge refering the mechanism of action of MSCs and their safe and effective potencies at a specific disease stage makes MSCs as an ideal therapeutic candidate. Although still the data to be obtained from future the large scale randomised controlled clinical trials conduct remains an underexplored research area in the field, we suggest that under the light of the available evidence today, MSCs can be used as add-on therapy with promising effectiveness and safety to control, and even treat the COVID-19 infection with regenerative, anti-inflammatory, anti-fibrotic, immunomodulatory and reparative characteristics.

Conflict of interest

The authors declare that they have no conflict of interest.

Abbreviations

ACE2	angiotensin-converting enzyme 2
ARDS	acute respiratory distress syndrome
CoV	Corona viruses
COVID-19	Coronavirus Disease 2019
CP	convalescent plasma
CRP	C-reactive protein
CRS	cytokine release syndrome
CT	Chest computerized tomography
HCQ	Hydroxychloroquine
HIV	human immunodeficient virus
Ig	Immunoglobulin
IL	Interleukin
MCP-1	monocyte chemoattractant protein-1
MERS-CoV	middle East respiratory syndrome-coronavirus
MIP-lα	macrophage inflammatory protein-1 alpha
MOD	multiorgan dysfunction
TNF-α	tumor necrosis factor alpha

Author details

Duygu Koyuncu Irmak[1,2*] and Erdal Karaoz[1,3]

1 Department of Histology and Embryology, Faculty of Medicine, Istinye University, Istanbul, Turkey

2 Stem Cell and Tissue Engineering R&D Center, Istinye University, Istanbul, Turkey

3 Liv Hospital, Stem Cell and Regenerative Therapies Center (LivMedCell), Istanbul, Turkey

*Address all correspondence to: duygu.irmak@istinye.edu.tr

References

[1] Wu Z, McGoogan JM, Characteristics of and Important Lessons from the Coronavirus Disease 2019 (COVID-19) Outbreak in China: Summary of a Report of 72 314 Cases from the Chinese Center for Disease Control and Prevention. JAMA. 2020; 323: 1239-1242. DOI

[2] Wang L, Wang Y, Ye D, Liu Q. Review of the 2019 novel coronavirus (SARS-CoV-2) based on current evidence. Int J Antimicrob Agents. 2020 Jun;55(6):105948. doi: 10.1016/j.ijantimicag.2020.105948. Epub 2020 Mar 19. Erratum in: Int J Antimicrob Agents. 2020;56(3):106137

[3] Chrzanowski W, Kim SY, McClements L. Can Stem Cells Beat COVID-19: Advancing Stem Cells and Extracellular Vesicles Toward Mainstream Medicine for Lung Injuries Associated With SARS-CoV-2 Infections. Frontiers in Bioengineering and Biotechnology. 2020; 8: 554. DOI:10.3389/fbioe.2020.00554

[4] Andersen KG, Rambaut A, Lipkin WI, Holmes, EC, Garry RF. et al. The proximal origin of SARS-CoV-2. Nat Med 2000; 26: 450-452 DOI: 10.1038/s41591-020-0820-9

[5] Bari E, Ferrarotti I, Torre ML, Corsico AG, Perteghella S. Mesenchymal stem/stromal cell secretome for lung regeneration: The long way through "pharmaceuticalization" for the best formulation. J Control Release. 2019;309:11-24. DOI: 10.1016/j.jconrel.2019.07.022

[6] Sengupta V, Sengupta S, LazoJr A, Woods P, Nolan A, et.al.Exosomes Derived from Bone Marrow Mesenchymal Stem Cells as Treatment for Severe COVID-19 Stem Cells and Development. 2020; 29: 12, DOI: 10.1089/scd.2020.0080

[7] Kong D, Liu X, Li X, Hu J, Li X, Xiao J. et.al. Mesenchymal stem cells significantly improved treatment effectsof Linezolid on severe pneumonia in a rabbit model. Bioscience Reports. 2019; 39 doi.org/10.1042/BSR20182455

[8] Hossein-khannazer N, Shokoohian B, Shpichka A. et.al. Novel therapeutic approaches for treatment of COVID-19. Journal of Molecular Medicine. 2020; 98(6). DOI: 10.1007/s00109-020-01927-6.

[9] Xu X, Chen P, Wang J, et al. Evolution of the novel coronavirus from the ongoing Wuhan outbreak and modeling of its spike protein for risk of human transmission. Sci China Life Sci. 2020; 63:457-460. DOI: 10.1007/s11427-020-1637-5.

[10] Song W, Gui M, Wang X, Xiang Y. Cryo-EM structure of the SARS coronavirus spike glycoprotein in complex with its host cell receptor ACE2. PLOS Pathog. 2018; 14:e1007236. DOI: 10.1371/journal.ppat.1007236

[11] Peiris JS, Yuen KY, Osterhaus AD, Stohr K. The severe acute respiratory syndrome. N Engl J Med. 2003; 349:25:2431-2441. DOI: 10.1056/NEJMra032498CrossRefGoogle Scholar

[12] Akkoc T. COVID-19 and Mesenchymal Stem Cell Treatment; Mystery or Not. Adv Exp Med Biol. 2020;1298:167-176. doi: 10.1007/5584_2020_557

[13] Kakodkar P, Kaka N, Baig M. A Comprehensive Literature Review on the Clinical Presentation, and Management of the Pandemic Coronavirus Disease 2019 (COVID-19). Cureus 2020; 12:4:e7560. DOI 10.7759/cureus.7560

[14] Zhu N, Zhang D, Wang W, Li X. et.al. China Novel Coronavirus

Investigating and Research Team. A Novel Coronavirus from Patients with Pneumonia in China, 2019. N Engl J Med. 2020; 20;382-8:727-733. DOI: 10.1056/NEJMoa2001017.

[15] Chu H, Chan JF, Wang Y, Yuen TT, Chai Y, Hou Y, et.al. Comparative Replication and Immune Activation Profiles of SARS-CoV-2 and SARS-CoV in Human Lungs: An Ex Vivo Study With Implications for the Pathogenesis of COVID-19. Clin Infect Dis. 2020;71(6):1400-1409. DOI: 10.1093/cid/ciaa410.

[16] Kampf G, Todt D, Pfaender S, Steinmann E. Persistence of coronaviruses on inanimate, surfaces and their inactivation with biocidal agents. J Hosp Infect. 2020; 104:246-251 DOI:10.1016/j.jhin.2020.01.022

[17] Otter JA, Donskey C, Yezli S, Douthwaite S, et.al. Transmission of SARS and MERS coronaviruses and influenza virus in healthcare settings: the possible role of dry surface contamination. J Hosp Infect. 2016; 92:235-250. DOI:10.1016/j.jhin.2015.08.027

[18] vanDoremalen N, Bushmaker T, Morris DH, et al. Aerosol and surface stability of SARS-CoV- 2 as compared with SARS-CoV-1. N Engl J Med. 2020:382(16):1564-1567. DOI: 10.1056/NEJMc2004973.

[19] Report of the WHO-China joint mission on coronavirus disease 2019 (COVID-19) . 2020; Accessed: Sep, 2020: https://www.who.int/docs/default-source/coronaviruse/whochina-joint-mission-on-covid-19-final-report.pdf

[20] Guan W, Ni Z, Hu Y, et al. Clinical characteristics of coronavirus disease 2019 in China . N Engl J Med. 2020; 15:6 e0234764 DOI: 10.1056/NEJMoa2002032

[21] Wang D, Hu B, Hu C, et al. Clinical characteristics of 138 hospitalized patients with 2019 novel coronavirus-infected pneumonia in Wuhan, China. JAMA. 2020; 323:1061-1069. DOI: 10.1001/jama.2020.1585

[22] Chen N, Zhou M, Dong X, et al. Epidemiological and clinical characteristics of 99 cases of 2019 novel coronavirus pneumonia in Wuhan, China: a descriptive study. Lancet. 2020; 395:507-513. DOI: 10.1016/S0140-6736(20)30211-7

[23] Shi H, Han X, Jiang N, et al.: Radiological findings from 81 patients with COVID-19 pneumonia in Wuhan, China: a descriptive study. Lancet Infect Dis. 2020, 20:425-434. 10.1016/S1473-3099(20)30086-4

[24] Huang C, Wang Y, Li X, et al. Clinical features of patients infected with 2019 novel coronavirus in Wuhan, China. Lancet. 2020: 395:497-506. DOI: 10.1016/S0140-6736(20)30183-5

[25] Xu T, Chen C, Zhu Z, et al. Clinical features and dynamics of viral load in imported and non-imported patients with COVID-19. Int J Infect Dis. 2020;94:68-71 DOI: 10.1016/j.ijid.2020.03.022

[26] Zhang X, Cai H, Lian J, et al. Epidemiological, clinical characteristics of cases of SARS-CoV-2 infection with abnormal imaging findings. Int J Infect Dis. 2020;94:81-87 DOI: 10.1016/j.ijid.2020.03.040

[27] Wu C, Chen X, Cai Y, et al. Risk factors associated with acute respiratory distress syndrome and death in patients with coronavirus disease 2019 pneumonia in Wuhan, China. JAMA Intern Med. 2020; 180(7):934-943. doi: 10.1001/jamainternmed.2020.0994. Erratum in: JAMA Intern Med. 2020 Jul 1;180(7):1031.

[28] Chen G, Wu D, Guo W, et al. Clinical and immunologic features in

severe and moderate coronavirus disease 2019. J Clin Invest. 2020; 130:5:2620-2629. DOI: 10.1172/JCI137244.

[29] Pedersen SF, Ho YC. SARS-CoV-2: a storm is raging. J Clin Invest. 2020;130:2202-22051. DOI: 10.1172/JCI137647

[30] Zhang W, Zhao Y, Zhang F, et al. The use of anti-inflammatory drugs in the treatment of people with severe coronavirus disease 2019 (COVID-19): the perspectives of clinical immunologists from China. Clin Immunol. 2020;214:108393.DOI: 10.1016/j.clim.2020.108393

[31] Huang C et al. 2020 Clinical features of patients infected with 2019 novel coronavirus in Wuhan, China. The Lancet 395, 497-506. DOI: 10.1016/S0140-6736(20)30183-5

[32] Zhou F et al. Clinical course and risk factors for mortality of adult inpatients with COVID-19 in Wuhan, China: a retrospective cohort study. Lancet. 2020; 395: 1054-1062. DOI:10.1016/S0140-6736(20) 30566-3

[33] Hu H, Ma F, Wei X, Fang Y. Coronavirus fulminant myocarditis saved with glucocorticoid and human immunoglobulin. Eur. Heart J. 2020; 16: ehaa190. DOI:10.1093/eurheartj/ehaa190

[34] Ruan Q, Yang K, Wang W, Jiang L, Song J. Clinical predictors of mortality due to COVID-19 based on an analysis of data of 150 patients from Wuhan, China. Intensive Care Med. 2020 ; 46: 846-848. DOI:10.1007/s00134-020-05991-x

[35] Wu C et al. Risk factors associated with acute respiratory distress syndrome and death in patients with coronavirus disease 2019 pneumonia in Wuhan, China. JAMA Internal Med.2020; 180, 934-943. DOI:10.1001/jamainternmed.2020.0994

[36] NIH . Management of COVID-19. 2020: Availablefrom: www.covid19treatmentguidelines.nih.gov/ Accessed: 5 Jan 2021

[37] Cennimo DJ. Coronavirus disease 2019 (COVID- 19) guidelines: CDC interim guidance on coronavirus disease 2019 (COVID-19). 2020: Available at: https://emedicine.medscape.com/article/2500114-guidelines.Accessed 5 Jan 2021.

[38] Poston JT, Patel BK, Davis AM. Management of critically ill adults with COVID-19. JAMA. 2020; 323, 1839-1841. DOI: 10.1001/jama.2020.4914

[39] Li MY, Li L, Zhang Y, Wang XS. Expression of the SARS-CoV-2 cell receptor gene ACE2 in a wide variety of human tissues. Infectious Dis. Poverty 2020; 9, 45. DOI: 10.1186/s40249-020-00662-x

[40] Hamming I, Timens W, Bulthuis ML, et.al. Tissue distribution of ACE2 protein, the functional receptor for SARS coronavirus: a first step in understanding SARS pathogenesis. J. Pathol. 2004; 203, 631-637. DOI: 10.1002/path.1570

[41] Uhlen M et al. Proteomics. Tissue-based map of the human proteome. Science 2015; 347, 1260419. DOI: 10.1126/science.1260419

[42] Goulter AB, Goddard MJ, Allen JC, Clark KL. ACE2 gene expression is up-regulated in the human failing heart. BMC Med. 2004; 2: 19. DOI: 10.1186/1741-7015-2-19

[43] Danilczyk U, Penninger JM. Angiotensinconverting enzyme II in the heart and the kidney. Circul. Res. 2006; 98, 463-471. DOI: 10.1161/01.RES.0000205761.22353.5f

[44] Lai CC, Shih TP, Ko WC, Tang HJ, Hsueh PR. Severe acute respiratory syndrome coronavirus 2 (SARS-CoV-2)

and coronavirus disease-2019 (COVID-19): the epidemic and the challenges. Int. J. Antimicrob. Agents 2020: 55 105924. DOI: 10.1016/j.ijantimicag

[45] Special Expert Group for Control of the Epidemic of Novel Coronavirus Pneumonia of the Chinese Preventive Medicine Association. An update on the epidemiological characteristics of novel coronavirus pneumonia (COVID-19). Zhonghua Liu Xing Bing Xue Za Zhi. 2020; 10;41(2):139-144. Chinese. DOI: 10.3760/cma.j.issn.0254-6450.2020.02.002

[46] Anderson RM, Heesterbeek H, Klinkenberg D, Hollingsworth TD. How will country-based mitigation measures influence the course of the COVID-19 epidemic? Lancet. 2020; 1;395:10228:931-934. DOI: 10.1016/S0140-6736(20)30567-5

[47] Wang D, Hu B, Hu C, et al. Clinical characteristics of 138 hospitalized patients with 2019 novel coronavirus-infected pneumonia in Wuhan, China. JAMA. 2020; 323:1061-1069. DOI: 10.1001/jama.2020.1585

[48] Chen H, Guo J, Wang C, et al. Clinical characteristics and intrauterine vertical transmission potential of COVID-19 infection in nine pregnant women: a retrospective review of medical records. Lancet. 2020; 395:809-815. DOI: 10.1016/S0140-6736(20)30360-3.

[49] Clinical management of COVID-19 is: interim guidance. 2020. Available at:https://www.who.int/publications/i/item/clinical-management-of-covid-19. Accessed:Feb2, 2021

[50] Dong L, Hu S, Gao J. Discovering drugs to treat coronavirus disease 2019 (COVID-19). Drug Discov Ther. 2020; 14:58-60 DOI: 10.5582/ddt.2020.01012.

[51] Fara A, Mitrev Z, Rosalia RA, Assas BM. Cytokine storm and COVID-19: a chronicle of pro-inflammatory cytokines. Open Biol. 2020; 10: 200160. DOI: 10.1098/rsob.200160

[52] Cron RQ, Behrens EM. Cytokine Storm Syndrome. Switzerland AG: Springer Nature; 2019. ISBN 978-3-030-22094-5

[53] Agha EE, Kramann R, Schneider RK, et al. Mesenchymal Stem Cells in Fibrotic Disease. Cell Stem Cell, 2017; 21:2: 166-177. DOI:10.1016/j.stem.2017.07.011.

[54] Tian S, Hu W, Niu L, Liu H, Xu H, Xiao SY. Pulmonary Pathology of Early-Phase 2019 Novel Coronavirus (COVID-19) Pneumonia in Two Patients With Lung Cancer. J Thorac Oncol. 2020;15(5):700-704. DOI: 10.1016/j.jtho.2020.02.010.

[55] Ulrich H, Pillat MM. CD147 as a Target for COVID-19 Treatment: Suggested Effects of Azithromycin and Stem Cell Engagement. Stem Cell Rev Rep. 2020;16(3):434-440. DOI: 10.1007/s12015-020-09976-7

[56] Shimabukuro-Vornhagen A, Gödel P, Subklewe M, et.al. Cytokine release syndrome. J Immunother Cancer. 2018; 6:1:56. DOI: 10.1186/s40425-018-0343-9

[57] Crayne CB, Albeituni S, Nichols KE, Cron RQ. The Immunology of Macrophage Activation Syndrome. Front Immunol. 2019;10:119. DOI: 10.3389/fimmu.2019.00119.

[58] Zhang Y et al. Analysis of serum cytokines in patients with severe acute respiratory syndrome Infect. Immun. 2004; 72: 4410-4415. DOI:10.1128/IAI.72.8.4410-4415.2004

[59] Min CK et al. Comparative and kinetic analysis of viral shedding and immunological responses inMERS patients representing a broad spectrum

of disease severity. Sci. Rep. 2016; 6: 25359. DOI:10.1038/srep25359

[60] Borrok MJ, Luheshi NM, Beyaz N, et al. Enhancement of antibodydependent cell-mediated cytotoxicity by endowing IgG with FcαRI (CD89) binding. mAbs. 2015;7:743-751. DOI: 10.1080/19420862.2015.1047570

[61] Chatenoud L, Ferran C, Reuter A, et al. Systemic reaction to the anti-T-cell monoclonal antibody OKT3 in relation to serum levels of tumor necrosis factor and interferon-gamma.NEngl JMed. 1989;320: 1420-1421. DOI: 10.1007/s00281-017-0629-x.

[62] Channappanavar R, Perlman S. Pathogenic human coronavirus infections: causes and consequences of cytokine storm and immunopathology. Semin Immunopathol. 2017;39:529-539. DOI: 10.1007/s00281-017-0629-x

[63] Cifaldi L, Prencipe G, Caiello I, et al. Inhibition of natural killer cell cytotoxicity by interleukin-6: implications for the pathogenesis of macrophage activation syndrome. Arthritis Rheumatol. 2015;67:3037-3046. DOI: 10.1002/art.39295

[64] Li T, Xie J, He Y, et al. Long-term persistence of robust antibody and cytotoxic T cell responses in recovered patients infected with SARS coronavirus. PLoS One. 2006;1:e24. DOI: 10.1371/journal.pone.0000024

[65] Xu Z, Shi L, Wang Y, et al. Pathological findings of COVID-19 associated with acute respiratory distress syndrome. Lancet Respir Med. 2020;8:420-422. DOI:https://doi.org/10.1016/S2213-2600(20)30076-X

[66] Tian S, Hu W, Niu L, Liu H, Xu H, Xiao S. Pulmonary pathology of early-phase 2019 novel coronavirus (COVID-19) pneumonia in two patients with lung cancer. J ThoracOncol. 2020;15:700-704. DOI: 10.1016/j.jtho.2020.02.010

[67] Chen N, Zhou M, Dong X, et al. Epidemiological and clinical characteristics of 99 cases of 2019 novel coronavirus pneumonia in Wuhan, China: a descriptive study. Lancet. 2020;395:507-513. DOI:https://doi.org/10.1016/S0140-6736(20)30211-7

[68] Ben Addi A, Lefort A, Hua X, Libert F, Communi D, Ledent C, et al. Modulation of murine dendritic cell function by adenine nucleotides and adenosine: involvement of the A(2B) receptor. European journal of immunology. 2008; 38: 1610-1620. DOI: 10.1002/eji.200737781.

[69] Lu X, Pan J, Tao J, Guo D. SARS-CoV nucleocapsid protein antagonizes IFN-beta response by targeting initial step of IFN-beta induction pathway, and its C-terminal region is critical for the antagonism. Virus Genes. 2011; 42:37-45. DOI: 10.1007/s11262-010-0544-x.

[70] Mathern DR, Heeger PS. Molecules Great and Small: The Complement System. Clin J Am Soc Nephrol. 2015; 10: 1636-1650. DOI: 10.2215/CJN.06230614

[71] Traggiai E, Becker S, Subbarao K, Kolesnikova L, Uematsu Y, Gismondo MR, et al. An efficient method to make human monoclonal antibodies from memory B cells: potent neutralization of SARS coronavirus. Nat Med. 2004; 10: 871-875. DOI: 10.1038/nm1080

[72] Tang B, Bragazzi NL, Li Q, Tang S, Xiao Y, Wu J. An updated estimation of the risk of transmission of the novel coronavirus (2019-nCov). Infect Dis Model. 2020; 5:248-255. DOI: 10.1016/j.idm.2020.02.001

[73] World Health Organization (WHO) “Solidarity” clinical trial for

COVID-19 treatments.2020. Available at: https://www.who.int/emergencies/diseases/novel-coronavirus-2019/global-research-on-novel-coronavirus-2019-ncov/solidarity-clinical-trial-for-covid-19-treatments Accessed: 10 Feb 2021

[74] Lamers MM, Beumer J, van der Vaart J, Knoops K, Puschhof J, et.al. SARS-CoV-2 productively infects human gut enterocytes. Science. 2020;369:6499::50-54. DOI: 10.1126/science.abc1669.

[75] Hamming I, Timens W, Bulthuis ML, Lely AT, et.al. Tissue distribution of ACE2 protein, the functional receptor for SARS coronavirus. A first step in understanding SARS pathogenesis. J Pathol. 2004;203(2):631-637. DOI: 10.1002/path.1570.

[76] World Health Organization (WHO) Clinical management of COVID-19: interim guidance, 27 May 2020 Available at: https://apps.who.int/iris/handle/10665/332196 Document No: WHO/2019-nCoV/clinical/2020.5

[77] Wang M, Cao R, Zhang L, et al.: Remdesivir and chloroquine effectively inhibit the recently emerged novel coronavirus (2019-nCoV) in vitro. Cell Res. 2020; 30:269-271. DOI: 10.1038/s41422- 020-0282-0].

[78] Stebbing J, Phelan A, Griffin I, Tucker C, et.al. COVID-19: combining antiviral and anti-inflammatory treatments. Lancet InfectDis 2020; 400-402. DOI: 10.1016/S1473-3099(20)30132-8

[79] Iyer M, Jayaramayya K, Subramaniam MD, et.al. COVID-19: an update on diagnostic and therapeutic approaches. BMB Rep. 2020;53:4:191-205. DOI: 10.5483/BMBRep.2020.53.4.080.

[80] Chu CM, Cheng VC, Hung IF, Wong MM, Chan KH, Chan KS, et.al. HKU/UCH SARS Study Group. Role of lopinavir/ritonavir in the treatment of SARS: initial virological and clinical findings. Thorax. 2004;59(3):252-256. DOI: 10.1136/thorax.2003.012658.

[81] Dong L, Hu S, Gao J. Discovering drugs to treat coronavirus disease 2019 (COVID-19) . Drug Discov Ther. 2020;14:58-60. DOI: 10.5582/ddt.2020.01012].

[82] Cao B, Wang Y, Wen D, et al.: A trial of lopinavir-ritonavir in adults hospitalized with severe Covid-19. N Engl J Med. 2020; 382:1787-1799 DOI: 10.1056/NEJMoa2001282

[83] Yan R, Zhang Y, Li Y, Xia L, Guo Y, Zhou Q. Structural basis for the recognition of SARS-CoV-2 by full-length human ACE2. Science. 2020 Mar 27;367(6485):1444-1448. DOI: 10.1126/science.abb2762

[84] Wang, K., Chen, W., Zhou, Y. S., et al. SARS-CoV-2 invades host cells via a novel route: CD147-spike protein. BioRxiv preprint. 2020; DOI:10.1101/2020.03.14.988345]

[85] Ishiyama EY, Gallagher BP, Averill AD, et.al. Upregulation of angiotensin-converting enzyme 2 after myocardial infarction by blockade of angiotensin II receptors. Hypertension. 2004; 43:970-976. DOI:10.1161/01.HYP.0000124667.34652.1a

[86] Furuhashi M, Moniwa N, Mita T, et al. Urinary angiotensin-converting enzyme 2 in hypertensive patients may be increased by olmesartan, an angiotensin II receptor blocker. AmJ Hypertens. 2015; 28:15-21. DOI:10.1093/ajh/hpu086

[87] Yao X, Ye F, Zhang M, Cui C. et.al. In Vitro Antiviral Activity and Projection of Optimized Dosing Design of Hydroxychloroquine for the Treatment of Severe Acute Respiratory Syndrome Coronavirus

2 (SARS-CoV-2). Clin Infect Dis. 2020;71(15):732-739. DOI: 10.1093/cid/ciaa237.

[88] Dodd, R.Y. Emerging pathogens and their implications for the blood supply and transfusion transmitted infections. Br. J. Haematol. 2012;159, 135-142. DOI: 10.1111/bjh.12031.

[89] Hung IF, To KK, Lee CK, Lee KL, Chan K, Yan WW, Liu R, Watt CL, et.al. Convalescent plasma treatment reduced mortality in patients with severe pandemic influenza A (H1N1) 2009 virus infection. Clin Infect Dis. 2011;52:4:447-456. DOI: 10.1093/cid/ciq106.

[90] Mair-Jenkins J, Saavedra-Campos M, Baillie JK, Cleary P, Khaw FM, et.al. Convalescent Plasma Study Group. The effectiveness of convalescent plasma and hyperimmune immunoglobulin for the treatment of severe acute respiratory infections of viral etiology: a systematic review and exploratory meta-analysis. J Infect Dis. 2015;211(1):80-90. DOI: 10.1093/infdis/jiu396.

[91] Zhang J, Xie B, Hashimoto K. Current status of potential therapeutic candidates for the COVID-19 crisis. Brain Behav Immun. 2020;87:59-73. DOI: 10.1016/j.bbi.2020.04.046.

[92] Roback JD, Guarner J. Convalescent Plasma to Treat COVID-19: Possibilities and Challenges. JAMA. 2020;323(16):1561-1562. DOI:10.1001/jama.2020.4940

[93] Felsenstein S, Herbert JA, McNamara PS, Hedrich CM. COVID-19: Immunology and treatment options. Clin Immunol. 2020;215:108448. DOI: 10.1016/j.clim.2020.108448

[94] Saghazadeh A, Rezaei N. Towards treatment planning of COVID-19: Rationale and hypothesis for the use of multiple immunosuppressive agents: Anti-antibodies, immunoglobulins, and corticosteroids. Int Immunopharmacol. 2020;84:106560. DOI: 10.1016/j.intimp.2020.106560.

[95] Pittenger MF, Mackay AM, Beck SC. et.al. Multilineage potential of adult human mesenchymal stem cells. Science. 1999;284(5411):143-147. DOI: 10.1126/science.284.5411.143.

[96] Yadav P, Vats R, Bano A, Bhardwaj R. Mesenchymal stem cell immunomodulation and regeneration therapeutics as an ameliorative approach for COVID-19 pandemics. Life Sci. 2020;263:118588. DOI: 10.1016/j.lfs.2020.118588.

[97] Dominici M, Le Blanc K, Mueller I, Slaper-Cortenbach I, Marini F, et.al. Minimal criteria for defining multipotent mesenchymal stromal cells. The International Society for Cellular Therapy position statement. Cytotherapy. 2006;8(4):315-317. DOI: 10.1080/14653240600855905.

[98] Pittenger MF, Discher DE, Péault BM, Phinney DG. et.al. Mesenchymal stem cell perspective: cell biology to clinical progress. NPJ Regen Med. 2019;4:22. DOI: 10.1038/s41536-019-0083-6.

[99] Hunt CL, Her Y, Law L, et al. Five generations of cell preparation: a translational framework for categorizing regenerative stem cell therapies. J Am Acad Regen Med. 2017;1(1);246-250.DOI:10.4081/jaarm.2017.7239

[100] Caplan AI. Mesenchymal Stem Cells: Time to Change the Name! Stem Cells Transl Med. 2017 Jun;6(6):1445-1451. DOI: 10.1002/sctm.17-0051.

[101] Yadav P, Vats R, Bano A, Bhardwaj R. Mesenchymal stem cell immunomodulation and regeneration therapeutics as an ameliorative approach for COVID-19 pandemics.

Life Sci. 2020 Dec 15;263:118588. doi: 10.1016/j.lfs.2020.118588.

[102] Ullah I, Subbarao RB, Rho GJ. Human mesenchymal stem cells - current trends and future prospective. Biosci Rep. 2015;35(2):e00191. DOI: 10.1042/BSR20150025.

[103] Galipeau J, Sensébé L. Mesenchymal Stromal Cells: Clinical Challenges and Therapeutic Opportunities. Cell Stem Cell. 2018 Jun 1;22(6):824-833. DOI: 10.1016/j.stem.2018.05.004.

[104] Hipp J, Atala A. Sources of stem cells for regenerative medicine. Stem Cell Rev. 2008;4(1):3-11. doi: 10.1007/s12015-008-9010-8.

[105] Caplan AI, Correa D. The MSC: an injury drugstore. Cell Stem Cell. 2011;9(1):11-15. DOI: 10.1016/j.stem.2011.06.008.

[106] Pittenger MF, Mackay AM, Beck SC, et.al. Multilineage potential of adult human mesenchymal stem cells. Science. 1999;284(5411):143-147. DOI: 10.1126/science.284.5411.143.

[107] Karaöz E, Çetinalp Demircan P, Erman G, Güngörürler E, Eker Sarıboyacı A. Comparative Analyses of Immunosuppressive Characteristics of Bone-Marrow, Wharton's Jelly, and Adipose Tissue-Derived Human Mesenchymal Stem Cells. Turk J Haematol. 2017;34(3):213-225. DOI: 10.4274/tjh.2016.0171.

[108] Le Blanc K, Rasmusson I, Sundberg B, Götherström C, Hassan M, Uzunel M, Ringdén O. Treatment of severe acute graft-versus-host disease with third party haploidentical mesenchymal stem cells. Lancet. 2004;363:9419:1439-1441. DOI: 10.1016/S0140-6736(04)16104-7.

[109] Yilmaz S, Inandiklioglu N, Yildizdas D, et.al. Mesenchymal stem cell: does it work in an experimental model with acute respiratory distress syndrome? Stem Cell Rev Rep. 2013;9(1):80-92. doi: 10.1007/s12015-012-9395-2.

[110] Uccelli A, Moretta L, Pistoia V. Mesenchymal stem cells in health and disease. Nat Rev Immunol. 2008;8(9):726-736. DOI: 10.1038/nri2395.

[111] Le Blanc K, Mougiakakos D. Multipotent mesenchymal stromal cells and the innate immune system. Nat Rev Immunol. 2012;12(5):383-396. DOI: 10.1038/nri3209. PMID: 22531326.

[112] Wang LT, Ting CH, Yen ML, Liu KJ, Sytwu HK, Wu KK, Yen BL. Human mesenchymal stem cells (MSCs) for treatment towards immune- and inflammation-mediated diseases: review of current clinical trials. J Biomed Sci. 2016;23(1):76. DOI: 10.1186/s12929-016-0289-5.

[113] Le Blanc K, Rasmusson I, Sundberg B, et al. Treatment of severe acute graft-versus-host disease with third party haploidentical mesenchymal stem cells. Lancet. 2004;363:1439-1441.

[114] Zhao Q, Zhang L, Wei Y, Yu H, Zou L. et.al. Systematic comparison of hUC-MSCs at various passages reveals the variations of signatures and therapeutic effect on acute graft-versus-host disease. Stem Cell Res Ther. 2019;10(1):354. doi: 10.1186/s13287-019-1478-4.

[115] Horwitz EM, Le Blanc K, Dominici M, et.al. International Society for Cellular Therapy. Clarification of the nomenclature for MSC: The International Society for Cellular Therapy position statement. Cytotherapy. 2005;7(5):393-395. doi: 10.1080/14653240500319234.

[116] Murphy MB, Moncivais K, Caplan AI. Mesenchymal stem cells:

environmentally responsive therapeutics for regenerative medicine. Exp Mol Med. 2013 Nov 15;45(11):e54. doi: 10.1038/emm.2013.94

[117] Chow L, Johnson V, Impastato R, Coy J, Strumpf A, Dow S. Antibacterial activity of human mesenchymal stem cells mediated directly by constitutively secreted factors and indirectly by activation of innate immune effector cells. Stem Cells Transl Med. 2020;9(2):235-249. doi: 10.1002/sctm.19-0092.

[118] Ni K et al. Human mesenchymal stein cells alleviate bleomycininduced pulmonary fibrosis in humanized mice. J Immunol. 2017;198 (suppl 1):82.21. doi: 10.1165/rcmb.2017-0326OC

[119] Tzouvelekis A, Toonkel R, et.al. Mesenchymal Stem Cells for the Treatment of Idiopathic Pulmonary Fibrosis. Front Med (Lausanne). 2018 May 15;5:142. doi: 10.3389/fmed.2018.00142.

[120] Kritas SK, Ronconi G, et.al. Mast cells contribute to coronavirus-induced inflammation: new anti-inflammatory strategy. J Biol Regul Homeost Agents. 2020,;34(1):9-14. doi: 10.23812/20-Editorial-Kritas.

[121] YYe Q, Wang B, Mao J. The pathogenesis and treatment of the `Cytokine Storm' in COVID-19. J Infect. 2020;80(6):607-613. doi: 10.1016/j.jinf.2020.03.037.

[122] Available at: ClinicalTrials.gov. https://clinicaltrials.gov. Access: 16 Feb 2021

[123] Wang LT, Ting CH, et.al. Human mesenchymal stem cells (MSCs) for treatment towards immune- and inflammation-mediated diseases: review of current clinical trials. J Biomed Sci. 2016;23(1):76. doi: 10.1186/s12929-016-0289-5.

[124] Prockop DJ, Oh JY. Mesenchymal stem/stromal cells (MSCs): role as guardians of inflammation. Mol Ther. 2012;20(1):14-20. doi: 10.1038/mt.2011.211.

[125] Prockop DJ. The exciting prospects of new therapies with mesenchymal stromal cells. Cytotherapy. 2017;19(1): 1-8. doi: 10.1016/j.jcyt.2016.09.008.

[126] Connick P, Kolappan M, Crawley C, Webber DJ, Patani R, et.al. Autologous mesenchymal stem cells for the treatment of secondary progressive multiple sclerosis: an open-label phase 2a proof-of-concept study. Lancet Neurol. 2012;11(2):150-156. doi: 10.1016/S1474-4422(11)70305-2.

[127] Wilson JG, Liu KD, Zhuo H, et.al. Mesenchymal stem (stromal) cells for treatment of ARDS: a phase 1 clinical trial. Lancet Respir Med. 2015;3(1):24-32. doi: 10.1016/S2213-2600(14)70291-7.

[128] Hashmi S, Ahmed M, Murad MH, et.al. Survival after mesenchymal stromal cell therapy in steroid-refractory acute graft-versus-host disease: systematic review and meta-analysis. Lancet Haematol. 2016 Jan;3(1):e45–e52. doi: 10.1016/S2352-3026(15)00224-0.

[129] Fatima F, Ekstrom K, Nazarenko I, et.al. Non-coding RNAs in Mesenchymal Stem Cell-Derived Extracellular Vesicles: Deciphering Regulatory Roles in Stem Cell Potency, Inflammatory Resolve, and Tissue Regeneration. Front Genet. 2017;8:161. doi: 10.3389/fgene.2017.00161.

[130] Cruz FF, Rocco PRM. The potential of mesenchymal stem cell therapy for chronic lung disease. Expert Rev Respir Med. 2020;14(1):31-39. doi: 10.1080/17476348.2020.1679628.

[131] Abraham A, Krasnodembskaya A. Mesenchymal stem cell-derived extracellular vesicles for the treatment

of acute respiratory distress syndrome. Stem Cells Transl Med. 2020;9(1):28-38. doi: 10.1002/sctm.19-0205.

[132] Aggarwal S, Pittenger MF. Human mesenchymal stem cells modulate allogeneic immune cell responses. Blood. 2005;105(4):1815-1822. doi: 10.1182/blood-2004-04-1559.

[133] Chan MC, Kuok DI, Leung CY, Hui KP, Valkenburg SA, Lau EH, et.al. Human mesenchymal stromal cells reduce influenza A H5N1-associated acute lung injury in vitro and in vivo. Proc Natl Acad Sci U S A. 2016;113(13):3621-3626. doi: 10.1073/pnas.1601911113.

[134] Chen J, Hu C, Chen L, et.al. Clinical Study of Mesenchymal Stem Cell Treatment for Acute Respiratory Distress Syndrome Induced by Epidemic Influenza A (H7N9) Infection: A Hint for COVID-19 Treatment. Engineering (Beijing). 2020;6(10):1153-1161. doi: 10.1016/j.eng.2020.02.006.

[135] Golchin A, Farahany TZ, et.al. The Clinical Trials of Mesenchymal Stem Cell Therapy in Skin Diseases: An Update and Concise Review. Curr Stem Cell Res Ther. 2019;14(1):22-33. doi: 10.2174/1574888X13666180913123424.

[136] Leng Z, Zhu R, Hou W, et.al. Transplantation of ACE2- Mesenchymal Stem Cells Improves the Outcome of Patients with COVID-19 Pneumonia. Aging Dis. 2020;11(2):216-228. doi: 10.14336/AD.2020.0228.

[137] Li Y, Liu S, Zhang S. et.al. Current treatment approaches for COVID-19 and the clinical value of transfusion-related technologies. Transfus Apher Sci. 2020;59(5):102839. doi: 10.1016/j.transci.2020.102839.

[138] Shi Y, Wang Y, Li Q, et.al. Immunoregulatory mechanisms of mesenchymal stem and stromal cells in inflammatory diseases. Nat Rev Nephrol. 2018;14(8):493-507. doi: 10.1038/s41581-018-0023-5.

[139] Willis GR, Fernandez-Gonzalez A, et.al. Mesenchymal Stromal Cell Exosomes Ameliorate Experimental Bronchopulmonary Dysplasia and Restore Lung Function through Macrophage Immunomodulation. Am J Respir Crit Care Med. 2018;197(1):104-116. doi: 10.1164/rccm.201705-0925OC.

[140] Chen QH, Wu F, Liu L, Chen HB, et.al. Mesenchymal stem cells regulate the Th17/Treg cell balance partly through hepatocyte growth factor in vitro. Stem Cell Res Ther. 2020;11(1):91. doi: 10.1186/s13287-020-01612-y.

[141] Corcione A, Benvenuto F, Ferretti E, et.al. Human mesenchymal stem cells modulate B-cell functions. Blood. 2006;107(1):367-372. doi: 10.1182/blood-2005-07-2657.

[142] de Witte SFH, Luk F, Sierra, et.al. Immunomodulation By Therapeutic Mesenchymal Stromal Cells (MSC) Is Triggered Through Phagocytosis of MSC By Monocytic Cells. Stem Cells. 2018;36(4):602-615. doi: 10.1002/stem.2779.

[143] Prockop DJ. Concise review: two negative feedback loops place mesenchymal stem/stromal cells at the center of early regulators of inflammation. Stem Cells. 2013;31(10):2042-2046. doi: 10.1002/stem.1400.

[144] Lu Z, Chang W, Meng S, Xu X, et.al.Mesenchymal stem cells induce dendritic cell immune tolerance via paracrine hepatocyte growth factor to alleviate acute lung injury. Stem Cell Res Ther. 2019 Dec 4;10(1):372. doi: 10.1186/s13287-019-1488-2.

[145] Liu J, Li S, Liu J, Liang B, Wang X, et.al. Longitudinal characteristics of lymphocyte responses and cytokine profiles in the peripheral blood

of SARS-CoV-2 infected patients. EBioMedicine. 2020;55:102763. doi: 10.1016/j.ebiom.2020.102763.

[146] Chousterman BG, Swirski FK, Weber GF. Cytokine storm and sepsis disease pathogenesis. Semin Immunopathol. 2017;39(5):517-528. doi: 10.1007/s00281-017-0639-8

[147] Chen X, Zhao B, Qu Y, Chen Y, et.al. Detectable Serum Severe Acute Respiratory Syndrome Coronavirus 2 Viral Load (RNAemia) Is Closely Correlated With Drastically Elevated Interleukin 6 Level in Critically Ill Patients With Coronavirus Disease 2019. Clin Infect Dis. 2020;5;71(8):1937-1942. doi: 10.1093/cid/ciaa449.

[148] Shao M, Xu Q, Wu Z, Chen Y, et.al. Exosomes derived from human umbilical cord mesenchymal stem cells ameliorate IL-6-induced acute liver injury through miR-455-3p. Stem Cell Res Ther. 2020 Jan 23;11(1):37. doi: 10.1186/s13287-020-1550-0.

[149] Cruz FF, Rocco PRM. The potential of mesenchymal stem cell therapy for chronic lung disease. Expert Rev Respir Med. 2020;14(1):31-39. doi: 10.1080/17476348.2020.1679628.

[150] Iyer SS, Co C, Rojas M. Mesenchymal stem cells and inflammatory lung diseases. Panminerva Med. 2009;51(1):5-16.

[151] Lu Z, Chang W, Meng S, Xu X, Xie J, et.al. Mesenchymal stem cells induce dendritic cell immune tolerance via paracrine hepatocyte growth factor to alleviate acute lung injury. Stem Cell Res Ther. 2019;10(1):372. doi: 10.1186/s13287-019-1488-2.

[152] Chousterman BG, Swirski FK, Weber GF. Cytokine storm and sepsis disease pathogenesis. Semin Immunopathol. 2017 Jul;39(5):517-528. doi: 10.1007/s00281-017-0639-8.

[153] Monsel A, Zhu YG, Gennai S, Hao Q, et.al. Therapeutic Effects of Human Mesenchymal Stem Cell-derived Microvesicles in Severe Pneumonia in Mice. Am J Respir Crit Care Med. 2015 Aug 1;192(3):324-336. doi: 10.1164/rccm.201410-1765OC.

[154] Xu Z, Shi L, Wang Y, Zhang J, Huang L, et.al. Pathological findings of COVID-19 associated with acute respiratory distress syndrome. Lancet Respir Med. 2020;8(4):420-422. doi: 10.1016/S2213-2600(20)30076-X. Epub 2020 Feb 18. Erratum in: Lancet Respir Med. 2020 Feb 25.

[155] Predictive technology group addresses use of mesenchymal stem cells in treatment of secondary issues related to coronavirus. GlobeNewswire, Access at: March 17, 2020.Available at: https: //finance.yahoo.com/news/predictive-tech nology-group-addressesmesenchymal-154552966.html

[156] Krasnodembskaya A, Song Y, Fang X, et.al. Antibacterial effect of human mesenchymal stem cells is mediated in part from secretion of the antimicrobial peptide LL-37. Stem Cells. 2010;28(12):2229-2238. doi: 10.1002/stem.544.

[157] Sutton MT, Fletcher D, Ghosh SK, Weinberg A, van Heeckeren R, et.al. Antimicrobial Properties of Mesenchymal Stem Cells: Therapeutic Potential for Cystic Fibrosis Infection, and Treatment. Stem Cells Int. 2016;2016:5303048. doi: 10.1155/2016/5303048.

[158] Alcayaga-Miranda F, Cuenca J, Khoury M. Antimicrobial Activity of Mesenchymal Stem Cells: Current Status and New Perspectives of Antimicrobial Peptide-Based Therapies. Front Immunol. 2017;8:339. doi: 10.3389/fimmu.2017.00339.

[159] Ji F, Li L, Li Z, Jin Y, Liu W. Mesenchymal stem cells as a potential

treatment for critically ill patients with coronavirus disease 2019. Stem Cells Transl Med. 2020 Jul;9(7):813-814. doi: 10.1002/sctm.20-0083.

[160] Khoury M, Cuenca J, Cruz FF, et.al. Current status of cell-based therapies for respiratory virus infections: applicability to COVID-19. Eur Respir J. 2020;55(6):2000858. doi: 10.1183/13993003.00858-2020.

[161] Liang B, Chen J, Li T, Wu H, Yang W, Li Y, Li J, Yu C, Nie F, Ma Z, et.al. Clinical remission of a critically ill COVID-19 patient treated by human umbilical cord mesenchymal stem cells: A case report. Medicine (Baltimore). 2020 Jul 31;99(31):e21429. doi: 10.1097/MD.0000000000021429.

[162] Yao D, Ye H, Huo Z, Wu L, Wei S. Mesenchymal stem cell research progress for the treatment of COVID-19. J Int Med Res. 2020 Sep;48(9):300060520955063. doi: 10.1177/0300060520955063.,

[163] Bamba C, Singh SP, Choudhury S. Can mesenchymal stem cell therapy be the interim management of COVID-19? Drug Discov Ther. 2020 Jul 15;14(3):139-142. doi: 10.5582/ddt.2020.03032.

[164] Qu W, Wang Z, Hare JM, Bu G, Mallea JM, Pascual JM, Caplan AI, et.al. Cell-based therapy to reduce mortality from COVID-19: Systematic review and meta-analysis of human studies on acute respiratory distress syndrome. Stem Cells Transl Med. 2020;9(9):1007-1022. doi: 10.1002/sctm.20-0146.

[165] Bydon M, Dietz AB, Goncalves S. et.al. CELLTOP Clinical Trial: First Report From a Phase 1 Trial of Autologous Adipose Tissue-Derived Mesenchymal Stem Cells in the Treatment of Paralysis Due to Traumatic Spinal Cord Injury. Mayo Clin Proc. 2020 Feb;95(2):406-414. doi: 10.1016/j.mayocp.2019.10.008.

[166] Heldman AW, DiFede DL, Fishman JE, Zambrano JP, Trachtenberg BH, et.al. Transendocardial mesenchymal stem cells and mononuclear bone marrow cells for ischemic cardiomyopathy: the TAC-HFT randomized trial. JAMA. 2014 Jan 1;311(1):62-73. doi: 10.1001/jama.2013.282909.

[167] Saad A, Dietz AB, Herrmann SMS, Hickson LJ, Glockner JF, McKusick MA, et.al. Autologous Mesenchymal Stem Cells Increase Cortical Perfusion in Renovascular Disease. J Am Soc Nephrol. 2017 Sep;28(9):2777-2785. doi: 10.1681/ASN.2017020151.

[168] Dozois EJ, Lightner AL, Mathis KL, Chua HK, Kelley SR, Fletcher JG, et.al. Early Results of a Phase I Trial Using an Adipose-Derived Mesenchymal Stem Cell-Coated Fistula Plug for the Treatment of Transsphincteric Cryptoglandular Fistulas. Dis *Colon rectum*. 2019;62(5):615-622. doi: 10.1097/DCR.0000000000001333.

[169] Keller CA, Gonwa TA, Hodge DO, Hei DJ, Centanni JM, Zubair AC. Feasibility, Safety, and Toleranceof Mesenchymal Stem Cell Therapy for Obstructive Chronic Lung Allograft Dysfunction. Stem Cells Transl Med. 2018;7(2):161-167. doi: 10.1002/sctm.17-0198.

[170] Glassberg MK, Minkiewicz J, Toonkel RL, Simonet ES, Rubio GA, et.al. Allogeneic Human Mesenchymal Stem Cells in Patients With Idiopathic Pulmonary Fibrosis via Intravenous Delivery (AETHER): A Phase I Safety Clinical Trial. Chest. 2017;151(5):971-981. doi: 10.1016/j.chest.2016.10.061.

[171] Arentz M, Yim E, Klaff L, Lokhandwala S, Riedo FX, Chong M, Lee M. Characteristics and Outcomes of 21 Critically Ill Patients With COVID-19 in Washington State. JAMA. 2020 Apr 28;323(16):1612-1614. doi: 10.1001/jama.2020.4326.

[172] Kamen DL, Nietert PJ, Wang H, et.al. CT-04 safety and efficacy of allogeneic umbilical cord-derived mesenchymal stem cells (MSCs) in patients with systemic lupus erythematosus: results of an open-label phase I study. Lupus Sci Med. 2018; 5:46-47.

[173] Connick P, Kolappan M, Crawley C, Webber DJ, Patani R, et.al. Autologous mesenchymal stem cells for the treatment of secondary progressive multiple sclerosis: an open-label phase 2a proof-of-concept study. Lancet Neurol. 2012;11(2):150-156. doi: 10.1016/S1474-4422(11)70305-2.

[174] Hashmi S, Ahmed M, Murad MH, et.al. Survival after mesenchymal stromal cell therapy in steroid-refractory acute graft-versus-host disease: systematic review and meta-analysis. Lancet Haematol. 2016;3(1):e45–e52. doi: 10.1016/S2352-3026(15)00224-0.

[175] Yip HK, Fang WF, Li YC, et.al. Human Umbilical Cord-Derived Mesenchymal Stem Cells for Acute Respiratory Distress Syndrome. Crit Care Med. 2020;48(5):e391-e399. doi: 10.1097/CCM.0000000000004285.

[176] Li Z, Wu M, Guo J, et al. Caution on Kidney Dysfunctions of COVID-19 Patients. https://ssrn.com/abstract=3559601 or https://doi.org/10.2139/ssrn.3559601. Accessed 26 Dec 2020.

[177] Matthay MA, Calfee CS, Zhuo H, et.al. Treatment with allogeneic mesenchymal stromal cells for moderate to severe acute respiratory distress syndrome (START study): a randomised phase 2a safety trial. Lancet Respir Med. 2019 Feb;7(2):154-162. doi: 10.1016/S2213-2600(18)30418-1.

[178] Thakkar UG, Trivedi HL, Vanikar AV, Dave SD. Insulin-secreting adipose-derived mesenchymal stromal cells with bone marrow-derived hematopoietic stem cells from autologous and allogenic sources for type 1 diabetes mellitus. Cytotherapy. 2015;17(7):940-947. doi: 10.1016/j.jcyt.2015.03.608.

[179] Cho J, D'Antuono M, Glicksman M, Wang J, Jonklaas J. A review of clinical trials: mesenchymal stem cell transplant therapy in type 1 and type 2 diabetes mellitus. Am J Stem Cells. 2018 Oct 1;7(4):82-93.

[180] Xu P, Yang X. The Efficacy and Safety of Mesenchymal Stem Cell Transplantation for Spinal Cord Injury Patients: A Meta-Analysis and Systematic Review. Cell Transplant. 2019;28(1):36-46. doi: 10.1177/0963689718808471.

[181] Zebin L, Qian F, Jinlian M, Lishi Z, Yu Q, Tian C. et al. The nucleocapsid protein of SARS-CoV-2 abolished pluripotency in human induced pluripotent stem cells. bioRxiv. 2020. doi: 10.1101/2020.03.26.010694

[182] Irmak DK, Darıcı H, Karaöz E. Stem Cell Based Therapy Option in COVID-19: Is It Really Promising? J.Aging and disease, 2020; 11(5): 1174-1191 DOI: 10.14336/AD.2020.0608

[183] Abdi R, Fiorina P, Adra CN, Atkinson M, Sayegh MH. Immunomodulation by mesenchymal stem cells: a potential therapeutic strategy for type 1 diabetes. Diabetes. 2008;57(7):1759-1767. doi: 10.2337/db08-0180.

[184] Wada N, Gronthos S, Bartold PM. Immunomodulatory effects of stem cells. Periodontol 2000. 2013 Oct;63(1):198-216. doi: 10.1111/prd.12024.

[185] Mahla RS. Stem Cells Applications in Regenerative Medicine and Disease Therapeutics. Int J Cell

Biol. 2016;2016:6940283. doi: 10.1155/2016/6940283.

[186] Bhattacharya J, Matthay MA. Regulation and repair of the alveolar-capillary barrier in acute lung injury. Annu Rev Physiol. 2013;75:593-615. doi: 10.1146/annurev-physiol-030212-183756.

[187] Aghai ZH, Kode A, Saslow JG, Nakhla T, Farhath S, et.aI. Azithromycin suppresses activation of nuclear factor-kappa B and synthesis of pro-inflammatory cytokines in tracheal aspirate cells from premature infants. Pediatr Res. 2007;62(4):483-488. doi: 10.1203/PDR.0b013e318142582d.

[188] Bouwman JJ, Visseren FL, Bouter PK, Diepersloot RJ. Azithromycin inhibits interleukin-6 but not fibrinogen production in hepatocytes infected with cytomegalovirus and chlamydia pneumoniae. J Lab Clin Med. 2004 Jul;144(1):18-26. doi: 10.1016/j.lab.2004.03.012.

[189] Gielen V, Johnston SL, Edwards MR. Azithromycin induces anti-viral responses in bronchial epithelial cells. Eur Respir J. 2010 Sep;36(3):646-654. doi: 10.1183/09031936.00095809.

[190] Armitage J, Tan DBA, Troedson R, Young P et.al. Stromal cell infusion modulates systemic immunological responses in stable COPD patients: a phase I pilot study. Eur Respir J. 2018 Mar 1;51(3):1702369. doi: 10.1183/13993003.02369-2017.

[191] Galipeau J, Sensébé L. Mesenchymal Stromal Cells: Clinical Challenges and Therapeutic Opportunities. Cell Stem Cell. 2018 Jun 1;22(6):824-833. doi: 10.1016/j.stem.2018.05.004.

[192] Lee RH, Pulin AA, Seo MJ, Kota DJ, Ylostalo J, et.al. Intravenous hMSCs improve myocardial infarction in mice because cells embolized in lung are activated to secrete the anti-inflammatory protein TSG-6. Cell Stem Cell. 2009 Jul 2;5(1):54-63. doi: 10.1016/j.stem.2009.05.003.

[193] Krasnodembskaya A, Song Y, Fang X, et.al. Antibacterial effect of human mesenchymal stem cells is mediated in part from secretion of the antimicrobial peptide LL-37. Stem Cells. 2010;28(12):2229-2238. doi: 10.1002/stem.544.

[194] Hu S, Park J, Liu A, et al. Mesenchymal stem cell microvesicles restore protein permeability across primary cultures of injured human lung microvascular endothelial cells. Stem Cells Transl Med 2018; 7: 615-624.

[195] Court AC, Le-Gatt A, L uz-Crawford P, Parra E, Aliaga-Tobar V,et.al. Mitochondrial transfer from MSCs to T cells induces Treg differentiation and restricts inflammatory response. EMBO Rep. 2020 Feb 5;21(2):e48052. doi: 10.15252/embr.201948052.

[196] Islam MN, Das SR, Emin MT, Wei M, Sun L, et.al. Mitochondrial transfer from bone-marrow-derived stromal cells to pulmonary alveoli protects against acute lung injury. Nat Med. 2012;18(5):759-765. doi: 10.1038/nm.2736.

[197] Liotta F, Angeli R, Cosmi L, Filì L, Manuelli C, Frosali F, Mazzinghi B, et.al. Toll-like receptors 3 and 4 are expressed by human bone marrow-derived mesenchymal stem cells and can inhibit their T-cell modulatory activity by impairing Notch signaling. Stem Cells. 2008;26(1):279-289. doi: 10.1634/stemcells.2007-0454.

[198] Waterman RS, Tomchuck SL, Henkle SL, Betancourt AM. A new mesenchymal stem cell (MSC) paradigm: polarization into a pro-inflammatory

MSC1 or an Immunosuppressive MSC2 phenotype. PLoS One. 2010 Apr 26;5(4):e10088. doi: 10.1371/journal.pone.0010088.

[199] Lee JW, Krasnodembskaya A, McKenna DH, et.al. Therapeutic effects of human mesenchymal stem cells in ex vivo human lungs injured with live bacteria. Am J Respir Crit Care Med. 2013;187(7):751-760. doi: 10.1164/rccm.201206-0990OC.

[200] Monsel A, Zhu YG, Gennai S, Hao Q, Hu S, Ret.al. Therapeutic Effects of Human Mesenchymal Stem Cell-derived Microvesicles in Severe Pneumonia in Mice. Am J Respir Crit Care Med. 2015;192(3):324-336. doi: 10.1164/rccm.201410-1765OC.

[201] Curley GF, Ansari B, Hayes M, Devaney J, Masterson C, et.al. Effects of intratracheal mesenchymal stromal cell therapy during recovery and resolution after ventilator-induced lung injury. Anesthesiology. 2013 Apr;118(4):924-932. doi: 10.1097/ALN.0b013e318287ba08.

[202] Kim SY, Chrzanowski W. "Stem cell delivery systems and devices – spraying," in Stem Cell-Based Therapy for Lung Disease, eds J. Burgess and I. Heijink (Cham: Springer), 2019:241-253. doi: 10.1007/978-3-030-29403-8_13

[203] Kim SY, Joglekar MV, Hardikar AA, Phan TH, et.al. Placenta Stem/Stromal Cell-Derived Extracellular Vesicles for Potential Use in Lung Repair. Proteomics. 2019;19(17):e1800166. doi: 10.1002/pmic.201800166.

[204] Skolasinski S, Timm M, Meyer C, Zeeshan S, Naqwi A. Mortari, A. Lung bioengineering and direct pulmonary cell therapy using a novel airway spray device. Am. J. Respir. Crit. Care.Med. 2020:201:A7634.

Chapter 19

Repurposed Therapeutic Strategies towards COVID-19 Potential Targets Based on Genomics and Protein Structure Remodeling

Ashok K. Singh, Aakansha Singh and Ankit Kumar Dubey

Abstract

Target recognition is important for the identification of drugs with a high target specificity and/or for the development of existing drugs that could be replicated for the treatment of SARS-CoV-2 infections. Since SARS-CoV-2 is a pathogen recently discovered, no specific medicines have been identified or are available at present. The scientific community had proposed list of current drugs with therapeutic potential for COVID-19 on the basis of genomic sequence information coupled with protein structure modeling, posing an effective and productive therapeutic approach for repurposing existing drugs. The possible therapeutics for the treatment of COVID-19 involves a wide range of alternatives, encompassing nucleic acid-based treatments directed at the expression of genes of viruses, cytokine therapy, genetic engineered and vectored antibodies, and different formulations of vaccines. The future prospective in the treatment approaches the exploration of antiviral therapy, such as screening of prevailing molecules or libraries, testing of existing broad-spectrum antiviral medications, modern drug discovery focused on genomic knowledge and biochemical properties of various coronaviruses to create new targeted drugs.

Keywords: SARS-CoV-2, drug repurposing, molecular docking, mRNA vaccine, monoclonal Antibodies

1. Introduction

The challenge of the epidemic outbreak has reached alarming levels, shocking national healthcare systems to unpreparedness and causing international deployment. No drug therapy has been found to be effective in the treatment of the virus, despite COVID-19 being declared a global pandemic by the World Health Organization (WHO). In contrast, several randomized controlled trials conducted towards treatment have not yet provided practical guidance on therapeutic choices and pharmacologic therapy. Several successful research tests for therapy are currently underway. Other emerging, non-conventional drug discovery approaches include alternative ways to discover potent anti-SARS-CoV2 drugs that are quicker and less expensive. In addition, while drugs for COVID-19 are being repurposed and discovered, new drug delivery systems will play a major role in developing effective delivery systems that have the potential to attack viruses, enhance physico-chemical characteristics, and avoid possible drug resistance that contributes to superior therapies. The best way to produce pharmaceutical drugs that cure SARS-CoV-2 is to find potential molecules from the medicines available for sale [1].

Coronavirus disease 19 (COVID-19) is a remarkably highly contagious and pathogenic infectious disease caused by severe acute respiratory syndrome- coronavirus-2 (SARS-CoV-2), which originated in Wuhan, China in December 2019 and spread worldwide. The infectibility of these viruses could only be in the wild before the outbreak of extreme acute respiratory syndrome (SARS) in 2002 and middle-eastern respiratory syndrome (MERS) in 2012 as spotted by the world. While the disease dissipated across the globe throughout the natural environment, the mode of transmission to humans from the wild was insignificant and still unknown. Analysis of the whole genome sequence of the bats, however, was shown to be 96% similar with a severe acute respiratory syndrome-like (SARS-like) bat virus and 79.5% comparable with SARS-CoV, indicating that it is the possible route of transmission to humans [2]. There are four genera of CoVs: Alphacoronavirus, Betacoronavirus (βCoV), Gammacoronavirus, and Deltacoronavirus. Two new βCoVs, extreme acute respiratory syndrome CoV (SARS-CoV) and Middle East respiratory syndrome CoV (MERS-CoV), have appeared over the past 12 years, and these viruses can cause significant human illnesses. The absence of adequate drug treatment and related elevated morbidity and death rates of these two CoVs, as well as their ability to cause epidemics, illustrate the need for innovative drug development for the prevention of diseases of CoV [3].

2. Genomic characterization of SARS-CoV-2

The size of the genome of the coronavirus ranges from 26 to 32 kb and contains 6 to 11 open reading frames (ORFs) encoding polyproteins with 9680 amino acids [4]. About 80 percent of the SARS-CoV-2 genome has been studied to be similar to the previous human coronavirus (SARS-like bat CoV) while, notable differences in SARS-CoV and SARS-CoV-2 genome have been reported in various studies, such as the lack of 8a protein and perturbations in the number of amino acids in 8b and 3c protein in SARS-CoV-2 [5]. The SARS-CoV2 genome is a polycistronic single-stranded RNA (+ssRNA) with a 5′-cap structure and 3′-poly-A tail (~30 kb), utilized as a template for translating polyproteins (pp1a/pp1ab) into the replication/transcription machinery (RTM) of a double membrane vesicle (**Figure 1**) (6) [6]. RTM subsequently synthesizes a nested set of subgenomic RNAs (sgRNAs) in a discontinuous manner. These subgenomic messenger RNAs (mRNAs) have standard 5′-leader and 3′-terminal sequences between open reading frames (ORFs) on transcription regulatory sequences, where transcription termination and subsequent acquisition of a leader RNA occurs. Such minus-strand sgRNAs serve as models for subgenomic mRNA growth. At least six ORFs comprise the genome and subgenomes of a standard CoVs [7].

For the ORFs from the 5′ end, a region of about 20 kb corresponds to the two ORFs; ORF1a and ORF1b encoding 11 and 5 non-structural proteins: nsp1 to nsp11 and nsp12 to 16, respectively. The largest SARS CoV2 ORF1 gene (about two-thirds of the total length of the gene) contains −1 frameshift between ORF1a and ORF1b, resulting in the formation of two conserved polypeptide domains: pp1a and pp1ab. The ribosomal frameshift is involved in the translation of ORF1a directly from the RNA genome, near to the bottom of ORF1, which contains one ORF1ab polypeptide. There are ORFs encoding a few to more than ten structural/non-structural proteins downstream from the ORF1ab [8]. In ORF1ab as well as in other ORFs, CoVs

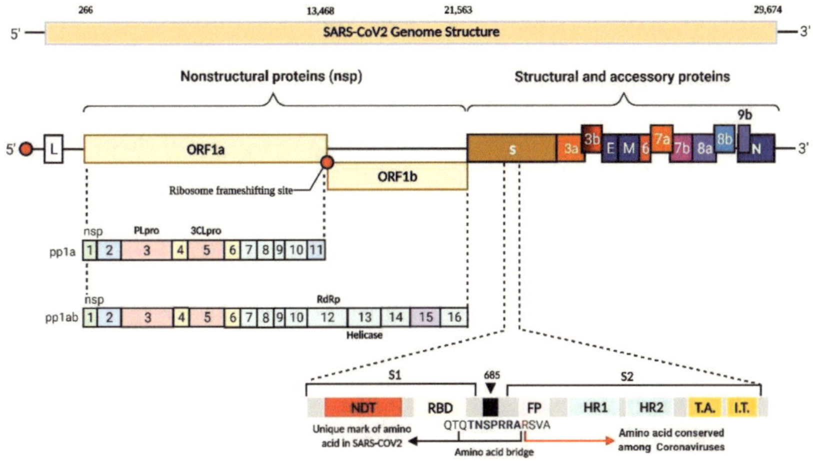

Figure 1.
Genomic organization of SARS-CoV-2. Schematic genomic structure of SARS-CoV-2 based on the SARS-CoV-2 Wuhan-Hu-1. The genome is categorized into two domains: Non-structural proteins and structural and accessory proteins. The S protein contains an S1 and S2 subunit, which are divided by the S cleavage site. Abbreviations: ORF, open reading frame; S, spike; E, envelope; M, membrane; N, nucleocapsid; NTD, N-terminal domain; RBD, receptor-binding domain; FP, fusion peptide; HR1 & 2, heptad repeat 1 and heptad repeat 2, containing the core binding motif in the external subdomain; TA, transmembrane anchor; IT, intracellular tail.

often code different non-structural proteins, particularly near the 3′ end, although the specifics of the exact genes in the SARS-CoV-2 genome are still unclear primarily due to overlapping genes encoded in a different coding frame [9]. Two viral proteases, papain-like protease (PLpro) and 3C-like protease (3CLpro), are cleaved by the large replicase polyprotein 1a (pp1a) and pp1ab encoded by the 5 terminal open reading frame 1a/b (ORF1a/b) to produce non-structural proteins (NSPs) [10]. The NSPs contain two viral cysteine proteases (nsp3), chymotrypsin like, 3C like, or main protease (nsp5), RNA-dependent RNA polymerase (nsp12), helicase (nsp13) and others that may be involved in SARS-CoV-2 transcription and replication. [4]. In addition, four major structural proteins are coded by ORFs on a third of the genome near the 3′ terminus: spike (S), membrane (M), envelope (E), and nucleocapsid (N) proteins (**Figure 2**). Different CoVs encode unique structural and accessory proteins, such as HE protein, 3a/b protein, and 4a/b protein, in addition to these four major structural proteins. The sgRNAs of CoVs is translated back from both these structural and accessory proteins [11–13].

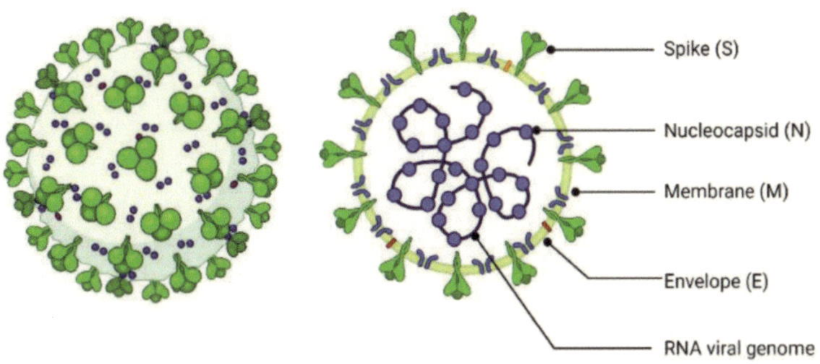

Figure 2.
The virion structure of SARS-CoV-2. The spike (S), envelope (E), membrane (M) proteins form the envelope of the CoV, and the nucleocapsid (N) proteins form the capsid to pack the genomic RNA.

3. Structural insights of potential SARS-CoV-2 proteins

The structural research was initiated by studying in silico modeling Wuhan-Hu1 market seafood pneumonia virus genome [14, 15]. Focused on reported studies on SARS-CoV-2, we highlighted the number of nsp structures of this virus available: the papain-like protease (PLpro, nsp3; PDB code: 7D47), the main protease (3CLpro, nsp5; PDB code: 6LZE), the RNA-dependent RNA polymerase (RdRp, nsp12) in complex with cofactors nsp7 and nsp8 (PDB code: 6M71), the helicase (nsp 13; PDB code: 6ZSL), the Spike glycoprotein (S) (PDB code: 6XR8) and the RNA binding domain of nucleocapsid (N) phosphoprotein (PDB code: 6VYO).

3.1 SARS CoV2 nsp3 PLpro

For SARS-CoV2, the papain-like proteinase (PLpro) domain is included in nsp3 (1945 amino acids; located in the polyprotein, from 818 to 2819 aa), a 217.28 kDa membrane-associated replicase product [16]. Nsp3 consists of two transmembrane regions and approximately 10–16 recognizable domains, nine of which are conserved, responsible for cleavages at the polyprotein replicate's N-terminus and assembly of viral-induced double-membrane cytoplasmic vesicles and viral replication, with nsp4 (**Figure 3**). It prevents the holding of NF-kappa-B signals. The inhibition of IRF3 host phosphorylation and dimerization and subsequent nuclear translocation was antagonized with type 1 interferon innate immune stimulation [17]. Additionally, PLpro has a deubiquitinating/deISGyling activity and processes cellular substrates from both 'Lys-48'-and' Lys-63′-linked polyubiquitin chains [18]. The role of Nsp3 is important to CoV replication and its domains include several predicted or demonstrated RNA replication accessories, such as ssRNA binding and unwinding domains, as well as those for which no separate function has yet been determined [19], cleaves ISG15 in vitro preferentially from substrates and utilizes host ADP-ribosylation to bind ADP-ribose [20].

3.2 SARS CoV2 nsp5 M^{pro}

The SARS-CoV-2 nsp5 contains 306 amino acids (located in the replicase polyprotein pp1ab, 3264 to 3569 aa), a 33.8-kDa main protease (M^{pro}), which is also referred to as 3C-like protease ($3CL^{pro}$) [21, 22]. The active site in SARS-CoV2 M^{pro} organized in between Domain I (8–99 aa) and Domain II (100–183 aa) was shown to be structurally similar to SARS-CoV M^{pro}. Both domains contribute one residue to the catalytic dyad (His41 and Cys145), linked to the helical domain IIII (200–306 aa)

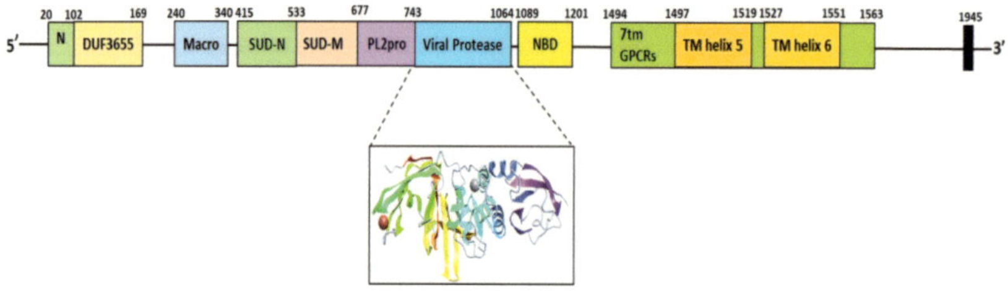

Figure 3.
Overview of the SARS-CoV2 nsp3 structural and genomic organization along with crystal structure of SARS-CoV-2 papain-like protease (PLpro). (PDB ID: 7D47). Abbreviations: DUF3655, protein of unknown function; macro, macro domain; SUD-N, SARS-unique domain binding G-quadruplexes; SUD-M, single-stranded poly(a) binding domain; PL2pro, coronavirus polyprotein cleavage domain; viral protease, papain like viral protease; NBD, nucleic-acid binding domain; 7tm GPCRs, seven-transmembrane G protein-coupled receptor superfamily; TM helix 5&6, transmembrane helix 5&6.

by a long loop region (184–199 aa) (**Figure 4**) [6]. Several co-crystalized SARS-M^{pro} structures bound with inhibitors, 11a and 11b (6LZE), I2 (2D2D), N1 (1WOF), N3 (2AMQ), and N9 (2AMD), revealed the position of S1, S2, and S4 subsites, especially in the active site close to His41 and Cys145, which is crucial for substrate recognition containing the core sequence [ILMVF]-Q-|-[SGACN] along with Tyr161 and His163 in the substrate-binding pocket [23]. Studies have estimated that the M^{pro} pp1ab protein has at least 11 conserved restriction sites, beginning with its autolytic cleavage site and even able to bind ADP-ribose-1′ [24, 25].

3.3 SARS CoV2 nsp12 RdRp

The SARS-CoV-2 nsp12 is a key component of the replication/transcription machinery sharing a strong structural homology with nsp12 of SARS-CoV, indicating that its function and mode of action may be well conserved [26]. SARS-CoV-2 nsp12, is a 106.7 kDa molecular weight protein with a chain length of 932 amino acids (located on the replicase polyprotein 1ab, 4393 to 5324 aa.), also referred to as RNA dependent RNA polymerase (RdRp) [27], has the capacity to synthesize the entire (−) RNA chains as a positive sense RNAs, as templates for additional genomic RNA (gNR) and subgenomic RNAs generation (sgRNAs) of the virus [21]. RNA-dependent RNA polymerases (RdRps) are a multi-domain protein that catalyzes polymerization of RNA-template (phosphodiesters formation between ribonucleotides), in the presence of divalent metal ions and thus play a major role in the viral replication and transcription of the SARS-CoV2 [28, 29]. The SARS-CoV-2 nsp12 (S1 to Q932) exists in complex with cofactors nsp7 (S1 to Q83) and nsp8 (A1 to Q198) heteromer with the second nsp8 attached to the distinct binding site. nsp12 contains the right-hand RdRp domain (S367 to F920) and the nidovirus-specific N-terminal β hairpin (D29 to K50) and extension domain (D60 to R249) which adopts the nidovirus RdRp-associated nucleotidyltransferase (NiRAN) architecture (**Figure 5**). The RdRp domain is divided into 3 sub-domains; the finger subdomain (L366–A581 and K621–G679), the palm subdomain (T582–P620 and T680–Q815), and the thumb subdomain (H816–E920) [30]. The nsp7-nsp8 heterodimer binding site is well conserved in the palm domain and overlaps with the functional domains of the preserved polymerase regions (fingers and thumb domains). In addition, seven preserved motifs (A-G) arranged in the polymerase active site domain, involved in template and nucleotide binding and catalysis, were also revealed by SARS-CoV-2 nsp12 structure [31]. Motif A contains the residue of classical divalent ion-binding glutamate (D) in position (618) & (623) of the conserved sequence

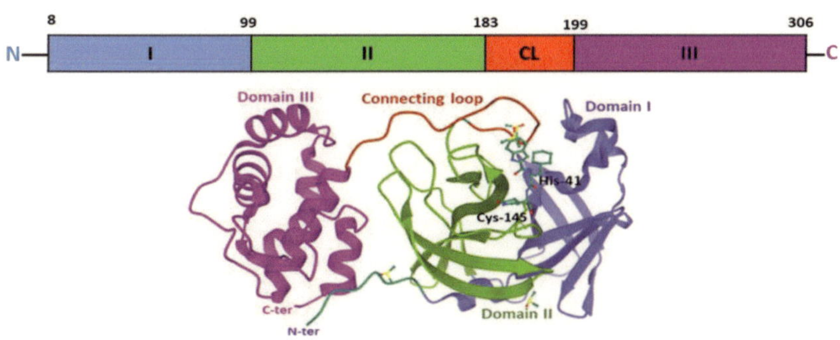

Figure 4.
Structural representation of SARS-CoV-2 M^{pro} monomer (PDB ID: 6LZE) (ribbon representation) composed of: N-terminal domain I (cornflower blue), domain II (green), and C-terminal domain III (pink). Substrate recognition site in (green and red) and catalytic dyad residues, His41 and Cys145 are highlighted and labeled.

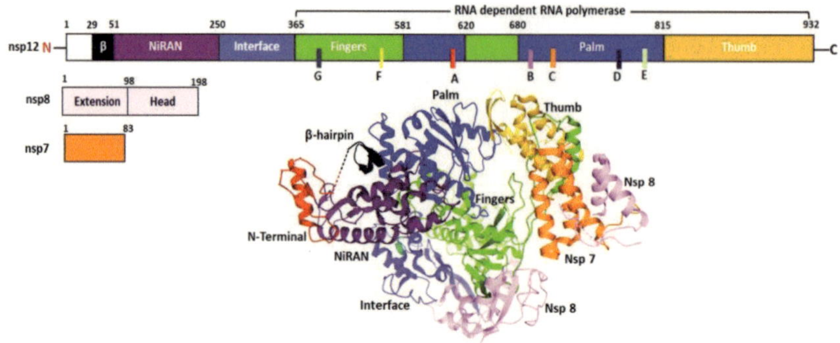

Figure 5.
Domain organization of COVID-19 virus nsp12 and structural ribbon representation of the SARS-Cov-2 RNA-dependent RNA polymerase in complex with cofactors nsp7-nsp8 (PDB ID: 6M71) displaying domains, conserved motifs (A-G), and protein regions in the structure. A broad N-terminal extension (red) consisting of the NiRAN domain (violet) and the interface domain (cornflower blue) adjacent to the polymerase domain comprises SARS-CoV nsp12-nsp7(orange)-nsp8 (light pink) complex. The interdomain borders are labeled with residue numbers.

611-TPHLMGW**D**YPKC**D**RAM-626. In motif C, (753- FSMMIL**SDD**AVVCFN-767), the catalytic residues of 759-SDD-761 (amino acids 759,760 and 761 are positioned between two β strands. Many other catalytic residues such as 317-**GDD**-319 and 327-**GDD**-329 are also conserved among other viruses [32].

3.4 SARS CoV2 nsp13 helicase

SARS-CoV-2 nsp13 is a 66.85 KDa protein, with a chain length of 601 aa. (located replicase polyprotein pp1ab, from 5325 to 5925 aa), also referred to as the Helicase [33]. SARS-CoV Nsp13 is a key enzyme in the disassembly of double stranded oligonucleotides into single strand using hydrolyzed energy of NTPs [34], having a N-terminal zinc-binding domain (ZBD) containing 3 zinc-finger motifs consisting of 2 tandem C-terminal RecA-like helicase domains (RecA1 and RecA2) and bridging stalk and 1B domains (**Figure 6**). The RecA-like domains catalyze the unwinding of the double stranded RNA and the NTP hydrolysis translocation of the complex. The stalk domain acts as a connection between the domain RecA-like/1B and the ZBD, which acts as an interface with other replicative machinery components [35, 36]. Nsp13 is strongly conserved among nidoviruses (percentage

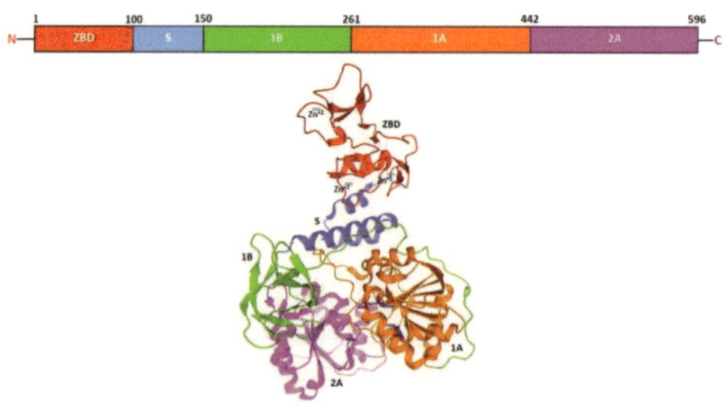

Figure 6.
Domain representation of SARS-CoV2 nsp13 and the structural ribbon representation of the SARS-CoV-2 helicase (PDB ID: 6ZSL). The interdomain borders are labeled with residue numbers. The colors of the protein domains are indicated in panel a (ZBD-red, stalk-cyan blue, 1B-green, 1A-orange and 2A-pink). Three zinc atoms are shown as black spheres. The NTPase active site (violet) consists of six residues-Lys288, Ser289, Asp374, Glu375, Gln404 and Arg567.

similarity of 99.8% with SARS-CoV, the only 1 amino acid substitution I570 V) consists of five domains that fold in a triangular pyramid shape [37]. These domains hold incredibly high conservation of protein sequences along with its essential role in viral replication, thus making it a vital target for a wide variety of therapeutics to target this viral family [38]. Helicase exhibits various enzymatic roles, including not only hydrolysis of NTPs required by the capping process, but also removal of 50–30 directionally RNA duplexes and 50-triphosphatase RNA activity. In addition, the association of Helicase nsp13 with RdRp Nsp12 promotes RNA unwinding activity and is a crucial viral replication enzyme, in all coronaviruses [39].

3.5 Spike glycoprotein (S)

The newly discovered SARS-CoV2 S-glycoprotein is a glycosylated trimer, each protomer with a chain length of 1260 amino acids (residues 14–1273), with a molecular weight of 141.1 kDa, consisting of two subunits, the surface subunit S1 and the transmembrane unit S2 [40, 41]. The surface subunit S1 is composed of 672 amino acids (residues 14–685) and differentiated into four divisions: N-terminal domain (NTD), a C-terminal domain (CTD, also known as the receptor-binding domain, RBD), and two subdomains (SD1 and SD2). The transmembrane S2 subunit is composed of 588 amino acids (residues 686–1273) and contains an N-terminal hydrophobic fusion peptide (FP), two heptad repeats (HR1 and HR2), a transmembrane anchor (TA), and an intracellular tail (IT), arranged as FP-HR1-HR2-TA-IT (**Figure 7**). A polybasic amino acid bridge (–QTQT-**NSPRRAR**-SVA-), essential for viral targeting studies, links S1 and S2 together (**Figure 1**). The SARS-CoV-2 S glycoprotein shares similar structural, topological and mechanistic features with other class I fusion proteins, including HIV envelope (Env) glycoprotein and influenza virus haemagglutinin (HA), as a standard class I viral fusion protein [42]. However, using crystallography, the actual structure of this protein can be studied. The Protein Data Bank (PDB) model of the glycoprotein shows various regions that are vital for the infection process compose the subunits [43]. Spike glycoprotein of

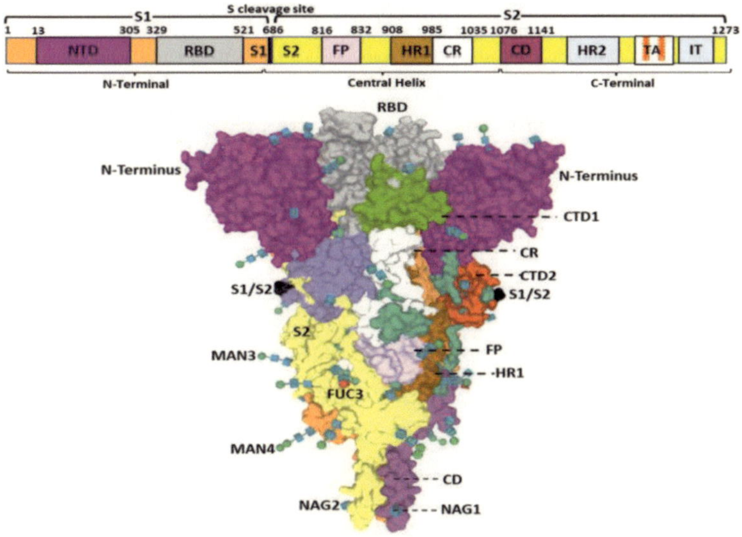

Figure 7.
Crystal structure of SARS-CoV 2 spike protein (S) PDB ID: 6XR8. Different domains of the spike protein that includes; signal sequence (SS), the N-terminal domain (NTD), receptor-binding domain (RBD), subdomain 1 and 2 (SD1&2), protease cleavage sites (S1/S2/S2′), fusion peptide (FP), heptad repeat 1 and 2 (HR1&2), central helix (CH), connector domain (CD), transmembrane anchor (TA), and intracellular tail (IT).

the Wuhan coronavirus is specified to be modified by homologous recombination which is supposed to be a combination of the SARS-CoV bat and the not identified Beta-CoV bat. The fluorescent study shows SARS-CoV-2 still uses the same ACE2 (angiotensin-converting enzyme 2) receptor and the entrance pathway previously used by SARS-CoV [44]. Both receptor binding expressed on the cell membranes of receptive cells and membrane fusion are responsible for the S protein. However, in the assembly and budding of viral particles, the proteins M and E are involved [9].

3.6 Nucleocapsid (N)

SARS-CoV-2's N (Nucleocapsid) protein is a putative RNA-binding protein responsible for gathering the viral RNA genome for encapsulation in the viral membrane into compact ribonucleoprotein (RNP) complexes [45]. N is the structural unit present in the nucleocapsid of the SARS-CoV-2 genome, 46 kDa protein and comprises of 419 amino acids (aa) containing three distinctly diverse domains: The N-terminal domain (NTD)/RNA-binding domain (46–174 aa), the serine/arginine-rich (SR-rich; 184–197 aa) linker region (LKR; 175–254 aa) and the C-terminal domain (CTD; 255–364 aa) (**Figure 8**) [46]. Both domains (NTD & CTD) are flanked by an inherently disordered region IDR, which is the central linker region (LKR) with a Ser/Arg (SR)-rich area containing alleged phosphorylation sites [47, 48]. An asymmetric unit crystal configuration of the N-terminal RNA nuclear protein binding field showed the sandwiched fold shared by the CoV N-NTD with the same right hand (loop) - (β-sheet core) - (loop), with the order β1-η1-β2- β3- β4- β5- β6- β7. The core β-sheet consists of five β-strands with just 3_{10} helix ahead of strand β2 and a β-strand between the strands β2 and β 5. The β-hairpin is functionally important in mutational analysis of amino acid residues at the RNA binding N-terminal domain of SARS-CoV2 [49]. The structures of the N-CTD RNA binding domain highlight the reserved architecture of 3_{10} helix acidic coil containing a β-sheet core of 5 antiparallel β-sheets, and an expanded β3–4 hairpin with the order η1-α1-α2-η2-α3-α4-β1-β2-α5-η3. Generally, the RNA binding domain of the N protein is essentially simple and sometimes defined as a right hand-like shape with a protruding fundamental finger, basic palm and acidic wrist [50].

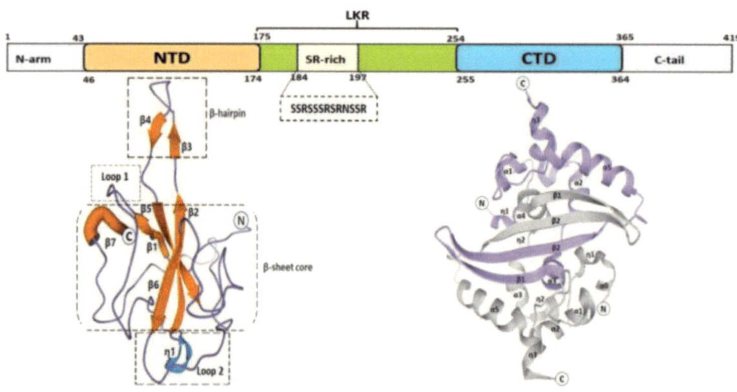

Figure 8.
Schematic representation of SARS-CoV-2 Nucleocapsid (N) protein domains. Three intrinsically disordered regions, i.e., N-arm, linker region (LKR) and C-tail, and the N-terminal domain (NTD) and C-terminal domain (CTD) are illustrated. The charged Ser/Arg (SR)-rich motif (colored light yellow) is shown. Cartoon view of the N protein NTD domain (PDB ID: 6M3M), a monomer, colored by the number variants at different positions, and CTD (PDB ID: 7C22), a heterodimer with one monomer colored gray and the other colored blue indicating various regions within the structure as observed in SARS-CoV-2 genomes.

4. Repurposing therapeutics towards SARS-CoV-2 potential targets

Therapeutics facilities aid physicians and scientist to help patients with the better cure for the disease and develop a vaccine. The production of novel therapeutics and vaccination is now at the earliest possible time to curb the epidemic. In addition, continuous attempts are being made at regional, national, and person levels to recognize the host, genomics, epidemiological interactions, and propagation modes of SARS-CoV-2 in order to control the epidemic. Scientists worldwide are actively working to establish an optimal antiviral agent and vaccine against SARS-CoV-2 [51]. One way of preventing this issue is to test two or three drugs with minimal prolixity that operate on various cellular signals with viral replication. A further approach that helps researchers to curb the variety of individual antimicrobials for emerging and re-emerging infectious diseases is the high-performance screening of host-virus interaction level composite libraries for synergistic combinations [52, 53]. Nevertheless, the screening of experimental small molecule drugs in combinations and other potent anti-SARS-CoV-22 agents with new and improved key characteristics can be effective which can be helpful in COVID-19 therapy. Potential medicines include previously used or tested medicines for diagnosing diseases and medicines recently discovered or developed. In most cases, the benefits of drug repurposing are safety evaluation, preclinical monitoring, and in some cases the development processes would not take much time and thus reduce the time needed for drug development. The chances of failure with repurposed drugs would be smaller as the early steps of medication efficacy and safety testing have already been completed and the treatment has already been shown to be sufficiently effective in a preclinical and human model [54]. Antiviral therapies are being investigated towards treatment of COVID-19 because the SARS-CoV-2 replication of leads to wide variation of the clinical manifestations. As significant functional proteins of SARS-CoV-2, Nsps and other structural and accessory proteins are involved in transcription of RNA, synthesis of protein, post-translational modification, viral duplication and contagion of the host. Among them, PLpro (nsp3), 3CLpro (nsp5), RdRp (nsp12), Helicase (nsp13), Spike glycoprotein (S) and Nucleocapsid (N) are the most important targets for the development of small-molecule inhibitors due to the enzyme active site and clear biological functions [55].

4.1 Protease inhibitors

Protease inhibitors are drugs that inhibit the activity of protease enzyme responsible for viral development, infection, and replication by cleaving it into smaller fragments. They bind to the active site of the enzyme, mediate and block the maturation of freshly formed virions [51]. Two major targets: PLpro and 3-CLpro in the replicase 1a and 1ab domain are essential component for virus reproduction and regulation of host cell response thus being the important target for the SARS-CoV-2 inhibitors (**Figure 9**). Ribavirin (SCH-18908) [NCT00578825], an antiviral drug acts on the replicase protein, preventing binding of the nucleotides, resulting in reduced viral replication or the formation of defective virions. Lopinavir [NCT04321174] and Ritonavir [NCT04330690], are protease inhibitors used to treat HIV infections by inhibiting the HIV protease enzyme to form an inhibitor-enzyme complex and proteolytic cleavage of the viral polyprotein precursors [3]. Darunavir [NCT01448707], another (HIV-1) nonpeptidic protease inhibitor with the inhibition activity of the dimerization and catalytic activity of HIV-1 protease. Saquinavir [DB01232] inhibiting HIV1/2 protease-mediated lysis of HIV gag and pol polyproteins was found cytotoxically active at conc. Above 50 μM [56]. Rupintrivir (DB05102) a broad-spectrum

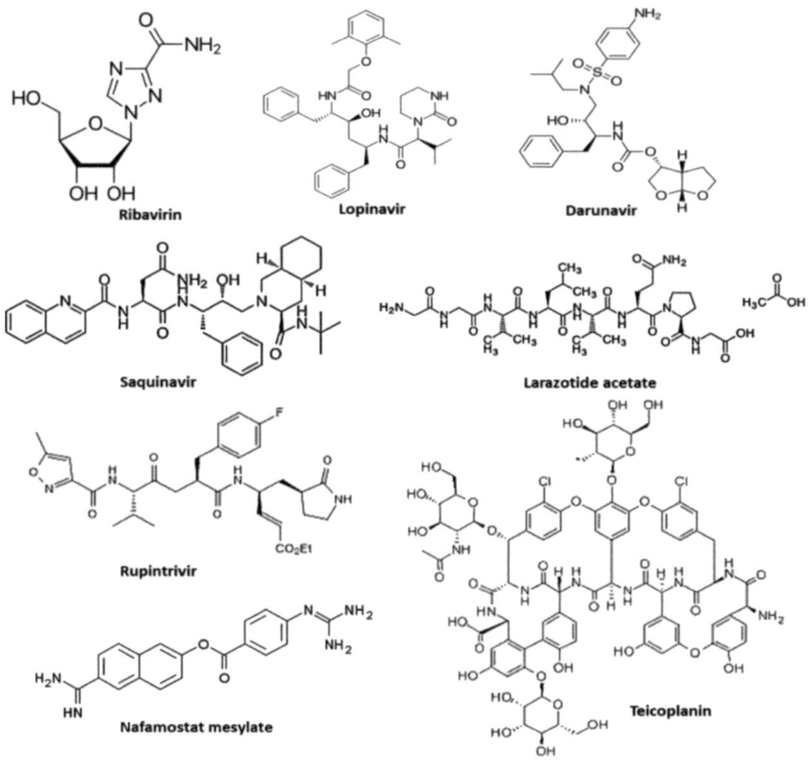

Figure 9.
Repurposed protease inhibitors for COVID-19 treatment.

antiviral agent is a potent 3C-Like protease inhibitor against norovirus, picornavirus, and coronavirus proteases in development against human rhinoviral (HRV) infections that has been recently co-crystallized with its target [57]. Larazotide acetate (AT1001) (NCT03569007) a paracellular permeability peptide inhibitor has been studied for the treatment of autoimmune diseases such as type I diabetes mellitus, gastrointestinal diseases and disorders. Studies have revealed that AT1001 potentially binds to the M^{pro} catalytic domain showing up intermolecular interactions [58]. Teicoplanin (DB06149), a glycopeptide antibiotic widely used to treat bacterial infections, has been reported to be active against SARS-CoV-2 in *in-vitro* studies inhibiting peptidoglycan polymerization, resulting in inhibition of bacterial cell wall synthesis and cell death [59, 60]. Nafamostat mesylate [NCT04418128], a clinical proven and synthetic serine protease inhibitor has been identified to inhibit the activity SARS-CoV-2 by targeting TMPRSS2-dependent host cell entry [61, 62]. However, *in-vitro* studies of active phytochemical compounds from the natural sources have revealed the SARS-CoV-2 proteolytic and inhibitory activity; Phaitanthrin D (*Isatis indigotica Fort*), Baicalin (*Scutellaria baicalensis*), Piceatannol (*Vitis vinifera*), Platycodin D (*Platycodon grandiflorus*), Betulonal (*Cassine xylocarpa*), 2b-Hydroxy-3,4-secofriedelolactone-27-oic acid (*Viola diffusa*), Cleistocaltone A (*Cleistocalyx operculatus*), Phyllaemblinol (*Phyllanthus emblica*) etc. [55].

4.2 Replicase inhibitors

RdRp is a critical non-structural protein component of the SARS-CoV-2 genome that uses a metal-ion-dependent mechanism to catalyze viral RNA synthesis. However, due to its comprehensive knowledge about the different domains and its functions, strong preservation among evolutionary RNA viruses and the lack of homologous sequences in mammalian cells; the ease progress and consequent access to biochemical assays to quickly detect large collections of compounds [63]. Remdesivir (GS-5734) [NCT04252664], a nucleoside analogue acts on the replicase polyprotein 1ab of SARS-CoV-2 genome preventing RNA polymerase function resulting in ending the transcription of RNA and reduces the production of viral RNA. Penciclovir [NCT00820534], another nucleoside analogue, synthetic acyclic guanine derivative with antiviral activity targets the RdRp inhibiting the DNA synthesis of virus-infected cells and terminating viral replication (**Figure 10**). β-D-N4-hydroxycytidine, an orally bioavailable, broad-spectrum antiviral ribonucleoside analogous to multiple RNA viruses like influenza, CoV, equine encephalitis and Ebola viruses have been found in *in-vitro* studies of antiviral effect on SARS-CoV-2 primarily through mutagenesis of viral RNA [64, 65]. Cefuroxime, an anti-bacterial drug is prescribed in patients with COVID-19, as a potential inhibitor with the ability of binding tightly to the active site of the enzyme, with a highest ICM score of −41.30, and mfscore of −63.04, which when compared to Remdesivir had a score of −27.4 and a mfscore of −113 [66] The natural products and derivatives with anti-virus, anti-inflammation and anti-tumor effects exhibited high binding affinity to RdRp, such as 14-deoxy-11,12-didehydroandrographolide (*Andrographis paniculate*), Gnidicin (*Gnidia lamprantha*), 2b,30b-dihydroxy-3,4-seco-friedelolactone-27-lactone (*V. diffusa*), Theaflavin 3,30-di-O-gallate (*Camellia sinensis*), Betulonal (*C. xylocarpa*), 1,7-dihydroxy-3- methoxyxanthone (*Swerti apseudochinensis*) [67].

SARS-CoV-2 replication enzyme, helicase has the properties of unwinding and splitting DNA and RNA into two single-stranded nucleic acids and these

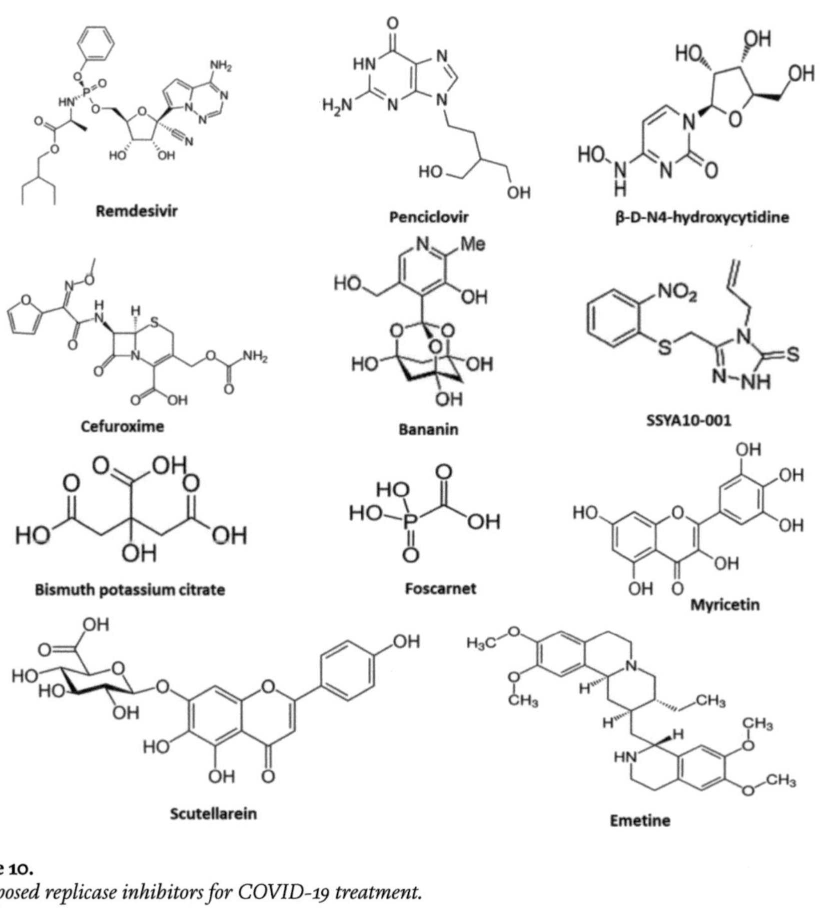

Figure 10.
Repurposed replicase inhibitors for COVID-19 treatment.

characteristic of the enzyme marks it as a potential target to be studied [68]. Bananins have been shown to inhibit SARS-CoV ATPase activity leading to inhibition of viral replication *in-vitro* with IC50 values far less than 10 mM [69] Bismuth salt, such as Bismuth potassium citrate (BPC) has been observed to dose-dependently inhibit both the NTPase and RNA helicase activities of SARS-CoV-2 nsp13. Further studies indicates that SARS-CoV-2 nsp13 may be a valuable target for antivirals, which could be beneficial in attempting to regulatory mechanism of this life-threatening virus [70]. Foscarnet, a class of antiviral drug approved for the treatment of HIV/AIDS-related cytomegalovirus (CMV) infections and herpes, functions as a pyrophosphate molecule by binding to viral DNA polymerase and preventing the elongation of the DNA chain [71]. *In vitro* studies have revealed that SSYA10–001, a small inhibitor molecule of SARS-CoV helicase, has an antiviral effect on several coronaviruses by likely targeting a conserved binding pocket in nsp13 domain and can lead the production of successful wide spectrum anti-coronavirus drugs including SARS-CoV-2 [72]. Scutellarein isolated from *Scutellaria baicalensis* has been historically used in the treatment of inflammation and respiratory diseases, and myricetin present in fruits such as cranberry and vegetables such as *Calamus scipionum* and garlic. Were found to inhibit SARS-CoV helicase (nsp13) via inhibition of ATPase activity being a potential phytochemical inhibitor [73, 74]. Emetine could be re-purposed to treat COVID-19 based on the *in-vitro* antiviral activity against SARS-CoV-2 and its ability to shield chicken embryos from IBV [75].

4.3 Structural protein inhibitors

For the entry of coronavirus into a host cell, transmembrane Spike (S) glycoprotein is essential. Fusion of the membrane and activation of the virus entry require cleavage at the S1–S2 junction and because of their vital role in the interaction between the virus and the cell receptor, spike protein can be an important potential target for antiviral agents [76]. The receptors that mediate the fusion of the S protein of SARS-CoV2 into the host cell are angiotensin converting enzyme-2 (ACE-2) and type 2 transmembrane protease serine (TMPRSS2). Cleavage via TMPRSS2 the fusion of the S protein to the ACE-2 receptor is achieved and thus are the potential drug targets in the SARS-CoV-2 therapeutics [51]. Umifenovir (Arbidol) [NCT04350684], an antiviral drug has been found to block and effectively prevent the trimerization and cell adherence and entry of SARS-CoV-2 spike glycoprotein interacting with the key residues in the target domain indicating as the potential target [77]. Griffithsin, a lectin protein has demonstrated antiviral properties and can potently inhibit viral entry and prevent binding to the S glycoprotein both in vitro and in vivo SARS-CoV infection with limited cytotoxic effects. Previous studies have shown griffithsin to inhibit MERS-CoV infectivity in *in vitro* assays without any noticeable cytotoxicity [78]. Camostat mesylate [NCT04608266] can feasible therapeutic choice for COVID-19 as it decreases the unregulated release of cytokine observed in extreme COVID-19, regardless of its antiviral function, because TMPRSS2 expression is necessary for vigorous secretion of cytokine when mice are exposed to polyIC [79]. Bromhexine hydrochloride [NCT04355026] (BRH) inhibits the viral entry of transmembrane protease serine 2 (TMPRSS2) and is potentially known to be protective against SARS-CoV-2 [80]. Eriodictyol, a *Herba santa* flavanone, is a popular herbal medicine used to cure asthma and colds. In silico studies predicts, eriodictyol binds to almost all targeted proteins with good energy and has shown its relevance for COVID 19 therapy [81].

SARS-CoV-2 nucleocapsid (N) protein is a multifunctional protein that plays a key role in the assembly of the virus and its transcription of the RNA. During

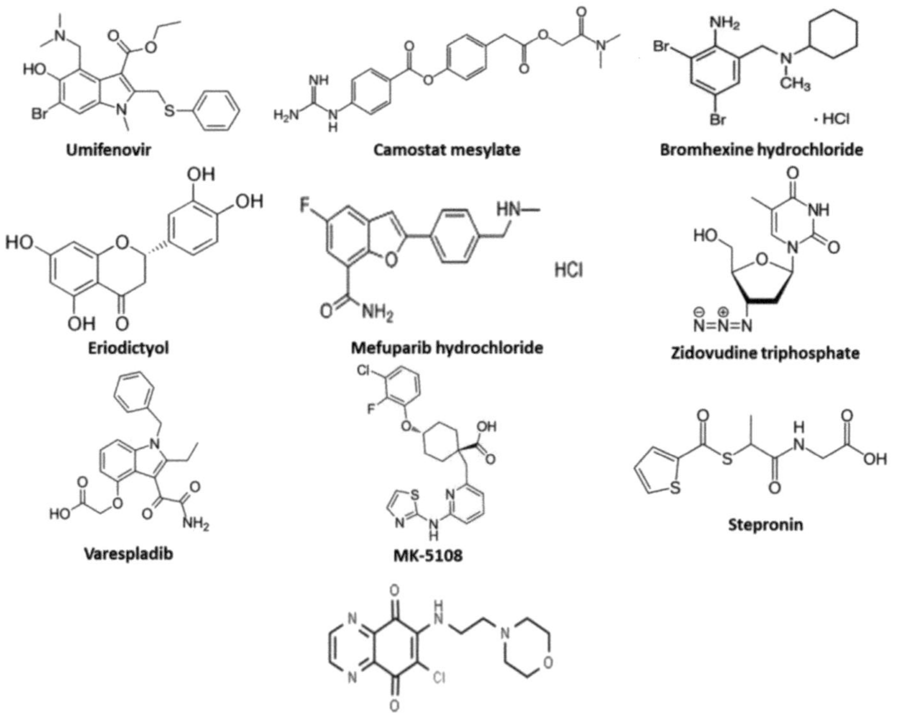

Figure 11.
Repurposed structural and accessory protein inhibitors for COVID-19 treatment.

the packing of the RNA genome, the N protein is critical in the creation of helical ribonucleoproteins, controlling viral RNA synthesis during replication and transcription. Infected host cells and their cellular functions are also regulated by the N protein [82]. Previous studies identified a special ribonucleotide-binding pocket composed of strongly conserved residues in the NTD by solving the complex structure of CoV NP-NTD bound with ribonucleotide monophosphate. Compounds that bind to this RNA-binding pocket may inhibit normal NP function and may be used to regulate CoV diseases. 6-chloro-7-(2-morpholin-4-yl-ethylamino) quinoxaline-5,8-dione (H3) (**Figure 11**) revealed inhibitory activity on the RNA-binding of NP [83]. Mefuparib hydrochloride, CVL218, a Poly [ADP-ribose] polymerase 1 (PARP1) inhibitor have shown to exhibit effective inhibitory activity against SARS-CoV-2 replication without apparent cytopathic effect in *in-vitro* and *in-silico* studies [84]. Zidovudine triphosphate, an anti-HIV drug, acts as a potential inhibitor of the N-terminal domain of SARS-CoV2 N-protein based on docking and simulation research, and can be considered to repurpose for therapeutic options to fight COVID-19 [85]. Out of 13 molecules analyzed for the molecular simulation study on SARS-CoV-2 nucleocapsid protein, 3 (Varespladib, MK-5108, Stepronin) have been found to be show inhibitory activity on SARS-CoV-2 N protein with high docking score [86].

5. Vaccines approved for emergency use authorization (EUA)

Various vaccines across the globe are in the progress of development against COVID-19, while the efficacy, productive and stability of most of them is still unclear. The latest report from the World Health Organization states about 69

S.No.	Candidate	Developer	Type	Approval Status (EUA)
1	BNT162b2	Pfizer–BioNTech	mRNA	FDA Approved
2	mRNA-1273	ModernaTX, Inc.	mRNA	FDA Approved
3	Sputnik-V	Gamaleya	Ad26, Ad5	EMA Approved
4	ChAdOx1 nCoV19	Oxford-AstraZeneca	Non-Replicating Viral Vector	WHO Approved
5	Covaxin (BBV152 A, B, C)	Serum Institute, Bharat Biotech	Inactivated	ICMR Approved (India)
6	CoronaVac	Sinovac	Inactivated	Approval limited (China, Indonesia)
7	Convidicea (Ad5-nCoV)	CanSino Biologics	Viral vector	Approval limited (China)
8	EpiVacCorona	Vector Institute	Protein vaccine	Approved for Early use (Russia)
9	Sinopharm	Sinopharm	Inactivated	Approval limited
10	BBIBP-CorV	Beijing Institute of Biological Products-Sinopharm	Inactivated	Approval limited

Table 1.
Vaccines against COVID-19 approved for emergency use authorization.

vaccine candidates in the progress of clinical trial and about 181 candidates in pre-clinical development [87]. About 7% of vaccinations in the state of preclinical trials performed are based on practice. Hereby, we list the current status of several vaccines across the globe approved by Food and Drug Administration (FDA), European Medicine Agency (EMA), World Health Organization (WHO), Indian Council of Medical Research (ICMR) and other countries medical advisory boards under progress of development for the emergency use authorization (EUA) in order to curb the pandemic (**Table 1**).

6. Conclusion

The principle of drug repurposing is very beneficial and may have proven success, although this may differ with the severity as well as the subjects in whom therapy is performed. In the case of vaccinations, several vaccines have shown promising effects throughout the globe and the proceeding steps will soon provide hope for the early commercial launch of COVID-19 vaccines. Since the structural organization and genomic constitution of the SARS-CoV-2 is similar to that of SARS-CoV, antiviral drugs and other therapeutic measures employed to control the disease at the time can be utilized in order to control this epidemic condition. However, the rate and amount of research and clinical COVID-19/SARS-CoV-2 studies to improve potential treatments and therapies for this disorder will surely help us in order to curb the disease soon. Consequently, the design and production of SARS-CoV-2 vaccines is similarly critical in comparison to the development of new medicines and clinical trials of old drugs. Experience from SARS-CoV and MERS-CoV suggests that there is a major focus on creating animal models that can summarize different forms of human disease and assess the safety and efficacy of vaccines.

Author details

Ashok K. Singh[1*], Aakansha Singh[2] and Ankit Kumar Dubey[3]

1 Pennsylvania State University, Penn State College of Medicine, Hershey, PA, USA

2 CSIR-Central Drug Research Institute, Lucknow, Uttar Pradesh, India

3 Department of Biotechnology, Indian Institute of Technology Madras, Tamil Nadu, India

*Address all correspondence to: indianashoksingh@gmail.com

'Biotechnology to Combat COVID-19' is a collaborative project with Biotechnology Kiosk

References

[1] Omolo, C.A., Soni, N., Fasiku, V.O., Mackraj, I., Govender, T., Update on therapeutic approaches and emerging therapies for SARS-CoV-2 virus. *European Journal of Pharmacology.* 2020; 883, 173348. https://doi.org/10.1016/j.ejphar.2020.173348

[2] Wu, D., Wu, T., Liu, Q., & Yang, Z. The SARS-CoV-2 outbreak: What we know. *International Society for Infectious Diseases*. 2020; *94*, 44-48. https://doi.org/10.1016/j.ijid.2020.03.004

[3] Zumla, A., Chan, J. F., Azhar, E. I., Hui, D. S., & Yuen, K. Y. Coronaviruses - drug discovery and therapeutic options. *Nature reviews. Drug discovery*. 2016; *15*(5), 327-347. https://doi.org/10.1038/nrd.2015.37

[4] Kumar S., Nyodu R., Maurya V.K., Saxena S.K. (2020) Morphology, Genome Organization, Replication, and Pathogenesis of Severe Acute Respiratory Syndrome Coronavirus 2 (SARS-CoV-2). In: Saxena S. (eds) Coronavirus Disease 2019 (COVID-19). Medical Virology: From Pathogenesis to Disease Control. Springer, Singapore. https://doi.org/10.1007/978-981-15-4814-7_3

[5] Shereen, M.A., Khan, S., Kazmi, A., Bashir, N., Siddique, R., COVID-19 infection: Origin, transmission, and characteristics of human coronaviruses. *Journal of Advanced Research* 2020; 24, 91-98. https://doi:10.1016/j.jare.2020.03.005

[6] Mirza, M.U., Froeyen, M. Structural elucidation of SARS-CoV-2 vital proteins: Computational methods reveal potential drug candidates against main protease, Nsp12 polymerase and Nsp13 helicase. *Journal of Pharmaceutical Analysis* 2020;10, 320-328. https://doi:10.1016/j.jpha.2020.04.008

[7] van Boheemen, S., de Graaf, M., Lauber, C., Bestebroer, T. M., Raj, V. S., Zaki, A. M., Osterhaus, A. D., Haagmans, B. L., Gorbalenya, A. E., Snijder, E. J., & Fouchier, R. A. (2012). Genomic characterization of a newly discovered coronavirus associated with acute respiratory distress syndrome in humans. *mBio*, *3*(6), e00473-12. https://doi.org/10.1128/mBio.00473-12

[8] Zhou, P., Yang, X.-L., Wang, X.-G., Hu, B., Zhang, L., Zhang, W., Si, H.-R., Zhu, Y., Li, B., Huang, C.-L., Chen, H.-D., Chen, J., Luo, Y., Guo, H., Jiang, R.-D., Liu, M.-Q., Chen, Y., Shen, X.-R., Wang, X., Zheng, X.-S., Zhao, K., Chen, Q.-J., Deng, F., Liu, L.-L., Yan, B., Zhan, F.-X., Wang, Y.-Y., Xiao, G.-F., Shi, Z.-L., 2020. A pneumonia outbreak associated with a new coronavirus of probable bat origin. Nature 579, 270-273. https://doi:10.1038/s41586-020-2012-7

[9] Nakagawa, S., Miyazawa, T., 2020. Genome evolution of SARS-CoV-2 and its virological characteristics. Inflammation and Regeneration 40. https://doi:10.1186/s41232-020-00126-7

[10] Chan, J.F.-W., Kok, K.-H., Zhu, Z., Chu, H., To, K.K.-W., Yuan, S., Yuen, K.-Y., 2020. Genomic characterization of the 2019 novel human-pathogenic coronavirus isolated from a patient with atypical pneumonia after visiting Wuhan. Emerging Microbes & Infections 9, 221-236. https://doi:10.1080/22221751.2020.1719902

[11] Khailany, R. A., Safdar, M., & Ozaslan, M. (2020). Genomic characterization of a novel SARS-CoV-2. *Gene reports*, *19*, 100682. https://doi.org/10.1016/j.genrep.2020.100682

[12] NCBI-Reference-Sequence. SARS coronavirus Tor2, complete genome. 2020.(Accession No.: NC_004718)

[13] NCBI-Reference-Sequence. Middle East respiratory syndrome-related coronavirus isolate HCoV-EMC/2012,

complete genome. 2020. (Accession No.: NC_019843)

[14] NCBI-Reference-Sequence. Severe acute respiratory syndrome coronavirus 2 isolate Wuhan-Hu-1, complete genome. 2020. (Accession No. NC_045512.2).

[15] Wu, F., Zhao, S., Yu, B., Chen, Y. M., Wang, W., Song, Z. G., Hu, Y., Tao, Z. W., Tian, J. H., Pei, Y. Y., Yuan, M. L., Zhang, Y. L., Dai, F. H., Liu, Y., Wang, Q. M., Zheng, J. J., Xu, L., Holmes, E. C., & Zhang, Y. Z. (2020). A new coronavirus associated with human respiratory disease in China. *Nature*, *579*(7798), 265-269. https://doi.org/10.1038/s41586-020-2008-3.

[16] NCBI-Reference-Sequence- nsp3 [Severe acute respiratory syndrome coronavirus 2] (Accession No.: YP_009725299.1)

[17] Lei, X., Dong, X., Ma, R., Wang, W., Xiao, X., Tian, Z., Wang, C., Wang, Y., Li, L., Ren, L., Guo, F., Zhao, Z., Zhou, Z., Xiang, Z., Wang, J. (2020). Activation and evasion of type I interferon responses by SARS-CoV-2. *Nature communications*, *11* (1), 3810. https://doi.org/10.1038/s41467-020-17665-9

[18] Shin, D., Mukherjee, R., Grewe, D., Bojkova, D., Baek, K., Bhattacharya, A., Schulz, L., Widera, M., Mehdipour, A. R., Tascher, G., Geurink, P. P., Wilhelm, A., van der Heden van Noort, G. J., Ovaa, H., Müller, S., Knobeloch, K. P., Rajalingam, K., Schulman, B. A., Cinatl, J., Hummer, G., ... Dikic, I. (2020). Papain-like protease regulates SARS-CoV-2 viral spread and innate immunity. *Nature*, *587*(7835), 657-662. https://doi.org/10.1038/s41586-020-2601-5

[19] Lei, J., Kusov, Y., & Hilgenfeld, R. (2018). Nsp3 of coronaviruses: Structures and functions of a large multi-domain protein. *Antiviral research*, *149*, 58-74. https://doi.org/10.1016/j.antiviral.2017.11.001

[20] Frick, D. N., Virdi, R. S., Vuksanovic, N., Dahal, N., & Silvaggi, N. R. (2020). Molecular Basis for ADP-Ribose Binding to the Mac1 Domain of SARS-CoV-2 nsp3. *Biochemistry*, *59* (28), 2608-2615. https://doi.org/10.1021/acs.biochem.0c00309

[21] NCBI-Reference-Sequence: 3C-like proteinase [Severe acute respiratory syndrome coronavirus 2] (Accession No.: YP_009725301.1)

[22] Zhu, G., Zhu, C., Zhu, Y., & Sun, F. (2020). Minireview of progress in the structural study of SARS-CoV-2 proteins. *Current research in microbial sciences*, *1*, 53-61. https://doi.org/10.1016/j.crmicr.2020.06.003

[23] Zhang, L., Lin, D., Sun, X., Curth, U., Drosten, C., Sauerhering, L., Becker, S., Rox, K., & Hilgenfeld, R. (2020). Crystal structure of SARS-CoV-2 main protease provides a basis for design of improved α-ketoamide inhibitors. *Science (New York, N.Y.)*, *368*(6489), 409-412. https://doi.org/10.1126/science.abb3405

[24] Dai, W., Zhang, B., Jiang, X. M., Su, H., Li, J., Zhao, Y., Xie, X., Jin, Z., Peng, J., Liu, F., Li, C., Li, Y., Bai, F., Wang, H., Cheng, X., Cen, X., Hu, S., Yang, X., Wang, J., Liu, X., ... Liu, H. (2020). Structure-based design of antiviral drug candidates targeting the SARS-CoV-2 main protease. *Science (New York, N.Y.)*, *368*(6497), 1331-1335. https://doi.org/10.1126/science.abb4489

[25] Jin, Z., Du, X., Xu, Y., Deng, Y., Liu, M., Zhao, Y., Zhang, B., Li, X., Zhang, L., Peng, C., Duan, Y., Yu, J., Wang, L., Yang, K., Liu, F., Jiang, R., Yang, X., You, T., Liu, X., Yang, X., ... Yang, H. (2020). Structure of M^{pro} from SARS-CoV-2 and discovery of its inhibitors. *Nature*, *582*(7811), 289-293. https://doi.org/10.1038/s41586-020-2223-y

[26] Pachetti, M., Marini, B., Benedetti, F. *et al.* Emerging SARS-CoV-2 mutation hot spots include a novel RNA-dependent-RNA polymerase variant. *J Transl Med* **18,** 179 (2020). https://doi.org/10.1186/s12967-020-02344-6

[27] NCBI-Reference-Sequence: RNA-dependent RNA polymerase [Severe acute respiratory syndrome coronavirus 2] (Accession No. YP_009725307.1)

[28] Venkataraman, S., Prasad, B., & Selvarajan, R. (2018). RNA Dependent RNA Polymerases: Insights from Structure, Function and Evolution. *Viruses*, *10*(2), 76. https://doi.org/10.3390/v10020076

[29] Subissi, L., Posthuma, C. C., Collet, A., Zevenhoven-Dobbe, J. C., Gorbalenya, A. E., Decroly, E., Snijder, E. J., Canard, B., & Imbert, I. (2014). One severe acute respiratory syndrome coronavirus protein complex integrates processive RNA polymerase and exonuclease activities. *Proceedings of the National Academy of Sciences of the United States of America*, *111*(37), E3900–E3909. https://doi.org/10.1073/pnas.1323705111

[30] Gao, Y., Yan, L., Huang, Y., Liu, F., Zhao, Y., Cao, L., Wang, T., Sun, Q., Ming, Z., Zhang, L., Ge, J., Zheng, L., Zhang, Y., Wang, H., Zhu, Y., Zhu, C., Hu, T., Hua, T., Zhang, B., Yang, X., ... Rao, Z. (2020). Structure of the RNA-dependent RNA polymerase from COVID-19 virus. *Science (New York, N.Y.)*, *368*(6492), 779-782. https://doi.org/10.1126/science.abb7498

[31] Hillen, H. S., Kokic, G., Farnung, L., Dienemann, C., Tegunov, D., & Cramer, P. (2020). Structure of replicating SARS-CoV-2 polymerase. *Nature*, *584* (7819), 154-156. https://doi.org/10.1038/s41586-020-2368-8

[32] Naqvi, A., Fatima, K., Mohammad, T., Fatima, U., Singh, I. K., Singh, A., Atif, S. M., Hariprasad, G., Hasan, G. M., & Hassan, M. I. (2020). Insights into SARS-CoV-2 genome, structure, evolution, pathogenesis and therapies: Structural genomics approach. *Biochimica et biophysica acta. Molecular basis of disease*, *1866*(10), 165878. https://doi.org/10.1016/j.bbadis.2020.165878

[33] NCBI-Reference-Sequence: helicase [Severe acute respiratory syndrome coronavirus 2] (Accession No.: YP_009725308.1)

[34] White, M. A., Lin, W., & Cheng, X. (2020). Discovery of COVID-19 Inhibitors Targeting the SARS-CoV2 Nsp13 Helicase. *bioRxiv: the preprint server for biology*, 2020.08.09.243246. https://doi.org/10.1101/2020.08.09.243246

[35] Hao, W., Wojdyla, J. A., Zhao, R., Han, R., Das, R., Zlatev, I., Manoharan, M., Wang, M., & Cui, S. (2017). Crystal structure of Middle East respiratory syndrome coronavirus helicase. *PLoS pathogens*, *13*(6), e1006474. https://doi.org/10.1371/journal.ppat.1006474

[36] Chen, J., Malone, B., Llewellyn, E., Grasso, M., Shelton, P., Olinares, P., Maruthi, K., Eng, E. T., Vatandaslar, H., Chait, B. T., Kapoor, T. M., Darst, S. A., & Campbell, E. A. (2020). Structural Basis for Helicase-Polymerase Coupling in the SARS-CoV-2 Replication-Transcription Complex. *Cell*, *182*(6), 1560-1573.e13. https://doi.org/10.1016/j.cell.2020.07.033

[37] Jia, Z., Yan, L., Ren, Z., Wu, L., Wang, J., Guo, J., Zheng, L., Ming, Z., Zhang, L., Lou, Z., & Rao, Z. (2019). Delicate structural coordination of the Severe Acute Respiratory Syndrome coronavirus Nsp13 upon ATP hydrolysis. *Nucleic acids research*, *47*(12), 6538-6550. https://doi.org/10.1093/nar/gkz409

[38] Littler, D. R., MacLachlan, B. J., Watson, G. M., Vivian, J. P., & Gully, B. S. (2020). A pocket guide on how to structure SARS-CoV-2

drugs and therapies. *Biochemical Society transactions*, *48*(6), 2625-2641. Advance online publication. https://doi.org/10.1042/BST20200396

[39] Romano, M., Ruggiero, A., Squeglia, F., Maga, G., & Berisio, R. (2020). A Structural View of SARS-CoV-2 RNA Replication Machinery: RNA Synthesis, Proofreading and Final Capping. *Cells*, *9*(5), 1267. https://doi.org/10.3390/cells9051267

[40] NCBI-Reference-Sequence: surface glycoprotein [Severe acute respiratory syndrome coronavirus 2] (Accession No. YP_009724390.1)

[41] Wrapp, D., Wang, N., Corbett, K.S., Goldsmith, J.A., Hsieh, C.-L., Abiona, O., Graham, B.S., Mclellan, J.S., 2020. Cryo-EM structure of the 2019-nCoV spike in the prefusion conformation. *Science* 367, 1260-1263. https://doi:10.1126/science.abb2507

[42] Duan, L., Zheng, Q., Zhang, H., Niu, Y., Lou, Y., Wang, H., 2020. The SARS-CoV-2 Spike Glycoprotein Biosynthesis, Structure, Function, and Antigenicity: Implications for the Design of Spike-Based Vaccine Immunogens. Frontiers in Immunology 11. https://doi:10.3389/fimmu.2020.576622

[43] Andersen, K.G., Rambaut, A., Lipkin, W.I., Holmes, E.C., Garry, R.F., 2020. The proximal origin of SARS-CoV-2. Nature Medicine 26, 450-452. https://doi:10.1038/s41591-020-0820-9

[44] Ji, W., Wang, W., Zhao, X., Zai, J., Li, X., 2020. Cross-species transmission of the newly identified coronavirus 2019-nCoV. Journal of Medical Virology 92, 433-440. https://doi:10.1002/jmv.25682

[45] Cascarina, S. M., & Ross, E. D. (2020). A proposed role for the SARS-CoV-2 nucleocapsid protein in the formation and regulation of biomolecular condensates. *FASEB journal: official publication of the Federation of American Societies for Experimental Biology*, *34*(8), 9832-9842. https://doi.org/10.1096/fj.202001351

[46] Rahman, M. S., Islam, M. R., Alam, A., Islam, I., Hoque, M. N., Akter, S., Rahaman, M. M., Sultana, M., & Hossain, M. A. (2020). Evolutionary dynamics of SARS-CoV-2 nucleocapsid protein and its consequences. *Journal of medical virology*, 10.1002/jmv.26626. Advance online publication. https://doi.org/10.1002/jmv.26626

[47] Nikolakaki, E., & Giannakouros, T. (2020). SR/RS Motifs as Critical Determinants of Coronavirus Life Cycle. *Frontiers in molecular biosciences*, *7*, 219. https://doi.org/10.3389/fmolb.2020.00219

[48] Peng, Y., Du, N., Lei, Y., Dorje, S., Qi, J., Luo, T., Gao, G. F., & Song, H. (2020). Structures of the SARS-CoV-2 nucleocapsid and their perspectives for drug design. *The EMBO journal*, *39*(20), e105938. https://doi.org/10.15252/embj.2020105938

[49] Kang, S., Yang, M., Hong, Z., Zhang, L., Huang, Z., Chen, X., He, S., Zhou, Z., Zhou, Z., Chen, Q., Yan, Y., Zhang, C., Shan, H., & Chen, S. (2020). Crystal structure of SARS-CoV-2 nucleocapsid protein RNA binding domain reveals potential unique drug targeting sites. *Acta pharmaceutica Sinica. B*, *10*(7), 1228-1238. https://doi.org/10.1016/j.apsb.2020.04.009

[50] Zhou, R., Zeng, R., Von Brunn, A., Lei, J., 2020. Structural characterization of the C-terminal domain of SARS-CoV-2 nucleocapsid protein. Molecular Biomedicine 1. https://doi.org/10.1186/s43556-020-00001-4

[51] Dubey, A.K., Singh, A., Prakash, S., Kumar, M., Singh, A.K., Race to arsenal COVID-19 therapeutics: Current alarming status and future directions.

Chemico-Biological Interactions. 2020; 109298. https://doi:10.1016/j.cbi.2020.109298

[52] W. Sun, P.E. Sanderson, W. Zheng, Drug combination therapy increases successful drug repositioning, Drug Discov. Today 21 (7) (2016) 1189-1195. https://doi.org/10.1016/j.drudis.2016.05.015.

[53] W. Zheng, W. Sun, A. Simeonov, Drug repurposing screens and synergistic drug-combinations for infectious diseases, Br. J. Pharmacol. 175 (2) (2018) 181-191. https://doi.org/10.1111/bph.13895.

[54] Pandey, A., Nikam, A. N., Shreya, A. B., Mutalik, S. P., Gopalan, D., Kulkarni, S., Padya, B. S., Fernandes, G., Mutalik, S., & Prassl, R. (2020). Potential therapeutic targets for combating SARS-CoV-2: Drug repurposing, clinical trials and recent advancements. *Life sciences*, *256*, 117883. https://doi.org/10.1016/j.lfs.2020.117883

[55] Wu, C., Liu, Y., Yang, Y., Zhang, P., Zhong, W., Wang, Y., Wang, Q., Xu, Y., Li, M., Li, X., Zheng, M., Chen, L., & Li, H. (2020). Analysis of therapeutic targets for SARS-CoV-2 and discovery of potential drugs by computational methods. *Acta pharmaceutica Sinica. B*, *10*(5), 766-788. https://doi.org/10.1016/j.apsb.2020.02.008

[56] Mahdi, M., Mótyán, J. A., Szojka, Z. I., Golda, M., Miczi, M., & Tőzsér, J. (2020). Analysis of the efficacy of HIV protease inhibitors against SARS-CoV-2's main protease. *Virology journal*, *17*(1), 190. https://doi.org/10.1186/s12985-020-01457-0

[57] Pinzi L., Tinivella A., Caporuscio F., Rastelli G. (2020). Drug repurposing and polypharmacology to fight SARS-CoV-2 through the inhibition of the main protease. *Nat. Commun*. [Preprint]. https://doi.org/10.21203/rs.3.rs-27222/v1

[58] Di Micco, S., Musella, S., Scala, M.C., Sala, M., Campiglia, P., Bifulco, G., Fasano, A., (2021). In silico Analysis Revealed Potential Anti-SARS-CoV-2 Main Protease Activity by the Zonulin Inhibitor Larazotide Acetate. *Frontiers in Chemistry* 8. https://doi.org/10.3389/fchem.2020.628609

[59] Baron, S. A., Devaux, C., Colson, P., Raoult, D., & Rolain, J. M. (2020). Teicoplanin: an alternative drug for the treatment of COVID-19?. *International journal of antimicrobial agents*, *55*(4), 105944. https://doi.org/10.1016/j.ijantimicag.2020.105944

[60] Zhang, J., Ma, X., Yu, F., Liu, J., Zou, F., Pan, T., Zhang, H., (2020). Teicoplanin potently blocks the cell entry of 2019-nCoV. https://doi.org/10.1101/2020.02.05.935387

[61] McKee DL, Sternberg A, Stange U, Laufer S, Naujokat C. Candidate drugs against SARS-CoV-2 and COVID-19. *Pharmacol Res*. 2020;157:104859. https://dx.doi.org/10.1016%2Fj.phrs.2020.104859

[62] Hoffmann, M., Schroeder, S., Kleine-Weber, H., Müller, M. A., Drosten, C., & Pöhlmann, S. (2020). Nafamostat Mesylate Blocks Activation of SARS-CoV-2: New Treatment Option for COVID-19. *Antimicrobial agents and chemotherapy*, *64*(6), e00754-20. https://doi.org/10.1128/AAC.00754-20

[63] Picarazzi, F., Vicenti, I., Saladini, F., Zazzi, M., & Mori, M. (2020). Targeting the RdRp of Emerging RNA Viruses: The Structure-Based Drug Design Challenge. *Molecules (Basel, Switzerland)*, *25*(23), 5695. https://doi.org/10.3390/molecules25235695v

[64] Sheahan, T. P., Sims, A. C., Zhou, S., Graham, R. L., Pruijssers, A. J., Agostini, M. L., Leist, S. R., Schäfer, A., Dinnon, K. H., 3rd, Stevens, L. J., Chappell, J. D., Lu, X., Hughes, T. M., George, A. S., Hill, C. S., Montgomery,

S. A., Brown, A. J., Bluemling, G. R., Natchus, M. G., Saindane, M., ... Baric, R. S. (2020). An orally bioavailable broad-spectrum antiviral inhibits SARS-CoV-2 in human airway epithelial cell cultures and multiple coronaviruses in mice. *Science translational medicine*, *12*(541), eabb5883. https://doi.org/10.1126/scitranslmed.abb5883

[65] Baby, K., Maity, S., Mehta, C. H., Suresh, A., Nayak, U. Y., & Nayak, Y. (2020). Targeting SARS-CoV-2 RNA-dependent RNA polymerase: An *in silico* drug repurposing for COVID-19. *F1000Research*, *9*, 1166. https://doi.org/10.12688/f1000research.26359.1

[66] Durojaiye, A. B., Clarke, J. D., Stamatiades, G. A., & Wang, C. (2020). Repurposing cefuroxime for treatment of COVID-19: a scoping review of *in silico* studies. *Journal of biomolecular structure & dynamics*, 1-8. Advance online publication. https://doi.org/10.1080/07391102.2020.1777904

[67] Xie, T., Song, S., Li, S., Ouyang, L., Xia, L., & Huang, J. (2015). Review of natural product databases. *Cell proliferation*, *48*(4), 398-404. https://doi.org/10.1111/cpr.12190

[68] Borgio, J. F., Alsuwat, H. S., Al Otaibi, W. M., Ibrahim, A. M., Almandil, N. B., Al Asoom, L. I., Salahuddin, M., Kamaraj, B., & AbdulAzeez, S. (2020). State-of-the-art tools unveil potent drug targets amongst clinically approved drugs to inhibit helicase in SARS-CoV-2. *Archives of medical science: AMS*, *16*(3), 508-518. https://doi.org/10.5114/aoms.2020.94567

[69] Habtemariam, S., Nabavi, S. F., Banach, M., Berindan-Neagoe, I., Sarkar, K., Sil, P. C., & Nabavi, S. M. (2020). Should We Try SARS-CoV-2 Helicase Inhibitors for COVID-19 Therapy?. *Archives of medical research*, *51*(7), 733-735. https://doi.org/10.1016/j.arcmed.2020.05.024

[70] Shu, T., Huang, M., Wu, D., Ren, Y., Zhang, X., Han, Y., Mu, J., Wang, R., Qiu, Y., Zhang, D. Y., & Zhou, X. (2020). SARS-Coronavirus-2 Nsp13 Possesses NTPase and RNA Helicase Activities That Can Be Inhibited by Bismuth Salts. *Virologica Sinica*, *35*(3), 321-329. https://doi.org/10.1007/s12250-020-00242-1

[71] Haji Abdolvahab, M., Moradi-Kalbolandi, S., Zarei, M., Bose, D., Majidzadeh-A, K., & Farahmand, L. (2021). Potential role of interferons in treating COVID-19 patients. *International immunopharmacology*, *90*, 107171. https://doi.org/10.1016/j.intimp.2020.107171

[72] Adedeji, A. O., Singh, K., Kassim, A., Coleman, C. M., Elliott, R., Weiss, S. R., Frieman, M. B., Sarafianos, S. G. (2014). Evaluation of SSYA10-001 as a replication inhibitor of severe acute respiratory syndrome, mouse hepatitis, and Middle East respiratory syndrome coronaviruses. *Antimicrobial agents and chemotherapy*, *58*(8), 4894-98. https://doi.org/10.1128/AAC.02994-14

[73] Mani, J. S., Johnson, J. B., Steel, J. C., Broszczak, D. A., Neilsen, P. M., Walsh, K. B., & Naiker, M. (2020). Natural product-derived phytochemicals as potential agents against coronaviruses: A review. *Virus research*, *284*, 197989. https://doi.org/10.1016/j.virusres.2020.197989

[74] Yu, M. S., Lee, J., Lee, J. M., Kim, Y., Chin, Y. W., Jee, J. G., Keum, Y. S., & Jeong, Y. J. (2012). Identification of myricetin and scutellarein as novel chemical inhibitors of the SARS coronavirus helicase, nsP13. *Bioorganic & medicinal chemistry letters*, *22*(12), 4049-4054. https://doi.org/10.1016/j.bmcl.2012.04.081

[75] Kumar, R., Khandelwal, N., Chander, Y., Riyesh, T., Gulati, B.R., Pal, Y., Tripathi, B.N., Barua, S., Kumar, N., 2020. Emetine as an

antiviral agent suppresses SARS-CoV-2 replication by inhibiting interaction of viral mRNA with eIF4E: An *in vitro* study. *bioRxiv* https://doi.org/10.1101/2020.11.29.401984

[76] Wondmkun, Y. T., & Mohammed, O. A. (2020). A Review on Novel Drug Targets and Future Directions for COVID-19 Treatment. *Biologics: targets & therapy*, *14*, 77-82. https://doi.org/10.2147/BTT.S266487

[77] Vankadari N. (2020). Arbidol: A potential antiviral drug for the treatment of SARS-CoV-2 by blocking trimerization of the spike glycoprotein. *International journal of antimicrobial agents*, *56*(2), 105998. https://doi.org/10.1016/j.ijantimicag.2020.105998

[78] Cai, Y., Xu, W., Gu, C., Cai, X., Qu, D., Lu, L., Xie, Y., & Jiang, S. (2020). Griffithsin with A Broad-Spectrum Antiviral Activity by Binding Glycans in Viral Glycoprotein Exhibits Strong Synergistic Effect in Combination with A Pan-Coronavirus Fusion Inhibitor Targeting SARS-CoV-2 Spike S2 Subunit. *Virologica Sinica*, *35*(6), 857-860. https://doi.org/10.1007/s12250-020-00305-3

[79] Hoffmann, M., Hofmann-Winkler, H., Smith, J. C., Krüger, N., Sørensen, L. K., Søgaard, O. S., Hasselstrøm, J. B., Winkler, M., Hempel, T., Raich, L., Olsson, S., Yamazoe, T., Yamatsuta, K., Mizuno, H., Ludwig, S., Noé, F., Sheltzer, J. M., Kjolby, M., & Pöhlmann, S. (2020). Camostat mesylate inhibits SARS-CoV-2 activation by TMPRSS2-related proteases and its metabolite GBPA exerts antiviral activity. *bioRxiv : the preprint server for biology*, 2020.08.05.237651. https://doi.org/10.1101/2020.08.05.237651

[80] Li, T., Sun, L., Zhang, W., Zheng, C., Jiang, C., Chen, M., Chen, D., Dai, Z., Bao, S., & Shen, X. (2020). Bromhexine Hydrochloride Tablets for the Treatment of Moderate COVID-19: An Open-Label Randomized Controlled Pilot Study. *Clinical and translational science*, *13*(6), 1096-1102. https://doi.org/10.1111/cts.12881

[81] Deshpande, R. R., Tiwari, A. P., Nyayanit, N., & Modak, M. (2020). In silico molecular docking analysis for repurposing therapeutics against multiple proteins from SARS-CoV-2. *European journal of pharmacology*, *886*, 173430. https://doi.org/10.1016/j.ejphar.2020.173430

[82] Kumar, A., Parveen, A., Kumar, N., Bairy, S., Kaushik, V., Chandola , C., et al. (2020). Characterization of nucleocapsid (N) protein from novel coronavirus SARS-CoV-2. Preprints 2020, 2020050413. https://doi:10.20944/preprints202005.0413.v1

[83] Chang, C. K., Jeyachandran, S., Hu, N. J., Liu, C. L., Lin, S. Y., Wang, Y. S., Chang, Y. M., & Hou, M. H. (2016). Structure-based virtual screening and experimental validation of the discovery of inhibitors targeted towards the human coronavirus nucleocapsid protein. *Molecular bioSystems*, *12*(1), 59-66. https://doi.org/10.1039/c5mb00582e

[84] Senger, M. R., Evangelista, T., Dantas, R. F., Santana, M., Gonçalves, L., de Souza Neto, L. R., Ferreira, S. B., & Silva-Junior, F. P. (2020). COVID-19: molecular targets, drug repurposing and new avenues for drug discovery. *Memorias do Instituto Oswaldo Cruz*, *115*, e200254. https://doi.org/10.1590/0074-02760200254

[85] Kwarteng, A., Asiedu, E., Sakyi, S. A., & Asiedu, S. O. (2020). Targeting the SARS-CoV2 nucleocapsid protein for potential therapeutics using immuno-informatics and structure-based drug discovery techniques. *Biomedicine & pharmacotherapy = Biomedecine & pharmacotherapie*, *132*, 110914. https://doi.org/10.1016/j.biopha.2020.110914

[86] Kandwal, S., & Fayne, D. (2020). Repurposing drugs for treatment of SARS-CoV-2 infection: computational design insights into mechanisms of action. *Journal of biomolecular structure & dynamics*, 1-15. Advance online publication. https://doi.org/10.1080/07391102.2020.1825232

[87] Covid-19 vaccines. (n.d.). Retrieved February 17, 2021, from https://www.who.int/emergencies/diseases/novel-coronavirus-2019/covid-19-vaccines

Chapter 20

Role of Anti-Viral Drugs in Combating SARS-CoV-2

Sweta Kamboj, Rohit Kamboj, Shikha Kamboj, Rohit Dutt, Reeva Chabbra and Priyanka Kriplani

Abstract

Viruses are the eventual assertion of parasitism, they not only take nutriments from the host cell, apart from that they direct its metabolic machinery to amalgamate novel virus particle and to diminish the ability of flu viruses to reproduce in an individual antiviral drugs are used. When used as directed, antiviral drugs may help to lessen the duration of flu symptoms and may reduce the severity of common flu symptoms. Antiviral drugs are the class of drugs which comes under the antimicrobials, and that also accommodates the larger group i.e. of antibiotics. They are broad-spectrum in nature and can be effective against a wide range of viruses. They can be used as a single drug as well as in combination of drugs. Antiviral drugs are dissimilar from the antibiotics, they do not demolish their target pathogen ideally they obstruct development of pathogen. To the greatest extent antiviral drugs currently accessible are delineate to deal with herpes viruses, covid-19, HIV, the hepatitis b and c viruses herpes simplex, small pox, picornavirus and influenza a and b viruses etc. Scientists are searching to drag out the range of antiviral to the other families of pathogens. They mainly act by inhibiting the attachment of viruses on cells, prevent genetic reproduction of virus, prevent viral protein production and vital for production of virus. The emanation of antiviral is generally the outcome about an appreciably expanded skills or proficiency of the generative, microscopic and atomic activity of organisms, allowing biomedical analyst to acknowledge the structure, mechanism of action and activity of viruses, significant progress within the procedure for come across the current drugs. Coronavirus 2019 (COVID 19) is highly infectious disease triggered by SARS-CoV-2 (severe acute respiratory syndrome) coronavirus 2 causing nearly 2.9 million deaths worldwide. With the emergence of SARS-CoV-2, the repurposing of antiviral drugs has come into picture.

Keywords: Parasitism, Broad spectrum, Genetic development of virus, Target pathogen, Viral protein production

1. Introduction

Severe Acute Respiratory Syndrome Coronavirus also known as SARS- CoV, a medical condition arises due to viral infection of SARS-CoV. It was proved to be major threat to human civilization in 21st century was declared as pandemic by World Health Organization in March 2020 as the exposure of this syndrome affected the human life cycle poorly causing deaths at an average of 10 percent of the affected population globally. This was first emerges in the Wuhan (a state of China) in December 2019 and later on feast globally by the transmission from affected person to the other person through physical contact [1, 2] and later on when it was established and discovered, the first preventive measure was social distancing which came into force February 2020 according to WHO guidelines and other coronavirus like MERS (Middle east respiratory syndrome) in 2017 and Covid-19 which emerges before 2020.

1.1 Symptoms of SARS

Symptoms of COVID-19 are homogenous to influenza to some extent, and it also causes a pneumonia type symptom, which has been seen in many patients throughout the world. The patients who have fallen ill are reported to suffered cough mainly with sputum, high temperature of the body, difficulties while breathing, headache and sore throat, shaking chills, and diarrhea.

1.2 Structure of coronavirus

SARS-CoV belongs to Coronaviridae family having spherical enveloped particle containing positive stranded RNA that binds to nucleocapsid present inside the membrane protein having glycoprotein spike in the envelop [3, 4] further explained in **Figure 1**.

1.3 Phases of development of SARS

As a virus, it also confiscates the host body system and then multiplies via viral attachment, fusion, penetration; uncoating, transcription, translation, and virion release [5].

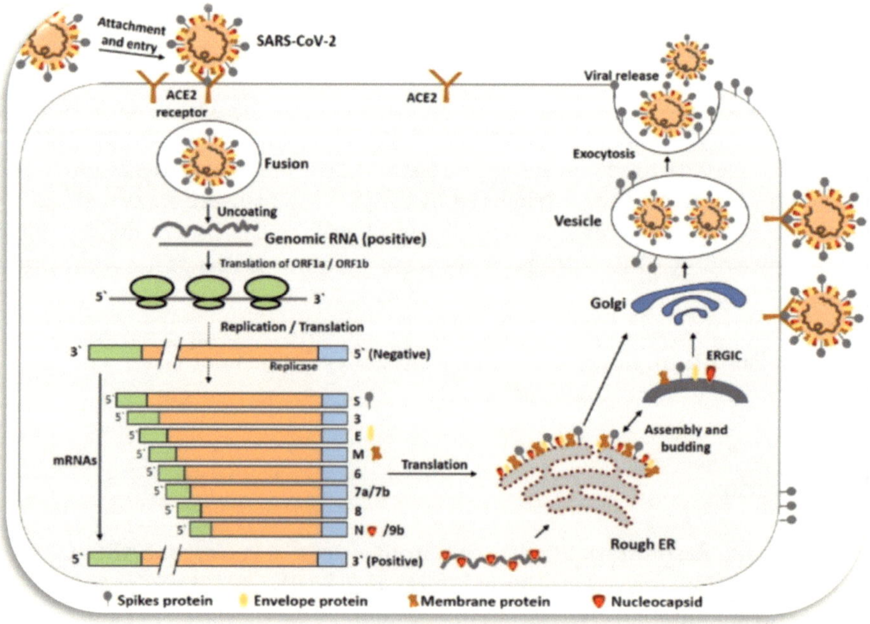

Figure 1.
Mechanism action of coronavirus.

Pathway used to combat SARS through direct inhibition of coronavirus either by inhibiting the vital viral protein corresponds to genome reproduction or else by impeding viral entry into eukaryotic cells. In second place, by modulating immune system either by boosting the immediate response or by inhibiting the inflammatory response [6].

2. Antiviral drugs

Although viral infections have been disclosed since earliest times, it was only during the nineteenth century that scientists were able to isolate "the filterable particles", later called viruses. Viruses are the infectious agent that reproduces only inside the living cell and they can infect all types of living cells and direct the cell to produce more viruses. They are smaller than the bacteria's. The entire infectious virus particle, called a virion, consists of the nucleic acid and an outer shell of protein. Antiviral drugs are classified as the medicines which are mainly used to treat viral infection. Many of the antiviral drugs target the specific viruses and they are considered as the broad spectrum drugs. Most viral infections rectify spontaneously in immunocompetent individuals. The objective of antiviral therapy is to diminish the symptoms and infectivity additionally to shorten the duration of illness [7]. These drugs react by arresting the viral replication cycle at numerous stages. Most of the antiviral drugs currently available are used to treat infections caused by HIV, herpes viruses, hepatitis Band C viruses, and influenza A and B viruses, and C viruses, and influenza A and B viruses etc. Designing effective and safe antiviral drugs is difficult as viruses use host cells to replicate. It is back-breaking to find targets for drugs that would affect only viruses leaving host cells. Viral variation is also one of the reasons posing difficulty in the development aof antiviral drugs and vaccines. Furthermore, antiviral drugs are classified as non-retroviral and retroviral drugs which act on the different types of viruses and stop their further growth or their replication and these results in the cure of viral disease [8]. Coronavirus 2019 (COVID 19) is highly infectious disease triggered by SARS-CoV-2 (severe acute respiratory syndrome coronavirus 2 causing nearly 2.9 million deaths worldwide Currently, a variety of antiviral drugs are in clinical trails to treat SARS-CoV-2 which inhibit viral replication.

3. Classification of viruses

3.1 ICTV classification

The ICTV evolves the current classification system and wrote guidelines that put a bigger weight on certain virus properties to maintain family consistency. A unified taxonomy has been accepted. Solitary a little part of the entire variety of viruses has been studied. Till 2019 ICTV explained 9 kingdoms, 4 realms, 2 subphyla, 16 phyla, 36 classes, 55 orders, 9 suborders, 168 families, 10 sub-families, 1421 genera, 68 subgenera and 6589 species of viruses [9].

The general taxonomic structure of ranges of taxon and the suffixes used in taxonomic names are mentioned under. Till 2019, the ranks of sub realm, subkingdom and subclass are unemployed whereas all ranks are in usage.

Realm (*-viria*), Subrealm (*vira*), Kingdom (*-virae*), Subkingdom (*-virites*), Phylum (*-viricota*), Subphylum (*-viricotina*), Class (*-viricetes*), Subclass (*-viricetidae*), Order (*-virales*), Suborder (*-virineae*), Family (*-viridae*), Subfamily (*-virinae*), Genus (*-virus*), Subgenus (*-virus*) [10].

3.2 Baltimore classification

This is based on the mechanism of mRNA production. Viruses produce proteins from their genomes and replicate themselves. Viral genome can be single-stranded (ss) and or double stranded (ds). ssRNA viruses may be either antisense (−) or sense (+) [11]. Viruses are classified in seven groups:

i. ssDNA viruses (+strand or sense) DNA (e.g., Parvovirus)

ii. dsDNA viruses (e.g., Adenovirus, Poxvirus)

iii. dsRNA viruses (Reovirus)

iv. (+) ssRNA viruses (+ strand or sense) RNA (e.g. Coronavirus,Picornavirus)

v. (−) ssRNA viruses (+ strand or antisense) RNA (e.g.Orthomyxovirus, Rhabdovirus)

vi. dsDNA-RT viruses DNA with RNA intermediate in life cycle (e.g., Hepadnavirus)

vii. ssRNS-RT viruses (+strand or sense) RNA with DNA intermediate in life cycle (eg. Retroviruses)

3.3 Based on their shape

Viruses are present in various sizes and shapes (**Figure 2**), but are composed of two vital components i.e., a core of genetic material, either RNA or DNA and a protein coat, capsid. A virion comes in four different shapes i.e. spherical, helical,

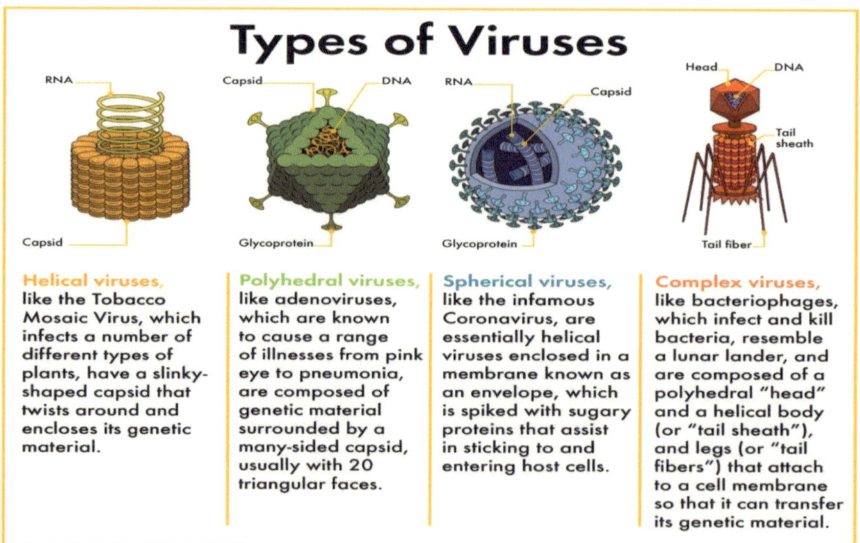

Figure 2.
Types of viruses.

polyhedral and complex Coronaviruses have positive stranded RNA (+ssRNA) with crown like structure possessing spike glycoproteins on the envelop [12].

4. Evolution

A virus is a tiny parasite, infectious substance of small size and basically structure that can multiply only in living cells of plants, animals or bacteria etc. The name is derived from a Latin word meaning "poison." Highly viruses have either RNA or DNA as their genetic material. The nucleic acid of viruses may be single or double stranded. The complete infectious virus element, called a virion, comprises of the nucleic acid and an outer shell is made up of protein [13]. Identifying evolving viruses are those that are freshly appeared or have recently expanded in predominance and/or geographical range uncovers several vital vague patterns. Primary virtually all emerging viruses have RNA more readily than DNA genomes. RNA viruses are more customarily familiar than DNA viruses. Additionally, almost all emergent viruses have an animal reservoir, such that the process of viral emergence can frequently be categorized as cross-species transmission. The extremely substantial exception for the rule is that cross-species transmission is central to viral emergence is HCV, which was first identified in 1989 but which is expected to have a considerably extended history in human populations [14]. In numerous cases, the specific cause of emergence, why the virus has traversed from animals and obsessed by humans can be assigned to ecological factors, involving to alterations in land use and deforestation. Although a multitude of such factors exist, either variations in the proximity of the donor and recipient populations, so that humans have an amplified coincidental of exposure to animal pathogens and variations in the size and density of the donor and recipient populations result in increase in both the exposure and the probability that continued networks of transmission will be established once a virus has inserted into a new species. Although biologists have assembled huge amount of knowledge how present day viruses evolve. When investigating the evolutionary history of most organisms, scientists can look at fossil record and homogenous historic evidence. While many of the viruses do not have the single ancestors. Generally recognizing the significance of ecology, it is also possible that genetic factors, whether in the host or further probably the virus, contribute to the process of disease emergence. As observed with other RNA viruses, SARS-CoV-2 is undergoing genetic mutations while adapting to new individual hosts. Several variants are reported, however only few are affecting public health. In United Kingdom, VOC 202012 (B.1.1.7 lineage) was described in December 2020 followed by B.1.351 lineage (501Y.V2) in South Africa. B.1.1.248/B.1.1.28/P1 (or 501Y.V3) was reported in Brazil in January 2021 and recently in California B.1.427/B.1.429 is discovered. As per WHO, 7 variants are of interest viz. B.1.525, B.1.526, B.1.427/B.1.429, B.1.1.28.2 alias P2, B.1.1.28.3, alias P.3 and B.1.616 [15].

5. How virus replicate

As viruses are obligate pathogen they cannot replicate on their own but they need the host to replicate and produce multiple copies of them. This typically occurs by the virus inserting its genetic material in host cells, co-opting the proteins to create viral replicates, until the cell bursts from the high volume of new viral particles.

There are six fundamental stages that are essential for viral replication (**Figure 3**).

1. Attachment

2. Penetration

3. Uncoating

4. Replication

5. Assembly

6. Virion Release

1. Attachment: This stage involves the interaction between the virus and host cell surface, there they interact with receptors peculiar to them and their host cells. This is also known as the tropism of a virus.

2. Penetration: The attachment to the specific receptor can produce conformational changes in the viral capsid protein that lead the way to the viral and cellular membranes fusing. Some DNA viruses can also undertake into the host cell through receptor-mediated endocytosis.

3. Uncoating: Once inside the cell, the first step is uncoating. This process requires the viral capsid degrading, either by the action of viral or host enzymes and release of genomic information takes place. This enables the start of replication through transcription or translation for RNA or DNA viral genomic information, respectively. The result of the replication step is the synthesis of the viral genome and proteins.

4. Replication: this process is different both in RNA and DNA viruses and also in viruses with dissimilar nucleic acid polarity. This procedure terminates in de novo synthesis of genome and viral proteins.

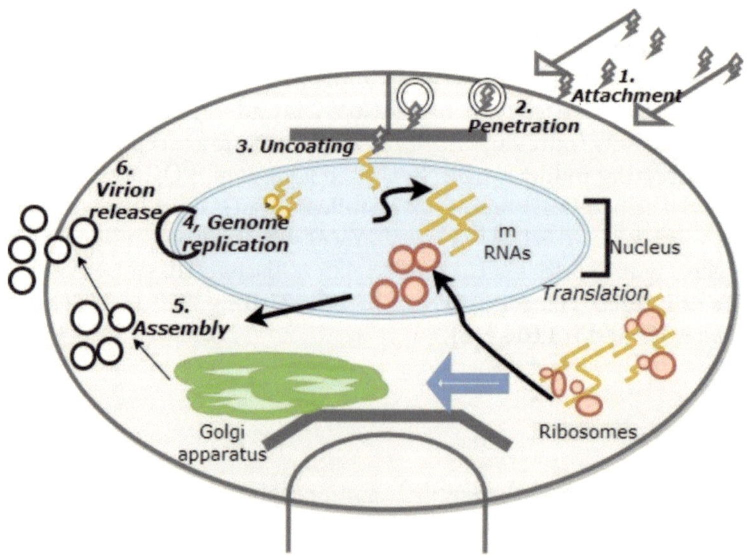

Figure 3.
Stages of viral replication.

5. Assembly: After de novo synthesis of viral proteins and genome, which can be altered post-transcriptionally, viral proteins are wrapped with newly replicated viral genome into new virions that are unconfined from host cells. This process is called maturation.

6. Virion Release: There are two mechanisms of viral freeing: lysis or budding. After virion release some viral proteins remain within the host's cell membrane, which acts as potential targets for circulating antibodies [16].

CoVs are positive stranded RNA enveloped viruses. Upon entry into the host, viral RNA replication begins with synthesis of polyprotein 1a/1ab(pp1a/pp1ab). By the synthesis of subgenomic RNAs sequences and replication-transcription complex, transcription occurs. Termination of transcription occurs at transcription regulatory sequences. Six open reading frames (ORF) are present on CoV genome. Frameshift between ORF 1a and ORF1b helps in production of both pp1a and pp1ab polypeptides which are further processed by chymotrypsin like protease (3CLpro) or main protease or may include papain like proteases which produces non-structural proteins (NSPs 1–16). Besides ORF1a and ORF1b, other ORFs encode structural proteins including nuclecapsid proteins, membrane, envelope, spike and accessory proteic chains [17]. Dedicated sgRNAs translate accessory and structural proteins. Researchers have also reported NSPs in stalling hosts immunity [18]. The envelop plays crucial role in viral pathogenesis as it encourages viral release and assembly [19].

5.1 Classification of antiviral drugs

Anti-viral drugs and their activity mention in **Table 1**.

A. Antiviral Drugs (Non-Retroviral).

1. Anti-herpes drugs
   - Acyclovir
   - Idoxuridine
   - Valacylovir
   - Famcicylovir
   - Cidofovir
   - Penciclovir
2. Anti-influenza virus drugs
   - Amantadine
   - Rimantadine
   - Oseltamivir
   - Zanamivir

Sr. No.	Name of Drugs	Description	Absorption	Metabolism	Protein Binding	Clearance	Dose	Toxicity
1.	Acyclovir	Acyclovir is a nucleotide analog antiviral drug	oral bioavailability of acyclovir is 10–20%	<15% oxidized to 9-carboxymethoxymethylguanine, 1% 8-hydroxylated to 8-hydroxy-acyclovir	9–33% protein bound in plasma	Renal clearance is 248 mL/min/ 1.73 m	200 mg 5 times a day oral (15 mg/ kg/day) 5–10 mg/kg 8 hourly by slow i.v. infusion 5% topical application 6 times a day;	agitation, coma, seizures, lethargy, reduced kidney function
2.	Penciclovir	Penciclovir is a synthetic acyclic guanine derivative	Following single or repeat application of the 1% cream at a dose of 180 mg penciclovir daily.	Hepatic	Less than 20%.	Total plasma clearance of 39.3 L. $hr.^{-1}$	1% cream at a dose of 180 mg	Headache, abdominal pain, increased serum lipase, nausea, dyspepsia, dizziness, and hyperbilirubinemia
3.	Amantadine	An antiviral that is used in the prophylactic or symptomatic treatment of influenza A	well absorbed orally from the gastrointestinal tract	It is metabolized to a small extent (5–15%) by acetylation.	67% bound to plasma proteins	0.2–0.3 L/hr./kg	100 mg BD, elderly—half dose children 5 mg/kg/ day	cardiac, respiratory, renal or central nervous system toxicity, arrhythmia, tachycardia and hypertension
4.	Rimantadine	An RNA synthesis inhibitor that is used as an antiviral agent	Well absorbed, with the tablet and syrup formulations being equally absorbed after oral administration	Glucuronidation and hydroxylation are the major metabolic pathways.	40%	Less than 25% of the dose excreted in the urine as unchanged drug	100 mg BD elderly 100 mg OD 5 mg/kg/day	agitation, hallucinations, cardiac arrhythmia and death

Sr. No.	Name of Drugs	Description	Absorption	Metabolism	Protein Binding	Clearance	Dose	Toxicity
5.	Lamivudine	A reverse transcriptase inhibitor and zalcitabine analog in which a sulfur atom replaces the 3′ carbon of the pentose ring	Absolute bioavailability in 12 adult patients was 86% ± 16% (mean ± SD) for the 150-mg tablet and 87% ± 13% for the oral solution	The only known metabolite of lamivudine is the trans-sulfoxide metabolite. This biotransformation is catalyzed by sulfotransferases.	<36% bound to plasma protein	Total clearance is 398.5 ± 69.1 mL/min	For chronic hepatitis B—100 mg OD For HIV infection—150 mg BD	headache, nausea, malaise and fatigue, nasal signs and symptoms, diarrhea, and cough
6.	Ribavirin	Ribavirin is a synthetic guanosine nucleoside and antiviral agent that interferes with the synthesis of viral mRNA	The oral bioavailability is 64% following a single oral dose administration of 600 mg ribavirin	It is phosphorylated by adenosine kinase to ribavirin mono-, di-, triphosphate metabolites. After activation and function, it undergoes metabolic pathways where it is reversibly phosphorlyated or degraded via deribosylation and amide hydrolysis to yield a triazole carboxylic acid metabolite	No protein binding	total apparent clearance rate of 1200 mg is 26 L/h	200 mg QID (children 10 mg/kg/day);	flu-like symptoms, depression, suicide, insomnia, irritability
7.	Zidovudine	A dideoxynucleoside compound in which the 3′-hydroxy group on the sugar moiety has been replaced by an azido group	Rapid and nearly complete absorption from the gastrointestinal tract. Systemic bioavailability of zidovudine capsules and solution is approximately 65% (range, 52 to 75%)	Hepatic. Metabolized by glucuronide conjugation to major, inactive metabolite, 3′-azido-3′-deoxy-5′- O-beta-D-glucopyranuronosylthymidine (GZDV)	30–38%	1.85 +/− 0.47 L/hr./kg	Adults 300 mg BD Children 180 mg/m2 (max 200 mg) BD.	fatigue, headache, nausea, and vomiting

Sr. No.	Name of Drugs	Description	Absorption	Metabolism	Protein Binding	Clearance	Dose	Toxicity
8.	Didanosine	Didanosine is a potent inhibitor of HIV replication, acting as a chain-terminator of viral DNA by binding to reverse transcriptase	Rapidly absorbed (bioavailability 30–40%) with peak plasma concentrations appearing within 0.5 and 1.5 hrs	Rapidly metabolized intracellularly to its active moiety, 2,3-dideoxyadenosine-5-triphosphate (ddA-TP). It is then further metabolized hepatically to yield hypoxanthine, xanthine, and uric acid	Low (<5%)	Renal clearance	400 mg/day 250 mg/day 1 hour before or 2 hours after meals	pancreatitis, peripheral neuropathy, diarrhea, hyperuricemia and hepatic dysfunction
9.	Nevirapine	A potent, non-nucleoside reverse transcriptase inhibitor (NNRTI	The absolute bioavailability in healthy adults following a single dose administration is 93 ± 9% for a 50 mg tablet and 91 ± 8% for an oral solution	nevirapine is extensively biotransformed via cytochrome P450 3A4 metabolism to several hydroxylated metabolites.	60% bound to plasma protein	Renal clearance	200 mg/day oral to be increased after 2 weeks to 200 mg BD	edema, erythema nodosum, fatigue, fever, headache, insomnia, nausea, pulmonaryinfiltrates, rash, vertigo, vomiting, and weight decrease
10.	Ritonavir	Ritonavir is an HIV protease inhibitor that interferes with the reproductive cycle of HIV. Although it was initially developed as an independent antiviral agent	Following oral administration, peak concentrations are reached after approximately 2 hours and 4 hours	Ritonavir circulates in the plasma predominantly as unchanged drug. Five metabolites have been identified. The cytochrome P450 enzymes CYP3A and CYP2D6 are the enzymes primarily involved in the metabolism of ritonavir.	~98–99%	The apparent oral clearance at steady-state is 8.8 ± 3.2 L/h	600 mg BD to be taken with meal	hepatotoxicity, pancreatitis, and allergic reactions/ hypersensitivity
11.	Indinavir	A potent and specific HIV protease inhibitor that appears to have good oral bioavailability	Rapidly absorbed	Hepatic. Seven metabolites have been identified, one glucuronide conjugate and six oxidative metabolites	60%	Less than 20% of indinavir is excreted unchanged in the urine	800 mg TDS	Symptoms of overdose include myocardial infarction and angina pectoris.

Sr. No.	Name of Drugs	Description	Absorption	Metabolism	Protein Binding	Clearance	Dose	Toxicity
12.	Efavirenz	It is a non-nucleoside reverse transcriptase inhibitor (NNRTI) and is used as part of highly active antiretroviral therapy (HAART)	EFV is readily *absorbed* and achieves peak serum concentration (Cmax) of 4.07 mcg/ml 3–5 hours following 600 mg standard adult oral dose.	Efavirenz is principally metabolized by the cytochrome P450 system to hydroxylated metabolites with subsequent glucuronidation	99.5–99.75%	Nearly all of the urinary excretion of the radiolabeled drug was in the form of metabolites	600 mg OD on empty stomach	The most common adverse effects with efavirenz therapy are central nervous system symptoms, rash and hepatitis
13.	Raltegravir	Raltegravir is an antiretroviral drug	Absorbed from the gastrointestinal tract	Hepatic (UGT1A1)	83%	9% of total dose	600 mg BD to be taken with meal	CNS toxicitySS

Table 1.
Anti-viral drugs and their activity [17–21].

3. Anti-hepatitis virus drugs

A. For hepatitis B

- Lamivudine
- Tenofovir

b. For hepatitis C

- Ribavirin
- Interferon alpha

B. Anti-Retrovirus Drugs.

1. Nucleoside reverse transcriptase Inhibtors (Nrtis)

- Zidovudine
- Didanosine
- Stavudine
- Lamivudine

2. Non-Nucleoside Reverse Transcriptase Inhibitor (Nnrtis).

- Nevirapine
- Efavirenz
- Delavirdine

3. Protease inhbitor (PIs)

- Ritonavir
- Atazanavir
- Indinavir
- Nelfinavir

4. Entry inhibitor

- Enfuviritide

5. Ccr-5 receptor inhibitor

- Maraviroc

6. Integrase inhibtor

    • Raltegravir

6. Mechanism of action of non- retroviral drugs

6.1 Anti-Herpes drugs

The recognition of acyclovir and penciclovir has leaded the way evolution of a fortunate systemic therapy for medicating herpes simplex virus infection. Acyclovir is a nucleotide analogue antiviral which is used to treat against herpes simplex. It is generally used as the first line drug in the treatment viruses. Acyclovir is converted into acyclovir monophosphate due to the action of viral thymidine kinase. Acyclovir monophosphate is further converted to the diphosphate form by guanylate kinase. Acyclovir diphosphate is become acyclovir triphosphate by help of nucleoside diphosphate kinase. Acyclovir triphosphate effectively binds to viral DNA polymerase than cellular DNA polymerase and enters into DNA where 2′ and 3′ carbon leads to DNA chain termination. Acyclovir stronger affinity for viral DNA polymerase did not allow other bases to bind it, making them inactive [20].

Dose and Preparation: 200 mg 5 times a day oral (15 mg/kg/day), 5–10 mg/kg 8 hourly by slow i.v. infusion, 5% topical application 6 times a day; ZOVIRAX 200 mg tab, 250 mg/vial for i.v. injection; CYCLOVIR 200 mg tab, 5% skin cream; HERPEX 200 mg tab, 3% eye ointment, 5% skin cream; OCUVIR 200, 400, 800 mg tab, 3% eye ointment, ACIVIR-DT 200, 400, 800 mg tab.

Toxicity: Symptoms of overdose include agitation, coma, seizures, lethargy, and precipitation in renal tubules. These symptoms are more unsophisticated in patients given high doses without monitoring of fluid and electrolyte balance or reduced kidney function.

6.2 Anti-influenza virus drugs

- As per CDC four antiviral drigs are approved by FDA against influenza virus.
- Relenza (zanamivir)
- Tamiflu (oseltamivir phosphate)
- Rapivab (peramivir)
- Xofluza (baloxavir marboxil)
- Amantadine and rimantadine were approved long back ago to cure influenza A virus infection. But new strains of influenza like 2009 H1N1 are resistant to these drugs. Zanamivir acts by inhibition of influenza virus neuraminidase thereby altering particle release and aggregation. It renders the virus inactive by making it unable to break into host cells and infect others [21].

Dose and Preparation: Therapeutic Dose 10 Mg Bd By Inhalation; Prophylactic Dose 10 Mg Od; Relenza 5 Mg Per Actuation Powder Inhaler.

Toxicity: The toxicology studies illustrated that zanamivir has very little toxicity and no drug-specific toxicities were observed in animal toxicity studies.

Arbidol which is popularly used to cure influenza is reported to inhibit SARS-CoV-2 [22]. Similarly, Favipiravir, an anti-influenza drug, also is undergoing clinical trials against COVID19 [23].

6.3 Anti-hepatitis virus drugs

To date, two classes of antiviral drugs have been accepted by the Food and Drug Administration for the treatment of hepatitis B, and nucleos(t)ide analogs (lamivudine, telbivudine, adefovir, tenofovir [TDF] and for hepatitis C, immunomodulators (interferon [IFN]-α and pegylated-interferon [PEG-IFN]-α). Lamivudine, a synthetic nucleoside analogue, is phosphorylated intracellularly to lamivudine triphosphate, 5′-triphosphate metabolite. The nucleoside analogue is inserted into viral DNA by HBV polymerase and HIV reverse transcriptase leading to DNA chain termination. Interferons are glycoproteins synthesized by host cells in response to viral infection and some other inducers. These are effective against DNA and RNA virus and have a no-specific inhibitory effect on the viral replication against a wide variety of unrelated viruses [24].

Dose and Preparation: For Chronic Hepatitis B 100 Mg Od; For Hiv Infection 150 Mg Bd (Along With Other Antiretroviral Drugs); Lamivir 150 Mg Tab, 150 Mg/5 Ml Solution; Lamivir-Hbv 100 Mg Tab; Heptavir, Lamidac, Lamuvid 100, 150 Mg Tabs.

Toxicity: The most common reported adverse reactions in adults were headache, nausea, malaise and fatigue, nasal signs and symptoms, diarrhea, and cough etc.

Remdesivir which was developed to treat Hepatitis C has also demonstrated antiviral activity against SARS-CoV-2 [25]. As per results of controlled, randomized clinical trials, remdesivir has shortened the time of recovery in adults employed to treat hospitilized COVID-19 patients [26–30]. However, remdesivir potential against new SARS-CoV-2 variants is under trail and should be monitored.

Ribavirin used to cure COVID-19 [31] approved to cure respiratory syncytial virus and HCV leads to anemia at higher dose [32]. Ribavirin is administered intravenously at a dose of 500 mg, 2–3 times a day [33].

Some Antiretroviral Combinations:

1. Lamivudine 150 Mg + Zidovudine 300 Mg Table (1 Tab Bd); Combivir, Cytocom, Duovir, Lamuzid, Zidolam Table.

2. Lamivudine 150 Mg + Stavudine 30 Mg Or 40 Mg Table (1 Tab Bd); Lamivir-S, Lamostad, Virolis Table.

3. Lamivudine 150 Mg + Zidovudine 300 Mg + Nevirapine 200 Mg Table (1 Tab Bd); Duovir-N, Cytocom-N, Nexivir-Z.

7. Mechanism of action of retroviral drugs.

7.1 Nucleoside reverse transcriptase inhibitors (NRTIS)

The nucleotide/nucleoside reverse transcriptase inhibitors are the first class of antiretroviral drugs approved by FDA. NRTIS are taken up by host cells and phosphorylated and activated by cellular kinases. NRTIS lack 3′-hydroxyl group at the 2'deoxyribosyl moiety and have nucleotide/nucleoside as base. They prevent the formation of 3′-5′-phosphodiester bond in DNA chains thus preventing the replication of virus. An important aspect these drugs is that they inhibit the production of either negative or positive strands of DNA if incorporated during DNA- dependent DNA synthesis or RNA-dependent DNA synthesis [34].

Dose and Preparation: Didanosine: 400 Mg/Day (For >60 Kg Bw), 250 Mg/Day (< 50 Kg Bw); 1 Hour Before or 2 Hours After Meals; Dinex Ec, Dd Retro, Virosine Dr. 250, 400 Mg Tabs. Zidovudine (Azidothymidine, AZT): Adults 300 mg BD; Children 180 mg/m2 (max 200 mg) BD. Retrovir, Zidovir 100 Mg Cap 300 Mg Tab, 50 Mg/5 Ml Syr, Zidomax, Zydowin 100 Mg Cap, 300 Mg Tab (To Be Taken With Plenty Of Water).

Toxicity: Symptoms of overdose include fatigue, headache, nausea, and vomiting. LD_{50} is 3084 mg/kg (orally in mice).

7.2 Non-nucleoside reverse transcriptase inhibitor (NNRTIS)

These are second class of reverse transcriptase inhibitors. They act by binding to reverse transcriptase and create hydrophobic pocket proximal to active site. This pocket generates novel spatial configuration of substrate binding site to decrease the overall activity of polymerase. By producing different configuration, synthesis of DNA slows down. NNRTIS are not effective against HIV-2 reverse transcriptase, because of non-competitive inhibitor action.

Dose and Preparation: Nevirapine: 200 mg/day oral to be increased after 2 weeks to 200 mg BD; Nevimune, Nevivir, Nevipan, Neviretro 200 Mg.

Toxicity: Symptoms of overdose include edema, erythema nodosum, fatigue, fever, headache, insomnia, nausea, pulmonary infiltrates, rash, vertigo, vomiting, and weight decrease. The most common adverse reaction is rash.

8. Protease inhbitor (PIs)

The HIV viral proteinase enzyme which always fragment the replicative and structural proteins which evolve from major HIV genes mormally as gag and pol, is restrain by Ritonavir. Ritonavir inhibits the cleavage of gag-pol polyprotein leading in non-infectious immature viral particles. Ritonavir is also potent inhibitor of cytochrome P450 CYP3A4 isoenzyme which is present in both liver and small intestine. It is type II ligand which binds into CYP3A4 and further irreversibly to heme iron via thiazole nitrogen linkage which reduces proteins redox potential and impedes its reduction with cytochrome P450 reductase, redox partner. Ritonavir may edge cellular transport and efflux of other protease inhibitor via MRP efflux channel and P-glycoprotein.

Ritonavir/ Lopinavir is FDA approved therapy to treat HIV and is also reported to treat COVID19. However in patients with severe COVID-19, this combination showed no benefit [35].

PREPARATIONS: RITOVIR 250 mg tab, RITOMUNE, RITOMAX 100 mg cap.

Entry inhibitors obstruct HIV entry into CD4 cells in organism cells. They act in a different way other than nucleoside reverse transcriptase inhibitors, protease inhibitors and non-nucleoside reverse transcriptase inhibitors which function after they it has infected CD4 cells. They work by taking themselves to proteins which is composed of amino acids on superficial side of CD4 cells, the proteins present on surface of CD4 cells or on the surface of HIV. The proteins on HIV outer coat must bind to proteins present on the surface of CD4. Entry proteins inhibit the above process.

PREPARATION: - Efavirenz: is available as 600 mg tab, also FFERVEN, VIRANZ, and EVIRENZ, 200 mg cap, 600 mg tab.

9. Conclusion

In this review we have concluded that the treatment of the viral infection and current covid 19 includes the combination therapy of antiviral drugs and the immune modeling drugs. Use of the antiviral drugs for the treatment of viral infection prevents from illness and as well as mortality rate. Lot of clinical trails are going on to prove their efficacy against SARS-CoV-2 and will definitely prove to be fruitful and help to save the human community.

Author details

Sweta Kamboj[1*], Rohit Kamboj[1], Shikha Kamboj[2], Rohit Dutt[3], Reeva Chabbra[4] and Priyanka Kriplani[1]

1 Guru Gobind Singh College of Pharmacy, Yamuna Nagar, Haryana, India

2 Guru Jambheshwar University of Science and Technology, Hisar, India

3 School of Medical and Allied Sciences, G.D. Goenka University, Gurugram, India

4 Maharshi Dayanand University, Rohtak, Haryana, India

*Address all correspondence to: Swetakamboj20@gmail.com

'Biotechnology to Combat COVID-19' is a collaborative project with Biotechnology Kiosk

References

[1] Liu J, Xie W, Wang Y, Xiong Y, Chen S, Han J, Wu Q. A comparative overview of COVID-19, Mers and Sars. IJS. 2020;81:1-8. DOI: 10.1016/j.ijsu.2020.07.032

[2] Lodish H, Berk A, Zipursky SL, Matsudaira P, Baltimore D, Darnell J. Viruses: Structure, Function, and Uses. Molecular Cell Biology 4th edition [Internet]. W. H. Freeman; 2000 [cited 2021 Apr 23]

[3] Salvati AL, De Dominicis A, Tait S, Canitano A, Lahm A, Fiore L. Mechanism of Action at the molecular level of the antiviral drug 3(2H)-Isoflavene against Type 2 Poliovirus. AAC. 2004;48(6):2233-2243. DOI:10.1128/AAC.48.6.2233-2243.2004

[4] Shiraki K, Daikoku T, Takemoto M, Himaki T, Kuramoto T. Mechanism of action of antiviral drugs. NR. 2012;70(4):545-551.

[5] Huraux JM, Ingrand D, Agut H, Devillechabrolle A. Prospects and current data in antiviral chemotherapy. RPC. 1989;45(3):99-105.

[6] Krammer F, Sars-Cov-2 vaccines in development. N. 2020;586:516-27

[7] Jenssen H, Hamill P, Hancock REW. Peptide antimicrobial agents.CMR. 2006;19(3):491-11. DOI: 10.1128/CMR.00056-05

[8] Takeda M, Khamdang S, Narikawa S, Kimura H, Kobayashi Y, Yamamoto T, Cha SH, Sekine T, Endou H: Human organic anion transporters and human organic cation transporters mediate renal antiviral transport. JPET. 2002;300(3):918-24

[9] Wada S, Tsuda M, Sekine T, Cha SH, Kimura M, Kanai Y, Endou H: Rat multispecific organic anion transporter 1 (rOAT1) transports zidovudine, acyclovir, and other antiviral nucleoside analogs. JPET. 2000;294(3):844-9.

[10] Hull R, Rima B. Viruses taxonomy and classification: naming of virus species. AV. 2020;165:2733-36.

[11] Shiraki K. Antiviral drugs against alphaherpesvirus. AEMB. 2018;1045:103-22. DOI: 10.1007/978-981-10-7230-7-6

[12] Shie J-J, Fang J-M. Development of effective anti-influenza drugs: congeners and conjugates - a review. JBS. 2019;26(1):84. DOI: 10.1186/s12929-019-0567-0

[13] Research C for DE and. Influenza (Flu) Antiviral Drugs and Related Information. FDA. [Internet]. 2020. Available from: https://www.fda.gov/drugs/information-drug-class/influenza-flu-antiviral-drugs-and-related-information [Accessed2021-April-23]

[14] Vilas Boas LCP, Campos ML, Berlanda RLA, de Carvalho Neves N, Franco OL. Antiviral peptides as promising therapeutic drugs. CMLS. 2019;76(18):3525-42. DOI: 10.1007/s00018-019-03138-w

[15] De Clercq E, Ferir G, Kaptein S, Neyts J. Antiviral Treatment of Chronic Hepatitis B Virus (HBV) Infections. V. 2010;2(6):1279-05. DOI: 10.3390/v2061279

[16] Qiu L-P, Chen L, Chen K-P. Antihepatitis B therapy: a review of current medications and novel small molecule inhibitors. FCP. 2014;28(4):364-81. DOI: 10.1111/fcp.12053

[17] Chan JF, Kok KH, Zhu Z, Chu H, To KK, Yuan S, Yuen KY. Genomic characterization of the 2019 novel human-pathogenic coronavirus isolated

from a patient with atypical pneumonia after visiting Wuhan. EMI. 2020;9(1):221-36. DOI: 10.1080/22221751.2020.1719902

[18] Lei J, Kusov Y, Hilgenfeld R. Nsp3 of coronaviruses: Structures and functions of a large multi-domain protein. AR. 2018;149:58-4. DOI: 10.1016/j.antiviral.2017.11.001

[19] Song W, Gui M, Wang X, Xiang Y. Cryo-EM structure of the SARS coronavirus spike glycoprotein in complex with its host cell receptor ACE2. PP. 2018 14(8): e1007236. DOI: 10.1371/journal.ppat.1007236

[20] Patel PH, Zulfiqar H. Reverse Transcriptase Inhibitors. In: StatPearls. StatPearls Publishing; 2021. Accessed 2021 April 23. http://www.ncbi.nlm.nih.gov/books/NBK551504/

[21] Pokorna J, Machala L, Rezacova P, Konvalinka J. Current and novel inhibitors of HIV protease. V. 2009;1(3):1209-39. DOI: 10.3390/v1031209

[22] Cao J et al. Clinical Features and Short-term Outcomes of 102 Patients with coronavirus disease 2019 in Wuhan, China, CID : an official publication of the Infectious Diseases Society of America. 2020; The United States 2020; 71(15):748-55. DOI: 10.1093/cid/ciaa243

[23] Li G, De Clercq E. Therapeutic options for the 2019 novel coronavirus (2019-nCoV). NRDD. 2020;19(3): 149-50. DOI: org/10.1038/d41573-020-00016-0

[24] Agbowuro AA, Huston WM, Gamble AB, Tyndall JDA. Protease and protease inhibitors in infectious diseases. MRR. 2017;38(4):1295-31. DOI: org/10.1002/med.21475

[25] Wang M, Cao R, Zhang L, Yang X, Liu J, Xu M, Shi Z, Hu Z, Zhong W, Xiao G. Remdesivir and chloroquine effectively inhibit the recently emerged novel coronavirus (2019-nCoV) in vitro. CR. 2020;30(3):269-71. DOI. org/10.1038/s41422-020-0282-0

[26] Beigel JH, Tomashek KM, Dodd LE, Mehta AK, Zingman BS, Kalil AC, Hohmann E, Chu HY, Luetkemeyer A, Kline S, Lopez de Castilla D, Finberg RW, Dierberg K, Tapson V, Hsieh L, Patterson TF, Paredes R, Sweeney DA, Short WR, Touloumi G, Lye DC, Ohmagari N, Oh MD, Ruiz-Palacios GM, Benfield T, Fätkenheuer G, Kortepeter MG, Atmar RL, Creech CB, Lundgren J, Babiker AG, Pett S, Neaton JD, Burgess TH, Bonnett T, Green M, Makowski M, Osinusi A, Nayak S, Lane HC., ACTT-1 Study Group Members. Remdesivir for the Treatment of Covid-19 - Final Report. NEJM. 2020;383(19):1813-26. DOI:10.1056/NEJMoa2007764.

[27] Goldman JD, Lye DCB, Hui DS, Marks KM, Bruno R, Montejano R, Spinner CD, Galli M, Ahn MY, Nahass RG, Chen YS, SenGupta D, Hyland RH, Osinusi AO, Cao H, Blair C, Wei X, Gaggar A, Brainard DM, Towner WJ, Muñoz J, Mullane KM, Marty FM, Tashima KT, Diaz G, Subramanian A., GS-US-540-5773 Investigators. Remdesivir for 5 or 10 Days in Patients with Severe Covid-19. NEJM. 2020 383(19):1827-37. DOI: 10.1056/NEJMoa2015301

[28] Spinner CD, Gottlieb RL, Criner GJ, Arribas López JR, Cattelan AM, Soriano Viladomiu A, Ogbuagu O, Malhotra P, Mullane KM, Castagna A, Chai LYA, Roestenberg M, Tsang OTY, Bernasconi E, Le Turnier P, Chang SC, SenGupta D, Hyland RH, Osinusi AO, Cao H, Blair C, Wang H, Gaggar A, Brainard DM, McPhail MJ, Bhagani S, Ahn MY, Sanyal AJ, Huhn G, Marty FM., GS-US-540-5774 Investigators. Effect of Remdesivir vs Standard Care on Clinical Status at 11

Days in Patients With Moderate COVID-19: A Randomized Clinical Trial. JAMA. 2020 324(11):1048-57. DOI: 10.1001/jama.2020.16349.

[29] Rabi YM, Murthy S, Webb S. COVID-19: A novel coronavirus and a novel challenge for critical care, ICM. 2020;1-4

[30] Li G, De Clercq E. Therapeutic options for the 2019 novel coronavirus (2019-nCoV), NR DD. 2020;19(3):149-50. DOI: doi.org/10.1038/d41573-020-00016-0

[31] Dong L, Hu S, Gao J. Discovering drugs to treat coronavirus disease 2019 (COVID-19), DDT. 2020;14(1):58-60. DOI: 10.5582/ddt.2020.01012

[32] Holec AD, Mandal S, Prathipati PK, Destache CJ. Nucleotide reverse transcriptase inhibitors: A Thorough review, present status and future perspective as HIV therapeutics. CHIVR. 2017;15(6):411-24. DOI.: 10.2174/1570162X15666171120110145

[33] Arts EJ, Hazuda D. HIV-1 antiretroviral drug therapy. CPHPM. 2012;2(4): a007161. DOI: org/10.1101%2Fcshperspect.a007161

[34] Shi S, Nguyen PK, Cabral HJ, Diez-Barroso R, Derry PJ, Kanahara SM, Kumar VA. Development of peptide inhibitors of HIV transmission. BM. 2016;1:109-21. DOI: org/10.1016/j.bioactmat.2016.09.004.

[35] Cao B, Wang Y, Wen D, Liu W, Wang J, Fan G, Ruan L, Song B, Cai Y, Wei M, Li X, Xia J, Chen N, Xiang J, Yu T, Bai T, Xie X, Zhang L, Li C, Yuan Y, Chen H, Li H, Huang H, Tu S, Gong F, Liu Y, Wei Y, Dong C, Zhou F, Gu X, Xu J, Liu Z, Zhang Y, Li H, Shang L, Wang K, Li K, Zhou X, Dong X, Qu Z, Lu S, Hu X, Ruan S, Luo S, Wu J, Peng L, Cheng F, Pan L, Zou J, Jia C, Wang J, Liu X, Wang S, Wu X, Ge Q, He J, Zhan H, Qiu F, Guo L, Huang C, Jaki T, Hayden FG, Horby PW, Zhang D, Wang C. A trial of lopinavir-ritonavir in adults hospitalized with severe covid-19. NEJM. 2020;382(19):1787-99. DOI: 10.1056/NEJMoa2001282

Chapter 21

Targeting Mononuclear Phagocytes to Treat COVID-19

Brandt D. Pence and Theodore J. Cory

Abstract

Coronavirus disease 2019 (COVID-19) and its etiological agent severe acute respiratory syndrome coronavirus-2 (SARS-CoV-2) have caused considerable illness and death worldwide. The innate immune system seems to play a principal in the disease, as a hallmark of severe COVID-19 is excessive inflammation. Monocytes and macrophages are important innate immune cells that become pro-inflammatory and promote adaptive immune responses during viral infection. In this chapter we present evidence linking these cells to severity of COVID-19. Namely, monocytes and macrophages infiltrate the infected tissue during the early stages of infection and show pro-inflammatory responses that appear to be linked to those predicting tissue pathology during disease. Additionally, studies in isolated cells demonstrate that monocytes and macrophages respond by producing pro-inflammatory cytokines when directly stimulated by SARS-CoV-2. While most anti-inflammatory pharmaceutical treatments for COVID-19 have focused on systemic infiltration, some of the most promising have known or suspected effects on monocyte and macrophage inflammatory responses. Therefore, targeting these cells to treat severe COVID-19 is a promising strategy for this important disease.

Keywords: COVID-19, SARS-CoV-2, monocytes, macrophages, innate immunity

1. Introduction

A novel highly pathogenic coronavirus emerged in Hubei Province, China in the latter months of 2019. The government of the People's Republic of China informed the World Health Organization of the outbreak of the virus, which was preliminarily named novel coronavirus 2019 (2019-nCov), on 31 December 2019. Early observational studies found high incidences of fever, cough, and fatigue in hospitalized patients with diagnosed infection, and pneumonia, acute respiratory distress syndrome, and higher plasma pro-inflammatory cytokine levels were also common in those admitted to the Intensive Care Unit [1]. Comorbidities including older age and diabetes were found to be associated with worse outcomes [2].

Patient samples were utilized to isolate a betacoronavirus which was distinct from previous highly pathogenic coronaviruses such as Severe Acute Respiratory Syndrome Coronavirus (SARS-CoV) and Middle East Respiratory Syndrome Coronavirus (MERS-CoV), which caused epidemic outbreaks in 2002–2003 [3] and 2012 [4] respectively. Molecular epidemiology studies on 2019-nCov found that the new virus shared approximately 80% sequence identity to SARS-CoV, and further that it shared ~96% sequence identity to the known bat coronavirus RaTG13 [5], suggesting a potential bat origin. Later papers have suggested transmission to humans through an intermediate host, with leading candidates including Malayan pangolins and minks [6], but to date no natural viral reservoir or intermediate host has been found despite extensive surveys. Although there has been some speculation as to a laboratory origin of 2019-nCov, this is generally rejected by most in the scientific community [7–10], and to date there is no compelling evidence of a human origin for the virus.

In March 2020, the World Health Organization declared a worldwide pandemic of Coronavirus Disease-2019 (COVID-19), the disease of which 2019-nCov is the etiological agent. Likewise in that month, the International Committee on Taxonomy of Viruses (ICTV) officially named the new virus the Severe Acute Respiratory Coronavirus-2 (SARS-CoV-2) [11], and this nomenclature will be utilized throughout the rest of the chapter. To date, SARS-CoV-2 and COVID-19 have caused tremendous morbidity and mortality worldwide, with deaths from COVID-19 numbering more than 3 million as of mid-April 2021 [12].

1.1 Clinical indicators of COVID-19

COVID-19 generally presents with some combination of cough, fever, and/or dyspnea, with less prevalent symptoms including diarrhea, myalgia, and nausea/vomiting [13]. Clinical immunology indicators of severe COVID-19 also include lymphopenia and thrombocytopenia [13] as well as significant elevations of circulating pro-inflammatory cytokines and other inflammation markers such as C-reactive protein [14]. Chest CT scans detect ground glass opacities and pneumonia in a substantial fraction of COVID-19 patients with severe disease [13, 15]. Severe COVID-19 can progress to acute respiratory distress syndrome [16] and can lead to death.

Multiple co-morbidities are associated with severity of COVID-19. Among these, advanced age is the strongest predictor of morbidity and mortality [17], and increased disease severity is also linked with pre-existing diabetes [18] and severe asthma [17]. In addition to the pulmonary system, SARS-CoV-2 has been found to infect other organ systems including the cardiovascular, central nervous, and gastrointestinal tract systems [19], therefore a variety of other symptoms can occur during COVID-19. A subset of COVID-19 patients develop persistent symptoms which last for weeks or months, which has been described as post-acute COVID-19 syndrome or colloquially as "long COVID" [20]. The etiology of long COVID is unknown, but does not appear to be associated with persistence of replication-competent SARS-CoV-2 [21].

2. Overview of the immune system

2.1 Adaptive immune system

The vertebrate immune system is generally divided into two complementary arms. The adaptive immune system is highly specialized and recognizes specific protein motifs corresponding to individual pathogens. Adaptive immunity is primarily mediated by T and B lymphocytes, with T cells further divided into cytotoxic T cells (CD8+) and several classes of helper T cells (CD4+). Cytotoxic T cells recognize infected cells through interactions of the T cell receptor (TCR) with antigen-bound class I major histocompatibility complex (MHC) molecules, and kill these cells via release of cytotoxins such as perforins and granzymes. Likewise, helper T cells recognize pathogens through interactions of their TCR with antigen-bound class II MHC molecules on antigen presenting cells, and serve to instruct activation of B cells or CD8+ T cells through the release of various cytokines. Finally, B cells produce pathogen-specific antibodies, which bind extracellular pathogens to allow them to be neutralized by a variety of methods. Adaptive immune responses are highly important during SARS-CoV-2 infection and are key to successful clearance of the virus from the host. However, these aspects of immunity during COVID-19 are otherwise beyond the scope of this chapter, and we can point readers to a recent review article on this subject [22].

2.2 Innate immune system

Unlike adaptive immunity, innate immunity is not specific to individual pathogens, but is instead a host system which allows for conserved responses to broad classes of pathogens. A key facet of the innate immune response is inflammation, which allows for the destruction and removal of infected or damaged cells, as well as tissue cleanup and infiltration of additional immune effector cells to the site of infection. A key component of innate immunity is inflammation. Chemokines and pro-inflammatory cytokines respectively attract innate immune cells to the site of infection and activate them, thereby promoting their various effector functions. Neutrophils are early responder cells which perform phagocytosis of pathogens and kill microorganisms via the release of soluble anti-microbial molecules and neutrophil extracellular traps. Dendritic cells take up pathogens and damaged cell components via phagocytosis and migrate to the lymph nodes, where they present antigen on class II MHC to activate CD4+ T cells. Likewise, macrophages can perform similar antigen presenting functions, and are also key orchestrators of the immune response via the release of cytokines and chemokines. A variety of other cell types are active during an innate immune response to pathogens such as SARS-CoV-2, and we point readers to a recent review on this topic [23].

2.3 Monocytes

The remainder of this chapter will principally focus on the contributions of monocytes and macrophages to COVID-19. These are innate immune cells of myeloid lineage. Monocytes arise in the bone marrow from common myeloid progenitor cells, which are also the precursor to erythrocytes, mast cells, and neutrophils among other cell types [24]. Monocytes circulate in the bloodstream and perform important innate immune effector functions, including antigen presentation, phagocytosis, and immune signaling through cytokine production [25]. Monocytes recognize broad classes of pathogen (e.g., gram-negative bacteria, dsRNA viruses, etc.) via pathogen binding to cell surface and intracellular pattern recognition receptors (PRRs) and respond by phagocytosis and/or cytokine production to further orchestrate the immune response [25].

In humans, three traditional monocyte phenotypes are widely recognized: classical ($CD14^{+}CD16^{-}$), intermediate ($CD14^{+}CD16^{+}$), and non-classical ($CD14^{dim}CD16^{+}$) [26]. Classical monocytes make up the bulk of circulating monocytes (>80%) and are highly phagocytic and potent cytokine producers. Intermediate monocytes are enriched for antigen presenting MHC molecules and produce cytokines under PRR binding, and non-classical monocytes have patrolling and wound healing functions and are less responsive to PRR binding compared to classical monocytes [27]. However, intermediate and non-classical monocytes are also associated with increased basal inflammation and are increased in circulation in a number of chronic diseases [27], thereby suggesting that proportional increases in $CD16^{+}$ monocyte populations may be reflective of detrimental innate immune responses.

2.4 Macrophages

Macrophages are tissue mononuclear phagocytes that participate in innate immune defense and stimulation of the adaptive immune system. During an inflammatory event, peripheral monocytes invade tissue and differentiate to macrophages to carry out host defense, tissue remodeling, and cellular signaling activities. Tissue enrichment of monocyte-derived macrophages is therefore a hallmark of many infections and contributes to immunopathology during acute disease [28–30]. Additionally, many long-lived tissue resident macrophages are not monocytic in origin and instead arise during embryonic development [31]. Tissue resident macrophages often have distinct nomenclature (e.g. Kupffer cells – liver; microglia – brain; osteoclasts – bone) and can perform highly diverse functions depending on tissue environment.

Macrophages are phenotypically heterogeneous and can be polarized along the inflammatory spectrum to mediate diverse functions which are pro-inflammatory (e.g., T cell stimulation) or anti-inflammatory (e.g., wound healing) in nature [32]. Macrophages are often classified as M1/pro-inflammatory or M2/anti-inflammatory depending on their polarization signals and their expression of cell surface or intracellular markers, which is recognized to be an oversimplification but persists due to the utility of studying these phenotypes, especially *in vitro*.

Within the tissue, macrophages play principal roles in phagocytosis of dead cells, cell debris, and extracellular pathogens, and additionally present antigens to CD4+ T cells to activate adaptive immune responses [33]. Macrophages also recognize pathogens through PRR binding and produce cytokines and chemokines to orchestrate the immune response, including both initiation and resolution of inflammation, the latter of which is key to successful tissue repair.

3. Monocytes and macrophages in COVID-19

A substantial body of evidence now demonstrates the importance of immune function during COVID-19 [22, 23]. Here we will focus on the potential contributions of monocytes and macrophages to severe COVID-19, especially as it pertains to the hyperinflammatory environment characteristic of severe disease [34–36]. A large number of cytokines have been shown to be upregulated during COVID-19 and associated with poor outcomes, including interleukin (IL)-1α, IL-1β, IL-2, IL-6, IL-8, IL-10, IL-17A, IL-33, monocyte chemoattractant protein-1 (MCP-1), granulocyte colony stimulating factor (G-CSF), interferon (IFN)-γ, IFNγ-inducible protein (IP10), and tumor necrosis factor-α (TNFα) among others [37–43].

3.1 Monocyte infiltration into infected tissue

The infiltration of monocytes and subsequent increase in monocyte-derived macrophages is a hallmark of infection severity for a number of viruses [28–30]. Several observations have now suggested that this is also the case in COVID-19. A variety of single cell RNA sequencing studies have noted increases in monocytes and macrophages in collected bronchoalveolar lavage fluid that are associated with severe disease [44–46]. Notably, infiltrating monocyte-derived macrophages seem ultimately to be the principal contributors to disease severity, rather than resident alveolar macrophages [45, 47, 48]. Likewise, several post-mortem analyses of patients who died due to COVID-19 have found significant numbers of monocytes and monocyte-derived macrophages in tissues, especially lungs [49–52].

A key drawback to observational human studies is that they cannot empirically determine whether monocyte infiltration and macrophage increases are due to SARS-CoV-2 infection itself, due to the ethical issues with infecting human subjects with the virus itself in a prospective manner. Animal studies are often used in such instances, and this is complicated in COVID-19 research by the general non-susceptibility of traditional laboratory mouse models to infection by SARS-CoV-2. This is due to significant sequence differences between mouse and human angiotensin converting enzyme 2 (ACE2), the principal receptor for SARS-CoV-2 [53].

Nevertheless, while standard mouse models are not susceptible to viral infection, a large number of other laboratory animals have been established as models of COVID-19. Experimental infection in these animals invariably leads to monocyte and macrophage infiltration into pulmonary tissue, as has been shown to date with human ACE2-expressing transgenic mice [54, 55], Syrian hamsters [56], rhesus macaques [57–59], and African green monkeys [60] among others. Given the associations with disease shown in human sequencing and pathology studies, as well as the empirical evidence from animal studies demonstrating monocyte/macrophage infiltration during infection, it appears clear that these cells are responding to localized tissue infection during COVID-19. However, the functions being mediated by monocytes and macrophages during the course of SARS-CoV-2 infection are not yet entirely clear.

3.2 Phenotypic shifts and hyperinflammation

In addition to infiltration into infected tissues, various observational studies have shown shifts in monocyte and macrophage phenotypes towards hyperinflammatory states in COVID-19. One of the most consistent changes noted in COVID-19 immune profiling studies is a decrease in monocyte expression of human leukocyte antigen (HLA)-DR, an MHC class II protein. HLA-DR downregulation has been seen in other inflammatory conditions such as sepsis and is linked to disease severity [61]. In COVID-19, HLA-DR downregulation is a prominent feature [38, 45, 62–66], and could signify immune exhaustion in virus-stimulated cells that could lead to impaired inflammation and antigen presentation, and therefore to defects in adaptive immune responses.

Likewise, both monocytes [67–70] and lung macrophages [44, 45, 71] produce increased levels of pro-inflammatory cytokines during acute SARS-CoV-2 infection as noted in human observational studies. Pro-inflammatory macrophage responses have also been noted in the lungs of experimentally infected non-human primates [60, 72, 73], thereby linking macrophage inflammation to infection with SARS-CoV-2 itself (and not some other biological factor). Therefore, it appears that SARS-CoV-2 infection causes inflammatory responses in macrophages and monocytes, although the immediate proximal cause of this response cannot be identified solely via immune cell phenotype profiling.

3.3 Responses to direct infection

Both macrophage infiltration to infected tissues and resulting hyperinflammation in these cells can be explained by indirect mechanisms (e.g., infected cells activating monocytes/macrophages via cytokine signaling). However, several *in vitro* studies have demonstrated that monocytes and macrophages react to infection with SARS-CoV-2 by mounting pronounced inflammatory responses [74–76]. It is likely that infection of these cells is abortive (i.e., does not produce additional infectious virus) [74, 75, 77], so these responses may be mediated by viral protein binding to cellular receptors rather than by recognition of replicating viral RNA.

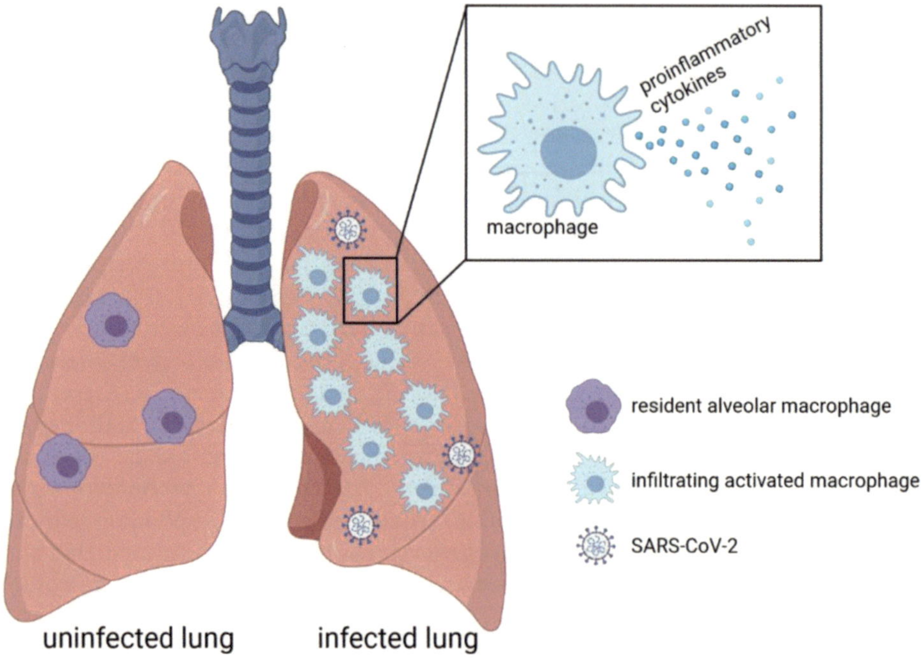

Figure 1.
Schematic of lung macrophage populations during COVID-19. Uninfected lungs (left) maintain a resident population of alveolar macrophages. During SARS-CoV-2 infection (right), infiltrating monocyte-derived macrophages become activated and produce pro-inflammatory cytokines. Created with BioRender.com.

Additionally, immunometabolic activation has been demonstrated in infected monocytes, which upregulate glycolytic activation [78] and accumulate intracellular lipid droplets [79] when exposed to SARS-CoV-2. Metabolic reprogramming is a hallmark of innate immune activation [80], and thus may be a mechanism by which myeloid cells mount their initial inflammatory responses to SARS-CoV-2. A schematic of lung macrophage populations with and without SARS-CoV-2 infection is shown in **Figure 1**.

4. Targeting monocytes and macrophages

Targeting monocytes and macrophages as a strategy to improve outcomes in people infected with SARS-CoV-2 has been an area of considerable interest since the beginning of the COVID-19 pandemic. As key effectors of the innate immune system, they play an important role orchestrating the immune response to SARS-CoV-2. This approach has been primarily focused on systemic anti-inflammatories, although a number of other strategies are under investigation. While a variety of small molecule and biologic based strategies have been investigated to treat COVID-19, there has been a relative dearth of strategies which have been shown to improve disease outcomes.

4.1 Dexamethasone

One such drug which has been recommended for use in critically ill COVID-19 subjects is the corticosteroid dexamethasone. A number of trials, most notably the RECOVERY trial have investigated the use of dexamethasone in individuals receiving advanced care for COVID-19, and have shown that the drug may of therapeutic utility for severe cases [81]. This trial showed that in ventilated patients and patients receiving supplemental oxygen, that administration of IV dexamethasone resulted in a significant increase in 28-day mortality. Interestingly, however, the same results were not observed for individuals not receiving supplemental oxygen.

Among other mechanisms, one way by which corticosteroids decrease inflammation is by modulating cytokine release from monocytes and macrophages [82]. This can include, among other cytokines, IL-8, GM-CSF, and TNF-α [82, 83]. By modulating cytokine production in monocytes and macrophages, dexamethasone may lessen the strong cytokine storm that occurs in many people infected with SARS-CoV-2 [84].

4.2 Baricitinib

Baricitinib is a JAK 1 and 2 inhibitor which has currently received an emergency use authorization to be used in combination with remdesivir for the treatment of COVID-19. Previously, it had been approved for the treatment of rheumatoid arthritis [85]. In patients with COVID-19, in combination with remdesivir it has been shown to be superior to remdesivir alone in improving clinical status, especially in ventilated individuals [86]. Baricitinib likely functions in COVID-19 by decreasing the release of inflammatory cytokines from immune cells, including macrophages.

Non-human primate studies of baricitinib has shown that it can decrease the production of pro-inflammatory cytokines in lung macrophages, including TNF-α, IL-6, and IL-1β [72]. These modulations in cytokine expression from macrophages also blunted neutrophil influx into the lungs of these animals, which likely represents the mechanism by which the drug improves COVID-19 outcomes.

4.3 Tocilizumab

Tocilizumab is a monoclonal antibody therapeutic which has been approved for the treatment of rheumatoid arthritis [87]. Its mechanism of action is to act as an antagonist for the interleukin-6 receptor. By blocking this receptor, it is able to decrease signal transduction of this pathway and decrease the host inflammatory response. During the COVID-19 pandemic, it has gained considerable interest as a therapeutic for COVID-19. Its use is recommended as a single IV dose in combination with dexamethasone in patients who are critically ill in the ICU and receiving mechanical ventilation [88] . The evidence supporting the use of tocilizumab in COVID-19 is somewhat mixed, with some studies showing no benefit in the disease [89].

Macrophages are key producers of IL-6, and the IL-6 receptor is expressed on the surface of macrophages [90]. In COVID-19, some patients experience an overly strong cytokine response, commonly referred to as a cytokine storm, or hyperinflammation. Treatment with tocilizumab may be able to decrease this strong inflammatory response through blunting IL-6 signaling [91].

4.4 Non-steroidal anti-inflammatory drugs (NSAIDs)

To date, there has been considerable controversy to the potential benefit of NSAIDs for the treatment of COVID-19. These drugs inhibit the activity of the cyclooxygenase isoforms 1 and 2 [92]. In March of 2020, the French Minister of Health raised concerns based on case reports in the country showing individuals with worsened symptoms after the administration of NSAIDs [93]. This was further supported by previous studies in lower respiratory infections suggesting that NSAID usage could worsen disease outcomes. These studies, however, were relatively weak, and additional research is likely necessary to determine the effect of these drugs on respiratory infections [94]. There is some evidence that suggests that NSAIDs may be able to decrease the production of pro-inflammatory cytokines including TNF-α from macrophages, which may represent a potential mechanism of action of any potential benefits for the treatment of COVID-19 [95].

5. Conclusions

COVID-19 is an emergent and ongoing disease with substantial public health and sociological implications. It is clear that inflammation underlies severe COVID-19, and so the biological mechanisms by which this occurs are of substantial interest. Monocytes and macrophages are important innate immune cells that appear to play central roles in COVID-19, as they infiltrate infected tissues and produce pro-inflammatory cytokines during infection. Some current biologic and non-steroidal anti-inflammatory therapies which may be efficacious in treating COVID-19 have known effects on macrophages and monocytes. However, these have primarily been used systemically, so the utility of directly targeting mononuclear phagocytes as a therapeutic for COVID-19 remains in need of investigation. A brief summary of evidence for anti-inflammatory drugs used to treat COVID-19 is presented in **Table 1** below.

Future studies are needed to define the molecular mechanisms by which monocytes and macrophages respond to SARS-CoV-2, either due to direct infection or due to signaling from nearby infected cells. A fuller understanding of how myeloid cells become activated during COVID-19 will allow for more targeted therapies to be developed. These may be more efficacious than the current systemic anti-inflammatory treatments outlined in Section 4 above, as they would represent evidence-based strategies for treating hyperinflammation during severe COVID-19.

Treatment	Proposed mechanism	Evidence	References
Corticosteroids	Decreased cytokine release	Weak	[81]
Baricitinib	JAK inhibitor	Modest	[72, 86]
Tocilizumab	IL-6R inhibitor	Mixed	[88, 89]
NSAIDs	Unclear for COVID-19	Weak	[93]

Table 1.
Targeting COVID-19 with anti-inflammatory drugs.

Author details

Brandt D. Pence[1]* and Theodore J. Cory[2]

1 College of Health Sciences, University of Memphis, Memphis, TN, USA

2 Department of Clinical Pharmacy and Translational Science, College of Pharmacy, University of Tennessee Health Science Center, Memphis, TN, USA

*Address all correspondence to: bdpence@memphis.edu

References

[1] Huang C, Wang Y, Li X, Ren L, Zhao J, Hu Y, et al. Clinical features of patients infected with 2019 novel coronavirus in Wuhan, China. Lancet. 2020;395:497-506. DOI: 10.1016/S0140-6736(20)30183-5

[2] Wang D, Hu B, Hu C, Zhu F, Liu X, Zhang J, et al. Clinical characteristics of 138 hospitalized patients with 2019 novel coronavirus-infected pneumonia in Wuhan, China. JAMA. 2020;323:1061-9. DOI: 10.1001/jama.2020.1585

[3] Rota PA, Oberste MS, Monroe SS, Nix WA, Campagnoli R, Icenogle JP, et al. Characterization of a novel coronavirus associated with severe acute respiratory syndrome. Science (80-). 2003;300:1394-9. DOI: 10.1126/science.1085952

[4] Zaki AM, van Boheemen S, Bestebroer TM, Osterhaus ADME, Fouchier RAM. Isolation of a Novel Coronavirus from a Man with Pneumonia in Saudi Arabia. N Engl J Med. 2012;367:1814-20. DOI: 10.1056/nejmoa1211721

[5] Zhou P, Yang X Lou, Wang XG, Hu B, Zhang L, Zhang W, et al. A pneumonia outbreak associated with a new coronavirus of probable bat origin. Nature. 2020;579:270-3. DOI: 10.1038/s41586-020-2012-7

[6] Zhao J, Cui W, Tian BP. The Potential Intermediate Hosts for SARS-CoV-2. Front Microbiol. 2020;11:580137. DOI: 10.3389/fmicb.2020.580137

[7] Andersen KG, Rambaut A, Lipkin WI, Holmes EC, Garry RF. The proximal origin of SARS-CoV-2. Nat Med. 2020;26:450-2. DOI: 10.1038/s41591-020-0820-9

[8] Rasmussen AL. On the origins of SARS-CoV-2. Nat Med. 2021;27:9. DOI: 10.1038/s41591-020-01205-5

[9] Lundstrom K, Seyran M, Pizzol D, Adadi P, El-Aziz TMA, Hassan SS, et al. Viewpoint: Origin of SARS-CoV-2. Viruses. 2020;12:1203. DOI: 10.3390/v12111203

[10] Burki T. The origin of SARS-CoV-2. Lancet Infect Dis. 2020;20:1018-9. DOI: 10.1016/S1473-3099(20)30641-1

[11] Gorbalenya AE, Baker SC, Baric RS, de Groot RJ, Drosten C, Gulyaeva AA, et al. The species Severe acute respiratory syndrome-related coronavirus: classifying 2019-nCoV and naming it SARS-CoV-2. Nat Microbiol. 2020;5:536-44. DOI: 10.1038/s41564-020-0695-z

[12] Worldometer. COVID-19 coronavirus pandemic [Internet]. 2021 [cited 2021 Apr 21];Available from: https://www.worldometers.info/coronavirus/

[13] Goyal P, Choi JJ, Pinheiro LC, Schenck EJ, Chen R, Jabri A, et al. Clinical Characteristics of Covid-19 in New York City. N Engl J Med. 2020;382:2372-4. DOI: 10.1056/nejmc2010419

[14] Fu L, Wang B, Yuan T, Chen X, Ao Y, Fitzpatrick T, et al. Clinical characteristics of coronavirus disease 2019 (COVID-19) in China: A systematic review and meta-analysis. J Infect. 2020;80:656-65. DOI: 10.1016/j.jinf.2020.03.041

[15] Guan W, Ni Z, Hu Y, Liang W, Ou C, He J, et al. Clinical Characteristics of Coronavirus Disease 2019 in China. N Engl J Med. 2020;382:1708-20. DOI: 10.1056/nejmoa2002032

[16] Wang A, Gao G, Wang S, Chen M, Qian F, Tang W, et al. Clinical characteristics and risk factors of acute respiratory distress syndrome (ARDS) in COVID-19 patients in Beijing, China: A retrospective study. Med Sci Monit.

2020;26:e925974. DOI: 10.12659/MSM.925974

[17] Williamson EJ, Walker AJ, Bhaskaran K, Bacon S, Bates C, Morton CE, et al. Factors associated with COVID-19-related death using OpenSAFELY. Nature. 2020;584:430-6. DOI: 10.1038/s41586-020-2521-4

[18] Lighter J, Phillips M, Hochman S, Sterling S, Johnson D, Francois F, et al. Obesity in Patients Younger Than 60 Years Is a Risk Factor for COVID-19 Hospital Admission. Clin Infect Dis. 2020;71:896-7. DOI: 10.1093/cid/ciaa415

[19] Zaim S, Chong JH, Sankaranarayanan V, Harky A. COVID-19 and Multi-Organ Response. Curr Probl Cardiol. 2020; DOI: https://doi.org/10.1016/j.cpcardiol.2020.100618

[20] Nalbandian A, Sehgal K, Gupta A, Madhavan M V., McGroder C, Stevens JS, et al. Post-acute COVID-19 syndrome. Nat Med. 2021; DOI: 10.1038/s41591-021-01283-z

[21] Datta SD, Talwar A, Lee JT. A Proposed Framework and Timeline of the Spectrum of Disease Due to SARS-CoV-2 Infection: Illness beyond Acute Infection and Public Health Implications. JAMA. 2020;324:2251-2. DOI: 10.1001/jama.2020.22717

[22] Sette A, Crotty S. Adaptive immunity to SARS-CoV-2 and COVID-19. Cell. 2021;184:861-80. DOI: 10.1016/j.cell.2021.01.007

[23] Schultze JL, Aschenbrenner AC. COVID-19 and the human innate immune system. Cell. 2021; DOI: 10.1016/j.cell.2021.02.029

[24] De Kleer I, Willems F, Lambrecht B, Goriely S. Ontogeny of myeloid cells. Front Immunol. 2014;5:423. DOI: 10.3389/fimmu.2014.00423

[25] Jakubzick C V., Randolph GJ, Henson PM. Monocyte differentiation and antigen-presenting functions. Nat Rev Immunol. 2017;17:349-62. DOI: 10.1038/nri.2017.28

[26] Ziegler-Heitbrock L, Ancuta P, Crowe S, Dalod M, Grau V, Hart DN, et al. Nomenclature of monocytes and dendritic cells in blood. Blood2010;116:e74-80.

[27] Kapellos TS, Bonaguro L, Gemünd I, Reusch N, Saglam A, Hinkley ER, et al. Human monocyte subsets and phenotypes in major chronic inflammatory diseases. Front Immunol. 2019;10:2035. DOI: 10.3389/fimmu.2019.02035

[28] Lee SMY, Dutry I, Peiris JSM. Editorial: Macrophage heterogeneity and responses to influenza virus infection. J Leukoc Biol. 2012;92:1-4. DOI: 10.1189/jlb.0312130

[29] Abassi Z, Knaney Y, Karram T, Heyman SN. The Lung Macrophage in SARS-CoV-2 Infection: A Friend or a Foe? Front Immunol. 2020;11:1312. DOI: 10.3389/fimmu.2020.01312

[30] Kaur M, Bell T, Salek-Ardakani S, Hussell T. Macrophage adaptation in airway inflammatory resolution. Eur Respir Rev. 2015;24:510-5. DOI: 10.1183/16000617.0030-2015

[31] Epelman S, Lavine KJ, Beaudin AE, Sojka DK, Carrero JA, Calderon B, et al. Embryonic and adult-derived resident cardiac macrophages are maintained through distinct mechanisms at steady state and during inflammation. Immunity. 2014;40:91-104. DOI: 10.1016/j.immuni.2013.11.019

[32] Murray PJ. Macrophage Polarization. Annu Rev Physiol. 2017;79:541-66. DOI: 10.1146/annurev-physiol-022516-034339

[33] Gordon S, Plüddemann A. Tissue macrophages: Heterogeneity and

functions. BMC Biol. 2017;15:53. DOI: 10.1186/s12915-017-0392-4

[34] Fajgenbaum DC, June CH. Cytokine Storm. N Engl J Med. 2020;383:2255-73. DOI: 10.1056/nejmra2026131

[35] Merad M, Martin JC. Pathological inflammation in patients with COVID-19: a key role for monocytes and macrophages. Nat Rev Immunol. 2020;20:355-62. DOI: 10.1038/s41577-020-0331-4

[36] Jiang L, Tang K, Levin M, Irfan O, Morris SK, Wilson K, et al. COVID-19 and multisystem inflammatory syndrome in children and adolescents. Lancet Infect Dis. 2020;20:e276-88. DOI: 10.1016/S1473-3099(20)30651-4

[37] Del Valle DM, Kim-Schulze S, Huang HH, Beckmann ND, Nirenberg S, Wang B, et al. An inflammatory cytokine signature predicts COVID-19 severity and survival. Nat Med. 2020;26:1636-43. DOI: 10.1038/s41591-020-1051-9

[38] Giamarellos-Bourboulis EJ, Netea MG, Rovina N, Akinosoglou K, Antoniadou A, Antonakos N, et al. Complex Immune Dysregulation in COVID-19 Patients with Severe Respiratory Failure. Cell Host Microbe. 2020;27:992-1000.e3. DOI: 10.1016/j.chom.2020.04.009

[39] Almanzar N, Antony J, Baghel AS, Bakerman I, Bansal I, Barres BA, et al. A single-cell transcriptomic atlas characterizes ageing tissues in the mouse. Nature. 2020;583:590-5. DOI: 10.1038/s41586-020-2496-1

[40] Xiong Y, Liu Y, Cao L, Wang D, Guo M, Jiang A, et al. Transcriptomic characteristics of bronchoalveolar lavage fluid and peripheral blood mononuclear cells in COVID-19 patients. Emerg Microbes Infect. 2020;9:761-70. DOI: 10.1080/22221751.2020.1747363

[41] Quartuccio L, Fabris M, Sonaglia A, Peghin M, Domenis R, Cifù A, et al. Interleukin 6, soluble interleukin 2 receptor alpha (CD25), monocyte colony-stimulating factor, and hepatocyte growth factor linked with systemic hyperinflammation, innate immunity hyperactivation, and organ damage in COVID-19 pneumonia. Cytokine. 2021;140:155438. DOI: 10.1016/j.cyto.2021.155438

[42] Blanco-Melo D, Nilsson-Payant BE, Liu WC, Uhl S, Hoagland D, Møller R, et al. Imbalanced Host Response to SARS-CoV-2 Drives Development of COVID-19. Cell. 2020;181:1036-1045.e9. DOI: 10.1016/j.cell.2020.04.026

[43] Costela-Ruiz VJ, Illescas-Montes R, Puerta-Puerta JM, Ruiz C, Melguizo-Rodríguez L. SARS-CoV-2 infection: The role of cytokines in COVID-19 disease. Cytokine Growth Factor Rev. 2020;54:62-75. DOI: 10.1016/j.cytogfr.2020.06.001

[44] Liao M, Liu Y, Yuan J, Wen Y, Xu G, Zhao J, et al. Single-cell landscape of bronchoalveolar immune cells in patients with COVID-19. Nat Med. 2020;26:842-4. DOI: 10.1038/s41591-020-0901-9

[45] Xu G, Qi F, Li H, Yang Q, Wang H, Wang X, et al. The differential immune responses to COVID-19 in peripheral and lung revealed by single-cell RNA sequencing. Cell Discov. 2020;6:73. DOI: 10.1038/s41421-020-00225-2

[46] Shaath H, Vishnubalaji R, Elkord E, Alajez NM. Single-Cell Transcriptome Analysis Highlights a Role for Neutrophils and Inflammatory Macrophages in the Pathogenesis of Severe COVID-19. Cells. 2020;9:2374. DOI: 10.3390/cells9112374

[47] Wauters E, Van Mol P, Garg AD, Jansen S, Van Herck Y V., Vanderbeke L, et al. Discriminating mild from critical COVID-19 by innate and adaptive

immune single-cell profiling of bronchoalveolar lavages. Cell Res. 2021;

[48] Bost P, Giladi A, Liu Y, Bendjelal Y, Xu G, David E, et al. Host-Viral Infection Maps Reveal Signatures of Severe COVID-19 Patients. Cell. 2020;181:1475-1488.e12. DOI: 10.1016/j.cell.2020.05.006

[49] Song JW, Zhang C, Fan X, Meng FP, Xu Z, Xia P, et al. Immunological and inflammatory profiles in mild and severe cases of COVID-19. Nat Commun. 2020;11:3410. DOI: 10.1038/s41467-020-17240-2

[50] Nienhold R, Ciani Y, Koelzer VH, Tzankov A, Haslbauer JD, Menter T, et al. Two distinct immunopathological profiles in autopsy lungs of COVID-19. Nat Commun. 2020;11:5086. DOI: 10.1038/s41467-020-18854-2

[51] Beigmohammadi MT, Jahanbin B, Safaei M, Amoozadeh L, Khoshavi M, Mehrtash V, et al. Pathological Findings of Postmortem Biopsies From Lung, Heart, and Liver of 7 Deceased COVID-19 Patients. Int J Surg Pathol. 2020; DOI: 10.1177/1066896920935195

[52] Li S, Jiang L, Li X, Lin F, Wang Y, Li B, et al. Clinical and pathological investigation of patients with severe COVID-19. JCI Insight. 2020;5:e138070. DOI: 10.1172/jci.insight.138070

[53] Hoffmann M, Kleine-Weber H, Schroeder S, Krüger N, Herrler T, Erichsen S, et al. SARS-CoV-2 cell entry depends on ACE2 and TMPRSS2 and is blocked by a clinically proven protease inhibitor. Cell. 2020; DOI: 10.1016/j.cell.2020.02.052

[54] Winkler ES, Bailey AL, Kafai NM, Nair S, McCune BT, Yu J, et al. SARS-CoV-2 infection of human ACE2-transgenic mice causes severe lung inflammation and impaired function. Nat Immunol. 2020;21:1327-35. DOI: 10.1038/s41590-020-0778-2

[55] Bao L, Deng W, Huang B, Gao H, Liu J, Ren L, et al. The pathogenicity of SARS-CoV-2 in hACE2 transgenic mice. Nature. 2020;583:830-3. DOI: 10.1038/s41586-020-2312-y

[56] Sia SF, Yan L, Chin AWH, Fung K, Choy K, Wong AYL, et al. Pathogenesis and transmissio of SARS-CoV-2 in golden hamsters. Nature. 2020; DOI: 10.1038/s41586-020-2342-5

[57] Song TZ, Zheng HY, Han JB, Jin L, Yang X, Liu FL, et al. Delayed severe cytokine storm and immune cell infiltration in SARS-CoV-2-infected aged Chinese rhesus macaques. Zool Res. 2020;41:503-16. DOI: 10.24272/j.issn.2095-8137.2020.202

[58] Shan C, Yao YF, Yang X Lou, Zhou YW, Gao G, Peng Y, et al. Infection with novel coronavirus (SARS-CoV-2) causes pneumonia in Rhesus macaques. Cell Res. 2020;30:670-7. DOI: 10.1038/s41422-020-0364-z

[59] Chandrashekar A, Liu J, Martino AJ, McMahan K, Mercad NB, Peter L, et al. SARS-CoV-2 infection protects against rechallenge in rhesus macaques. Science. 2020;369:812-7. DOI: 10.1126/science.abc4776

[60] Speranza E, Williamson BN, Feldmann F, Sturdevant GL, Pérez-Pérez L, Meade-White K, et al. Single-cell RNA sequencing reveals SARS-CoV-2 infection dynamics in lungs of African green monkeys. Sci Transl Med. 2021;13:eabe8146. DOI: 10.1126/scitranslmed.abe8146

[61] Kim OY, Monsel A, Bertrand M, Coriat P, Cavaillon JM, Adib-Conquy M. Differential down-regulation of HLA-DR on monocyte subpopulations during systemic inflammation. Crit Care. 2010;14:R61. DOI: 10.1186/cc8959

[62] Gatti A, Radrizzani D, Viganò P, Mazzone A, Brando B. Decrease of Non-Classical and Intermediate

Monocyte Subsets in Severe Acute SARS-CoV-2 Infection. Cytom Part A. 2020;97:887-90. DOI: 10.1002/cyto.a.24188

[63] Laing AG, Lorenc A, del Molino del Barrio I, Das A, Fish M, Monin L, et al. A dynamic COVID-19 immune signature includes associations with poor prognosis. Nat Med. 2020;26:1623-35. DOI: 10.1038/s41591-020-1038-6

[64] Payen D, Cravat M, Maadadi H, Didelot C, Prosic L, Dupuis C, et al. A Longitudinal Study of Immune Cells in Severe COVID-19 Patients. Front Immunol. 2020;11:580250. DOI: 10.3389/fimmu.2020.580250

[65] Spinetti T, Hirzel C, Fux M, Walti LN, Schober P, Stueber F, et al. Reduced Monocytic Human Leukocyte Antigen-DR Expression Indicates Immunosuppression in Critically Ill COVID-19 Patients. Anesth Analg. 2020;131:993-9. DOI: 10.1213/ANE.0000000000005044

[66] Schulte-Schrepping J, Reusch N, Paclik D, Baßler K, Schlickeiser S, Zhang B, et al. Severe COVID-19 Is Marked by a Dysregulated Myeloid Cell Compartment. Cell. 2020;182:1419-1440.e23. DOI: 10.1016/j.cell.2020.08.001

[67] Varchetta S, Mele D, Oliviero B, Mantovani S, Ludovisi S, Cerino A, et al. Unique immunological profile in patients with COVID-19. Cell Mol Immunol. 2020; DOI: 10.1038/s41423-020-00557-9

[68] Su Y, Chen D, Yuan D, Lausted C, Choi J, Dai CL, et al. Multi-Omics Resolves a Sharp Disease-State Shift between Mild and Moderate COVID-19. Cell. 2020;183:1479-1495.e20. DOI: 10.1016/j.cell.2020.10.037

[69] Guo C, Li B, Ma H, Wang X, Cai P, Yu Q, et al. Single-cell analysis of two severe COVID-19 patients reveals a monocyte-associated and tocilizumab-responding cytokine storm. Nat Commun. 2020;11:3924. DOI: 10.1038/s41467-020-17834-w

[70] Kahn R, Schmidt T, Golestani K, Mossberg A, Gullstrand B, Bengtsson AA, et al. Mismatch between circulating cytokines and spontaneous cytokine production by leukocytes in hyperinflammatory COVID-19. J Leukoc Biol. 2021;109:115-20. DOI: 10.1002/JLB.5COVBCR0720-310RR

[71] Carvelli J, Demaria O, Vély F, Batista L, Chouaki Benmansour N, Fares J, et al. Association of COVID-19 inflammation with activation of the C5a–C5aR1 axis. Nature. 2020;588:146-50. DOI: 10.1038/s41586-020-2600-6

[72] Hoang TN, Pino M, Boddapati AK, Viox EG, Starke CE, Upadhyay AA, et al. Baricitinib treatment resolves lower-airway macrophage inflammation and neutrophil recruitment in SARS-CoV-2-infected rhesus macaques. Cell. 2021;184:460-475.e21. DOI: 10.1016/j.cell.2020.11.007

[73] Aid M, Busman-Sahay K, Vidal SJ, Maliga Z, Bondoc S, Starke C, et al. Vascular Disease and Thrombosis in SARS-CoV-2-Infected Rhesus Macaques. Cell. 2020;183:1354-1366.e13. DOI: 10.1016/j.cell.2020.10.005

[74] Zheng J, Wang Y, Li K, Meyerholz DK, Allamargot C, Perlman S. Severe Acute Respiratory Syndrome Coronavirus 2–Induced Immune Activation and Death of Monocyte-Derived Human Macrophages and Dendritic Cells. J Infect Dis. 2020;jiaa753. DOI: 10.1093/infdis/jiaa753

[75] Yang D, Chu H, Hou Y, Chai Y, Shuai H, Lee ACY, et al. Attenuated interferon and proinflammatory response in SARS-CoV-2-infected human dendritic cells is associated with viral antagonism of STAT1

phosphorylation. J Infect Dis. 2020;222:734-45. DOI: 10.1093/infdis/jiaa356

[76] Codo AC, Davanzo GG, Monteiro L de B, de Souza GF, Muraro SP, Virgilio-da-Silva JV, et al. Elevated Glucose Levels Favor SARS-CoV-2 Infection and Monocyte Response through a HIF-1α/Glycolysis-Dependent Axis. Cell Metab. 2020;32:437-446.e5. DOI: 10.1016/j.cmet.2020.07.007

[77] Boumaza A, Gay L, Mezouar S, Bestion E, Diallo AB, Michel M, et al. Monocytes and macrophages, targets of SARS-CoV-2: the clue for Covid-19 immunoparalysis. J Infect Dis. 2021;

[78] Ajaz S, McPhail MJ, Singh KK, Mujib S, Trovato FM, Napoli S, et al. Mitochondrial metabolic manipulation by SARS-CoV-2 in peripheral blood mononuclear cells of patients with COVID-19. Am J Physiol Physiol. 2021;320:C57-65. DOI: 10.1152/ajpcell.00426.2020

[79] da Silva Gomes Dias S, Soares VC, Ferreira AC, Sacramento CQ, Fintelman-Rodrigues N, Temerozo JR, et al. Lipid droplets fuel SARS-CoV-2 replication and production of inflammatory mediators. PLoS Pathog. 2020;16:e1009127. DOI: 10.1371/journal.ppat.1009127

[80] O'Neill LAJ, Kishton RJ, Rathmell J. A guide to immunometabolism for immunologists. Nat Rev Immunol. 2016;16:553-65. DOI: 10.1038/nri.2016.70

[81] The RECOVERY Collaborative Goup. Dexamethasone in Hospitalized Patients with Covid-19. N Engl J Med. 2021;384:693-704. DOI: 10.1056/nejmoa2021436

[82] Culpitt S V., Rogers DF, Shah P, De Matos C, Russell REK, Donnelly LE, et al. Impaired inhibition by dexamethasone of cytokine release by alveolar macrophages from patients with chronic obstructive pulmonary disease. Am J Respir Crit Care Med. 2003;167:24-31. DOI: 10.1164/rccm.200204-298OC

[83] Gratchev A, Kzhyshkowska J, Köthe K, Muller-Molinet I, Kannookadan S, Utikal J, et al. Mφ1 and Mφ2 can be re-polarized by Th2 or Th1 cytokines, respectively, and respond to exogenous danger signals. Immunobiology. 2006;211:473-86. DOI: 10.1016/j.imbio.2006.05.017

[84] Vaninov N. In the eye of the COVID-19 cytokine storm. Nat Rev Immunol. 2020;20:277. DOI: 10.1038/s41577-020-0305-6

[85] Markham A. Baricitinib: First Global Approval. Drugs. 2017;77:697-704. DOI: 10.1007/s40265-017-0723-3

[86] Kalil AC, Patterson TF, Mehta AK, Tomashek KM, Wolfe CR, Ghazaryan V, et al. Baricitinib plus Remdesivir for Hospitalized Adults with Covid-19. N Engl J Med. 2021;384:795-807. DOI: 10.1056/nejmoa2031994

[87] Dhillon S, Oldfield V, Plosker GL. Tocilizumab a review of its use in the management of rheumatoid arthritis. Drugs. 2009;69:609-32. DOI: 10.2165/00003495-200969050-00007

[88] Salama C, Han J, Yau L, Reiss WG, Kramer B, Neidhart JD, et al. Tocilizumab in Patients Hospitalized with Covid-19 Pneumonia. N Engl J Med. 2021;384:20-30. DOI: 10.1056/nejmoa2030340

[89] Stone JH, Frigault MJ, Serling-Boyd NJ, Fernandes AD, Harvey L, Foulkes AS, et al. Efficacy of Tocilizumab in Patients Hospitalized with Covid-19. N Engl J Med. 2020;383:2333-44. DOI: 10.1056/nejmoa2028836

[90] Melody M, Nelson J, Hastings J, Propst J, Smerina M, Mendez J, et al.

Case report: Use of lenzilumab and tocilizumab for the treatment of coronavirus disease 2019. Immunotherapy. 2020;12:1121-6. DOI: 10.2217/imt-2020-0136

[91] Mehta P, McAuley DF, Brown M, Sanchez E, Tattersall RS, Manson JJ. COVID-19: consider cytokine storm syndromes and immunosuppression. Lancet. 2020;395:1033-4. DOI: 10.1016/S0140-6736(20)30628-0

[92] Vane JR, Botting RM. Mechanism of action of nonsteroidal anti-inflammatory drugs. Am J Med. 1998;104:2S–8S. DOI: 10.1016/S0002-9343(97)00203-9

[93] Day M. Covid-19: ibuprofen should not be used for managing symptoms, say doctors and scientists. BMJ. 2020;368:m1086. DOI: 10.1136/bmj.m1086

[94] Vaja R, Chan JSK, Ferreira P, Harky A, Rogers LJ, Gashaw HH, et al. The COVID-19 ibuprofen controversy: A systematic review of NSAIDs in adult acute lower respiratory tract infections. Br J Clin Pharmacol. 2021;87:776-84. DOI: 10.1111/bcp.14514

[95] Jae YC. Immunomodulatory effect of nonsteroidal anti-inflammatory drugs (NSAIDs) at the clinically available doses. Arch Pharm Res. 2007;30:64-74. DOI: 10.1007/bf02977780

Chapter 22

Convalescent Plasma: An Evidence-Based Old Therapy to Treat Novel Coronavirus Patients

Saurabh Kumar, Chandra Devi, Subhabrata Sarkar, Vivek Kumar Garg, Priyanka Choudhary, Madhu Chopra, Vinit Sharma and Ravi Prakash

Abstract

Novel Coronavirus (nCoV-2019) is a highly infectious viral outbreak that has so far infected more than 110 million people worldwide. Fast viral transmission and high infection rates have severely affected the entire population, especially the old aged and comorbid individuals leaving significantly less time to find some effective treatment strategy. In these challenging times, convalescent plasma (CP) therapy came as a ray of hope to save humankind. It is a form of passive immunization that has been used to treat various infectious diseases since 1890, including the 1918 Spanish flu, 2002/03 SARS-CoV, 2009 H1N1, 2012 MERS-CoV, and 2014 Ebola outbreak. The transfusion includes administration of CP containing a high value of neutralizing antibodies against the virus in hospitalized patients. This chapter summarizes the potential outcome of CP therapy in the treatment of nCoV-2019 patients.

Keywords: nCoV-2019, CP therapy, viral infection, neutralizing antibody

1. Introduction

Convalescent plasma (CP) is defined as a blood plasma that is withdrawn from an individual who had encountered some infectious disease and had recovered with a required amount of antibodies against the disease [1]. It is a way of passive immunization [2]. The concept has been widely used in medical sciences, especially in the case of infectious disease outbreaks. It is an old therapy used since late 1800 [3]. In Germany (1890), researchers treated diphtheria patients with sera from immunized animals. Afterward, the patients were treated with the sera from the recovered ones [4, 5]. The wide use of CP therapy was established during the Spanish influenza outbreak between 1918 to 1920 [6]. Humanity faces a great survival challenge when a new infectious disease emerges and becomes a pandemic. We do not have much to do in such cases, and we mostly rely on our scientific or medical fraternity. Therefore, during such a pandemic/epidemic, there is an urgent need to have a quick, available therapeutic option [3]. A study estimates that on an average basis, there have been 5.3 newly emerged viruses between 1940 to 2004, which includes 60–70% of viruses having an animal origin and have potential to the infect humans [7]. In such circumstances where there are very few options available for the treatment, and when a patient condition is worsening, CP therapy has always been an excellent choice for clinicians. Humans can get exposed to these viruses by different means of exposure, and generally, these are considered "unavoidable or by chance." In viruses, the major therapeutic challenges arise because of the high degree of genetic changes, which may be due to mutation or genomic instability [8].

In December 2019, a new virus emerged in the Huanan Seafood market and resulted in a dreadful outbreak in China, and the virus rapidly spread to more than 200 countries globally [9]. Further sequence-based analysis of respiratory tract samples identified a novel strain, which was distinct from the other known coronavirus strains, subsequently named Severe Acute Respiratory Syndrome Coronavirus 2 (SARS-CoV-2), and the disease caused by SARS-CoV-2 infection was designated as novel coronavirus-2019 (nCoV-2019) by the World Health Organization (WHO) [10]. The emergence of novel coronavirus came up as a big challenge for the concerned authorities of the various country [11]. Clinicians had no clue regarding its treatment approaches that made the situation even worse [12]. Soon, on March 11, 2020, WHO declared it a pandemic. In its initial days, the unavailability of any potential drug/therapy resulted in an exponential increase in infections.

For more than a century, this therapy has been widely explored against various outbreaks. During the 2002/3 SARS-CoV outbreak, 2012 Middle East Respiratory Syndrome (MERS-CoV) outbreak, and H1N1 pandemic (2009), CP therapy was successfully explored [13–16]. Similarly, for the 2013/14 Ebola virus infection treatment, CP therapy was recommended as an empirical treatment approach [17]. Based on previous experiences and similarities in terms of virological and clinical characteristics among the SARS-CoV, MERS-CoV, and nCoV-2019 [18], CP therapy was explored for its efficacy in the battle against newly emerged (nCoV-2019) pandemic. In February 2020, for the first time, a group of researchers from China reported and published the usefulness of CP in nCoV-2019 severe patients in Journals like JAMA [17] and PNAS [16]. CP therapy can be used as a prophylaxis for various infectious diseases, primarily when an outbreak occurs.

Many studies showed a significant correlation between CP therapy and improved clinical symptoms. In a preliminary study involving 5 critically ill nCoV-2019 patients, 400 mL CP administration (high neutralizing antibody (NAb) titer >40) resulted in improved clinical characteristics [17]. A similar study with 10 critically ill patients who received 200 mL of CP (one dose; NAb>1:640) significantly improved clinical symptoms within 3 days and viremia resolution within 7 days [16]. Altuntas et al. carried out a CP-based study on 888 patients, reported that CP administration reduced the ICU stay ($p = 0.001$) and MV support ($p = 0.02$) [19]. However, there is some uncertainty with large-scale CP transfusion. A PLACID trial published on 464 patients found that CP therapy did not reduce the progression to severe illness or 28-day mortality (19% treatment Vs. 18% control group) [20]. A clinical trial on 228 patients reported no significant benefits in symptoms and overall mortality between the intervention (10.93%) and the placebo group (11.43%) [21]. Similarly, a review article that studied 20 articles reflected that the efficacy of CP therapy in nCoV-2019 patients is uncertain [22]. Therefore, the US FDA recommended the use of CP as an investigational product [23]. Here, in this chapter, we have explored CP therapy potentials on nCoV-2019 based on available literature.

2. Methods

Relevant review search was done using keywords "nCoV-2019 or COVID-19, Convalescent Plasma or Plasma therapy". The search engine included electronic databases like PubMed, Google Scholar, and ClinicalTrials.gov.

3. History of convalescent plasma

This therapy is not new for nCoV-2019, as physicians used this therapy more than a century ago [24]. Convalescent plasma has been used historically for a long time to develop passive immunity in patients suffering from various bacterial and viral diseases such as measles [25], mumps [26], and poliomyelitis [27] by transferring plasma carrying NAb from previously recovered patients. Although antibiotics have replaced CP usage in bacterial diseases, it remains a useful tool for novel viral infections for which the vaccine is not available.

A literature study reported that serotherapy was used during the Spanish flu (influenza A) pandemic in 1918–1920 for the first time, but this therapy was also used before the Spanish flu pandemic [3]. Serotherapy was tried as a therapeutic treatment in a poliomyelitis outbreak in New York in 1916 [28]. In 1916 (Tunis), some researchers again performed this therapy for the measles [6]. Hess AF in 1915 applied serotherapy to treat mumps and successfully prevented the testicular complications in the affected patients [29]. However, the credit goes to the Italian Francesco Cenci, who for the first time used convalescent serum as a therapeutic means to save the children that were exposed to measles [30]. Cenci performed this experiment by withdrawing 600 mL blood from a patient who recovered from measles after 21 days. After that, he administered this therapy to four children aged 4–8 years [30]. The results were overwhelming as the children did not contract measles following the treatment. Since the mortality rate in measles was high, ranging from 6–7%, this prophylactic therapy lasted for a long time [31]. There was again a measles outbreak in December 1906 in Italy where this therapy was administrated in forty sick children, and all the patients recovered successfully. One children had severe symptoms, but after therapy, the child showed milder symptoms. Luigi Concetti performed a similar therapy in 1900 on two children affected with diphtheria in Rome, Italy [6, 32]. After that, CP therapy was used for treating many diseases like MERS, Ebola, SARS etc. (**Table 1**) [33].

During H1N1 influenza epidemics in 2009, CP therapy was given to the patients who were in critical conditions and were presented to the hospitals with severe respiratory problems. The patients showed reduced viral load in the respiratory system and there was also decreased cytokine response and mortality rate [14]. CP therapy was also used in the Ebola epidemic in 2013 in West Africa regions [34]. SARS-CoV in 2002/2003 and MERS-CoV in 2012, the two outbreaks with

Disease (epidemic/pandemic)	Country	Year
Diphtheria	Italy	1900
Measles	Italy	1906
Mumps (epidemic)	USA	1915
Poliomyelitis	USA	1916
Measles (epidemic)	Tunis	1916
Influenza A (pandemic)	Spain	1918
SARS1 (epidemic)	China	2002/3
MERS (endemic)	Middle East	2012
Ebola (pandemic)	West Africa	2013
COVID-19 (pandemic)	China	2019

Table 1.
Use of CP therapy during various diseases outbreak.

high mortality occurred in early 21st century [35]. In South Korea, MERS became endemic, and there was an urgent need for CP therapy as the mortality rate was very high, and there was no effective treatment available [35]. Eighty patients of SARS-CoV in Hong Kong were given early administration of convalescent plasma, and they demonstrated an increased prognosis and got early discharge from the hospital [15]. A study in Taiwan showed that the administration of CP in 3 patients reduced the viral load [36].

4. Significance of convalescent plasma therapy during SARS-CoV and MERS-CoV outbreaks

Earlier, CP therapy was used to treat similar coronavirus outbreaks, i.e., SARS and the MERS in the last two decades (**Table 2**).

4.1 SARS-CoV outbreak

The first outbreak of the twentieth century that surfaced from China in 2002 led to severe respiratory illness and pneumonia-like symptoms in patients. A case study published in 2003 reports that CP administration as an adjunctive treatment along-with ribavirin and prednisolone in a 57-year-old SARS patient on Day 14 reduces the viral load and fever within a few days. Further, a better resolution of a basal lung infiltrate was seen in chest X-ray post- convalescent plasma treatment [40]. A group of Hong-Kong-based researchers, Soo et al. (2004) and Cheng et al. (2005), first reported using convalescent plasma as an emergency therapy to contain this outbreak. They found that patients treated with steroids and CP had low mortality and got early discharge from the hospitals compared to patients treated with steroids alone [15, 37, 41].

Further, they have found that patients with early administration of convalescent plasma (before 14 days of symptoms onset) have shorter hospital stay and have less mortality ($p = 0.08$) than those who received convalescent plasma after 14 days [15]. A similar study by Yeh et al. reports about the beneficial effect of CP administration in SARS infected Health-workers who were severely ill and showed no response to available antiviral treatments. The CP administration in them resulted in a reduced viral load and fever within a day, followed by resolution of pulmonary infiltrates and a time-dependent increase in anti-SARS-CoV IgM and IgG antibodies [36]. In conclusion, early administration of convalescent plasma led to better patient outcomes in terms of fast recovery, short hospital stays, reduction in viral load, and improvement in clinical symptoms.

4.2 MERS-CoV outbreak

This outbreak took place due to another strain of respiratory illness causing coronaviruses, referred to as MERS, pointing to its origin from central-east Asia (Arabian countries). From the prior experience of using CP during SARS-CoV outbreak, passive immunotherapy by administering NAb in patients serves as a vital tool in battle with this disease. Chan et al. in 2012, found that convalescent sera of previously recovered SARS patients have cross-reactive NAb that can work effectively against novel coronavirus strains [42]. Corti et al. in 2015, based on anecdotal evidence, studied the prevalence of MERS specific antibodies in dromedary camels from the middle east (Oman) and European countries (Netherland and Chile). They found that all Omanian camels in their study group had MERS-CoV-specific NAb in their serum compared to European animals,

Sr. No.	Title of the study	Year	Indication	Outcomes	References
1.	Retrospective comparison of convalescent plasma with continuing high-dose methylprednisolone treatment in SARS patients	2004	SARS	Low mortality was observed in patients treated with convalescent plasma with no adverse effects	[37]
2.	Use of convalescent plasma therapy in SARS patients in Hong Kong	2005	SARS	Low mortality rate and a better outcome was observed in patients treated with convalescent plasma	[15]
3.	Experience of using convalescent plasma for severe acute respiratory syndrome among healthcare workers in a Taiwan hospital	2005	SARS	Fast recovery with reduced viral load was observed in patients treated with convalescent plasma	[36]
4.	Middle East respiratory syndrome coronavirus neutralising serum antibodies in dromedary camels: a comparative serological study	2013	MERS	MERS-CoV specific neutralizing antibodies were found in serum Omanian camels	[38]
5.	Efficacy of antibody-based therapies against Middle East respiratory syndrome coronavirus (MERS-CoV) in common marmosets	2017	MERS	Reduction in viral load and severity in marmosets treated with convalescent plasma	[39]

Table 2.
List of studies describing the significance of CP therapy during SARS-CoV and MERS-CoV outbreaks.

highlighting the importance of passive immunotherapy upon successfully detecting the transmission source. These antibodies of CP have the potential to neutralize the MERS-CoV if administered in the patients [38]. The effectiveness of CP was also reported by van Dorelman et al. in 2017, in common marmosets infected with MERS-CoV. They found that marmosets treated with hyperimmune plasma and m336 (monoclonal antibodies) showed a reduction in viral load and overall severity [39]. However, the use of MERS-CoV antibodies is very challenging, as some studies report that they are produced at a low level and are short-lived in mild infections [43, 44].

5. Mechanism of action of convalescent plasma

Convalescent plasma to be donated contains specific antibodies for particular infectious diseases or pathogens. These antibodies possess neutralization activity. This activity is achieved in different ways: either by impeding the binding of viral particles with the endosomes, by hindering the viral protein proteolytic cleavage, by blocking the release of viral progeny, or by inhibiting the viral surface glycoproteins from invading the human cells [45]. A report published by Lu *et al.* suggests that when a neutralizing antibody (NAb-3BNC117) was passively administered on mice model, it helped block NAb helped block the new infection, enhanced clearance of the infected cells, and accelerated the HIV-1 infected cell clearance [46].

The other mode of action includes antibody-dependent-cellular-phagocytosis (ADCP), complement system activation, and antibody-dependent cellular-mediated cytotoxicity (ADCC). CP antibodies induce clearance of virus-infected cells by ADCP. A cross-talk is established among the CP antibodies, which helps in eliciting the Fc-dependent effector functions. The activated complement system helps eliminate the virus by two means. First, by direct means i.e., through complement dependent cytotoxicity. Second, indirect means, i.e., by phagocytosis, help clear the associated complement targets. In the case of nCoV-2019, the recovered patients may develop serum antibody response (IgG) against various virus epitopes [1]. This IgG competes with the angiotensin-converting enzyme-2 receptor (ACE-2) to bind with the virus receptor-binding domain (RBD) and may neutralize the nCoV-2019 infection. Therefore, in this case, the binding domain acts as both, i.e., the epitope for antibody and a binding site for the receptor enzyme [2]. Literature suggests that when CP therapy is administered at an early stage of nCoV-2019 infection, the therapeutic effect may be more effective [47]. In most viral infections, the peak of viremia starts appearing in the early first week of the illness. However, between days 10–14 or early in some cases, the host primary immune response starts exerting its potential effect [47].

6. Use of CP therapy on nCoV-2019 patients

In the absence of any specific treatment of nCoV-2019 and vaccines with proven long-term results, CP administration comes to the rescue for an effective treatment for critically ill nCoV-2019 patients (**Tables 3** and **4**). This is a kind of passive immunization method where CP from a recovered nCoV-2019 individual is obtained and uses them on diseased individuals to resolve the symptoms and reduce disease course by suppressing the viremia [18]. The use of passive immunotherapy is a widely used approach to combat various infectious diseases, which consisted of various formulations such as whole blood, pooled human sera containing immunoglobulin and convalescent plasma. Plasma collected through apheresis with subsequent CP transfusion is the most commonly used passive immunotherapy approach to battle against pandemics happened earlier [24]. Theoretically, a person who got infected from an infectious disease, upon recovery, blood is screened for NAb specific to the causative pathogen suffered earlier. The convalescent plasma containing a high-titer NAb is used as a therapy to maximize the capacity to neutralize an infecting pathogen (**Figure 1**) [56].

Studies from the current nCoV-2019 pandemic suggested that it elicits a robust immune response resulting in cytokine storm which generates high levels of IgM and IgG mostly that persists for months even after the symptom disappears. Thus, a large window period and maximum chances of successful extraction of high titer anti-SARS-CoV-2 immunoglobulins act as a boon to utilize it as passive immunotherapy [57, 58]. Further studies have elaborated on NAb response. More severe disease may lead to higher antibody response levels [58], and antibody level decreases considerably within the first 90 days after symptom start among individuals suffered from the mild disease [59].

SN	Trial No.	Title	Type	Country	Phase	Status	Sample size	Primary/Secondary outcome measures		Trial result (based on publications posted on clinicaltrials.gov)
								Primary	Secondary	
1	NCT04343261	Convalescent Plasma in the Treatment of COVID 19	Interventional	United States	Phase 2	Completed	48	Mortality, viral load, serum antibody titer.	—	Early administration of CP with sufficient antibody titer is safer and helpful in recovery and survival of COVID-19 patients.
2	NCT04747158	COVID-19 Convalescent Plasma Therapy (TPCC)	Interventional (Clinical Trial)	Paraguay	Phase 2/3	Completed	350	Evaluation of the efficacy of CP therapy. To decrease mortality in the patients hospitalized with COVID-19 and who exhibit risk factor for clinical deterioration.	Disease severity, difference in the level of inflammatory marker viz. ferritin, D dimer, leukocytes. To check adverse effects and frequency of the patients' admission in ICU.	Updated safety data from 20000 COVID-19 patients suggests that early administration of CP is safer and helpful in reducing mortality.

SN	Trial No.	Title	Type	Country	Phase	Status	Sample size	Primary/Secondary outcome measures		Trial result (based on publications posted on clinicaltrials.gov)
								Primary	Secondary	
3	NCT04407208	Convalescent Plasma Therapy in Patients With COVID-19	Interventional	Indonesia	Phase 1	Completed	10	Assessment of C-Reactive Protein (CRP), D-dimer, Plaque reduction neutralization test (PNRT), International Normalized Ratio (INR), Oxygenation Index, X-ray of chest.	Duration of hospitalization, severe adverse events.	—
4	NCT04476888	Convalescent Plasma Treatment in COVID-19 (COLLATE)	Interventional (Clinical Trial), Non-Randomized	Pakistan	NA	Completed	110	Assessment of the stay period in hospital/ ICU/SCU, mortality, adverse effects after CP transfusion.	Clinical status of COVID-19 patient, level of serum ferritin, procalcitonin, C-reactive protein, D-Dimer, Complete blood count. X-ray observation of chest.	—
5	NCT04616976	COVID-19 With Convalescent Plasma	Observational	China	NA	Completed	78	Mortality of severe COVID-19 patients.	Viral shedding	—

SN	Trial No.	Title	Type	Country	Phase	Status	Sample size	Primary/Secondary outcome measures		Trial result (based on publications posted on clinicaltrials.gov)
								Primary	Secondary	
6	NCT04332835	Convalescent Plasma for Patients With COVID-19: A Randomized, Single Blinded, Parallel, Controlled Clinical Study (CP-COVID-19)	Single Blinded, Randomized, Controlled Clinical Study	Colombia	Phase 2 Phase 3	Completed	92	Alteration in the level of viral load, IgM and IgG COVID-19 antibody titer.	Proportion of the admission and duration of the stay in hospital/ ICU. Requirement and period of mechanical ventilation. Clinical status and mortality.	—
7	NCT04405310	Convalescent Plasma of Covid-19 to Treat SARS-COV-2 a Randomized Doble Blind 2 Center Trial (CPC-SARS)	Randomized Doble Blind 2 Center Trial	Mexico	Phase 2	Completed	42	Mortality	Duration of the stay in ICU, duration of mechanical ventilation and supplemental oxygen. Viral load, level of inflammatory markers viz. ferritine, D Dimer, IL-6, PCR, IL-8, IL-10. SOFA scaling.	NA Expected: Recovery of the patients with normal body temperature, reduced viral load, no progression to ARDS, and liberation of the patient from mechanical ventilation.

SN	Trial No.	Title	Type	Country	Phase	Status	Sample size	Primary/Secondary outcome measures		Trial result (based on publications posted on clinicaltrials.gov)
								Primary	Secondary	
8	NCT04458363	Convalescent Plasma in Pediatric COVID-19	Interventional, Feasibility Study	United States	Early Phase 1	Completed	3	Safety of CP in pediatric COVID-19 patients.	Mortality. Duration of the stay in hospital/ ICU. Requirement of respiratory support and duration of ventilation. Assessment of kidney dysfunction or/ and multisystem-organ failure. IL-6 level, circulating T cells diversity, ARS-CoV-2 Antibody Titer, andSARS-CoV-2 Neutralizing antibody titer.	—

SN	Trial No.	Title	Type	Country	Phase	Status	Sample size	Primary/Secondary outcome measures		Trial result (based on publications posted on clinicaltrials.gov)
								Primary	Secondary	
9	NCT04346446	Efficacy of Convalescent Plasma Therapy in Severely Sick COVID-19 Patients	Pilot Randomized Controlled Trial	India	Phase 2	Completed	29	Number of the patients without mechanical ventilation.	Mortality. Assessment of improvement in Pa02/Fi02 ratio and SOFA score. Need of Vasopressor. Duration of the stay in hospital/ICU. Time length of free of dialysis.	CP administration shortened the recovery, and improved respiratory parameters
10	NCT04381858	Convalescent Plasma vs. Human Immunoglobulin to Treat COVID-19 Pneumonia	Randomized Controlled Trial	Mexico	Phase 3	Completed	196	Period of hospitalization. PaO2/FiO2, severe ARDS evolution. Mortality and duration of invasive mechanical ventilation.	Time frame of RT-qPCR SARS-CoV-2 negative test.	—
11	NCT04542941	Assessment of Safety and Efficacy of CCP (COVIDIT)	Randomised Controlled Trial	Uganda	NA	Completed	136	Time frame of RT-PCR SARS-CoV-2 negative test.	Time frame of primary symptoms resolution. Assessment of clinical improvement of the patients and adverse events.	—

SN	Trial No.	Title	Type	Country	Phase	Status	Sample size	Primary/Secondary outcome measures		Trial result (based on publications posted on clinicaltrials.gov)
								Primary	Secondary	
12	NCT04389944	Amotosalen-Ultraviolet A Pathogen-Inactivated Convalescent Plasma in Addition to Best Supportive Care and Antiviral Therapy on Clinical Deterioration in Adults Presenting With Moderate to Severe COVID-19	Interventional	Switzerland	NA	Completed	15	Post CP treatment serious adverse events, Virologic clearance in nasopharyngeal swab and plasma of treated patients, Transfer to ICU in-hospital death	SARS-CoV-2 antibody titer to see the humoral immune response, Time of hospital discharge.	—

SN	Trial No.	Title	Type	Country	Phase	Status	Sample size	Primary/Secondary outcome measures		Trial result (based on publications posted on clinicaltrials.gov)
								Primary	Secondary	
13	NCT04547660	Convalescent Plasma for Severe COVID-19 Patients (PLACOVID)	Interventional, Randomized, Open-label	Brazil	Phase 3	Completed	160	Clinical improvement.	Mortality, hospital stay, PaO2/FiO2 ratio, duration of Mechanical ventilation, Lactate Dehydrogenase, Troponin I, C Reactive Protein, D-Dimers, Fibrinogen, Prothrombin Time, Activated Partial Thromboplastin Time, TNF-Alfa, Sequential Organ Failure, Safety, and Adverse Events, National Early Warning Score 2.	—
14	NCT04332380	Convalescent Plasma for Patients With COVID-19: A Pilot Study (CP-COVID-19)	Interventional, Pilot Study	Colombia	Phase 2	Completed	10	Change in Viral Load, IgM and IgG COVID-19 antibodies titers.	Duration of ICU and hospital stay, mechanical ventilation, Clinical status and mortality.	—

SN	Trial No.	Title	Type	Country	Phase	Status	Sample size	Primary/Secondary outcome measures		Trial result (based on publications posted on clinicaltrials.gov)
								Primary	Secondary	
15	NCT04356534	Convalescent Plasma Trial in COVID -19 Patients	Interventional, Randomized	Bahrain	NA	Completed	40	Assessment of requirement for invasive ventilation after CP transfusion	viral clearance, X-ray, C reactive protein, white cell count, lactate dehydrogenase, Procalcitonin measurement, D Dimer, Ferritin measurement, Troponin T, Brain naturetic peptide measurement, and mortality.	—
16	NCT04340050	COVID-19 Convalescent Plasma	Interventional	United States	Early Phase 1	Completed	10	Feasibility of administration of anti-SARS-CoV-2 CP. Respiratory support required by the patients 28 days after CP administration.	Cardiac arrest, Duration of ICU and hospital stay, mortality, duration without ventilator, survival	—
17	NCT04338360	Expanded Access to Convalescent Plasma for the Treatment of Patients With COVID-19	Expanded Access	United States	NA	Approved for marketing	5000 (expanded)	—	—	Administration of CP is safe in critically ill COVID-19 patients. No excessive mortality observed.

SN	Trial No.	Title	Type	Country	Phase	Status	Sample size	Primary/Secondary outcome measures		Trial result (based on publications posted on clinicaltrials.gov)
								Primary	Secondary	
18	NCT04321421	Hyperimmune Plasma for Critical Patients With COVID-19 (COV19-PLASMA)	Interventional (proof-of-concept)	Italy	NA	Completed	49	Death	Extubation timing, ICU stay period, CPAP weaning, viral load, and immune response.	—
19	NCT04441424	Convalescent Plasma Therapy on Critically-ill Novel Coronavirus (COVID-19) Patients	Interventional, Randomized	Iraq	NA	Completed	49	Mortality	Duration of the stay in hospitals.	CP therapy is effective if administered at early stage
20	NCT04569188	Convalescent Plasma in COVID-19 Elderly Patients (RESCUE)	Interventional	Italy	Phase 2	Completed	21	Death	Viral load	—
21	NCT04383535	Convalescent Plasma and Placebo for the Treatment of COVID-19 Severe Pneumonia (PLASM-AR)	Interventional, Randomized	Argentina	NA	Completed	333	Clinical Status	Clinical status, discharge from ICU and hospital, complete functional recovery, adverse events, negative PCR results, D-dimer, ferritin, neutralizing antibodies concentration in plasma, death.	The difference in clinical status and mortality between the two groups (CP treated vs. placebo) was not significant.

SN	Trial No.	Title	Type	Country	Phase	Status	Sample size	Primary/Secondary outcome measures		Trial result (based on publications posted on clinicaltrials.gov)
								Primary	Secondary	
22	NCT04392414	Hyperimmune Convalescent Plasma in Moderate and Severe COVID-19 Disease	Interventional, Randomized	Russian Federation	Phase 2	Completed	60	Normal body temperature post CP transfusion	Requirement of mechanical ventilation, oxygen therapy, days in ICU/ hospital, SARS-CoV-2 antibodies titer, plasma level of cytokines, requirement of cytokine storm inhibitor, CRP level, mortality rate.	—
23	NCT04375098	Efficacy and Safety of Early COVID-19 Convalescent Plasma in Patients Admitted for COVID-19 Infection	Interventional, Randomized	Chile	Phase 2	Completed	58	Hospitalization, Mechanical ventilation, death	1 year follow-up of: Median duration of fever, mechanical ventilation, ICU stay, viral clearance and admission length. Hospital mortality and 30 day mortality. Readmission rate.	—

SN	Trial No.	Title	Type	Country	Phase	Status	Sample size	Primary/Secondary outcome measures		Trial result (based on publications posted on clinicaltrials.gov)
								Primary	Secondary	
24	NCT04479163	Prevention of Severe Covid-19 in Infected Elderly by Early Administration of Convalescent Plasma With High-titers of Antibody Against SARS-CoV2	Interventional, Randomized	Argentina	NA	Completed	165	respiratory rate > 30 and/or an O2 sat < 93%	Severe respiratory disease, respiratory failure, death, requirement and duration of oxygen support.	Early infusion of high titer CP in mildly ill COVID-19 older adults resulted in slower progression of the disease with no adverse events.
25	NCT04492501	Investigational Treatments for COVID-19 in Tertiary Care Hospital of Pakistan	Interventional, Non-Randomized	Pakistan	NA	Completed	600	Survival	Period of hospitalization, time length to normalize symptoms, viral clearance, complications.	—
26	NCT04521309	SARS-CoV-2 Antibodies Based IVIG Therapy for COVID-19 Patients	Interventional, Randomized	Pakistan	Phase 1 Phase 2	Completed	50	Mortality, need of supplemental oxygen, days to shift from ICU to ward, hospital discharge, adverse events, CRP level, difference in neutrophil lymphocyte ratio.	Change in Ferritin levels, LDH, Sodium, Potassium, Chloride, Bicarbonate, chest X-ray findings fever, Anti-SARS-CoV-2 antibody titer	—

SN	Trial No.	Title	Type	Country	Phase	Status	Sample size	Primary/Secondary outcome measures		Trial result (based on publications posted on clinicaltrials.gov)
								Primary	Secondary	
27	NCT04442958	Effectiveness of Convalescent Immune Plasma Therapy	Interventional, Randomized	Turkey	NA	Completed	60	Level of ferritin, C Reactive Protein, D-Dimers, Fibrinogen, procalcitonin, Lymphocyte count	Arterial oxygenation, Partial Oxygen Saturation	—

Table 3.
List of completed CP based Clinical trials registered on ClinicalTrial.gov nCoV-2019 patients.

S. No.	Type of Study (group)	Country	Sample size	Volume of CP administered	Overall Mortality rates	Adverse events reported	Reported outcome
1	Multicentred/open-labelled/ uncontrolled trial- Gazitúa et al., 2020 [48]	Chile (NCT04384588)	192	200-mL (twice)	1). 7 day- 5.7% (95% CI: 10.0%) 2). 30 day- 16.1% (95% CI: 22.1%%)	11 (2.9%)	CP administration was found to be safe.
2	Retrospective study (expanded access)/Joyner et al., 2021 [49]	USA (NCT04338360)	3082	—	30 day- 26.9% (95% CI: 25.4–28.5%)	—	CP administration in hospitalized nCoV-2019 patients was found to be potentially beneficial
3	Case series/Xia et al., 2020 [50]	China	138	200–1200- mL (based on body weight and clinical condition)	2.2%	-No severe transfusion issues	CP transfusion can improve the clinical symptoms and mortality rate in nCoV-2019 severe patients
4	Multiceter trial/Abolghasemi et al., 2020 [51]	Iran (IRCT20200325046860N1)	189 (115 CP)	500 cc - one unit (another unit, if needed)	14.8%	-1 (0.87%) (transient mild fever and chill)	Early administration of CP may be more effective
5.	Multicenter/open-labeled/ expanded access/Joyner et al., 2020 [52]	USA	20,000	—	7 day- 12.96% (95% CI: 12.5–13.44%)	<1% serious adverse events	CP therapy is safe with no or little complications
6.	Retrospective/matched-control study/Shenoy et al., 2021 [53]	USA	526 (263 CP)	200–500 mL (one/ two units)	1). 7 day- 9.1% 2). 14 day-14.8% 3). 28 day- 25.5%	—	CP administration may provide immediate mortality benefits (at 7-day and 14-day, but not at 28-day)

S. No.	Type of Study (group)	Country	Sample size	Volume of CP administered	Overall Mortality rates	Adverse events reported	Reported outcome
7	multicenter randomized, double-blind, placebo-controlled clinical trial/ Simonovich VA et al., 2020 [54]	Argentina (NCT04383535)	333 (228 CP)	500 mL (IQ range, 415–600)	30 day-10.96%	11 (4.8% in CP group)	CP therapy in COVID-19 patients with severe pneumonia did not reduce mortality.
8	Prospective study/ Tworek et al., 2020 [55]	Poland	204 (102 CP)	200 mL (once or more depending upon the condition)	13.7%	—	CP therapy was found to be safe and effective in high risk nCoV-2019 patients
9	multicentre randomised (PLACID)/ Agarwal et al., 2020 [20]	India (CTRI/2020/04/024775)	464 (235 CP)	200 mL	19%	Non-life-threatening adverse events in some cases	CP therapy was not relayed to the reduction in all-cause mortality

Table 4.
Status of mortality rate after CP administration in hospitalized nCoV-19 patients (studies with sample size >100).

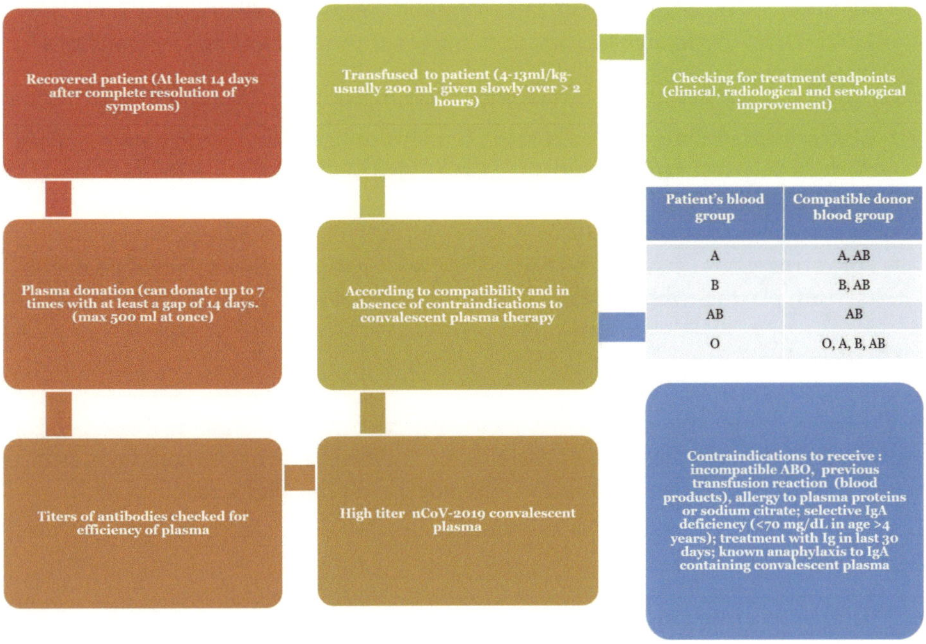

Figure 1.
Diagrammatic representation of the use of CP in nCoV-2019 patients.

6.1 Source/donor requirement

In order to overcome various challenges for enrolment of successful plasma donors during the outbreak different strategies such as social distancing, travel restrictions, and imposed lockdowns have been implemented. To recruit possible plasma contributors, this includes donor self-identification, social awareness utilizing social/formal/e-media outlets and clinician referral of individuals got previous exposure to the infection [60]. NAb titres can be examined in possible donor or CP units through ELISA/chemiluminescence assay or pseudovirus neutralization assays which are known as indirect methods or directly under biosafety level 3 conditions by using live SARS-CoV-2 neutralization assays. USFDA has permitted the use of CP therapy under the clause of EUA for hospitalised nCoV-2019 infected patients [61]. CP units were categorized as lower or higher antibody titre based on qualitative chemiluminescent immunoassay for detection of neutralizing IgG against SARS-CoV2 spike protein [60]. The collected plasma is treated for pathogen inactivation to avoid the risk of transfusion transmitted infections. A donor can donate CP weekly for several months till the antibody titers are high. There are several factors that restrict the donation, including the individuals who already received the CP for their nCoV-2019 treatment (minimum of 90 days) are not allowed to donate blood products.

6.2 Who can donate CP

- Person who has confirmed validated diagnostic record of SARS-CoV-2 infection.
- Physical examination, including the absence of fever and respiratory symptoms. Minimum of 14-day post-recovery with no symptoms.
- A person who meets the standard routine blood donation criteria. The donor and recipient should be ensured for ABO compatibility

- CP must be free of HIV, HCV, HBV syphilis, human T-cell lymphotropic virus 1 and 2, and *Trypanosoma cruzi* and any other transfusion/locally transmitted infections.

- CP from either male donors or from female donors with no pregnancy history is preferentially used to avoid any risk of TRALI (Transfusion Related Acute Lung Injury) [62].

- For retrospective testing and scientific investigations, donors blood products (serum, plasma, whole blood) should be saved at -80^0 C.

6.3 Plasma donation

Convalescent plasma donors may be identified during national disease-specific cohorts, during hospitalization of the patient, by the practitioners treating outpatients, and through various specific online/social helpline-networks.

6.3.1 FDA guidelines

The FDA recommends three approaches for the administration of CP. First is directed for the treatment of patients of nCoV-2019 through EUA. Second, patients with severe nCoV-2019 illness who are unable to participate in RCT through expanded access protocol. The third one involves clinical trials where clinicians are advised to enroll patients in the trials to examine the effectiveness of CP therapy in nCoV-2019 [63].

6.4 Dosage

Various dosage regimens were utilized in various hospital setups for the management of SARS-CoV2 infected patients. Universally 200 ml of convalescent plasma in 1 or 2 doses with an infusion rate of 100 to 200 ml/h are administered with an interval of 12 hr. apart. The dosage regimen is decided according to body weight and antibody titer [64]. Standard hospital procedures and recommendations should be followed for thawing and transfusion of plasma through a peripheral or central venous catheter.

6.5 Follow up

CP therapy is still an experimental model. For future scientific investigations and correlations, the blood products of the recipient should be stored (prior and after transfusion). As per published trials, the response post CP therapy is mainly assessed i.e., PaO2/FiO2 ratio clinically or through Ct scan or X-ray (radiological) of the infected organ. However, elicitation of nCoV-2019 antibody titer or increased ALC in recipients, as well as a decline in SARS-CoV2 viral load either in terms of absolute quantification or increase of cycle threshold (Ct) value, could be considered as surrogate endpoints [65].

7. Risk associated with the use of CP therapy

Major adverse events associated with CP transfusion are not much evident so far. However, risk assessment before/after the transfusion is important. Several studies/clinical trials have shown that the use of CP therapy in severely ill nCoV-2019 patients is safe and early administration with adequate anti-SARS-CoV-2-NAb titer is helpful in faster recovery and survival of nCoV-2019 patients [18, 66]. CP therapy is contraindicated in certain individuals such as those who are allergic to plasma protein or sodium citrate, patients with selective IgA deficiency (70 mg/dl in patients four years old or older), or the ones who received treatment with immunoglobulins in the last 30 days as it could lead to the development of serum sickness [67].

However, large U.S. national registry, through its interim report, showed that among over 100,000 hospitalized adults that had nCoV-2019 infection, low incidences of transfusion reactions were documented in the first 5,000, and 20,000 patients transfused with nCoV-2019 CP therapy, which is suggestive of the fact that transfusion of convalescent plasma is safe and poses no additional risk of complications among hospitalized patients with nCoV-2019 [52, 68]. An RCT compared the safety of convalescent plasma transfusion with fresh frozen plasma transfusion documented a comparatively less rates between the controls (7%) and CP (4%) group of patients and highlighted the safety profile of CP transfusion [69].

8. Conclusions

In the absence of any effective antiviral drug and vaccine (long term effect is not yet established) to prevent the infection, several approaches have been explored to reduce the duration of the disease course. One therapeutic approach that is being utilized globally is convalescent plasma therapy against nCoV-2019. Once the person recovers from nCoV-2019, the blood contains antibodies against the causative virus. In emergency situations, these antibodies can be given to other affected people to provide immediate immunity against the virus, reducing the severity and helping in faster recovery. FDA has not yet approved the use of CP as a treatment of nCoV-2019. It is administered under the EUA or an IND. However, further large-scale, world-wide controlled clinical trials are needed to prove the efficacy of the CP therapy for the current pandemic.

Acknowledgements

The authors would like to thank all the researchers/clinicians/healthcare workers or frontline workers for their dedication and valuable contribution towards the society in this hard time. We would also like to thank Dr. Akhilesh Gupta, Adviser & Head, STIP Secretariat, DST, Govt of India for motivating the corresponding author to write this article.

Conflict of interest

The authors declare no conflict of interest.

Acronyms and abbreviations

nCoV-2019	Novel Coronavirus
CP	Convalescent Plasma
SARS	Severe Acute Respiratory Syndrome Coronavirus
WHO	World Health Organization

MERS	Middle East Respiratory Syndrome
NAb	Neutralizing Antibody
ADCP	Antibody-Dependent-Cellular-Phagocytosis
ADCC	Antibody-Dependent-Cellular-Mediated Cytotoxicity
ACE-2	Angiotensin-Converting Enzyme-2 Receptor
RBD	Receptor-Binding Domain

Author details

Saurabh Kumar[1,2*], Chandra Devi[3], Subhabrata Sarkar[4], Vivek Kumar Garg[5], Priyanka Choudhary[6], Madhu Chopra[7], Vinit Sharma[8] and Ravi Prakash[9]

1 DST- Centre for Policy Research, Indian Institute of Science (IISc), Bengaluru, India

2 Department of Science and Technology (DST), New Delhi, India

3 Centre for Genetic Disorders, Institute of Science, Banaras Hindu University (BHU), Varanasi, India

4 Regional Virus Research and Diagnostic Lab Department of Virology, Postgraduate Institute of Medical Education and Research Chandigarh, India

5 CoViD Lab, Punjab Biotechnology Incubator (PBTI), Mohali, India

6 Department of Mycology and Plant Pathology, Banaras Hindu University (BHU), Varanasi, India

7 Department of Internal Medicine, Postgraduate Institute of Medical Education and Research (PGIMER), Chandigarh, India

8 Department of Anatomy, Postgraduate Institute of Medical Education and Research (PGIMER), Chandigarh, India

9 Touring Veterinary Officer Cum Nodal Officer, Class One Veterinary Hospital Nirmali, Supaul, Bihar, India

*Address all correspondence to: saurabh.kum1991@gmail.com

References

[1] Anudeep T, Jeyaraman M, Shetty DU, Raj H, Ajay S, Soma sundaram R, et al. Convalescent Plasma as a plausible therapeutic option in nCOVID-19–A Review. J Clin Trials. 2020;10:2167-0870.20. DOI: 10.35248/2167-0870.20.10.409

[2] Kumar S, Sharma V, Priya K. Battle against COVID-19: Efficacy of sConvalescent Plasma as an emergency therapy. Am J Emerg Med. 2020. DOI: 10.1016/j.ajem.2020.05.101

[3] Brown BL, McCullough J. Treatment for emerging viruses: Convalescent plasma and COVID-19. Transfus Apher Sci. 2020. DOI: 10.1016/j.transci.2020.102790

[4] Diorio C, Teachey DT, Bassiri H. Convalescent plasma for COVID-19: an old therapy for a novel pathogen. The Hematologist. 2020;17:. DOI: 10.1182/hem.V17.4.10407

[5] Behring K, Kitasato S. On the development of immunity to diphtheria and tetanus in animals. Dtsch Med Wochenschr. 1965;90:2183.

[6] Marson P, Cozza A, De Silvestro G. The true historical origin of convalescent plasma therapy. Transfus Apher Sci. 2020;59:102847. DOI: 10.1016/j.transci.2020.102847

[7] Stramer SL. Current perspectives in transfusion-transmitted infectious diseases: emerging and re-emerging infections. ISBT Sci Ser. 2014;9:30-36. DOI: 10.1111/voxs.12070

[8] Kumar S, Dwivedi D, Chopra M. COVID-19 Outbreak: Neurological Manifestations beyond Cough and Fever. CNS Neurol Disord Drug Targets. 2020. DOI: 10.2174/187152731966620 1120143654

[9] Kumar S, Kumar S, Karim A, Bisht K, Ghani A, Munda VS. Outbreak of Respiratory Infection: nCoV-2019 Current Status and Its Impact on Global Health. Current Respiratory Medicine Reviews. 2020;16:156-164. DOI: 10.2174/1573398X16999201203162129

[10] Coronaviridae Study Group of the International Committee on Taxonomy of Viruses., Gorbalenya A, Baker S, et al. The species severe acute respiratory syndrome related coronavirus: classifying 2019-nCoV and naming it SARS-CoV-2. Nat Microbiol. 2020;5:536-544. DOI: 10.1038/s41564-020-0695-z

[11] Kumar S. Novel coronavirus (COVID-19) outbreak: Hope and search for effective therapeutic agent. Lett Drug Des Discov. 2020;17:940-942. DOI: 10.2174/1570180817999200612095513

[12] Kumar S, Chopra M. COVID-19 vaccine development: need for a pre-planned vaccination program: Science Policy Forum. 2020. Available from: http://thesciencepolicyforum.org/articles/perspectives/vaccinedevelopment/. [Accessed: 2021-02-15]

[13] Ko J-H, Seok H, Cho SY, Ha YE, Baek JY, Kim SH, et al. Challenges of convalescent plasma infusion therapy in Middle East respiratory coronavirus infection: a single centre experience. Antivir Ther. 2018;23:617-622. DOI: 10.3851/IMP3243

[14] Hung IF, To KK, Lee C-K, Lee K-L, Chan K, Yan W-W, et al. Convalescent plasma treatment reduced mortality in patients with severe pandemic influenza A (H1N1) 2009 virus infection. Clin Infect Dis. 2011;52:447-456. DOI: 10.1093/cid/ciq106

[15] Cheng Y, Wong R, Soo Y, Wong W, Lee C, Ng M, et al. Use of convalescent plasma therapy in SARS patients in Hong Kong. Eur J Clin Microbiol Infect

Dis. 2005;24:44-46. DOI: 10.1007/s10096-004-1271-9

[16] Duan K, Liu B, Li C, Zhang H, Yu T, Qu J, et al. Effectiveness of convalescent plasma therapy in severe COVID-19 patients. Proc Natl Acad Sci USA. 2020;117:9490-9496. DOI: 10.1073/pnas.2004168117

[17] Shen C, Wang Z, Zhao F, Yang Y, Li J, Yuan J, et al. Treatment of 5 critically ill patients with COVID-19 with convalescent plasma. Jama. 2020;323:1582-1589. DOI: 10.1001/jama.2020.4783

[18] Chen L, Xiong J, Bao L, Shi Y. Convalescent plasma as a potential therapy for COVID-19. Lancet Infect Dis. 2020;20:398-400. DOI: 10.1016/S1473-3099(20)30141-9

[19] Altuntas F, Ata N, Yigenoglu TN, Bascı S, Dal MS, Korkmaz S, et al. Convalescent plasma therapy in patients with COVID-19. Transfus Apher Sci. 2020;102955. DOI: 10.1016/j.transci.2020.102955

[20] Agarwal A, Mukherjee A, Kumar G, Chatterjee P, Bhatnagar T, Malhotra P. Convalescent plasma in the management of moderate covid-19 in adults in India: open label phase II multicentre randomised controlled trial (PLACID Trial). BMJ. 2020;371:m3939. DOI: 10.1136/bmj.m3939.

[21] Simonovich VA, Burgos Pratx LD, Scibona P, Beruto MV, Vallone MG, Vázquez C, et al. A randomized trial of convalescent plasma in Covid-19 severe pneumonia. New England Journal of Medicine. 2020;384:619-629. DOI: 10.1056/NEJMoa2031304

[22] Piechotta V, Chai KL, Valk SJ, Doree C, Monsef I, Wood EM, et al. Convalescent plasma or hyperimmune immunoglobulin for people with COVID-19: a living systematic review. Cochrane Database Syst Rev. 2020;10:7. DOI: 10.1002/14651858.CD013600.pub2

[23] USFDA. Recommendations for Investigational COVID-19 Convalescent Plasma. 2021. Available from: https://www.fda.gov/vaccines-blood-biologics/investigational-new-drug-ind-or-device-exemption-ide-process-cber/recommendations-investigational-covid-19-convalescent-plasma. [Accessed: 2021-02-16]

[24] Marano G, Vaglio S, Pupella S, Facco G, Catalano L, Liumbruno GM, et al. Convalescent plasma: new evidence for an old therapeutic tool? Blood Transfus. 2016;14:152-157. DOI: 10.2450/2015.0131-15

[25] PARK WH, FREEMAN RG. The prophylactic use of measles convalescent serum. JAMA. 1926;87(8):556-558. DOI: 10.1001/jama.1926.02680080022009

[26] RAMBAR AC. Mumps: use of convalescent serum in the treatment and prophylaxis of orchitis. Am J Dis Child. 1946;71:1-13.

[27] Park WH. Therapeutic use of antipoliomyelitis serum in preparalytic cases of poliomyelitis. JAMA. 1932;99:1050-1053. DOI: 10.1001/jama.1932.02740650008003

[28] Wyatt H. Before the vaccines: medical treatments of acute paralysis in the 1916 New York epidemic of poliomyelitis. Open Microbiol J. 2014;8:144-147. DOI: 10.2174/1874285801408010144

[29] Hess AF. A protective therapy for mumps. Am J Dis Child. 1915;10:99-103. DOI: 10.1001/archpedi.1915.04110020024005

[30] Marks Hh, Thalhimer W. Prophylaxis Of Measles With Convalescent Serum: Principal Factors Influencing the Results. Am J Dis

Child. 1944;67:1-14. DOI: 10.1001/archpedi.1944.02020010008001

[31] Casadevall A, Scharff MD. Return to the past: the case for antibody-based therapies in infectious diseases. Clin Infect Dis. 1995;21:150-161. DOI: 10.1093/clinids/21.1.150

[32] Samad N, Sodunke TE, Al Banna H, Sapkota A, Fatema AN, Iskandar K, et al. Convalescent Plasma Therapy for Management of COVID-19: Perspectives and Deployment in the Current Global Pandemic. Risk Manag Healthc Policy. 2020;13:2707-2728. DOI: 10.2147/RMHP.S281388

[33] Arabi Y, Balkhy H, Hajeer AH, Bouchama A, Hayden FG, Al-Omari A, et al. Feasibility, safety, clinical, and laboratory effects of convalescent plasma therapy for patients with Middle East respiratory syndrome coronavirus infection: a study protocol. Springerplus. 2015;4:709. DOI: 10.1186/s40064-015-1490-9.

[34] Omilabu S, Salu O, Oke B, James A. The West African ebola virus disease epidemic 2014-2015: A commissioned review. Niger Postgrad Med J. 2016;23:49-56. DOI: 10.4103/1117-1936.186299.

[35] Ahire ED, Sonawane VN, Surana KR, Jadhav KR, Sonawane DD, Shah AA. Convalescent plasma therapy: A promising approach in the treatment of Covid-19. Int J Pharm Sci Res. 2020;11:4078-4086. DOI: 10.13040/IJPSR.0975-8232

[36] Yeh K-M, Chiueh T-S, Siu L, Lin J-C, Chan PK, Peng M-Y, et al. Experience of using convalescent plasma for severe acute respiratory syndrome among healthcare workers in a Taiwan hospital. J Antimicrob Chemother. 2005;56:919-922. DOI: 10.1093/jac/dki346.

[37] Soo Y, Cheng Y, Wong R, Hui D, Lee C, Tsang K, et al. Retrospective comparison of convalescent plasma with continuing high-dose methylprednisolone treatment in SARS patients. Clin Microbiol Infect. 2004;10:676-678. DOI: 10.1111/j.1469-0691.2004.00956.x.

[38] Reusken CB, Haagmans BL, Müller MA, Gutierrez C, Godeke G-J, Meyer B, et al. Middle East respiratory syndrome coronavirus neutralising serum antibodies in dromedary camels: a comparative serological study. Lancet Infect Dis. 2013;13:859-866. DOI: 10.1016/S1473-3099(13)70164-6.

[39] van Doremalen N, Falzarano D, Ying T, de Wit E, Bushmaker T, Feldmann F, et al. Efficacy of antibody-based therapies against Middle East respiratory syndrome coronavirus (MERS-CoV) in common marmosets. Antiviral research. 2017;143:30-37. DOI: 10.1016/j.antiviral.2017.03.025

[40] Wong V, Dai D, Wu A, Sung J. Treatment of severe acute respiratory syndrome with convalescent plasma. Hong Kong Med J. 2003;9:199-201.

[41] Wooding DJ, Bach H. Treatment of COVID-19 with convalescent plasma: lessons from past coronavirus outbreaks. Clin Microbiol Infect. 2020;26:1436-1446. DOI: 10.1016/j.cmi.2020.08.005

[42] Chan K-H, Chan JF-W, Tse H, Chen H, Lau CC-Y, Cai J-P, et al. Cross-reactive antibodies in convalescent SARS patients' sera against the emerging novel human coronavirus EMC (2012) by both immunofluorescent and neutralizing antibody tests. J Infect. 2013;67:130-140. DOI: 10.1016/j.jinf.2013.03.015

[43] Drosten C, Meyer B, Müller MA, Corman VM, Al-Masri M, Hossain R, et al. Transmission of MERS-coronavirus in household contacts.

N Engl J Med. 2014;371:828-835. DOI: 10.1056/NEJMoa1405858.

[44] Alrashid M, Taleb A, Hajeer A, Arabi Y. Prevalence of antibodies against the Middle East Respiratory Syndrome coronavirus, influenza A and B viruses among blood donors, Saudi Arabia. Ann Thorac Med. 2017;12:217-218. DOI: 10.4103/atm.ATM_143_17.

[45] Dai W, Gu H, Hao S. Potential benefits, mechanisms, and uncertainties of convalescent plasma therapy for COVID-19. Blood Science. 2020;2:71-75. DOI: 10.1097/BS9.0000000000000047

[46] Lu C-L, Murakowski DK, Bournazos S, Schoofs T, Sarkar D, Halper-Stromberg A, et al. Enhanced clearance of HIV-1–infected cells by broadly neutralizing antibodies against HIV-1 in vivo. Science. 2016;352:1001-1004. DOI: 10.1126/science.aaf1279

[47] Psaltopoulou T, Sergentanis TN, Pappa V, Politou M, Terpos E, Tsiodras S, et al. The emerging role of convalescent plasma in the treatment of COVID-19. Hemasphere. 2020;4:e409. DOI: doi: 10.1097/HS9.0000000000000409

[48] Gazitúa R, Briones JL, Selman C, Villarroel-Espíndola F, Aguirre A, González-Steigmaier R, et al. Convalescent Plasma in COVID-19. Mortality-Safety First Results of the Prospective Multicenter FALP 001-2020 Trial. medRxiv. 2020. DOI: 10.1101/2020.11.30.20218560

[49] Joyner MJ, Carter RE, Senefeld JW, Klassen SA, Mills JR, Johnson PW, et al. Convalescent plasma antibody levels and the risk of death from covid-19. N Engl J Med. 2021. DOI: 10.1056/NEJMoa2031893

[50] Xia X, Li K, Wu L, Wang Z, Zhu M, Huang B, et al. Improved clinical symptoms and mortality among patients with severe or critical COVID-19 after convalescent plasma transfusion. Blood. 2020;136:755-759. DOI: 10.1182/blood.2020007079

[51] Abolghasemi H, Eshghi P, Cheraghali AM, Fooladi AA, Moghaddam FB, Imanizadeh S, et al. Clinical efficacy of convalescent plasma for treatment of COVID-19 infections: Results of a multicenter clinical study. Transfus Apher Sci. 2020;59:102875. DOI: 10.1016/j.transci.2020.102875

[52] Joyner MJ, Bruno KA, Klassen SA, Kunze KL, Johnson PW, Lesser ER, et al. Safety update: COVID-19 convalescent plasma in 20,000 hospitalized patients. Mayo Clin Proc. 2020;95:1888-1897. DOI: 10.1016/j.mayocp.2020.06.028

[53] Shenoy AG, Hettinger AZ, Fernandez SJ, Blumenthal J, Baez V. Early mortality benefit with COVID-19 convalescent plasma: a matched control study. Br J Haematol. 2021;192:706-713. DOI: 10.1111/bjh.17272

[54] Simonovich VA, Burgos Pratx LD, Scibona P, Beruto MV, Vallone MG, Vázquez C, et al. A randomized trial of convalescent plasma in Covid-19 severe pneumonia. N **Engl J Med.** 2021;384:619-629. DOI: 10.1056/NEJMoa2031304

[55] Tworek A, Jaroń K, Uszyńska-Kałuża B, Rydzewski A, Gil R, Deptała A, et al. Convalescent plasma treatment is associated with lower mortality and better outcomes in high risk COVID-19 patients–propensity score matched case-control study. **Int J** Infect Dis. 2021. DOI: 10.1016/j.ijid.2021.02.054

[56] Casadevall A, Pirofski L-a. The convalescent sera option for containing COVID-19. J Clin Invest. 2020;130:1545-1548. DOI: 10.1172/JCI138003.

[57] Ni L, Ye F, Chen M-L, Feng Y, Deng Y-Q, Zhao H, et al. Characterization of anti-viral immunity in recovered individuals infected by

SARS-CoV-2. medRxiv. 2020. DOI: 10.1101/2020.03.17.20036640

[58] Wajnberg A, Amanat F, Firpo A, Altman DR, Bailey MJ, Mansour M, et al. Robust neutralizing antibodies to SARS-CoV-2 infection persist for months. Science. 2020;370:1227-1230. DOI: 10.1126/science.abd7728

[59] Ibarrondo FJ, Fulcher JA, Goodman-Meza D, Elliott J, Hofmann C, Hausner MA, et al. Rapid decay of anti–SARS-CoV-2 antibodies in persons with mild Covid-19. N Engl J Med. 2020;383:1085-1087. DOI: 10.1056/NEJMc2025179

[60] Ripoll JG, van Helmond N, Senefeld JW, Wiggins CC, Klassen SA, Baker SE, et al. Convalescent Plasma for Infectious Diseases: Historical Framework and Use in COVID-19. Clin Microbiol Newsl. 2021;43:23-32. DOI: 10.1016/j.clinmicnews.2021.02.001

[61] Bloch EM, Kleinman S, Tirnauer J, Feldweg A. Coronavirus disease 2019 (COVID-19): Convalescent plasma and hyperimmune globulin. 2020. Available from: https://www.uptodate.com/contents/coronavirus-disease-2019-covid-19-convalescent-plasma-and-hyperimmune-globulin. [Accessed: 2021-02-17]

[62] Epstein J, Burnouf T. Points to consider in the preparation and transfusion of COVID-19 convalescent plasma. Vox sanguinis. 2020;115:485-487. DOI: 10.1111/vox.12939

[63] USFDA. Investigational COVID-19 convalescent plasma: guidance for industry. 2021. Available from: https://www.fda.gov. [Accessed: 2021-02-16].

[64] Knudson CM, Jackson JB. COVID-19 convalescent plasma: phase 2. Transfusion. 2020;60:1332-1333. DOI: 10.1111/trf.15842

[65] Focosi D, Anderson AO, Tang JW, Tuccori M. Convalescent plasma therapy for COVID-19: state of the art. Clin Microbiol Rev. 2020;33:e00072–e00020. DOI: 10.1128/CMR.00072-20.

[66] Bloch EM, Shoham S, Casadevall A, Sachais BS, Shaz B, Winters JL, et al. Deployment of convalescent plasma for the prevention and treatment of COVID-19. J Clin Invest. 2020;130:2757-2765. DOI: 10.1172/JCI138745.

[67] Sandler SG, Mallory D, Malamut D, Eckrich R. IgA anaphylactic transfusion reactions. Transfus Med Rev. 1995;9:1-8. DOI: 10.1016/s0887-7963(05)80026-4.

[68] Joyner MJ, Wright RS, Fairweather D, Senefeld JW, Bruno KA, Klassen SA, et al. Early safety indicators of COVID-19 convalescent plasma in 5000 patients. J Clin Invest. 2020;130:4791-4797. DOI: 10.1172/JCI140200

[69] Bajpai M, Maheshwari A, Chabra K, Kale P, Gupta A, Gupta E, et al. Efficacy of Convalescent Plasma Therapy compared to Fresh Frozen Plasma in Severely ill COVID-19 Patients: A Pilot Randomized Controlled Trial. medRxiv. 2020. DOI: 10.1101/2020.10.25.20219337

Chapter 23

Potential Therapeutics Pathways in Solving the Challenges of the COVID-19 Pandemic

Tafirenyika Mafugu

Abstract

Millions of lives throughout the globe are under threat due to the COVID-19 pandemic. COVID-19 causes severe respiratory tract infections. In most countries COVID-19 Infections and deaths continue to soar despite the various measures put in place by the World Health Organization. These measures include limited mobility through lock down and banning international travelers. Furthermore, social distancing, wearing masks, frequent hand washing with soap and sanitizing were undertaken to slow down the rate of the virus spread. Only few countries like South Korea have been able to contain the virus to date. Our only hope is in biotechnology which have been used to develop diagnostic kits and more recently approved vaccines: vaccines by Pfizer-BioNTech and Moderna; AstraZeneca and Oxford University vaccine; Sputnik V vaccine; Sinopharm and the Beijing Institute of Biological Products vaccine. However, the vaccines are yet to reach the majority of the world population. Hence, there is need for concerted effort among governments and non-governmental organizations in all nations to develop the necessary infrastructures to step up vaccine production, and procurement as well as vaccination programmes. There is need for continued effort in biotechnology, to develop COVID-19 therapeutic drugs.

Keywords: COVID-19, social distancing, pandemic, diagnostic kits, prevention, biotechnology, vaccines

1. Introduction

The outbreak of the novel COVID-19 (SARS-CoV-2) which the World Health Organization declared a pandemic in March 2020 was first detected in Wuhan, China [1]. It has endangered millions of lives, especially individuals with chronic conditions such as high blood pressure and diabetes [2]. COVID-19 causes severe respiratory tract infections. This chapter focuses on the current status of coronavirus cases and deaths worldwide, and the underway efforts to develop a vaccine or a therapeutic drug to the pandemic.

2. The current status of coronavirus cases and deaths

On the 12th of December 2020, the World Health Organization (WHO) reports that there were 69 808 588 confirmed cases and 1 588 854 deaths worldwide [3]. From **Figure 1**. America and Europe had the highest number of confirmed daily

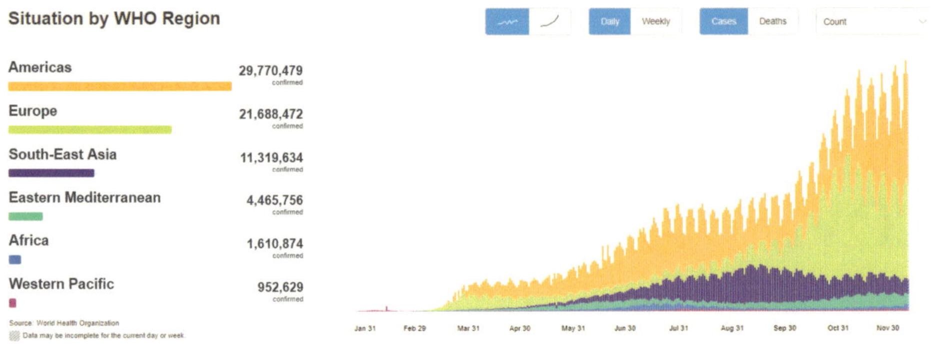

Figure 1.
Number of COVID-19 daily confirmed cases by WHO region from 31 January 2020 up to 30 November 2020 (WHO, 2020).

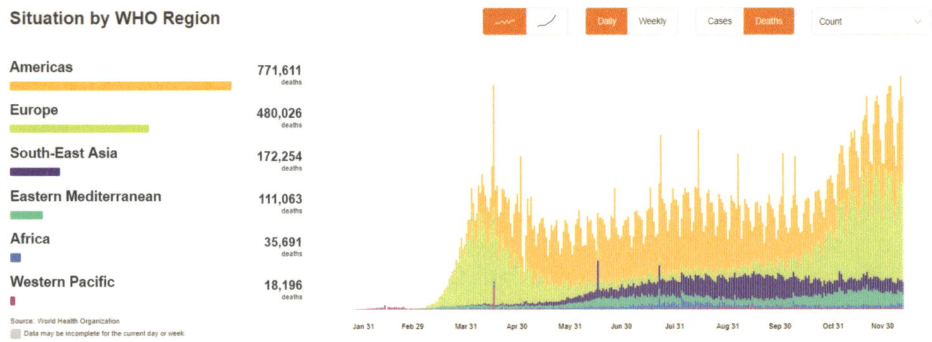

Figure 2.
Number of COVID-19 daily confirmed deaths by WHO region from 31 January 2020 up to 30 November 2020 (WHO, 2020).

COVID-19 cases of 29 770 479 and 21 688 472 respectively on the 30th of November 2020. The least numbers of daily confirmed cases are recorded in Africa (1 610 874) and the Western Pacific (952 629).

From **Figure 2**. America and Europe recorded the highest numbers of deaths by the 30th of November 2020 while Africa and the Western Pacific recorded the least numbers of deaths.

3. An overview of the successes and failures to contain the virus

The COVID-19 pandemic has affected the health, economy, and social mobility of people in countries around the world. Limited mobility through a lockdown and banning international travelers and social distancing, wearing face masks, and health officials and agencies undertook frequent hand washing with soap to slow down the rate of infection. These measures delay the spread of viral infections, reduce the acute pressure on hospital beds, frontline medical personnel, and resources [4]. The measures, thus, prevent the collapse of the national healthcare systems.

Countries like South Korea and Singapore were able to contain the virus due to the rapid and extensive tests carried out accompanied by preventive measures, including early school closures [5]. Furthermore, interviews were conducted by the South Korean government followed by cellphone contact tracing to track down the contacts of new coronavirus patients and ordered those contacts to self-isolate [6]. However, the United States of America's failure to contain COVID-19 is attributed to the slow rate of testing during the first onset of the pandemic due to the shortage of testing kits [7]. A huge proportion of the population in the USA has chronic conditions [8]. Hence, they easily succumb to the virus. Measures such as lockdown are important to slow down the rate of transmission. However, there is a need to develop a vaccine or a drug that can treat the coronavirus. It is hoped that Biotechnology companies will come with a suitable vaccine or therapeutic drug to ease the pressure of the pandemic.

4. Opportunities in the biotechnology industry

Biotechnology research is essential in the development of key interventions such as vaccines and drugs to fight off the pandemic [9]. The new pandemic opened up opportunities for medical specialists and biological researchers to look for different ways of managing and containing the spread of the virus using biotechnology. Rosales-Mendoza, Comas-García and Korban (2020, p.283) assert that the onset of Covid-19 opened up opportunities for researchers:

> *Under these unusual circumstances, academic researchers can work on pending manuscripts, analyze data, conduct experiments left behind on the back burner, and more importantly pursue new ideas for discovery: developing vaccines and monoclonal antibodies and screening antiviral compounds, such as secondary metabolites and peptides; thereby, actively participating in finding solutions to ongoing real-time global human and economic crises.*

More research groups in academia and in private industry are now offering free webinars to share and demonstrate new technologies or experimental protocols [9]. Young researchers will have valuable new opportunities to acquire and develop new skills and ideas to make the best out of this situation.

Efforts were made to develop diagnostic assays, prophylactic vaccines and therapeutics using biotechnology to combat the Covid-19 pandemic. Significant efforts have been made by biotechnology companies and organizations to develop new types of diagnostic kits, ventilators and therapeutic regimens or antivirals [1]. Several centres were made available for clinical trials.

Shortages of Test kits prompted Local companies such as CapeBio Technologies in South Africa to develop Covid-19 test kits that were more efficient than the imported kits [1]. To speed up the production of reagents and test kits for Covid-19, the organizations such Department of Science and Innovation, the South African Medical Research Council and the Technology Innovation Agency funded companies, organizations and researchers for Covid-19 projects. The University of the Witwatersrand collaborated with the University of Oxford and started the Ox1Cov-19 vaccine trial in South Africa in June 2020 [1]. Human Research Ethics Committee had to approve the vaccine to ensure the safety of participants. The Covid-19 pandemic has demonstrated that some developing countries such as South Africa have the biotechnological expertise needed to address their health challenges.

5. The role of plants in biotechnology

Plants can play an essential role in producing diagnostic reagents to identify infected and recovered individuals, vaccines to combat infection, and antivirals to treat symptoms [4]. Plants have been used as a platform for the production of plant-derived proteins as diagnostic reagents for more than 30 years [10]. Assays for the detection of the virus can either detect the virus genomic RNA or virus proteins. The RNA based assay lacks a universal positive control, which would allow standardization across different testing laboratories. Scientists are using biotechnology to develop a diagnostic control reagent for COVID-19 based on virus-like particles (VLPs) derived from Cowpea mosaic virus [11]. Thus, plant biotechnology is playing an important role in the development of diagnostic reagents. In addition, the plant is also being used to produce vaccines and antivirals that are being tested using mice. According to Capell et al., antiviral drugs interfere with the viral replication cycle and slow down the infection [4]. The slowed infection gives the immune system more time to respond to the virus.

6. Current efforts and successes in finding a lasting solution to the coronavirus pandemic

Healthcare professional researchers are trying different types of drugs existing in the market [2]. Such drugs have proven effective in the treatment of other respiratory illnesses. They are hopeful that some of the drugs may also be effective against COVID-19.

Lockdowns due to the COVID 19 pandemic can only be implemented for a reasonably short period as they disrupt industrial production, the global supply chain as well as international trade [2]. Hence, there is need to develop thereupetic drugs and vaccines through biotechnology.

As a result, the demand for the vaccine, drugs and other medical products is rising exponentially as the new COVID-19 cases rise throughout the world. The biotechnology industry, such as pharmaceutical companies and research organizations across the world have the challenge to develop vaccines and drug therapies to combat the spread of COVID-19 [2]. Different organizations are working together in tracking the pandemic, providing advice on essential interventions, distributing vital medical supplies to the needy [12].

Vaccines save millions of lives by boosting the immune system to produce the necessary antibodies that recognize and fight off the pathogens they target [12]. If the body is exposed to the pathogens later, the immune system immediately destroys them, preventing illness. Vaccines consist of small amounts of weakened harmless versions of the pathogen that cause the disease.

Several companies including non-governmental entities and the World Health Organization are working tirelessly to identify the vaccines and treatment drugs to prevent the spread of COVID-19 [1, 12, 13]. WHO is working in collaboration with different partners, with more than 50 COVID-19 vaccine in trials to speed up the pandemic response. A safe vaccine will first be distributed to people who are most at risk while the public health actions continue to suppress transmission and reduce mortality. The people who are at risk include health workers, older age groups and people with underlying medical conditions. It has not been established how long the vaccines will last in terms of protection. Therefore, all measures being taken now to reduce the transmission should continue.

The National Institute of Allergy and Infectious Diseases and the Coalition for Epidemic Preparedness Innovations – developed a vaccine using mRNA biotechnology with hopes to begin human tests of their product in April 2020 [14]. The Regional Centre for Biotechnology (RCB), a top research institute in Faridabad, India, is actively contributing to the global research efforts to combat the COVID-19 pandemic. RCB is conducting research activities such as potential inhibitors, markers and transmission reduction through the virucidal coating [14]. The virucidal coating will help destroy or deactivate the virus on different surfaces like glass, plastic and textiles, including cotton, nylon, and polyester that can potentially hinder the viral transmission [14]. Several companies have begun the development of vaccines and antiviral therapies.

The work previously done on medical countermeasures (MCMs) against other coronaviruses, including SARS, are being tested against the novel COVID-19. Various other antiviral drugs and biologics are being investigated, and several have entered clinical trials to test for efficacy and safety against COVID-19.

By the 18th of November 2020, Pfizer and BioNTech conclude phase 3 study of the covid-19 vaccine candidate. Their vaccine, BNT162b2, has proved to be 95% effective against COVID-19 beginning 28 days after the first dose. The vaccine has met the following conditions:

- Efficacy was consistent across age, gender, race and ethnicity demographics; observed efficacy in adults over 65 years of age was over 94%

- Safety data milestone required by the U.S. Food and Drug Administration (FDA) for Emergency Use Authorization (EUA) has been achieved

- Data demonstrate vaccine was well tolerated across all populations with over 43,000 participants enrolled; no serious safety concerns observed; the only Grade 3 adverse event greater than 2% in frequency was fatigue at 3.8% and headache at 2.0% [15].

The following plans are under way:

- Companies plan to submit within days to the FDA for EUA and share data with other regulatory agencies around the globe

- The companies expect to produce globally up to 50 million vaccine doses in 2020 and up to 1.3 billion doses by the end of 2021

- Pfizer is confident in its vast experience, expertise and existing cold-chain infrastructure to distribute the vaccine around the world [15].

The vaccines by Pfizer-BioNTech and Moderna are nucleic acid/genetic vaccines [16]. Nucleic acid/genetic vaccines use synthetic virus genes to initiate the immune response. The genetic material causes the body's cells to produce the antigen, which in turn stimulates the production of antibodies [16, 17]. Although the immune response is long-lasting, the genetic instructions are short-lived. Nucleic acid vaccine technology allows the creation of vaccines and prompt manufacture of thousands of doses once the viral genetic sequence is known [18].

Similarly, viral vector-based vaccines provide the body cells with genetic instructions [19]. They use a harmless virus to transport the instructions [19]. The body's cells produce the antigen, which triggers antibody production. The Covid-19 vaccine Sputnik and the vaccine made by AstraZeneca and Oxford University use this biotechnology [16].

The third type of vaccines is called Inactivated vaccines. Inactivated vaccines contain viruses with destroyed genetic material, but they can still stimulate the immune system to produce antibodies [20]. The vaccine by Sinopharm and the Beijing Institute of Biological Products use this biotechnology [16].

Finally, the Protein-based vaccines use either fragment of or the entire virus protein, which triggers an immune response. Coronavirus vaccines produced by Novavax, Sanofi and Bektop, use this biotechnology although they are currently not yet approved [16].

Once a vaccine has been produced, it is critical to identify the dose that best balances safety and efficacy. Age is also another important factor that should be considered since the immune functions decline with age leading to poor vaccine responses. Currently, it has not been proved whether older adults would need high doses of Covid-19 vaccine as is the case with influenza vaccines [21]. After passing all the trial phases, each vaccine must be licensed and then production must be increased to meet the global demands. It is critical to ensure that vaccines are affordable and accessible to both low income and middle-income countries for immunization programmes can be implemented.

Efforts are being made to use monoclonal antibodies in the treatment of COVID-19. Currently, cocktail REGN-CoV 2 and Lilly's LY-CoV555 which target the viral spike glycoprotein (S-protein) are under trial for the treatment of the coronavirus [22]. Eleven other monoclonal antibodies that target the S-protein are under trial [22]. Monoclonal antibodies are vital especially for the elderly who may not respond well to the vaccine.

Although there is no cure for COVID-19, patients have been found to benefit from the use of remdesivir [23]. However, the solidarity trials done in October 2020 indicated that the remdesivir and other drugs (hydroxychloroquine, lopinavir and interferon) had little or no effect on mortality and duration of hospital stay for patients in hospital[Who 2020]. The use of corticosteroids has been found to be effective against severe COVID-19 [24].

7. Conclusion

Biotechnology has raised hope to the world through the production of several vaccines. However, until there is an efficacious vaccine and an effective treatment drug that is accessible to everyone, we should keep in mind that SARS-CoV-2 or coronavirus is likely to remain a seasonal pathogen. The current measures that are in place to prevent the spread of infection should be maintained because it will take a long time for the vaccine to be accessible to all nations. The efforts that are being made to come up with more vaccines and therapeutic drugs should continue to be supported. The governments and the private sector should collaborate in providing the necessary funding to companies and researchers who are working tirelessly to develop new vaccines and treatment drugs.

Acknowledgements

I am very grateful to Dr. Cronje, who edited and improved the chapter. I am also grateful to the reviewers who provided constructive comments to improve the chapter. I am also very thankful to the funders who paid the publication fees.

Conflict of interest

The author declare no conflict of interest.

Author details

Tafirenyika Mafugu
University of the Free State, Phuthaditjhaba, South Africa

*Address all correspondence to: mafugut@ufs.ac.za

'Biotechnology to Combat COVID-19' is a collaborative project with Biotechnology Kiosk

References

[1] Ramalapa B. Biotechnology industry is key in Covid-19 fight [Internet]. 2020. Available from: https://www.iol.co.za/pretoria-news/biotechnology-industry-is-key-in-covid-19-fight-51062421 [Accessed: 2021-01-10].

[2] Chatterjee P. COVID-19 Pandemic Has Unveiled The Importance of Biotechnologists [Internet]. 2020. Available from: https://www.biotecnika.org/2020/05/biotechnologists-covid19-pandemic-role-of-biotech-industry/ [Accessed: 2021-01-05].

[3] World Health Organisation. WHO Coronavirus Disease (COVID-19) Dashboard [Internet]. 2020. Available from: https://covid19.who.int [Accessed: 2021-01-10].

[4] Capell T, Twyman RM, Armario-NajeraV, Ma JKC, Schillberg S, Christou P. Potential Applications of Plant Biotechnology against SARS-CoV-2. Trends in Plant Science. 2020; 25(7): 635-643.

[5] Healthline. How South Korea Successfully Battled COVID-19 While the U.S. Didn't [Internet]. 2020. Available from: https://www.healthline.com/health-news/what- south-korea-has-done-correctly-in-battling-covid-19 [Accessed: 2020-06-06].

[6] Thompson D. What's Behind South Korea's COVID-19 Exceptionalism [Internet]. 2020. Available from: https://www.theatlantic.com/ideas/archive/2020/05/ whats-south-koreas-secret/611215/ [Accessed 2020-06-04].

[7] Balogun JA. Lessons from USA delayed response to the COVID-19 pandemic. African Journal of Reproductive Health. 2020; 24: 14-21. Doi: 10.29063/ajrh2020/v24i1.2

[8] Buttorff C, Ruder T, Bauman M. Multiple Chronic Conditions in the United States. Santa Monica, CA: RAND Corporation; 2017.

[9] Rosales-Mendoza S, Comas-García M, Korban SS. Challenges and Opportunities for the Biotechnology Research Community during the Coronavirus Pandemic. Trends in Biotechnology. 2020; 38(8): 823-824.

[10] Schillberg S, Raven N, Spiegel H, Rasche S, Buntru M. Critical analysis of the commercial potential of plants for the production of recombinant proteins. Frontiers in Plant Science. 2019; 10: 720. Doi:org/10.3389/fpls.2019.00720.

[11] King DP, Montague N, Ebert K, Reid SM, Dukes JP, Schädlich L, et al. Development of a novel recombinant encapsidated RNA particle: evaluation as an internal control for diagnostic RT-PCR. Journal of Virological Methods. 2007; 146, 218-225. DOI: 10.1016/j.jviromet.2007.07.002

[12] World Health Organisation. COVID-19 vaccines [Internet]. 2020. Available from: https://www.who.int/emergencies/diseases/novel-coronavirus-2019/covid-19-vaccines[Accessed: 2020-12-10].

[13] Biotechnology Innovation organization. Biopharmaceutical innovators are leading the charge in fight against coronavirus [Internet]. 2020. Available from: https://www.bio.org/policy/human-health/vaccines-biodefense/coronavirus [Accessed: 2020-12-10].

[14] Broucke G. Biotechnology research to combat COVID-19 [Internet]. 2020. Available from: https://en.unesco.org/news/biotechnology-research-combat-covid-19 [Accessed: 2020-12-10].

[15] Pfizer. Pfizer and Biontech conclude phase 3 study of covid-19 vaccine candidate, meeting all primary efficacy

endpoints [Internet]. 2020. Available from: https://www.pfizer.com/news/press-release/press-release-detail/pfizer-and-biontech-conclude-phase-3-study-covid-19-vaccine [Accessed: 2020-12-12].

[16] Nortier C. To date, more than 15.9 million doses of Covid-19 vaccines have been administered in 37 countries. Almost half of all countries rely solely on the Covax facility for access to vaccines, and they may have to wait until 2022 for their shipment. We take a look at which vaccines have been dispensed, and where. Daily Maverick [Internet]. 2021. Available from: https://www.dailymaverick.co.za/article/2021-01-09-a-snapshot-of-global-covid-19-vaccines/[Accessed: 2021-01-13].

[17] Srivastava IK, Liu MA. Gene vaccines. Annals of Internal Medicine. 2003; 138(7):550-559. doi: 10.7326/0003-4819-138-7-200304010-00011.

[18] Fuller DH, Berglund P. Amplifying RNA vaccine development. New England Journal of Medicine. 2020; 382: 2469-2471.

[19] Rauch S, Jasny E, Schmidt K.E, Petsch B. New Vaccine Technologies to Combat Outbreak Situations. Frontiers in Immunology. 2018; 9: 1963. DOI=10.3389/fimmu.2018.01963

[20] Vohora D, Singh G, Editors. Pharmaceutical Medicine and Translational Clinical Research. London: Academic Press; 2018.

[21] DiazGranados CA, Dunning AJ, Kimmel M, et al. Efficacy of high-dose versus standard-dose influenza vaccine in older adults. New England Journal of Medicine. 2014; 371: 635-645.

[22] DeFrancesco L. COVID-19 antibodies on trial. Nature Biotechnology. 2020; 38: 1242-1252. doi: org/10.1038/s41587-020-0732-8.

[23] Wu KJ, Zimmer C, Corum J. Coronavirus Drug and Treatment Tracker [Internet]. 2020. Available from: https://www.nytimes.com/interactive/2020/science/coronavirus-drugs-treatments.html [Accessed: 2021-01-28].

[24] World Health Organisation. "Solidarity" clinical trial for COVID-19 treatment [Internet]. 2020. Available from: https://www.who.int/emergencies/diseases/novel-coronavirus-2019/global-research-on-novel-coronavirus-2019-ncov/solidarity-clinical-trial-for-covid-19-treatments [Accessed: 2021-01-28].

Chapter 24

Different Therapeutic Strategies to Tackle the Infection Associated with COVID-19

Meemansha Sharma, Thakur Uttam Singh, Madhu Cholenahalli Lingaraju and Subhashree Parida

Abstract

Covid-19 is a pandemic and the whole world is facing the loss in terms of morbidity and mortality of the human resources. Therefore, there is an urgent need for various therapeutic agents or drugs to treat the covid-19 patients. Although, vaccination process is under way, it is not possible to provide the vaccination to whole world in a short period. Therefore, it is an essential strategy to work on the various therapeutic aspects of covid-19 treatment. The present book chapter will discuss and review the various aspects of the treatment strategies of the covid-19. Further, we will provide an overview of the virus and host based potential therapeutic targets along with existing therapeutics which are effective against SARS-CoV-2 virus. Also, the novel vaccines are being developed against covid-19 deadly virus will be discussed.

Keywords: SARS-CoV-2, covid-19, therapeutics, pandemic

1. Introduction

The new covid-19 pandemic was reported in Wuhan, China in December, 2019 [1]. This disease is caused by corona virus also known as SARS-CoV-2 and characterized by severe acute respiratory distress syndrome [2]. As per the recent report of WHO on 20 December, 2020, there have been over 75 million cases and 1.6 million deaths reported worldwide since the start of the pandemic [3]. In 2002, SARS-CoV (Severe Acute Respiratory Syndrome Coronavirus) outbreak was reported in China then spread worldwide, whereas, MERS-CoV (Middle East Respiratory Syndrome Coronavirus) emerged in Saudi Arabia in 2012 with 37% mortality rate. Similar to SARS and MERS, newly identified severe acute respiratory syndrome coronavirus 2 (SARS-CoV-2) belongs to beta-coronaviridae family and showed close resemblance with them [4]. These three zoonotic viruses have pandemic potential and able to produce severe respiratory infection in humans [5].

The SARS-CoV-2 infection is transmitted through respiratory secretions either in droplet or aerosol form from one person to another [6]. Apart from respiratory secretions, urine, stool and close proximity with patients may be the sources for dissemination of SARS-CoV-2 [7, 8]. Based on phylogenetic studies, the genomic sequence of SARS-CoV-2 virus is 96% similar to bat corona viruses so these bats may be potential reservoir host for human corona virus [9]. However, there are no clear evidences which have suggested virus transmission directly from bats to human population [10]. Further, some studies suggested that pangolins can be considered as intermediate hosts between bats and human [11, 12]. Severe infectious covid-19 cases have rapidly progressed to dyspnoea, shock and acute respiratory distress [13]. In addition, the other organ dysfunctions have also been reported from patients including severe cardiac injury, acute renal, gastrointestinal, liver injury, neurological defect along with coagulation impairment and death [13].

It is important to understand the virus biology, and replication cycle to identify effective therapies against SARS-CoV-2, because most of therapies are directly targeting the stages in the virus life cycle. Highly pathogenic SARS-CoV-2 are enveloped, single-stranded positive sense RNA betacoronavirus with size ranging from 80–120 nm, and their genomes encode non-structural proteins (nsps), structural proteins, and several accessory proteins [14]. Genome of RNA virus contains ten open reading frames (ORF1–10) and has total 29,903 nucleotides [15]. Among the ten ORFs ORF2–10 generates four structural proteins S (spike), N (nucleocapsid), E (Envelop protein), M (Membrane protein) along with auxillary proteins. However, large replicase polyproteins (PP1a/b) encoded by ORF1ab further gets cleaved by proteolytic enzymes into non structural proteins (nsp1–16) [15].

The SARS-CoV-2 virus entry in host cell is mediated with attachment of the spike (S) glycoprotein with the host angiotensin-converting enzyme 2 (ACE2) receptor thereby infection process starts [16]. Further, virus S protein cleaved by the cathepsin L proteases which get activated in a pH- dependant manner allows the release of viral genome into host cell cytoplasm [17]. In addition, other host cell proteases like TMPRSS2 (Transmembrane Protease Serine Type-2) and TMPRSS11D (Airway trypsin like protease) participate in the cleavage of spike protein into its constituents (S1 and S2) which further lead to entry of virus genome into host cell through non endocytic pathway [18]. S1 subunit of spike protein possesses receptor binding domain (RBD) which binds with host receptors and S2 subunit favors fusion of viral membrane with host cell [19]. Once the virus genome released inside the host cell, then host ribosomes are involved in the process of translation of virus genome containing ORF1ab into replicase polyproteins PP1ab [20]. These PP1ab further cleaved by important viral proteases include 3CLpro (3 chymotrypsin like proteases) and PLpro (papain like proteases) to generate nsp2–16 [20]. These nsp2–16 are participated in virus replication and transcription complex, while virus structural proteins are translated from another ORF2–10 containing viral genome and contribute to outer structure of virus [21]. At last, the newly born virions are delivered outside the infected cell by exocytosis after completion of their structural assembling in the endoplasmic reticulum golgi bodies complex [22].

The WHO (world health organization) has declared covid-19 a public health emergency due to its high spreading potential across the world. Although, vaccine development trial has almost finished and vaccination drive is going to be started. However, till now there are no effective therapies or specific drug candidates against this communicable disease. Thus, it is required to understand detail biology of virus (SARS-CoV-2) to further elucidate novel drug therapeutics.

2. Therapeutic agents to tackle the covid-19 infection

2.1 ACE-2 modulators

Like SARS-CoV, it is confirmed that SARS-CoV-2 virus also interacts with ACE-2 human enzyme for entry and replication into the host cell. SARS-CoV-2 spike protein has high binding affinity with ACE-2 enzyme present in respiratory epithelial cell of host [23]. Hence, the therapeutics which inhibit spike protein-ACE-2 interaction would be considered effective therapy against SARS-CoV-2. ACE-2 enzyme is a zinc metalloproteinase which contains two domains in its structure which include amino terminal domain and carboxy terminal domain [5]. ACE-2 enzymes are exhibits in type-I and type-II alveolar cells of respiratory tract, liver, kidney, testes, heart and intestine [24]. Wu et al. [25] have found that ACE-2 enzymes are highly expressed in alveolar epithelial type-II cells in an around 83% which indicate these cell can be served as reservoir for virus. ACE-2 enzyme is a key regulator protein of RAS (Renin-Angiotensin System) system which contributes to vascular homeostasis [26]. In RAS system, angiotensinogen glycoprotein is cleaved by renin enzyme present in kidney to angiotensin-I, which has converted into angiotensin-II (Ang-II) by ACE-1. Further, Ang-II binds to angiotensin receptor (ATR1) and produces vasoconstriction, cell proliferation, inflammation, thrombosis and vascular constriction [27]. For the counterbalance of AngII- ATR_1 axis effect, AngII is cleaved by ACE-2 enzymes into Ang1–7 peptides [28]. These angiotensin peptides further act on MASR (mitochondrial assembly receptor) and exhibits protective effects such as anti-inflammatory, anti-apoptotic and vasodilatation. Rothlin and co-worker [29] have reported the protective effects of ACE inhibitors and angiotensin receptor blockers (ARBs). They have found that patients with Covid-19 infection are taking ACE inhibitors and angiotensin receptor blockers exhibited lower mortality as compared with non-user patients. Previous study revealed that SARS-CoV virus down-regulates the ACE-2 enzymes present in host cell surface and increased ACE enzyme activity which lead to severe lung injury [30]. Increased ACE enzyme activity has been observed in SARS-CoV-2 patients. Hence, it has been proposed that delivery of soluble ACE-2 recombinant protein compete with host ACE-2 enzymes for the SARS-CoV-2 spike protein and ultimately neutralize the virus load and further, protect the patients from lung injury. For this purpose, recombinant human ACE-2 such as APN01 and GK2586881 have been analyzed and found effective in patient suffered from acute severe respiratory syndrome (**Figure 1**) [31].

2.2 TMPRSS2 inhibitors

Transmembrane serine protease-2 (TMPRSS-2) is present in host epithelium cells of various tissues [32]. It is involved in the pathogenesis of SARS-CoV-2 through cleavage of spike protein and facilitates virus entry into host cell [33]. Matsuyama et al. [34] demonstrated that over-expressed protein TMPRSS-2 containing vero E6 cell lines are susceptible for SARS-CoV virus infection and used as pharmacological tool for SARS-CoV-2 research. Thus any drug candidate which inhibits TMPRSS-2 protease may be effective in SARS-CoV-2 infection. In this regard, *in vitro* study conducted against SARS-CoV-2 to check the efficacy of compound camostat mesylate blocked the spike mediated virus entry in caco-2 cells [35]. In addition, some repurposing studies have been conducted to evaluate the efficacy of other proteases inhibitors such as nafamostat, 4-(2 aminomethyl) benzenesulfonyl fluoride and mucolytic drug bromhexine which can offer new therapeutic option for this pandemic (**Figure 1**) [36, 37].

2.3 JAK–STAT inhibitors

In covid-19 infection, patients suffer from severe acute respiratory syndrome in which huge amounts of various cytokines are released from immune cells leading to multiorgan failure and death [38]. Moreover, JAK–STAT signaling pathway is involved in SARS-CoV-2 virus entry into host cell which has linked with AAK1 (Adaptor-associated protein kinase-1) related clathrin mediated endocytosis [39].

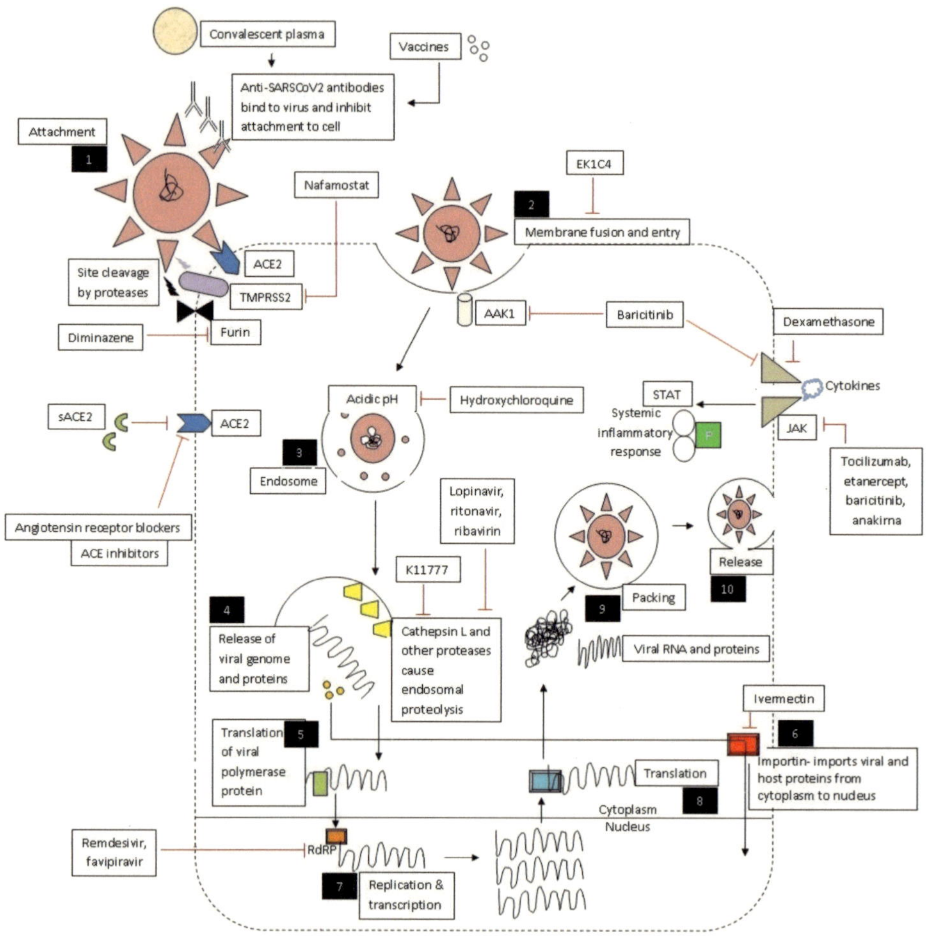

Figure 1.
Diagram showing the therapeutics approach to treat the infection of covid-19 patients.

Activation of JAK–STAT pathway through Ang-II/AT_1R may generate cytokines storm including IL-1, IL-2, IL-6, IL-7, IL-10 and TNF-α [39]. Thus, it may be suggested that JAK–STAT inhibitors could be potential therapeutics for the covid-19 infection. Further, Junior and co-workers [40] have shown that baricitinib, a JAK–STAT inhibitor, has potential to prevent generation of cytokines through inhibition of JAK–STAT signaling and also block the entry of SARS-CoV-2 via inhibiting AAK1 related clathrin mediated endocytosis (**Figure 1**).

2.4 Cathepsin L inhibitors

Cathepsin L is a cysteine protease reside in endosomes and works in acidic pH [41]. It cleaves S1 virus spike glycoprotein and facilitates three actions including virus entry into host cell, virus-host cell endosomal membrane fusion and RNA release. Serine protease (TMPRSS-2) acts on the surface of host cell membrane in neutral pH [42], whereas, cathepsin L mediates its action at host cell membrane as well as inside the endosomes in acidic pH [43]. Therefore, Liu and coworkers, [17] have proposed that the combined use of serine protease and cathepsin-L inhibitors could be effective therapeutics to prevent virus entry and their genome release inside the host cell thereby inhibit the virus replication. In addition, they have also mentioned some cathepsin-L inhibitors compounds which are found effective against coronavirus infection such as dec-RVKR-CMK, K11777, small molecule 5705213, MDL28170, SSAA09E1, EST, and oxocarbazate. Based on the proposed mechanism, it is reported that the combined use of TMPRSS-2 inhibitors including camostat and nafamostat mesylate along with cathepsin-L inhibitor E64d have shown inhibitory potential against SARS-CoV and SARS-CoV-2 infection in human epithelial cells (**Figure 1**) [44].

2.5 Furin inhibitors

Furin, is a human protease enzyme, present in multiple tissues and highly expressed in lungs [45]. It has been reported that SARS-CoV-2 virus contains furin like cleavage site (FCS) in its spike protein which has made covid-19 virus more pathogenic in nature as compared to other ancestors virus of coronaviridae family [46]. SARS-CoV-2 virus utilizes host furin protease for the cleavage of spike protein and gain entry into the host cell. Moreover, mortalities from SARS-CoV-2 infection have been reported in those patients compromised with cardiac disease, diabetes, obesity and hypertension and likely to be associated with higher circulating furin level [47]. Hence, scientists have drawn attention towards furin inhibitors to provide new therapeutic intervention against covid-19 infection (**Figure 1**).

2.6 Inhibitors of virus structural proteins and enzymes

Structural proteins and virus encoded enzymes of SARS-CoV-2 may be considered as important drug targets because these are responsible for virus survival and propagation. Researchers and pharmaceuticals companies have focused to develop short interfering RNA (siRNA) based therapeutics to target virus structural proteins and enzymes such as 3CL pro, PLpro and RNA dependant RNA polymerases to combat covid-19 infection [48]. Some previous studies revealed that siRNA therapeutics have already been designed against SARS-CoV and MERS viruses and found effective in outbreaks [49]. In addition, heptad repeat 1 region (HR1) present in the S protein involved in fusion and entry of virus could also be a good target for the development of fusion inhibitors against covid-19 [50]. Xia and co-workers, [51] have developed EK1C4 fusion inhibitors which target SARS-CoV-2 spike protein and found effective in HCoV-OC43 challenged mice. Recently in clinical trials, many chemical peptides, existing drugs and new drug candidates have been recognized through virtual and high throughput screening techniques against SARS-CoV-2 coded enzyme proteases [52]. Based on computational strategy, 6LU7PDB compound has been identified which acts as non-covalent inhibitor of 3CL pro enzyme in SARS-CoV-2 infection [53]. Some 3CL pro enzyme inhibitors antiviral drugs such as lopinavir and ritonavir have been found effective against SARS-CoV-2 virus infection [54]. In addition, some therapeutics are also identified which showed high binding affinity with SARS-CoV PLpro enzyme such as ribavirin, valganciclovir, beta-thymidine and some natural products like platycodin D, baicalin and catechin [55]. Moreover, RNA dependant RNA polymerase (RdRp) inhibitor antiviral drug remdesivir was approved by FDA for emergency treatment for covid-19 patients [56]. However, still its role is controversial for the treatment of covid-19 patients (**Figure 1**).

2.7 Inhibitors of cytokines

During covid-19 infection, higher amounts of cytokines have secreted from inflammatory cells and serve as potential therapeutic targets for drug development.

The major cytokines, IL-6, IL-1, TNF and interferons are generated during cytokine storm which cause the increased vascular permeability, vascular leakage along with dissemination of virus which may lead to fatal pneumonia and acute respiratory distress syndrome [57, 58]. However, many neutralizing strategy against these inflammatory mediators are being used to cope with this cytokine storm in covid-19 pandemic. Chi and co-workers, [59] reported the use of antibodies against IL-6 receptor (tocilizumab and sarilumab) for the treatment of covid-19 infection. Anti-TNF drug etanercept has shown favorable effect in covid-19 patients [60]. Moreover, another targeting approach against cytokine IL-1 is important because it is the major cytokine present in higher amount in alveolar lavage of covid-19 patients and secreted from inflammatory macrophages and monocytes [61]. Cavalli & coworkers, [62] have reported the use of anakirna in high dose and found safe in 72% patients suffered from covid-19 and ARDS with non-invasive ventilation outside the ICU. Furthermore, interferons (IFNs) have immunostimulant and antiviral effects and their use as a treatment along with some antiviral drugs have been found effective against MERS, SARS and IBV viruses (**Figure 1**) [63].

2.8 Antiviral drugs

As per the previous information related with SARS & MERS outbreak, many existing anti-viral drugs are being repurposed against SARS-CoV-2 virus in covid-19 pandemic. Remdesivir is a prodrug that converts into active metabolite and inhibits RNA dependant RNA polymerases (RdRp) thereby preventing the viral RNA synthesis [64]. It is prescribed against ebola virus infection and reported to have *in vitro* antiviral activity towards SARS and MERS coronaviruses [56]. Recently, it was reported that remdesivir prevents SARS-CoV-2 infection in human liver cancer cells [65]. Based on one clinical trial, remdesivir has been found clinically effective in 36 out of 53 patients suffered from covid-19 infection and receiving oxygen support [66]. In addition, many clinical trials are being carried out to check efficacy of remdesivir in covid-19 patients in various countries. Hung & co-workers, [67] have conducted clinical trial by using the combination of triple antiviral drug include lopinavir, ritonavir and ribavirin along with interferon which were found more promising compared to antiviral drug used alone in patient suffered from covid-19 infection. Another antiviral drug, favipiravir inhibits viral RNA polymerase enzyme and reported to have antiviral activity against many RNA viruses such as influenza, bunya and filoviruses [68]. However, to check the clinical efficacy of favipiravir in covid-19 patients various clinical trials have been performed in China and found favorable results (**Figure 1**) [13].

2.9 Corticosteroids

Corticosteroids are extensively used for SARS-CoV, MERS-CoV, H1N1 influenza, and ARDS that have similar pathological features with covid-19. But, their role in reducing mortality and improving these conditions remain controversial [69]. It was reported that corticosteroids did not improve the outcome during the SARS and MERS outbreaks, but delayed viral clearance and increased rates of secondary infections [70]. A systemic review and meta-analysis are conducted in covid-19 patients by van-Paassen et al. [71], their findings based on observational and clinical studies suggested the beneficial effects of corticosteroids on mortality rate and reduced ventilation support. However, delayed viral clearance and increased secondary infection have also been observed. Similarly, the study has been conducted in China in 201 patients confirmed with covid-19 pneumonia. In 62 patients who received methylprednisolone likely had decrease risk of death [72]. As per another report of Mishra & Mulani, [73] corticosteroids are not recommended in the late course of acute respiratory distress syndrome (ARDS) condition because their persistent use more than 2 weeks has increased risk of death in ARDS patients. It seems that corticosteroid treatment work like double edged sword in covid-19 fight, therefore duration of corticosteroid therapy needs to be clarified in clinical trials (**Figure 1**).

2.10 Convalescent plasma therapy

Convalescent plasma is obtained from donors who have recovered from covid-19 infection, possess antibodies against SARS-CoV-2 that may neutralize the virus and modify the immune response [74]. Convalescent plasma therapy offers short term protection strategy and generates immediate immune response in susceptible patients. This approach has already been used in earlier outbreak of corona viruses such as SARS and MERS [75]. In this corona pandemic, many clinical trials have also been conducted against SARS-CoV-2. Recently the clinical study conducted by Duan et al. [76] revealed that the convalescent plasma therapy was well tolerated and positively improved the clinical outcomes in severe covid-19 patients. Salazar et al. [77] reported the use of convalescent plasma therapy in 25 patients who had severe covid-19 disease and evaluated safety along with clinical outcomes at 14 day after the transfusion. They found clinical improvement in nine patients within seven days and other were discharged at day 14. Hence, convalescent plasma therapy has potential to treat covid-19 cases but some adverse events have also been reported such as allergic reaction, dyspnoea and acute lung injury [78] (**Figure 1**).

2.11 Ivermectin

Ivermectin is an broad spectrum antiparasitic drug and its antiviral activity has also been reported against number of viruses both *in vitro* and *in vivo* [79]. Recently, *in vitro* study revealed that ivermectin can inhibit SARS-CoV-2 replication by reducing viral RNA up to 5000 fold at 48 h. in culture cells [80]. However, the mechanism of action of ivermectin is not clearly known. Choudhry and Sharma, [81] have mentioned that ivermectin may act by creating acidic environment and blocking the importin IMP2/β1 mediated viral intranuclear import (**Figure 1**).

2.12 Hydroxychloroquine

Hydroxychloroquine has been prescribed since decades in the prevention and treatment of malaria as well as rheumatoid arthritis and systemic lupus erythematosus (SLE) like chronic inflammatory condition [82]. In SARS-CoV-2 pandemic, it was suggested that hydroxychloroquine may have potential to treat covid-19 affected patients [83]. Food and Drug Administration (FDA) has granted permission for emergency use of hydroxychloquine in the treatment of covid-19 patients during initial stage of pandemic [84]. Recently, many *in vitro* studies have been conducted and found that hydroxychloroquine possess inhibitory activity against SARS-CoV-2 [85, 86]. Further, several studies have been published regarding the use of hydroxychloroquine in covid-19 but results are conflicting. One population based cohort study conducted by Rentsch and coworkers, [87] stated that there was no difference observed in mortality of covid-19 patients who had already received hydroxychloroquine for the treatment of rheumatoid arthritis or systemic lupus erythematosus. Similarly, in an observational study in covid-19 hospitalized patients, hydroxychloroquine did not show any benefit over mortality reduction (**Figure 1**) [88].

2.13 Vaccines

Various vaccine developments are being carried out across the world due to urgent need to overcome this covid-19 pandemic. Now in covid-19 emergency, vaccines could only be considered as potent therapeutics against SARS-CoV-2 deadly virus which normalize social life and working environment as it was earlier before pandemic. For the effective vaccines development against SARS-CoV-2 virus, various components are being used which include inactive or live-attenuated viruses, virus-like particles, viral vectors, protein-based, DNA-based, and mRNA-based vaccines [89]. Till now various potential vaccine candidates have already been

Type/ plateform	Vaccine Construct	Developer	Clinical Stage & Current Status	References
Inactivated virus	Nucleic acid	National institute for communicable disease control and prevention, China	Phase-III	[91]
Inactivated virus	Novel corona virus inactivated vero cells	Bejing institute of biological products Sinopharma	Ongoing Phase-III	[92]
Inactivated virus	Whole virion inactivated SARS-CoV-2 antigen	Bharat Biotech, India	Phase-I / II (DCGI-CDSCO Approved for emergency use in India)	[93, 94]
DNA	S Protein	INOVIO Pharmaceuticals, with, International Vaccine Institute and Seoul National University Hospital of South Korea	Phase-I/ II (Phase–III study put on hold by FDA,US)	[95, 96]
RNA	LNP-encapsulated m-RNA	Moderna with national institute of allergy and infectious disease, USA	Phase-III [FDA issued Emergency Use Authorization (EUA)]	[97, 98]
RNA	Lipid nanoparticle encapsulated mRNA (BNT162b2)	BioNTech and Pfizer	Phase-III (FDA issued EUA)	[99]
Protein subunit	Full length SARS-CoV-2 glycoprotein nanoparticle vaccine	Novavax, USA	Phase-III (Planning to apply FDA EUA in April, 2021)	[100, 101]
Non replicating virus vector	ChAdOx1-S	University of Oxford with Astrazeneca (UK) and Serum Institute, India	Phase-III (Approved for emergency use in some selected countries)	[102, 103]
Non replicating virus vector	Adeno virus based	Gamaleya Research Institute (Sputnik U)	Phase-III (Approved for use in Russia)	[104]

Table 1.
List of various important vaccines which are developed or being in different development phases against covid-19 infection.

developed and undergone for vaccination shot which have completed their clinical evaluation phase successfully [90]. However, several new vaccines are still under clinical developmental phase (**Figure 1**). Some important vaccines which are being developed against SARS-CoV-2 virus are mention below in **Table 1**.

3. Conclusion

Covid-19 is a devastating situation to the whole world and this infection is the reason for the morbidity and mortality of millions of people around the globe. It has shown impact on the health, economy and social aspect of the general population. Various therapeutic agents like ACE-2, TMPRSS2, JAK–STAT, cathepsin L, furin inhibitors, antiviral drugs, corticosteroids and plasma therapy have been tried for the treatment of covid-19 infected patients; however, conflicting results are obtained during the various clinical trials in the use of some therapeutic agents. Further, various vaccination programmes through various vaccine candidates are under progress; nevertheless, it will take time to complete dosing the millions of people. Therefore, various therapeutic agents are in need and require research to tackle this SARS-CoV-2 infection.

Conflict of interest

The authors declare no conflict of interest.

Author details

Meemansha Sharma, Thakur Uttam Singh*, Madhu Cholenahalli Lingaraju and Subhashree Parida
Division of Pharmacology and Toxicology, ICAR-Indian Veterinary Research Institute, Izatnagar, Bareilly, Uttar Pradesh, India

*Address all correspondence to: tusingh80@gmail.com

References

[1] Zhu H, Wei L, Niu P. The novel coronavirus outbreak in Wuhan, China. Global health research and policy. 2020 Dec; 5(1):1-3.

[2] Mohanty SK, Satapathy A, Naidu MM, Mukhopadhyay S, Sharma S, Barton LM, Stroberg E, Duval EJ, Pradhan D, Tzankov A, Parwani AV. Severe acute respiratory syndrome coronavirus-2 (SARS-CoV-2) and coronavirus disease 19 (COVID-19)–anatomic pathology perspective on current knowledge. Diagnostic Pathology. 2020; 15(1):1-17.

[3] World Health Organization. COVID-19 weekly epidemiological update, 22 December 2020.

[4] Pal M, Berhanu G, Desalegn C, Kandi V. Severe acute respiratory syndrome coronavirus-2 (SARS-CoV-2): an update. Cureus. 2020; 12(3).

[5] Gil C, Ginex T, Maestro I, Nozal V, Barrado-Gil L, Cuesta-Geijo MÁ, Urquiza J, Ramírez D, Alonso C, Campillo NE, Martinez A. COVID-19: drug targets and potential treatments. Journal of Medicinal Chemistry. 2020; 63(21):12359-86.

[6] Lu CW, Liu XF, Jia ZF. 2019-nCoV transmission through the ocular surface must not be ignored. Lancet (London, England). 2020; 395(10224):e39.

[7] Saawarn B, Hait S. Occurrence, fate and removal of SARS-CoV-2 in wastewater: Current knowledge and future perspectives. Journal of Environmental Chemical Engineering. 2020; 104870.

[8] Dhiman R, Rakheja V, Saxena R. An Ophthalmologist's Insight Into The Viral Pandemics. Journal of Optometry. 2021 Jan 6.

[9] Flores-Alanis A, Sandner-Miranda L, Delgado G, Cravioto A, Morales-Espinosa R. The receptor binding domain of SARS-CoV-2 spike protein is the result of an ancestral recombination between the bat-CoV RaTG13 and the pangolin-CoV MP789. BMC research notes. 2020; 13(1):1-6.

[10] Kumar R, Lee MH, Mickael C, Kassa B, Pasha Q, Tuder R, Graham B. Pathophysiology and potential future therapeutic targets using preclinical models of COVID-19. ERJ Open Research. 2020; 6(4).

[11] Zhao J, Cui W, Tian BP. The potential intermediate hosts for SARS-CoV-2. Frontiers in Microbiology. 2020; 11.

[12] Zhang T, Wu Q, Zhang Z. Probable pangolin origin of SARS-CoV-2 associated with the COVID-19 outbreak. Current Biology. 2020; 30(7):1346-51.

[13] Zhang J, Xie B, Hashimoto K. Current status of potential therapeutic candidates for the COVID-19 crisis. Brain, Behavior, and Immunity. 2020 Apr 22.

[14] Prasad R. COVID-19: Current status, Challenges and Future Perspectives. 2020; 1-2.

[15] Kumar BK, Sekhar KV, Kunjiappan S, Jamalis J, Balaña-Fouce R, Tekwani BL, Sankaranarayanan M. Druggable targets of SARS-CoV-2 and treatment opportunities for COVID-19. Bioorganic Chemistry. 2020 Sep 8:104269.

[16] Baig MS, Alagumuthu M, Rajpoot S, Saqib U. Identification of a potential peptide inhibitor of SARS-CoV-2 targeting its entry into the host cells. Drugs in R&D. 2020; 20(3):161-9.

[17] Liu T, Luo S, Libby P, Shi GP. Cathepsin L-selective inhibitors:

A potentially promising treatment for COVID-19 patients. Pharmacology & Therapeutics. 2020 May 26:107587.

[18] Iwata-Yoshikawa N, Okamura T, Shimizu Y, Hasegawa H, Takeda M, Nagata N. TMPRSS2 contributes to virus spread and immunopathology in the airways of murine models after coronavirus infection. Journal of Virology. 2019; 93(6).

[19] Belouzard S, Millet JK, Licitra BN, Whittaker GR. Mechanisms of coronavirus cell entry mediated by the viral spike protein. Viruses. 2012; 4(6):1011-33.

[20] V'kovski P, Gerber M, Kelly J, Pfaender S, Ebert N, Lagache SB, Simillion C, Portmann J, Stalder H, Gaschen V, Bruggmann R. Determination of host proteins composing the microenvironment of coronavirus replicase complexes by proximity-labeling. Elife. 2019; 8:e42037.

[21] V'kovski P, Kratzel A, Steiner S, Stalder H, Thiel V. Coronavirus biology and replication: implications for SARS-CoV-2. Nature Reviews Microbiology. 2020;1-6.

[22] Saxena A. Drug targets for COVID-19 therapeutics: Ongoing global efforts. Journal of Biosciences. 2020; 45(1):1-24.

[23] Davidson AM, Wysocki J, Batlle D. Interaction of SARS-CoV-2 and other Coronavirus with ACE (Angiotensin-Converting Enzyme)-2 as their main receptor: therapeutic implications. Hypertension. 2020; 76(5):1339-49.

[24] Fu J, Zhou B, Zhang L, Balaji KS, Wei C, Liu X, Chen H, Peng J, Fu J. Expressions and significances of the angiotensin-converting enzyme 2 gene, the receptor of SARS-CoV-2 for COVID-19. Molecular Biology Reports. 2020; 47:4383-92.

[25] Wu C, Zheng S, Chen Y, Zheng M. Single-cell RNA expression profiling of ACE2, the putative receptor of Wuhan 2019-nCoV, in the nasal tissue. MedRxiv. 2020 Jan 1.

[26] Tikellis C, Thomas MC. Angiotensin-converting enzyme 2 (ACE2) is a key modulator of the renin angiotensin system in health and disease. International journal of peptides. 2012.

[27] Gómez J, Albaiceta GM, García-Clemente M, López-Larrea C, Amado-Rodríguez L, Lopez-Alonso I, Hermida T, Enriquez AI, Herrero P, Melón S, Alvarez-Argüelles ME. Angiotensin-converting enzymes (ACE, ACE2) gene variants and COVID-19 outcome. Gene. 2020; 762:145102.

[28] Sriram K, Insel PA. A hypothesis for pathobiology and treatment of COVID-19: The centrality of ACE1/ACE2 imbalance. British Journal of Pharmacology. 2020; 177(21):4825-44.

[29] Rothlin RP, Vetulli HM, Duarte M, Pelorosso FG. Telmisartan as tentative angiotensin receptor blocker therapeutic for COVID-19. Drug Development Research. 2020; 81(7): 768-770.

[30] Kuba K, Imai Y, Rao S, Gao H, Guo F, Guan B, Huan Y, Yang P, Zhang Y, Deng W, Bao L. A crucial role of angiotensin converting enzyme 2 (ACE2) in SARS coronavirus–induced lung injury. Nature Medicine. 2005; 11(8):875-9.

[31] Zhang H, Penninger JM, Li Y, Zhong N, Slutsky AS. Angiotensin-converting enzyme 2 (ACE2) as a SARS-CoV-2 receptor: molecular mechanisms and potential therapeutic target. Intensive Care Medicine. 2020; 46(4):586-90.

[32] Mukhopadhyay D, Mussa BM. Identification of novel hypothalamic microRNAs as promising therapeutics

for SARS-CoV-2 by regulating ACE2 and TMPRSS2 expression: an in silico analysis. Brain Sciences. 2020; 10(10):666.

[33] Kawase M, Shirato K, van der Hoek L, Taguchi F, Matsuyama S. Simultaneous treatment of human bronchial epithelial cells with serine and cysteine protease inhibitors prevents severe acute respiratory syndrome coronavirus entry. Journal of Virology. 2012; 86(12):6537-45.

[34] Matsuyama S, Nagata N, Shirato K, Kawase M, Takeda M, Taguchi F. Efficient activation of the severe acute respiratory syndrome coronavirus spike protein by the transmembrane protease TMPRSS2. Journal of Virology. 2010; 84(24):12658-64.

[35] Hoffmann M, Kleine-Weber H, Schroeder S, Krüger N, Herrler T, Erichsen S, Schiergens TS, Herrler G, Wu NH, Nitsche A, Müller MA. SARS-CoV-2 cell entry depends on ACE2 and TMPRSS2 and is blocked by a clinically proven protease inhibitor. Cell. 2020; 181(2):271-80.

[36] Shen LW, Mao HJ, Wu YL, Tanaka Y, Zhang W. TMPRSS2: A potential target for treatment of influenza virus and coronavirus infections. Biochimie. 2017;142:1-10.

[37] Maggio R, Corsini GU. Repurposing the mucolytic cough suppressant and TMPRSS2 protease inhibitor bromhexine for the prevention and management of SARS-CoV-2 infection. Pharmacological Research. 2020; 157:104837.

[38] Huang C, Wang Y, Li X, Ren L, Zhao J, Hu Y, Zhang L, Fan G, Xu J, Gu X, Cheng Z. Clinical features of patients infected with 2019 novel coronavirus in Wuhan, China. The Lancet. 2020; 395(10223):497-506.

[39] Seif F, Aazami H, Khoshmirsafa M, Kamali M, Mohsenzadegan M, Pornour M, Mansouri D. JAK inhibition as a new treatment strategy for patients with COVID-19. International Archives of Allergy and Immunology. 2020; 181(6):467-75.

[40] Júnior ML, de Souza LM, Dutra RE, de Melo Valente RG, Melo TS. Review on therapeutic targets for COVID-19: insights from cytokine storm. Postgraduate Medical Journal. 2020.

[41] Liu CL, Guo J, Zhang X, Sukhova GK, Libby P, Shi GP. Cysteine protease cathepsins in cardiovascular disease: from basic research to clinical trials. Nature Reviews Cardiology. 2018; 15(6):351-70.

[42] Meyer D, Sielaff F, Hammami M, Böttcher-Friebertshäuser E, Garten W, Steinmetzer T. Identification of the first synthetic inhibitors of the type II transmembrane serine protease TMPRSS2 suitable for inhibition of influenza virus activation. Biochemical Journal. 2013; 452(2):331-43.

[43] Ou X, Liu Y, Lei X, Li P, Mi D, Ren L, Guo L, Guo R, Chen T, Hu J, Xiang Z. Characterization of spike glycoprotein of SARS-CoV-2 on virus entry and its immune cross-reactivity with SARS-CoV. Nature Communications. 2020 Mar 27; 11(1):1-12.

[44] Hoffmann M, Schroeder S, Kleine-Weber H, Müller MA, Drosten C, Pöhlmann S. Nafamostat mesylate blocks activation of SARS-CoV-2: new treatment option for COVID-19. Antimicrobial Agents and Chemotherapy. 2020.

[45] Belen-Apak FB, Sarialioglu F. The old but new: Can unfractioned heparin and low molecular weight heparins inhibit proteolytic activation and cellular internalization of SARS-CoV2 by inhibition of host cell proteases. Medical Hypotheses. 2020; 142:109743.

[46] Wu C, Zheng M, Yang Y, Gu X, Yang K, Li M, Liu Y, Zhang Q, Zhang P, Wang Y, Wang Q. Furin: A Potential Therapeutic Target for COVID-19. Iscience. 2020; 23(10):101642.

[47] Fitzgerald K. Furin Protease: From SARS CoV-2 to Anthrax, Diabetes, and Hypertension. The Permanente Journal. 2020; 24.

[48] Uludağ H, Parent K, Aliabadi HM, Haddadi A. Prospects for RNAi therapy of COVID-19. Frontiers in Bioengineering and Biotechnology. 2020; 8:916.

[49] Ghosh S, Firdous SM, Nath A. siRNA could be a potential therapy for COVID-19. EXCLI Journal. 2020; 19:528.

[50] Huang Y, Yang C, Xu XF, Xu W, Liu SW. Structural and functional properties of SARS-CoV-2 spike protein: potential antivirus drug development for COVID-19. Acta Pharmacologica Sinica. 2020; 41(9):1141-9.

[51] Xia S, Liu M, Wang C, Xu W, Lan Q, Feng S, Qi F, Bao L, Du L, Liu S, Qin C. Inhibition of SARS-CoV-2 (previously 2019-nCoV) infection by a highly potent pan-coronavirus fusion inhibitor targeting its spike protein that harbors a high capacity to mediate membrane fusion. Cell Research. 2020; 30(4):343-55.

[52] Jin Z, Du X, Xu Y, Deng Y, Liu M, Zhao Y, Zhang B, Li X, Zhang L, Peng C, Duan Y. Structure of M pro from SARS-CoV-2 and discovery of its inhibitors. Nature. 2020; 582(7811):289-93.

[53] Macchiagodena M, Pagliai M, Procacci P. Identification of potential binders of the main protease 3CLpro of the COVID-19 via structure-based ligand design and molecular modeling. Chemical Physics Letters. 2020; 750:137489.

[54] Bhatnagar T, Murhekar MV, Soneja M, Gupta N, Giri S, Wig N, Gangakhedkar R. Lopinavir/ritonavir combination therapy amongst symptomatic coronavirus disease 2019 patients in India: Protocol for restricted public health emergency use. Indian Journal of Medical Research. 2020; 151(2):184.

[55] Wu C, Liu Y, Yang Y, Zhang P, Zhong W, Wang Y, Wang Q, Xu Y, Li M, Li X, Zheng M. Analysis of therapeutic targets for SARS-CoV-2 and discovery of potential drugs by computational methods. Acta Pharmaceutica Sinica B. 2020; 10(5):766-88.

[56] Malin JJ, Suárez I, Priesner V, Fätkenheuer G, Rybniker J. Remdesivir against COVID-19 and other viral diseases. Clinical microbiology reviews. 2020; 34(1).

[57] Monteleone G, Sarzi-Puttini PC, Ardizzone S. Preventing COVID-19-induced pneumonia with anticytokine therapy. The Lancet Rheumatology. 2020; 2(5):e255-6.

[58] Rahmati M, Moosavi MA. Cytokine-targeted therapy in severely ill COVID-19 patients: options and cautions. Mortality. 2020; 105954.

[59] Chi Zhang MD, Zhao Wu PD, Jia-Wen Li MD. The cytokine release syndrome (CRS) of severe COVID-19 and Interleukin-6 receptor antagonist Tocilizumab may be the key to reduce mortality. International Journal of Antimicrobial Agents. 2020; 105954(10.1016).

[60] Duret PM, Sebbag E, Mallick A, Gravier S, Spielmann L, Messer L. Recovery from COVID-19 in a patient with spondyloarthritis treated with TNF-alpha inhibitor etanercept. Annals of the Rheumatic Diseases. 2020; 79(9):1251-2.

[61] Calabrese LH, Calabrese C. Cytokine release syndrome and

the prospects for immunotherapy with COVID-19. Part 2: The role of interleukin 1. Cleveland Clinic Journal of Medicine. 2020 Jul 9. DOI: https://doi.org/10.3949/ccjm.87a.ccc044.

[62] Cavalli G, De Luca G, Campochiaro C, Della-Torre E, Ripa M, Canetti D, Oltolini C, Castiglioni B, Din CT, Boffini N, Tomelleri A. Interleukin-1 blockade with high-dose anakinra in patients with COVID-19, acute respiratory distress syndrome, and hyperinflammation: a retrospective cohort study. The Lancet Rheumatology. 2020; 2(6):e325-31.

[63] Nile SH, Nile A, Qiu J, Li L, Jia X, Kai G. COVID-19: Pathogenesis, cytokine storm and therapeutic potential of interferons. Cytokine & Growth Factor Reviews. 2020; 53:66-70.

[64] Eastman RT, Roth JS, Brimacombe KR, Simeonov A, Shen M, Patnaik S, Hall MD. Remdesivir: a review of its discovery and development leading to emergency use authorization for treatment of COVID-19. ACS Central Science. 2020; 6(5):672-83.

[65] McKee DL, Sternberg A, Stange U, Laufer S, Naujokat C. Candidate drugs against SARS-CoV-2 and COVID-19. Pharmacological research. 2020 Apr 29:104859.

[66] Grein J, Ohmagari N, Shin D, Diaz G, Asperges E, Castagna A, Feldt T, Green G, Green ML, Lescure FX, Nicastri E. Compassionate use of remdesivir for patients with severe Covid-19. New England Journal of Medicine. 2020 ;382(24):2327-36.

[67] Hung IF, Lung KC, Tso EY, Liu R, Chung TW, Chu MY, Ng YY, Lo J, Chan J, Tam AR, Shum HP. Triple combination of interferon beta-1b, lopinavir–ritonavir, and ribavirin in the treatment of patients admitted to hospital with COVID-19: an open-label, randomised, phase 2 trial. The Lancet. 2020; 395(10238):1695-704.

[68] Delang L, Abdelnabi R, Neyts J. Favipiravir as a potential countermeasure against neglected and emerging RNA viruses. Antiviral research. 2018; 153:85-94.

[69] Belete TM. An Up-to-Date Overview of Therapeutic Agents for the Treatment of COVID-19 Disease. Clinical pharmacology: advances and applications. 2020; 12:203.

[70] Zha L, Li S, Pan L, Tefsen B, Li Y, French N, Chen L, Yang G, Villanueva EV. Corticosteroid treatment of patients with coronavirus disease 2019 (COVID-19). Medical Journal of Australia. 2020; 212(9):416-20.

[71] van Paassen J, Vos JS, Hoekstra EM, Neumann KM, Boot PC, Arbous SM. Corticosteroid use in COVID-19 patients: a systematic review and meta-analysis on clinical outcomes. Critical Care. 2020; 24(1):1-22.

[72] Wu C, Chen X, Cai Y, Zhou X, Xu S, Huang H, Zhang L, Zhou X, Du C, Zhang Y, Song J. Risk factors associated with acute respiratory distress syndrome and death in patients with coronavirus disease 2019 pneumonia in Wuhan, China. JAMA Internal Medicine. 2020; 180(7):934-43.

[73] Mishra GP, Mulani J. Corticosteroids for COVID-19: the search for an optimum duration of therapy. The Lancet. Respiratory Medicine. 2021; 9(1):e8.

[74] Wang X, Guo X, Xin Q, Pan Y, Hu Y, Li J, Chu Y, Feng Y, Wang Q. Neutralizing antibodies responses to SARS-CoV-2 in COVID-19 inpatients and convalescent patients. Clinical Infectious Diseases. 2020.

[75] Bloch EM, Shoham S, Casadevall A, Sachais BS, Shaz B, Winters JL, Van Buskirk C, Grossman BJ, Joyner M, Henderson JP, Pekosz A. Deployment of convalescent plasma for the prevention and treatment of COVID-19.

The Journal of clinical investigation. 2020; 130(6):2757-65.

[76] Duan K, Liu B, Li C, Zhang H, Yu T, Qu J, Zhou M, Chen L, Meng S, Hu Y, Peng C. Effectiveness of convalescent plasma therapy in severe COVID-19 patients. Proceedings of the National Academy of Sciences. 2020;117(17):9490-6.

[77] Salazar E, Perez KK, Ashraf M, Chen J, Castillo B, Christensen PA, Eubank T, Bernard DW, Eagar TN, Long SW, Subedi S. Treatment of coronavirus disease 2019 (COVID-19) patients with convalescent plasma. The American Journal of Pathology. 2020; 190(8):1680-90.

[78] Trivedi N, Verma A, Kumar D. Possible treatment and strategies for COVID-19: review and assessment. European Review for Medical and Pharmacological Sciences. 2020; 24(23):12593-608.

[79] Padhy BM, Mohanty RR, Das S, Meher BR. Therapeutic potential of ivermectin as add on treatment in COVID 19: A systematic review and meta-analysis: Ivermectin in COVID-19: A meta-analysis. Journal of Pharmacy & Pharmaceutical Sciences. 2020; 23:462-9.

[80] Caly L, Druce JD, Catton MG, Jans DA, Wagstaff KM. The FDA-approved drug ivermectin inhibits the replication of SARS-CoV-2 in vitro. Antiviral Research. 2020; 178:104787.

[81] Choudhary R, Sharma AK. Potential use of hydroxychloroquine, ivermectin and azithromycin drugs in fighting COVID-19: trends, scope and relevance. New Microbes and New Infections. 2020:100684.

[82] dos Reis Neto ET, Kakehasi AM, de Medeiros Pinheiro M, Ferreira GA, Marques CD, da Mota LM, dos Santos Paiva E, Pileggi GC, Sato EI, Reis AP, Xavier RM. Revisiting hydroxychloroquine and chloroquine for patients with chronic immunity-mediated inflammatory rheumatic diseases. Advances in Rheumatology. 2020; 60(1):1-1.

[83] Jorge A. Hydroxychloroquine in the prevention of COVID-19 mortality. The Lancet Rheumatology. 2021; 3(1):e2-3.

[84] Juurlink DN. Safety considerations with chloroquine, hydroxychloroquine and azithromycin in the management of SARS-CoV-2 infection. Canadian Medical Association Journal. 2020; 192(17):E450-3.

[85] Wang M, Cao R, Zhang L, Yang X, Liu J, Xu M, Shi Z, Hu Z, Zhong W, Xiao G. Remdesivir and chloroquine effectively inhibit the recently emerged novel coronavirus (2019-nCoV) in vitro. Cell Research. 2020; 30(3):269-71.

[86] Yao X, Ye F, Zhang M, Cui C, Huang B, Niu P, Liu X, Zhao L, Dong E, Song C, Zhan S. In vitro antiviral activity and projection of optimized dosing design of hydroxychloroquine for the treatment of severe acute respiratory syndrome coronavirus 2 (SARS-CoV-2). Clinical Infectious Diseases. 2020; 71(15):732-9.

[87] Rentsch CT, DeVito NJ, MacKenna B, Morton CE, Bhaskaran K, Brown JP, Goldacre B. Effect of pre-exposure use of hydroxychloroquine on COVID-19 mortality: a population-based cohort study in patients with rheumatoid arthritis or systemic lupus erythematosus using the Open SAFELY platform. The Lancet Rheumatology, 2021; 3(1): e19-e27.

[88] Geleris J, Sun Y, Platt J, Zucker J, Baldwin M, Hripcsak G, Labella A, Manson DK, Kubin C, Barr RG, Sobieszczyk ME. Observational study of hydroxychloroquine in hospitalized patients with Covid-19. New England Journal of Medicine. 2020; 382(25):2411-8.

[89] Yadav T, Srivastava N, Mishra G, Dhama K, Kumar S, Puri B, Saxena SK. Recombinant vaccines for COVID-19. Human Vaccines & Immunotherapeutics. 2020; 16(12):2905-12.

[90] Krammer F. SARS-CoV-2 vaccines in development. Nature. 2020; 586(7830):516-27.

[91] Gao Q, Bao L, Mao H, Wang L, Xu K, Yang M, Li Y, Zhu L, Wang N, Lv Z, Gao H. Development of an inactivated vaccine candidate for SARS-CoV-2. Science. 2020; 369(6499):77-81.

[92] Tumban E. Lead SARS-CoV-2 Candidate Vaccines: Expectations from Phase III Trials and Recommendations Post-Vaccine Approval. Viruses. 2021;13(1):54

[93] Tregoning JS, Brown ES, Cheeseman HM, Flight KE, Higham SL, Lemm NM, Pierce BF, Stirling DC, Wang Z, Pollock KM. Vaccines for COVID-19. Clinical & Experimental Immunology. 2020; 202(2):162-92.

[94] COVAXIN® -India's first indigenous COVID-19 vaccine. Bharat Biotech. (http://www.bharatbiotech.com).

[95] Batty CJ, Heise MT, Bachelder EM, Ainslie KM. Vaccine formulations in clinical development for the prevention of severe acute respiratory syndrome coronavirus 2 infection. Advanced Drug Delivery Reviews. 2020 Dec 13.

[96] Inovio expects to begin late-stage COVID-19 vaccine study in second quarter. Thomson Reuters Foundation news, 10 Feb, 2021.

[97] Buschmann MD, Carrasco MJ, Alishetty S, Paige M, Alameh MG, Weissman D. Nanomaterial Delivery Systems for mRNA Vaccines. Vaccines. 2021; 9(1):65.

[98] Moderna announces primary efficacy analysis in phase 3 COVE study for its COVID-19 vaccine candidate and filing today with U.S. FDA for emergency use authorization. Moderna Press Release. November 30, 2020.

[99] Oliver SE, Gargano JW, Marin M, Wallace M, Curran KG, Chamberland M, McClung N, Campos-Outcalt D, Morgan RL, Mbaeyi S, Romero JR. The Advisory Committee on Immunization Practices' Interim Recommendation for Use of Pfizer-BioNTech COVID-19 Vaccine—United States, December 2020. Morbidity and Mortality Weekly Report. 2020 ; 69(50):1922.

[100] Dai L, Gao GF. Viral targets for vaccines against COVID-19. Nature Reviews Immunology. 2020;1-10.

[101] Novavax to seek EUA for covid-19 vaccine as early as april. Medscape Medical News, 26 Feb, 2021. (https://www.medscape.com/viewarticle/946422).

[102] Ng WH, Liu X, Mahalingam S. Development of vaccines for SARS-CoV-2. F1000Research. 2020; 9.

[103] WHO gives emergency use approval to AstraZeneca-Oxford's COVID-19 vaccine. Business Today. 15 Feb, 2021. (https://www.businesstoday.in/current/economy-politics/who-gives-emergency-use-approval-to-astrazeneca-oxford-covid-19-vaccines/story/431366.html)

[104] Nikhra V. Stages in COVID-19 Vaccine Development: The Nemesis, the Hubris, and the Elpis. International Journal Clinical Virology. 2020; 4:126-35.

Chapter 25

COVID-19 Researches: Where India Stands So Far?

Nikhil Srivastava and Gyaneshwer Chaubey

Abstract

By the end of the year 2019, in the month of November first pneumonia-like case of COVID-19 was detected in an individual aged 55 years in the Hubei Province of Central China. However the 'patient zero' or the first patient contracted with the disease is still unknown, but it is speculated that first contraction with virus occurred in Wuhan province of China. The rate by which the number of cases of the disease surged in China was remarkable and by the mid of January 2020 cases begin to appear in different parts of the world. WHO declared the COVID-19 outbreak a Public Health Emergency of International Concern by the end of January 2020. Researchers from different parts of the world continue to study the pathogenesis and spread pattern of this disease. This chapter emphasizes upon some of the prominent studies in the field of COVID-19 researches from India. It also focuses upon the *ACE2* gene polymorphism which has decreased the susceptibility against the virus amongst human population, and explains how at the molecular level ACE2 receptor concentration may affect the entry of the virus into the host cell. It also highlights the impact of the viral RNA on mitochondrial machinery of the host cell and how it instigates a pro-inflammatory response by declining the efficiency of immune system in whole. We also aim to highlight two potential drug candidates of COVID-19 and how these are performing against the virus according to several studies.

Keywords: COVID-19, India, ACE2, hydroxychloroquine, mitochondria

1. Introduction

India reported its first COVID-19 case on January 30th, 2020 which was about the same day when World Health Organization (WHO) declared this outbreak "a public health emergency of international concern" [1, 2]. Today, when India is reporting ~100,000 cases every day, an extreme load on healthcare system is proving to be a challenging situation for the middle-income nation [3]. World Health Organization (WHO) accounted first severe acute respiratory syndrome coronavirus (SARS-CoV) from 2002 to 2003, which spread through 26 countries across the world and was considered 'the first serious emergent disease of 21st century' [4]. The Coronavirus disease (COVID-19) spread in 2019–2020 is caused by a novel coronavirus designated as SARS-CoV-2 [5]. Coronaviruses belong to Coronaviridae family of the order Nidovirales whose members are large and enveloped containing a single-stranded (+) RNA as genetic material, these are considered the largest known RNA viruses with genome size of 25 to 32 kb and virions of 118–140 nm in diameter [6]. Within the family Coronaviridae there are two sub-families- Coronavirinae and Torovirinae further divided into six genera out of which members of the genus Betacoronavirus infects mostly mammals and genus Deltacoronavirus infect mammalian as well as avian hosts [7]. The COVID-19 causing SARS-CoV-2 belongs to genus Betacoronavirus [8].

As the surge in the number of cases started to be reported all across the world, major disparities on the basis of ethnicity, gender and populations were also noticed in different regions. The advancing age, and pre-existing medical conditions like diabetes, high blood pressure (BP), renal-associated diseases etc. increase the vulnerability of a person towards the severity in consequences of the disease [9, 10]. However, a surprising observation emanating from the pandemic is the rate of hospitalization of younger, ostensibly healthy individuals; which reflects that differences in the vulnerability of individuals to infection in the spectrum of COVID-19 symptoms remain to be understood [11]. This review will focus upon some of the studies leading to understanding the genomics of Indian populations and their vulnerabilities towards the SARS-CoV-2 infection, the studies relating to the mitochondrial impacts of the SARS-CoV-2 infection, molecular mechanisms through which ACE2 expression affects the viral pathogenesis and about two potential drug candidates of COVID-19.

This chapter provides an account on some of the major contributions towards the understanding the COVID-19 disease by Indian scientists and researchers.

2. ACE2 rs2285666 association with spatial distribution of COVID-19 in India

Host-pathogen interaction studies have revealed that ACE2 receptor present on the host cell works as a receptor for the spike glycoprotein of SARS-CoV-2 [12]. ACE2 is present on X-chromosome in humans, in which a polymorphism rs2285666 is shown to have significant disparity amongst Europeans and Asians

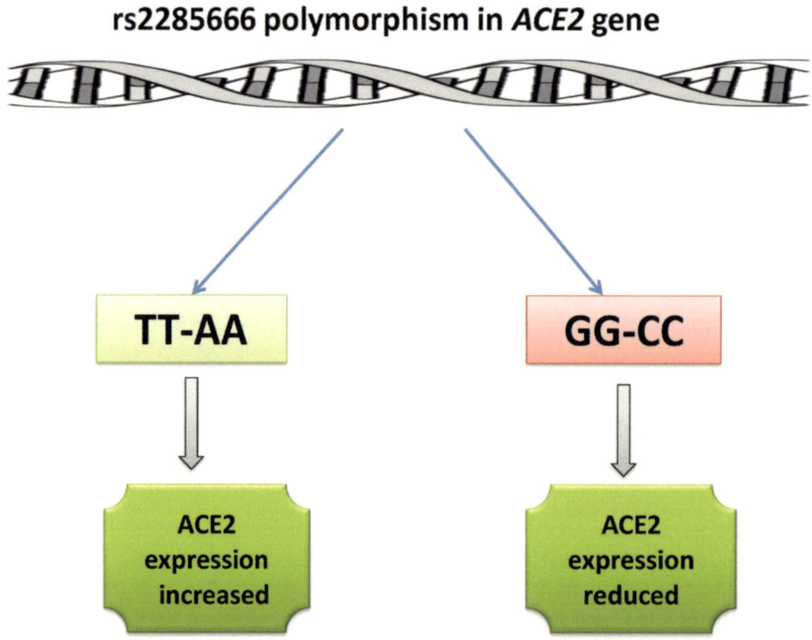

Figure 1.
Srivastava et al. have shown a direct correlation between the rs2285666 polymorphism and ACE2 gene expression.

[13, 14]. The decreased expression of ACE2 is frequently associated with increased susceptibility towards the severity of COVID-19 disease. Shrivastava et al. used this information as the principle of their study to find out the frequency of alternate allele (allele T on plus strand or allele A on minus strand) of this single nucleotide variation (SNV) in Indian populations and predict the cause of low infection rate as well as low Case Fatality Rate (CFR) in western states of India (**Figure 1**) [15].

In yet another study they showed that the overall genome of South Asians share greater genetic affinity with West Eurasians, however the ACE2 gene has greater genetic affinity with East Eurasians. The phylogenetic analysis of haplotypes distinctly classifies three types of haplotypes in order to identify the SNP which reveals greater affinity between South Asians and East Eurasians. Out of these three haplotypes- haplotype 3 (ht3) is shown to be harbored by East Eurasians and South Asians and derived from rs2285666 [16]. The ACE2 gene rs2285666 polymorphism is also shown to have association with type 2 diabetes mellitus (T2DM) in which A allele is associated with higher risk of T2DM [17]. The protective role of ACE2 in nephric tubules is shown in several studies, and its reduced expression contributes to the development and progression of kidney injury and diabetic nephropathy is explored by Reich et al. [18]. These studies strengthen the hypothesis of the association of rs2285666 (TT-plus strand or AA-minus strand), which increases the expression of ACE2 receptor protein with lower case fatality rate.

3. Molecular mechanisms of ACE2 expression during COVID-19

Angiotensin converting enzyme-2 (ACE2) receptors serve as medium for entry of SARS-CoV-2, the receptor is found attached in the plasma membrane of the cells in the heart, vessels, gut, lung, kidney, testis and brain and very rarely found solubilized in the circulation [19]. The function of ACE2 is to break down Ang II and form Ang 1-7, therefore ACE2 helps in checking the levels of Ang II and plays an important role in renin-angiotensin system (RAS) [20]. It is an established fact now that ACE2 expression is significantly down-regulated during COVID-19 which

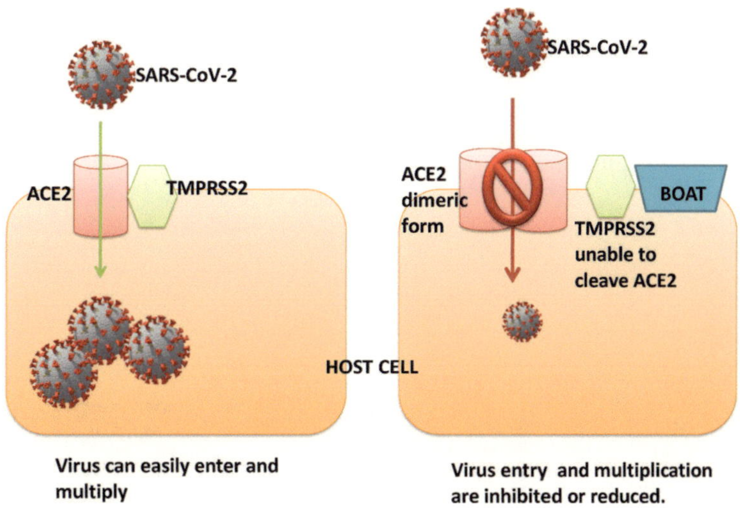

Figure 2.
Homo-dimerization of ACE2 receptor in case of higher expression levels of ACE2 gene results into decreased interaction and entry of virus into the host cell. BOAT transporter protein makes this process even more difficult, thereby decreasing the levels of viral multiplication.

results into abnormally increased levels of Ang II, which leaves critical organ systems susceptible to hyper-inflammation and failure [21, 22]. In an unpublished but important paper, it is significantly shown that the homo-dimerization of ACE2 as a result of its higher expression levels prevents binding of Spike protein (S-protein) complex of SARS-CoV-2 virus [23]. This study supports the hypothesis that ACE2 in its monomeric form, can bind to S-protein of the virus with greater preference. ACE2 acting as e-QTLs (Expression quantitative trait loci) due to natural genetic variations it results into homo-dimerized forms which lead to lowered cleavage by TMPRSS2 (**Figure 2**). The presence of broad neutral amino acid transporter, B0AT1 make the completion of this step even more difficult implied by the virus to get into the host cell. It is identified that natural variations in host genes like ADAM17, RPS6, HNRNPA1, SUMO1, NACA, BTF3 might help in bringing such homo-dimerizing structural variations in ACE2.

4. SARS-CoV-2, the highjacker of host mitochondria

A very interesting study focuses on yet another important aspect of COVID-19, that how 'the powerhouse of the cell' i.e. mitochondria are affected by the SARS-CoV-2 infection. The non-structural proteins of the virus are translated from two open reading frames (ORFs), ORF1a ORF3a, ORF6a, ORFF7a, ORF8a and ORF1b present in the genomic RNA of the virus. ORF1ab is responsible for the production of spike (S) protein, the envelope proteins (E), the membrane proteins (M), and the nucleocapsid proteins (N) of the viral structure [24–26]. Host mitochondria play a crucial role in the host immunity against the viral infection. The viral RNA genome portions and proteins localization into the mitochondria results into its dysfunction and production of mitochondria derived double-membranous vesicles (MDV) which work as a site of viral safe-house for unchecked replication (**Figure 3**). The viral pathogenesis is amplified as the hijacked mitochondria induce inflammatory responses and decrease the effectiveness of innate and adaptive immune responses [25].

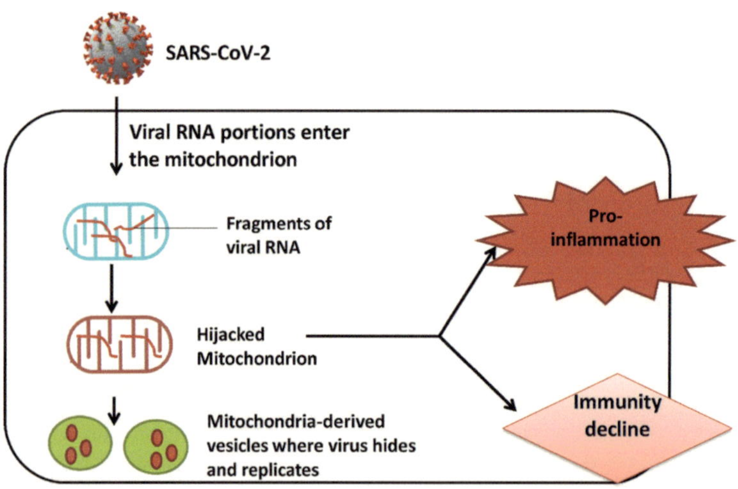

Figure 3.
There is an important role played by the host mitochondria in the host immunity against the viral infection. The MDV's (mitochondria derived double-membranous vesicles) formed from the hijacked mitochondria are the sites of unchecked viral replication.

5. Rapamycin and hydroxychloroquine: story of two repurposed drugs against the virus

SARS-CoV-2 spreads rapidly in comparison to its two cousins- SARS-CoV and MERS-CoV [27]. Therefore an effective drug development strategy is needed to control the faster spread of the disease, which is a time-consuming process. Repurposing or repositioning the already existing and approved drugs can help to shorten this time span and cost expenses. Rapamycin, which is an mTOR-inhibitor, is proposed to be a potential drug candidate against COVID-19 [28]. Rapamycin can play significant roles as a potential antibiotic in case of COVID-19, it can check the packaging of viral particles, prevent cytokine storms and also through its anti-aging and anti-obesity effects can be useful in this viral infection [28–30].

Hydroxychloroquine (HCQ), which is a much hyped candidate drug against COVID-19, has received a very straight forward judgment - it has no benefit in treatment of Covid-19 [31]. A group of medical doctors studied a population consisting of a total of 4984 patients with COVID-19, out of which 35.5% were provided with HCQ or its congeners and 62.01% were provided standard of care or had included antiviral medication. However, the estimated success of the treatment of both the groups was similar (77.45% and 77.87% respectively). This study shows that HCQ does not show any significant benefit in patients affected by COVID-19. Apart from many limitations in this study which includes patient cohort selection, variations in HCQ dosage etc. this study aligns with many studies regarding the ineffectiveness of the drug [32, 33].

6. Conclusion

COVID-19 is one of the most infectious diseases of 21st century which has already claimed to take lives of millions. The disease caused by the SARS-CoV-2 virus may affect a person symptomatically or asymptomatically. The range of symptoms may vary from mild to very high complications which may even lead to death. The people with already declined immunity with pre-occurring comorbidities like diabetes, cardiac-related ailments, and kidney-related problems are highly vulnerable towards the extreme effects of the disease. Strict actions like frequent hand-wash, use of face-masks and face-covers, use of hand sanitizers, at the community level are important to defeat this disease. Preventions and precautions are necessary to protect vulnerable and comorbid people from this viral infection along with normal people. The ICMR and Ministry of Health of the Government of India have provided several recommendations against the spread of COVID-19. India being one of the fastest growing nations amongst the South Asian countries needs to invest and believe more into research and development field, home to some prominent institutions of the region those are performing with their expanded capabilities towards the good cause of the nation. As of now, when every day approximately 100,000 cases of the disease are being observed in India, it is a need of time that people and government put more faith in science and medicine.

Acknowledgements

The authors would like to thank Anshika Srivastava and Pushp Ranjan for their comments, insightful suggestions and careful reading of the manuscript.

Conflict of interest

The authors declare no conflict of interest.

Author details

Nikhil Srivastava[1] and Gyaneshwer Chaubey[2*]

1 Department of Zoology, Institute of Science, Banaras Hindu University, India

2 Cytogenetics Laboratory, Department of Zoology, Institute of Science, Banaras Hindu University, India

*Address all correspondence to: gyaneshwer.chaubey@bhu.ac.in and nikhilsr2@gmail.com

References

[1] Mahalmani VM, Mahendru D, Semwal A, et al. COVID-19 pandemic: A review based on current evidence. Indian J Pharmacol. 2020;52(2):117-129. doi:10.4103/ijp.IJP_310_20

[2] Kaur S, Sonali S. India fights COVID-19. Psychol Trauma. 2020;12(6):579-581. doi:10.1037/tra0000615

[3] https://www.mohfw.gov.in/, accessed on 10 Oct 2020

[4] Weidmann M, Zanotto PM, Weber F, et al. High-efficiency detection of severe acute respiratory syndrome virus genetic material. J Clinical Microbiol. 2004;42(6):2771-2773. doi: 10.1128/jcm.42.6.2771-2773.2004.

[5] Zheng J. SARS-CoV-2: an Emerging Coronavirus that Causes a Global Threat. Int J Biol Sci. 2020;16(10):1678-1685. Published 2020 Mar 15. doi:10.7150/ijbs.45053

[6] Payne S. Family Coronaviridae. Viruses. 2017;149-158. doi:10.1016/B978-0-12-803109-4.00017-9

[7] Phan MVT, Ngo Tri T, Hong Anh P, Baker S, Kellam P, Cotten M. Identification and characterization of Coronaviridae genomes from Vietnamese bats and rats based on conserved protein domains. Virus Evol. 2018;4(2):vey035. Published 2018 Dec 15. doi:10.1093/ve/vey035

[8] Kim D, Lee JY, Yang JS, Kim JW, Kim VN, Chang H. The Architecture of SARS-CoV-2 Transcriptome. Cell. 2020;181(4):914-921.e10. doi:10.1016/j.cell.2020.04.011

[9] Abdi A, Jalilian M, Sarbarzeh PA, Vlaisavljevic Z. Diabetes and COVID-19: A systematic review on the current evidences. Diabetes Res Clin Pract. 2020;166:108347. doi:10.1016/j.diabres.2020.108347

[10] Huang S, Wang J, Liu F, et al. COVID-19 patients with hypertension have more severe disease: a multicenter retrospective observational study. Hypertens Res. 2020;43(8):824-831. doi:10.1038/s41440-020-0485-2

[11] Godri Pollitt, K.J., Peccia, J., Ko, A.I. et al. COVID-19 vulnerability: the potential impact of genetic susceptibility and airborne transmission. Hum Genomics 14, 17 (2020). doi:10.1186/s40246-020-00267-3

[12] Liu M, Wang T, Zhou Y, Zhao Y, Zhang Y, Li J. Potential Role of ACE2 in Coronavirus Disease 2019 (COVID-19) Prevention and Management. J Transl Int Med. 2020;8(1):9-19. doi:10.2478/jtim-2020-0003

[13] Asselta R, Paraboschi EM, Mantovani A, Duga S. ACE2 and TMPRSS2 variants and expression as candidates to sex and country differences in COVID-19 severity in Italy. Aging (Albany NY). 2020;12(11):10087-10098. doi:10.18632/aging.103415

[14] Cao Y, Li L, Feng Z, et al. Comparative genetic analysis of the novel coronavirus (2019-nCoV/SARS-CoV-2) receptor ACE2 in different populations. Cell Discov. 2020;6:11. Published 2020 Feb 24. doi:10.1038/s41421-020-0147-1

[15] Srivastava A, Bandopadhyay A, Das D, et al. Genetic Association of ACE2 rs2285666 Polymorphism With COVID-19 Spatial Distribution in India. Front Genet. 2020;11:564741. Published 2020 Sep 25. doi:10.3389/fgene.2020.564741

[16] Srivastava A, Pandey RK, Singh PP, et al. Most frequent South Asian haplotypes of ACE2 share identity by descent with East Eurasian populations.

PLoS One. 2020;15(9):e0238255. Published 2020 Sep 16. doi:10.1371/journal.pone.0238255

[17] Wu YH, Li JY, Wang C, Zhang LM, Qiao H. The ACE2 G8790A Polymorphism: Involvement in Type 2 Diabetes Mellitus Combined with Cerebral Stroke. J Clin Lab Anal. 2017;31(2):e22033. doi:10.1002/jcla.22033

[18] Reich HN, Oudit GY, Penninger JM, Scholey JW, Herzenberg AM. Decreased glomerular and tubular expression of ACE2 in patients with type 2 diabetes and kidney disease. Kidney Int. 2008;74(12):1610-1616. doi:10.1038/ki.2008.497

[19] Verdecchia P, Cavallini C, Spanevello A, Angeli F. The pivotal link between ACE2 deficiency and SARS-CoV-2 infection. Eur J Intern Med. 2020;76:14-20. doi:10.1016/j.ejim.2020.04.037

[20] Tikellis C, Thomas MC. Angiotensin-Converting Enzyme 2 (ACE2) Is a Key Modulator of the Renin Angiotensin System in Health and Disease. Int J Pept. 2012;2012:256294. doi:10.1155/2012/256294

[21] McLachlan C.S. The angiotensin-converting enzyme 2 (ACE2) receptor in the prevention and treatment of COVID-19 are distinctly different paradigms. Clin. Hypertens. 2020;26:14.

[22] Vaduganathan M, Vardeny O, Michel T, McMurray JJV, Pfeffer MA, Solomon SD. Renin-Angiotensin-Aldosterone System Inhibitors in Patients with Covid-19. N Engl J Med. 2020;382(17):1653-1659. doi:10.1056/NEJMsr2005760

[23] Sharma S, Singh I, et al. ACE2 Homo-dimerization, Human Genomic variants and Interaction of Host Proteins Explain High Population Specific Differences in Outcomes of COVID19. bioRxiv 2020.04.24.050534; doi: https://doi.org/10.1101/2020.04.24.050534

[24] Kim D, Lee JY, Yang JS, Kim JW, Kim VN, Chang H. The Architecture of SARS-CoV-2 Transcriptome. Cell. 2020;181(4):914-921.e10. doi:10.1016/j.cell.2020.04.011

[25] Singh KK, Chaubey G, Chen JY, Suravajhala P. Decoding SARS-CoV-2 hijacking of host mitochondria in COVID-19 pathogenesis. Am J Physiol Cell Physiol. 2020;319(2):C258-C267. doi:10.1152/ajpcell.00224.2020

[26] Tang X, Wu C, Li X, et al. On the origin and continuing evolution of SARS-CoV-2. Natl Sci Rev. 2020;nwaa036. Published 2020 Mar 3. doi:10.1093/nsr/nwaa036

[27] Singhal T. A Review of Coronavirus Disease-2019 (COVID-19). Indian J Pediatr. 2020;87(4):281-286. doi:10.1007/s12098-020-03263-6

[28] Husain, A., & Byrareddy, S. N. (2020). Rapamycin as a potential repurpose drug candidate for the treatment of COVID-19. Chemico-Biological Interactions, 331. https://doi.org/10.1016/j.cbi.2020.109282

[29] Omarjee L, Janin A, Perrot F, Laviolle B, Meilhac O, Mahe G. Targeting T-cell senescence and cytokine storm with rapamycin to prevent severe progression in COVID-19. Clin Immunol. 2020;216:108464. doi:10.1016/j.clim.2020.108464

[30] Zheng Y, Li R, Liu S. Immunoregulation with mTOR inhibitors to prevent COVID-19 severity: A novel intervention strategy beyond vaccines and specific antiviral medicines. J Med Virol. 2020;92(9):1495-1500. doi:10.1002/jmv.26009

[31] Pathak DSK, Salunke DAA, Thivari DP, et al. No benefit of

hydroxychloroquine in COVID-19: Results of Systematic Review and Meta-Analysis of Randomized Controlled Trials". Diabetes Metab Syndr. 2020;14(6):1673-1680. doi:10.1016/j.dsx.2020.08.033

[32] Rosenke K, Jarvis MA, Feldmann F, et al. Hydroxychloroquine Proves Ineffective in Hamsters and Macaques Infected with SARS-CoV-2. Preprint. bioRxiv. 2020;2020.06.10.145144. Published 2020 Jun 11. doi:10.1101/2020.06.10.145144

[33] Ibáñez S, Martínez O, Valenzuela F, Silva F, Valenzuela O. Hydroxychloroquine and chloroquine in COVID-19: should they be used as standard therapy?. Clin Rheumatol. 2020;39(8):2461-2465. doi:10.1007/s10067-020-05202-4

Section 7

Nano-Biotechnology

Chapter 26

Sensor Surface Design with NanoMaterials: A New Platform in the Diagnosis of COVID-19

Eliete A. Alvin, Anna V.B. e Borges, Rhéltheer de P. Martins, Marcela R. Lemes, Rafaela M. Barbosa, Carlo J.F. de Oliveira, Diógenes Meneses, Bruno G. Lucca, Noelio O. Dantas, Virmondes R. Junior, Renata P.A. Balvedi, Fabiane C. de Abreu, Marcos V. da Silva and Anielle C.A. Silva

Abstract

Mass testing for COVID-19 is essential to defining patient management strategies, choosing the best clinical management, and dimensioning strategies for controlling viral dissemination and immunization strategies. Thus, it is of utmost importance to search for devices that allow a quick and reliable diagnosis of low cost that can be transposed from the bench to the bedside, such as biosensors. These devices can help choose the correct clinical management to minimize factors that lead to infected patients developing more severe diseases. The use of nanomaterials to modify biosensors' surfaces to increase these devices' sensitivity and their biofunctionality enables high-quality nanotechnological platforms. In addition to the diagnostic benefits, nanotechnological platforms that facilitate the monitoring of anti-SARS-CoV-2 antibodies may be the key to determining loss of protective immune response after an episode of COVID-19, which leads to a possible chance of reinfection, as well as how they can be used to assess and monitor the success of immunization strategies, which are beginning to be administered on a large scale and that the extent and duration of their protection will need to be determined. Therefore, in this chapter, we will cover nanomaterials' use and their functionalities in the surface design of sensors, thus generating nanotechnological platforms in the various facets of the diagnosis of COVID-19.

Keywords: COVID-19, SARS-CoV-2, nanotechnological platforms, nanomaterials, biosensors, diagnosis, sensor surface design

1. Introduction

SARS-CoV-2 is a virus in the coronavirus family, discovered in December 2019 in Wuhan, China, and the cause of COVID-19 [1]. Coronaviruses (CoV) are RNA viruses and can cause anything from the common cold to more serious diseases with neurological, gastrointestinal, and pulmonary involvement [2]. They are zoonotic viruses;

that is, they can be transmitted between animals and people due to their ability to recombine their viral proteins between coronaviruses of different hosts [3].

COVID-19 was defined as Pandemic on March 11, 2020 (1), and by February 1, 2021, there are already 103,221,369 individuals infected worldwide, and the number of global deaths already exceeds 2,232,563 [4]. Before SARS-CoV-2, two other CoVs causing a pandemic disease were identified: the first was SARS-CoV in 2002, originating in Foshan (China), which caused Severe Acute Respiratory Syndrome (SARS); the second was MERS-CoV, which originated in the Arabian Peninsula in 2012, causing the Middle East Respiratory Syndrome (MERS) [5].

A significant bottleneck in COVID-19 is mass diagnosis. The real-time reverse-transcription polymerase chain reaction (RT-PCR) is the "gold standard" method for demonstrating the presence of SARS-CoV-2. This diagnosis is reliable; however, most countries have suffered from a lack of supplies and equipment and its high cost. IgM and IgG antibodies can be detected in the serum of patients with COVID-19, where their monitoring can indicate recent or late infection and the duration of the post-infection protective immune response.

The development of easy-to-use alternative platforms is encouraged with specific attention paid to sensitivity and simplicity to specifically detect targets at a very low concentration, in about minutes, enabling portable on-site screening upon further optimizations of the detection limit. However, the accuracy of these techniques depends on several factors; variations in these factors might significantly lower the sensitivity of detection.

Nanomaterials can be applied in several types of sensors due to their physical and chemical properties, making them possible to detect by colorimetric, fluorescence, magnetism, surface plasmon resonance, and electrochemical [6–10]. In electrochemical sensing, the conductive nanomaterials are interesting for application due to their well-known ability to improve the catalytic activity, the electron transfer speed, and the conductivity of the sensors. Furthermore, the superficial area and amplify the analytical signal can be increased by deposition of nanomaterials over electronic surfaces, enhancing the sensitivity regarding target analytes' detection. Therefore, the group has been working with several nanomaterials to develop sensors.

Therefore, in this book chapter, we describe case reports and proof-of-concept for a simple, label-free electrochemical sensor for the fast and direct detection of SARS-CoV-2 through the detection of the specific probe. Early and widespread testing has proven to reduce mortality rates and improve contact tracing. However, the value of testing is directly linked to the availability and accuracy of diagnostic tests as concerns grow. Additionally, we have demonstrated in this work the possibility of a biorecognition element between the target concentration and the viral load exploring different electrode materials and redox markers allows for improved sensor properties with higher effectiveness than the commercially available assay or traditional diagnostic methods.

2. Diagnosis of COVID-19: the old and the gold

Coronaviruses infect human cells mainly by binding proteins from viral spikes (spike proteins) to molecules of the angiotensin-converting enzyme 2 (ACE2), [11] widely expressed in human organs and tissues, such as nasal, bronchial epithelial cells, and pneumocytes. After entering the cell, viral replication occurs and the host cell's subsequent death, whether epithelial, endothelial, or immune cells [12].

Due to the increase in viral replication, the epithelial-endothelial barrier's integrity is compromised, accentuating the inflammatory response, causing edema and inflammatory infiltrates. Furthermore, it compromises coagulation pathways, increasing fibrin degradation products and alterations in leukocytes and red blood cells. Together with the inflammatory infiltrate, the resulting edema contributes to the ground-glass opacities seen in imaging studies and too low oxygenation [13].

Symptoms and clinical evolution depend on the triad: virus strain, host immunity, and pre-existing conditions, known as comorbidities, such as hypertension, obesity, diabetes, cardiovascular disease, chronic lung disease, chronic kidney disease, and malignancies [14]. Symptoms range from the most common in flu-like conditions, such as fever, cough, and shortness of breath, nausea, diarrhea, loss of smell and taste, and more severe symptoms such as pneumonia leukopenia, kidney failure, myocarditis, meningitis, and thromboembolic events [15].

The immune response against COVID-19 has been extensively investigated and is directly related to clinical evolution. The presence of lymphopenia and increased production of chemokines and proinflammatory cytokines have been demonstrated in patients with COVID-19, especially in the most severe cases, which can worsen tissue damage [16]. Serum levels of chemokines (IL-8) and proinflammatory cytokines (TNF-α, IL-1, IL-6, IFN-γ, IP-10, and MCP-1) are found in greater quantities patients with COVID- 19 severe when compared with individuals with mild disease. This fact indicates that the cytokine storm is associated with the severity of the disease and adverse outcomes, suggesting a possible role of hyperinflammatory responses in the pathogenesis of COVID-19 [16, 17].

Studies on the humoral immune response demonstrate that antibodies, such as IgA, IgM, and IgG against SARS-CoV-2, appear on the first day after the onset of symptoms [18, 19]. IgM levels appear on days 0 to 7, increasing on days 8 to 14 and reaching a plateau, while IgA levels increased from days 0 to 14, whereas IgG levels were detected on days 0 to 7, increased on days 8 to 14, continued to increase until the 15th to the 21st and reached a plateau on the 21st [18]. This kinetics of antibody levels indicates a rapid and almost simultaneous response of these three isotypes during the first weeks of infection by SARS-CoV-2, IgA and IgG remain with higher titers for a longer time when compared to IgM [20, 21].

The amount of antibodies in samples from patients with COVID-19 is dependent on the number of viral RNA present: the lower the viral load, the lower the level of antibodies present, and the severity of clinical evolution [19–21]. Initial data indicate a lower concentration of anti-SARS-CoV-2 antibodies in asymptomatic patients, but more quickly, while in mild symptomatic ones, there is a slower but more continuous production. Serious patients have high levels of antibodies, mainly IgA and IgG. However, there are still gaps about whether specific humoral and cellular immune memory persist and for how long [20]. Despite these limitations in understanding the long-term humoral immune response, the determination of IgA, IgM, and IgG antibodies are widely used in laboratory tests for the detection of COVID-19. Early diagnosis also allows the infected patient to have faster access to medical care and increases their chances of a better prognosis. It will enable the initiation of treatment when the viral load is in low concentrations.

Antibody determination is also important to monitor patients who have been vaccinated since immunization stimulates the immune system's production without having to be infected [22]. Results about vaccines against COVID-19 showed that vaccinated patients increased the production of specific antibodies and their affinity to levels similar to those observed in patients who recovered from COVID-19 [23–25]. Data show that a standardized quantification/determination of antibody levels may be sufficient to monitor vaccinated patients and estimate the quality and duration of this protection [24].

To date, quantitative real-time reverse-transcription polymerase chain reaction (RT-PCR), qRT-qPCR assay is the gold standard for the early detection of virus

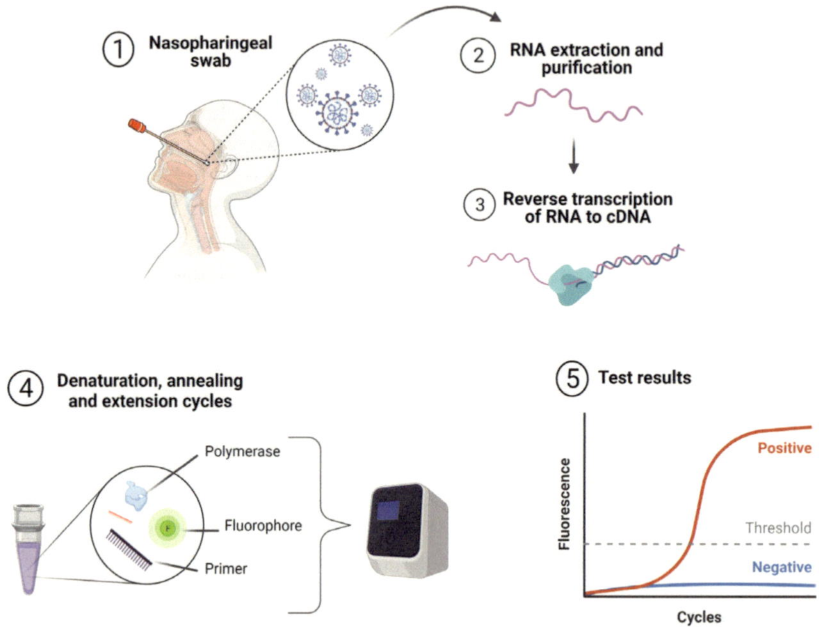

Figure 1.
Major steps of qRT-PCR as a diagnostic tool at COVID-19 (1) A patient suspected of COVID-19 undergoes collection of cells infected with SARS-CoV-2 through a nasopharyngeal swab. (2–3) Viral RNA is extracted and purified. The enzyme reverse transcriptase converts RNA into cDNA.

(major steps presented in **Figure 1**), but the CRISPR–Cas12-based lateral flow, Immunochromatographic, ELISA, loop-mediated isothermal amplification (LAMP) and other techniques has been developed and applied to screening or to confirm positive COVID-19 patients allowing prompt clinical and quarantine decisions this infection (**Table 1**).

To minimize the cost and logistical problems of sample collection and diagnostics, rapid diagnostic systems based on classical methodological approaches, such as immunochromatography, were quickly implemented in the detection of SARS-CoV-2 antigens or antibodies produced against it. However, the accuracy of these techniques depends on several factors. The bioavailability of the researched molecule, as viral genetic material, viral antigens, and various subclasses of antibodies, the stability of these biomolecules to the procedures of sample collection and transport to the diagnostic platforms, the possibility of storage for later evaluation are significant bottlenecks that have impaired mass testing, especially in developing countries and variations in these factors might significantly lower the sensitivity of detection. The degree of reliability is uncertain in many of them, and implementing a faster and accurate diagnosis system is essential to monitor the disease and define policies to control viral spread.

Biosensors are one of the most popular types of point-of-care devices in various diagnostics areas, which offer several advantages such as the low cost, the capability of miniaturization, and high sensitivity and selectivity. The transposition of the molecular and immunological diagnosis to miniaturization platforms like point-of-care systems implies a drastic reduction in the amount of sample needed, increases specificity, reliable measurements in real-time, and portability. The development of easy-to-use alternative platforms is encouraged with specific attention paid to sensitivity and simplicity to detect targets at a very low concentration in about minutes, enabling portable on-site screening upon further optimizing the detection limit.

Detection type	Sensitivity %	Specificity %	LOD	Biom. of the probe	Biom. target	Methodology	Detection time (m)	Nanomaterials	Database	References
Frosted glass opacity	86–98	25	—	—	—	Computed tomography	5–30	—	P/S/WS	[26, 27]
RT- PCR	90–100	100	0.15–100 copies/μL	Primers	Viral RNA	Real-time Transcript to Reverse	240–360	—	P/S/WS	[28, 29]
RT-dPCR	90	100	2 copies/reaction	Primers	Viral RNA	Real - time Transcripta to Reverse Digital PCR	—	—	P/S/WS	[30]
RT-LAMP	90–100	Low	100 copies/μL	Primers	Viral RNA	Isothermal amplification of the Transcript reversed	30–40	—	P/S/WS	[29, 31, 32]
CRISPR-cas12	95–100	100	10–100 copies/μL	gRNA	Viral RNA	gRNA binds to the target segment making precise cutting	45–75	—	P/S/WS	[33]
RT-RPA	98	100	7.659 copies/μL	Primers	Viral RNA	Real-time Transcript to Reverse Recombinase Polymerase Amplification	< 20	—	P/S	[34]
ELISA	86–100 *	89–100	—	Anti-antibody IgM	IgM	Indirect	60–300	—	P/S/WS	[31]
ELISA	86–100 *	89–100	—	Anti-antibody IgG	IgG	Indirect	60–300	—	P/S	[35]
ELISA	*	100	—	Antibody	Ag	Sandwich	60–300	—	P/S/WS	[31]
Lateral flow immunoassay	60–80	85–100	—	Ag	IgM	Immunoassay/Quick Test	2–20	—	P/S/WS	[31]

Detection type	Sensitivity %	Specificity %	LOD	Biom. of the probe	Biom. target	Methodology	Detection time (m)	Nanomaterials	Database	References
Lateral flow immunoassay	60–80	85–100	—	Ag	IgG	Immunoassay/Quick Test	2–20	—	P/S/WS	[31]
Lateral flow immunoassay	91.2 Swab 60.1 Sample solution	100	—	Antibody	Ag	Immunoassay/Quick Test	15–30	—	P/S/WS	[31, 36]
Chimiolumi nescence	82–97	75–87	—	Ag	IgM	Immunoassay/ Chemiluminescence	30–60	Magnetic microsphere	P/S/WS	[37, 38]
Chimiolumi nescence	82–97	75–87	—	Ag	IgG	Immunoassay/ Chemiluminescence	30–60	Magnetic microspheres	P/S/WS	[38, 39]

LOD: limit of detection, RPA: Recombinase Polymerase Amplification, Database: Pubmed (P), Scopus (S), and Web of Science (WS).
**Variable sensitivity according to kit and sample collection day.*

Table 1.
Comparison of methodologies applied to the diagnosis of (SARS)-CoV-2.

An overview of some methodologies applied to the diagnosis of (SARS)-CoV-2 is presented in **Table 1**. The ELISA-based test was used to validate the antibody–antigen interaction, or RT-PCR was used to validate the primer, particularly the complexity of the assays during inventory shortages, while cyclic voltammetry, electrochemical impedance spectroscopy, differential pulse voltammetry was used to characterize the electrode functionalization.

Multi sensors, lateral flow tests, mobile biosensors, and wearable biosensors are critical parts for precision medicine in COVID-19. Russell, S.M. et al., defined these biosensors' ideal characteristics using some prototypes from recent literature as examples [40]. Multi sensors, lateral flow tests, mobile biosensors, and wearable biosensors are crucial parts for precision medicine in COVID-19. We propose the ideal characteristics of these biosensors using some prototypes from recent literature as examples. Multi sensors, lateral flow tests, mobile biosensors, and wearable biosensors are crucial parts for precision medicine in COVID-19.

In his work, Fukumoto, T. et al. 2020 has developed a fast, easy to use, and inexpensive diagnostic method that is needed to help control the current outbreak of the new coronavirus based on microfluidic microdevices. A new detection kit - the 2019 Novel Coronavirus Detection Kit (nCoV-DK) - cuts detection time in half, eliminating RNA extraction and purification steps. The nCoV-DK test effectively detects SARS-CoV-2 in all types of samples, including saliva, while reducing the time required for detection and risk of human error [41].

Laghrib, F. et al., showed the leading current trends and strategies in diagnosing n-SARS-CoV-2 based on emerging and traditional assessment technologies for continuous innovation. Addressing recent biosensors trends to build a fast, reliable, more sensitive, accessible, friendly system with easily adaptable n-SARS-CoV-2 detection and monitoring technology [42]. Overall, we address and identify evidence from research that supports biosensors' use based on the premise that screening people for n-SARS-CoV-2 is the best way to stem its spread. The detection and notification of infectious pathogens in a fast, sensitive, and specific way is essential for managing the patient and surveillance of outbreaks. With their ability to diagnose in real-time with the high specificity of a low concentration sample, biosensors are much more reliable than the rapid test for coronavirus detection. The use of nano biosensors has been considered the most promising approach for detecting new n-SARSCoV-2 coronavirus disease. Meanwhile, the current work has also tried to improve biosensors' detection sensitivity, simplicity, and performance.

Hui, X. et al. 2020, showed in his work, G quadruplex-based Biosensor: A potential tool for SARS-CoV-2 detection to discover additional advantageous attributes of G-quadruplex as potential to be used in new biosensors, such as ligand binding enhanced and unique folding properties [43]. The newly developed G-quadruplex biosensors include electrochemical and optical biosensors that have shown better performance with potential applications with a wide detection range and a broad spectrum of pathogens SARS-CoV-2, the causative agent of COVID-19 disease. G-quadruplex is a non-canonical nucleic acid structure formed by the folding of guanine-rich DNA or RNA.

3. Platform with nanomaterials in the diagnosis of COVID-19: a brave new world

Biosensors are analytical devices that incorporate a biological recognition element capable of detecting the presence, activity, or concentration of the sample under analysis connected to a transducer. This biological element can be a microorganism, an antibody, oligonucleotides, lectins, biomolecule enzymes that can interact with the target substrate. About the transducer, it can be an electrode, fiber optic, or oscillating quartz [42, 44]. Thus, biosensors are one of the most popular types of point-of-care devices in various areas of diagnostics, which offer several advantages such as low cost, the capability of miniaturization, and high sensitivity and selectivity.

Immunosensors are analytical devices of the biosensor class, which detect and transmit information regarding biochemical changes involving integrating a biological element with an electronic interface [45, 46]. This integration can convert a biological signal into an electrical response that is proportional to the concentration of the analyte. Thus, these biosensors can recognize a specific antibody or antigen by forming an antigen–antibody immunocomplex. The recognition event is detected and converted, through a transducer, to a measurable signal (such as electrical current, for example). The primary transducers used in immunosensors are electrochemical, optical, and piezoelectric. Therefore, the incorporation of specific nanomaterial can be intensified by improving the biosensor's sensitivity and versatility.

Genosensors can also be used, a specific type of biosensor based on nucleic acid chemistry phenomena, such as the hybridization process [47]. Nucleic acids have been widely used in the development of biosensors for drug detection, identification of pathogenic microorganisms and other biological substances, and the diagnosis of diseases. The sensory technique through hybridization involves the immobilization of an oligonucleotide probe on the surface of a transducer and subsequent sensor exposure to a sample containing the complementary sequence (target oligonucleotide) with consequent hybridization. Complementary DNA (cDNA) is a DNA synthesized from a messenger RNA molecule in a reaction catalyzed by the enzyme reverse transcriptase. Thus, the incorporation of nanomaterials on the biosensor's surface ensures the enhancement of the electrochemical response.

Our group has been demonstrating through publications and patents expertise in the development of nanomaterials with specific properties, such as increased sensitivity of some devices, biocompatibility, and low genotoxicity, essential properties in developing nanotechnological platforms [48–53]. Toxicity is an important parameter in nanomaterials, but depending on synthesis methodologies it is possible to decrease toxicity. For example, Silva et al. demonstrated some toxicities of nanomaterials, some influenced by the crystalline phase, composition or type of material [54–61]. In relation to quantum dots, synthesis methodologies were developed, making it possible to increase cellular viability and specificity aiming at several applicability as biological probes [52, 53, 62–68].

The development of artificial intelligence software enables more accurate detection and quantification and low-cost analytical platforms [69, 70]. These nanotechnological platform [71] s can be used in large-scale production, with low cost and low consumption of samples and reagents [6, 72].

High-quality, low-cost nanotechnological platforms based on the detection of anti-SARS-CoV-2 antibodies may be the key to defining groups already exposed to the disease, even if asymptomatic, that have a potentially protective immune response, a crucial factor for delimitation priority immunization groups. Besides, we can determine the loss of protective immune response after an episode of COVID-19, which leads to a possible chance of reinfection. Some advantages are the amount of sample of interest, in the order of μL, simultaneous analysis of several analytes in the same device and miniaturization, being portable, light, and easy to use the equipment. Also, nanotechnological platforms can be used to assess and monitor the success of immunization strategies, which should soon begin to be administered on a large scale, and the extent and duration of their protection will need to be determined.

Several diagnostic methods have been reported, aiming at biomedical applications, especially in the diagnosis of covid-19, to detect the coronavirus in clinical, research, and public health laboratories. Based on biosensors for SARS-CoV-2, diagnostic methods presented have analytical performance and response times ranging from a few minutes to several hours, which make them promise for practical use in health care points, showing as a strong ally for control of endemics and pandemics.

An overview of current efforts to improve point-of-care diagnostic systems based on biosensors using different nanomaterials at COVID-19 is presented in **Table 2**.

Currently, diverse electrochemical biosensors have been lately developed for the detection of the SARS-CoV-2 using modified electrodes with metallic nanoparticle or nano-islands or nanostars, carbon nanofiber (CNF), using inorganic quantum dots, zinc oxide nanowires (ZnO NWs) or nanorods, bimetallic nanoparticles, Graphene Oxide (GO) nanosheet and other modifications show in **Table 2**. These nanomaterials showed excellent applications in biosensors because of their ease of functionalization, large surface area, stability, on the stable immobilization of probe molecules, the blocking reagent to minimize nonspecific binding, high electronic conductivity (accelerate the electron transfer), high carrier/charge mobility, and strong adsorption capability that increase the sensitivity of electrochemical platform due to their excellent unmatched properties followed by enhancement in the electrochemical response toward the selective detection of SARS-CoV-2.

Vadlamani, B S. et al., the synthesis of a TiO_2 functionalized with cobalt but susceptible electrochemical sensor based on nanotubes (Co-TNTs) for rapid detection of SARS-CoV-2 using peak detection (binding domain receptor (RBD)) present on the virus surface [83]. A simple, low-cost, one-step electrochemical anodization route was used to synthesize TNTs, followed by an incipient wetting method for cobalt functionalization of the TNT platform, which was connected to a potentiostat for data collection. This sensor specifically detected the S-RBD protein from SARS-CoV-2, even at very low concentrations (range 14 to 1400 nM (nanomolar)). Besides, our sensor showed a linear response in the detection of viral protein in the concentration range. Thus, our Co-TNT sensor is highly effective in detecting the SARS-CoV-2 S-RBD protein in approximately 30s.

Cuy and Zhou, 2019, showed in their review work that timely detection and diagnosis are urgently needed to guide epidemiological measures, infection control, antiviral treatment, and vaccine research [86]. In this review, biomarkers/indicators for diagnosis of coronavirus 2019 disease or detection of severe acute respiratory syndrome coronavirus 2 in the environment are summarized and discussed. However, antibody detection methods can be combined with real-time quantitative polymerase reverse transcriptase chain reaction to improve diagnostic sensitivity and specificity and boost vaccine research significantly. The deep throat saliva and induced sputum are desired for the RT-qPCR test or other early detection technologies. The ultra-sensitive and specific laboratory diagnostic method and portable devices are essential to control the rapidly evolving COVID-19 pandemic associated with SARS-CoV-2. Currently, computed tomography, RT-qPCR, and LFICS based on the colloid Au NPs (colloidal gold method) have been developed.

Based on the table results, we can verify that the biosensors that showed the best sensitivities are using carbon-based materials due to their conductive properties, metallic oxides (ZnO and TiO2) with supercapacitor properties, and nanocomposites (containing the capacitive and metallic systems).

In nanomaterials, the effects of size, morphology, and chemical structures have a strong influence on the optical, electrical, and magnetic properties. Thus, the tuning of these parameters allows maintaining the same material and intensifying the biosensors' responses. Another critical parameter is the synergism between

Detection type	Sensitivity %	Specificity %	LOD	RSD %	Biom. of probe	Biom. target	Methodology	Detection time (m)	Nanomaterials	Database	References
Electrochemical biosensor	—	—	—	—	cRNA	Viral RNA	Genosensors	—	—	P/S	[73]
Electrochemical biosensor	—	—	1 fg/mL	—	Antibodies with 1-pyrenobutyric acid N-hydroxysuccin-imide	Ag. Protein S	Field effect transistor FET	< 4	Grafeno leaves	P/S/WS	[74]
Electrochemical biosensor	—	—	—	—	Ag. Protein S	Antibody	Impedance Spectroscopy	—	Polyethylene terephthalate	P/S/WS	[75]
Electrochemical biosensor	Lowest PCR	—	20 ng/mL	—	Antibody Anti- Protein S	Ag. Protein S	Impedance Spectroscopy/ Cyclic voltammetry/ Square wave voltammetry	45	Graphene layer/1-Pyrene butyric acid N-hydroxysuccin-imide ester linker (PBASE)	P/S/WS	[76]
Electrochemical biosensor	100	90	1 ng/mL	4.2 for IgG and 3.3 for IgM	Ag. Protein S	IgM/IgG Antibodies	Paper platform	30	—	P/S	[77]
Ultra- sensitive electrochemical biosensor	High	High	3 aM	—	cDNA	Viral RNA	Differential pulse voltammetry/ Smartphone detection	181	Modified SPCE nanocomposite (Au @ SCX8-TB-RGO-AP-LPTarget/HT/CP/Au @ Fe3O4)	P/S/WS	[78]
Electrochemical biosensor Immunosensor	High	High	0.8 pg/mL	—	Ag. Protein N	Ag. Protein N	Square wave voltammetry	20	Carbon nanofiber	P/S	[79]

Detection type	Sensitivity %	Specificity %	LOD	RSD %	Biom. of probe	Biom. target	Methodology	Detection time (m)	Nanomaterials	Database	References
Electrochemical biosensor	High	High	6.5 pfu/mL	—	Antibody Anti-Protein S and N	Ag. Protein S and N in saliva	Immunosensor/ Differential pulse voltammetry	30	Magnetic nanoparticle/Black carbon	P/S/WS	[80]
Electrochemical biosensor	95	High	$1.68x10^{22}$ mg/mL	—	Antibody Anti-Protein S	Ag. Protein S	Differential pulse voltammetry	1	Gold nanoparticle/ Graphene oxide	P/S/WS	[81]
Electrochemical biosensor	High	High	—	—	Ag. Protein S	IgM/IgG Antibodies	Impedance Spectroscopy	30	Zinc oxide nanowires	P	[82]
Electrochemical biosensor	—	—	0.7 nM	—	Titanium dioxide/ Cobalt nanotube	Protein S-RBD	Amperometry	> 1	Titanium dioxide/ Cobalt nanotube	P/S/WS	[83]
Electrochemical biosensor	100	100	6.9 copies/µL	—	cDNA	Ag. Protein N	Genosensors/ Cyclic voltammetry	5	Graphene/Gold nanoparticle	P/WS	[84]
Multiplexed electrochemical platform	High	High	—	Average of 7.07	Protein S/Anti-IgM and IgG antibodies	IgM/IgG Antibodies Ag. Protein N	Immunossensor/ Differential pulse voltammetry/ Impedance Spectroscopy	> 1	Graphene	P/WS	[85]

LOD: Limit of Detection; RDS: Relative Squared Difference.
Database: Pubmed (P), Scopus (S) and Web of Science (WS).

Table 2.
Comparison of electrochemical biosensors for the detection of (SARS)-CoV-2.

nanomaterials, several biosensors using more than one type of nanomaterials to further improve sensitivity. Thus, unfortunately, this systematic study of the literature in biosensors does not exist, being difficult to compare the sensitivity properties using different materials and nanocomposites.

4. Conclusion

Therefore, this chapter showed use of systems in diagnosis COVID-19 and how the nanomaterials may enable an improvement in sensitivity when being incorporated in the surface design of sensors, thus generating nanotechnological platforms. The functional improvement of biosensors using nanomaterials has undoubted benefits, both from the point of view of biological samples, ease of technical execution, better distribution and application logistics and better cost–benefit, being able to direct a whole new generation of rapid diagnoses easily transposable to combat other human diseases. These nanotechnological platforms could be the revolution for the mass diagnosis of COVID-19, without implying an increase in investments since it is a low-cost diagnostic proposal. In this way, they can be immediately translated into clinical practice and used in all parts of the health chain used to combat COVID-19, given its simplicity of use, biosafety, and low cost. The use of nanotechnology to modify diagnostic platforms has a special impact as they generate patents, strengthen technology, and arouse worldwide interest for their technological robustness, which may impact the attraction of resources to countries through the export of these or other forms of sharing that be advantageous.

Acknowledgements

This work was supported by grants of CNPq, CAPES, FAPEAL, and FAPEMIG.

Conflict of interest

The authors declare no conflict of interest.

Author details

Eliete A. Alvin[1,2,3], Anna V.B. e Borges[4], Rhéltheer de P. Martins[5], Marcela R. Lemes[4], Rafaela M. Barbosa[4], Carlo J.F. de Oliveira[4], Diógenes Meneses[3], Bruno G. Lucca[6], Noelio O. Dantas[1], Virmondes R. Junior[4], Renata P.A. Balvedi[5], Fabiane C. de Abreu[3], Marcos V. da Silva[4] and Anielle C.A. Silva[1,2*]

1 Laboratory of New Nanostructured and Functional Materials, Physics Institute, Federal University of Alagoas, Maceió, AL, Brazil

2 Programa de Pós-Graduação da Rede Nordeste de Biotecnologia (RENORBIO), Federal University of Alagoas, Maceió, AL, Brazil

3 LEMAN, Institute of Chemistry and Biotechnology, Federal University of Alagoas, Maceió, AL, Brazil

4 Department of Microbiology, Immunology and Parasitology, Institute of Bilogical and Natural Sciences, Federal University of Triângulo Mineiro, Uberaba, MG, Brazil

5 Federal University of Triângulo Mineiro, Iturama, MG, Brazil

6 Institute of Chemistry, Federal University of Mato Grosso do Sul, Campo Grande, MS, Brazil

*Address all correspondence to: acalmeida@fis.ufal.br

References

[1] Organization, W.H. Novel Coronavirus (2019-nCoV) Situation Report – 1 2020.

[2] Benvenuto, D.; Giovanetti, M.; Ciccozzi, A.; Spoto, S.; Angeletti, S.; Ciccozzi, M. The 2019-new coronavirus epidemic: Evidence for virus evolution. J. Med. Virol. **2020**, *92*, 455-459, doi:10.1002/jmv.25688.

[3] Ji, W.; Wang, W.; Zhao, X.; Zai, J.; Li, X. Cross-species transmission of the newly identified coronavirus 2019-nCoV. J. Med. Virol. **2020**, *92*, 433-440, doi:10.1002/jmv.25682.

[4] Hopkings, J. COVID-19 dashboard by the Center for Systems Science and Engineering (CSSE) at Johns Hopkins University (JHU) 2020.

[5] Cui, J.; Li, F.; Shi, Z.L. Origin and evolution of pathogenic coronaviruses. Nat. Rev. Microbiol. 2019, *17*, 181-192.

[6] de França, C.C.L.; Meneses, D.; Silva, A.C.A.; Dantas, N.O.; de Abreu, F.C.; Petroni, J.M.; Lucca, B.G. Development of novel paper-based electrochemical device modified with CdSe/CdS magic-sized quantum dots and application for the sensing of dopamine. *Electrochim. Acta* **2021**, *367*, doi:10.1016/j.electacta.2020.137486.

[7] da Silva, M.P.G.; Candido, A.C.L.; de Araújo-Júnior, J.X.; Silva, A.C.A.; Dantas, N.O.; de Aquino, T.M.; de Abreu, F.C. Evaluation of the interaction of a guanylhydrazone derivative with cobalt ferrite nanoparticles and PAMAM electrochemical and UV/visible spectroscopic techniques. J. Solid State Electrochem. **2020**, *25*, 743-752, doi:10.1007/s10008-020-04848-z.

[8] de Lima França, C.C.; da Silva Terto, E.G.; Dias-Vermelho, M. V.; Silva, A.C.A.; Dantas, N.O.; de Abreu, F.C. The electrochemical behavior of core-shell CdSe/CdS magic-sized quantum dots linked to cyclodextrin for studies of the encapsulation of bioactive compounds. J. Solid State Electrochem. **2016**, *20*, 2533-2540, doi:10.1007/s10008-016-3221-8.

[9] Martins, B.R.; Barbosa, Y.O.; Andrade, C.M.R.; Pereira, L.Q.; Simão, G.F.; de Oliveira, C.J.; Correia, D.; Oliveira, R.T.S.; da Silva, M. V.; Silva, A.C.A.; et al. Development of an Electrochemical Immunosensor for Specific Detection of Visceral Leishmaniasis Using Gold-Modified Screen-Printed Carbon Electrodes. Biosensors **2020**, *10*, 81, doi:10.3390/bios10080081.

[10] Petroni, J.M.; Lucca, B.G.; da Silva Júnior, L.C.; Barbosa Alves, D.C.; Souza Ferreira, V. Paper-based Electrochemical Devices Coupled to External Graphene-Cu Nanoparticles Modified Solid Electrode through Meniscus Configuration and their Use in Biological Analysis. Electroanalysis **2017**, *29*, 2628-2637, doi:10.1002/elan.201700398.

[11] Hoffmann, M.; Kleine-Weber, H.; Schroeder, S.; Krüger, N.; Herrler, T.; Erichsen, S.; Schiergens, T.S.; Herrler, G.; Wu, N.H.; Nitsche, A.; et al. SARS-CoV-2 Cell Entry Depends on ACE2 and TMPRSS2 and Is Blocked by a Clinically Proven Protease Inhibitor. *Cell* **2020**, *181*, 271-280.e8, doi:10.1016/j.cell.2020.02.052.

[12] Sungnak, W.; Huang, N.; Bécavin, C.; Berg, M.; Queen, R.; Litvinukova, M.; Talavera-López, C.; Maatz, H.; Reichart, D.; Sampaziotis, F.; et al. SARS-CoV-2 entry factors are highly expressed in nasal epithelial cells together with innate immune genes. Nat. Med. **2020**, *26*, 681-687, doi:10.1038/s41591-020-0868-6.

[13] Xu, Z.; Shi, L.; Wang, Y.; Zhang, J.; Huang, L.; Zhang, C.; Liu, S.; Zhao, P.; Liu, H.; Zhu, L.; et al. Pathological findings of COVID-19 associated with acute respiratory distress syndrome. Lancet Respir. Med. **2020**, *8*, 420-422, doi:10.1016/S2213-2600(20)30076-X.

[14] Yang, J.; Zheng, Y.; Gou, X.; Pu, K.; Chen, Z.; Guo, Q.; Ji, R.; Wang, H.; Wang, Y.; Zhou, Y. Prevalence of comorbidities and its effects in coronavirus disease 2019 patients: A systematic review and meta-analysis. Int. J. Infect. Dis. **2020**, *94*, 91-95, doi:10.1016/j.ijid.2020.03.017.

[15] Esakandari, H.; Nabi-Afjadi, M.; Fakkari-Afjadi, J.; Farahmandian, N.; Miresmaeili, S.M.; Bahreini, E. A comprehensive review of COVID-19 characteristics. Biol. Proced. Online 2020, *22*, 19.

[16] Qin, C.; Zhou, L.; Hu, Z.; Zhang, S.; Yang, S.; Tao, Y.; Xie, C.; Ma, K.; Shang, K.; Wang, W.; et al. Dysregulation of immune response in patients with coronavirus 2019 (COVID-19) in Wuhan, China. *Clin. Infect. Dis.* **2020**, *71*, 762-768, doi:10.1093/cid/ciaa248.

[17] Huang, C.; Wang, Y.; Li, X.; Ren, L.; Zhao, J.; Hu, Y.; Zhang, L.; Fan, G.; Xu, J.; Gu, X.; et al. Clinical features of patients infected with 2019 novel coronavirus in Wuhan, China. *Lancet* **2020**, *395*, 497-506, doi:10.1016/S0140-6736(20)30183-5.

[18] Guo, L.; Ren, L.; Yang, S.; Xiao, M.; Chang, D.; Yang, F.; Dela Cruz, C.S.; Wang, Y.; Wu, C.; Xiao, Y.; et al. Profiling early humoral response to diagnose novel coronavirus disease (COVID-19). Clin. Infect. Dis. **2020**, *71*, 778-785, doi:10.1093/cid/ciaa310.

[19] Wang, Y.; Zhang, L.; Sang, L.; Ye, F.; Ruan, S.; Zhong, B.; Song, T.; Alshukairi, A.N.; Chen, R.; Zhang, Z.; et al. Kinetics of viral load and antibody response in relation to COVID-19 severity. J. Clin. Invest. **2020**, *130*, 5235-5244, doi:10.1172/JCI138759.

[20] Carsetti, R.; Zaffina, S.; Mortari, E.P.; Terreri, S.; Corrente, F.; Capponi, C.; Palomba, P.; Mirabella, M.; Cascioli, S.; Palange, P.; et al. Different Innate and Adaptive Immune Responses to SARS-CoV-2 Infection of Asymptomatic, Mild, and Severe Cases. *Front. Immunol.* **2020**, *11*, 3365, doi:10.3389/fimmu.2020.610300.

[21] Figueiredo-Campos, P.; Blankenhaus, B.; Mota, C.; Gomes, A.; Serrano, M.; Ariotti, S.; Costa, C.; Nunes-Cabaço, H.; Mendes, A.M.; Gaspar, P.; et al. Seroprevalence of anti-SARS-CoV-2 antibodies in COVID-19 patients and healthy volunteers up to 6 months post disease onset. *Eur. J. Immunol.* **2020**, *50*, 2025-2040, doi:10.1002/eji.202048970.

[22] CDC Vaccines: The Basics 2012.

[23] Anderson, E.J.; Rouphael, N.G.; Widge, A.T.; Jackson, L.A.; Roberts, P.C.; Makhene, M.; Chappell, J.D.; Denison, M.R.; Stevens, L.J.; Pruijssers, A.J.; et al. Safety and Immunogenicity of SARS-CoV-2 mRNA-1273 Vaccine in Older Adults. N. Engl. J. Med. **2020**, *383*, 2427-2438, doi:10.1056/NEJMoa2028436.

[24] Folegatti, P.M.; Ewer, K.J.; Aley, P.K.; Angus, B.; Becker, S.; Belij-Rammerstorfer, S.; Bellamy, D.; Bibi, S.; Bittaye, M.; Clutterbuck, E.A.; et al. Safety and immunogenicity of the ChAdOx1 nCoV-19 vaccine against SARS-CoV-2: a preliminary report of a phase 1/2, single-blind, randomised controlled trial. Lancet **2020**, *396*, 467-478, doi:10.1016/S0140-6736(20)31604-4.

[25] Xia, S.; Zhang, Y.; Wang, Y.; Wang, H.; Yang, Y.; Gao, G.F.; Tan, W.; Wu, G.; Xu, M.; Lou, Z.; et al. Safety and immunogenicity of an inactivated SARS-CoV-2 vaccine, BBIBP-CorV:

a randomised, double-blind, placebo-controlled, phase 1/2 trial. *Lancet Infect. Dis.* **2021**, *21*, 39-51, doi:10.1016/S1473-3099(20)30831-8.

[26] Wong, H.Y.F.; Lam, H.Y.S.; Fong, A.H.T.; Leung, S.T.; Chin, T.W.Y.; Lo, C.S.Y.; Lui, M.M.S.; Lee, J.C.Y.; Chiu, K.W.H.; Chung, T.W.H.; et al. Frequency and Distribution of Chest Radiographic Findings in Patients Positive for COVID-19. Radiology **2020**, *296*, E72–E78, doi:10.1148/radiol.2020201160.

[27] Udugama, B.; Kadhiresan, P.; Kozlowski, H.N.; Malekjahani, A.; Osborne, M.; Li, V.Y.C.; Chen, H.; Mubareka, S.; Gubbay, J.B.; Chan, W.C.W. Diagnosing COVID-19: The Disease and Tools for Detection. ACS Nano **2020**, *14*, 3822-3835, doi:10.1021/acsnano.0c02624.

[28] Leblanc, J.J.; Gubbay, J.B.; Li, Y.; Needle, R.; Arneson, S.R.; Marcino, D.; Charest, H.; Desnoyers, G.; Dust, K.; Fattouh, R.; et al. Since January 2020 Elsevier has created a COVID-19 resource centre with free information in English and Mandarin on the novel coronavirus COVID-19. The COVID-19 resource centre is hosted on Elsevier Connect, the company' s public news and information. **2020**.

[29] Corman, V.M.; Landt, O.; Kaiser, M.; Molenkamp, R.; Meijer, A.; Chu, D.K.; Bleicker, T.; Brünink, S.; Schneider, J.; Luisa Schmidt, M.; et al. Detection of 2019-nCoV by RT-PCR. Euro Surveill **2020**, *25*, 1-8.

[30] Lv, Y.; Wu, R.; Feng, K.; Li, J.; Mao, Q.; Yuan, H.; Shen, H.; Chai, X.; Li, L.S. Highly sensitive and accurate detection of C-reactive protein by CdSe/ZnS quantum dot-based fluorescence-linked immunosorbent assay. *J.* Nanobiotechnology **2017**, *15*, 35, doi:10.1186/s12951-017-0267-4.

[31] Rai, P.; Kumar, B.K.; Deekshit, V.K.; Karunasagar, I.; Karunasagar, I. Detection technologies and recent developments in the diagnosis of COVID-19 infection. Appl. Microbiol. Biotechnol. **2021**, *105*, 441-455, doi:10.1007/s00253-020-11061-5.

[32] Zhang, Y.; Odiwuor, N.; Xiong, J.; Sun, L.; Nyaruaba, R.O.; Wei, H.; Tanner, N.A. Rapid molecular detection of SARS-CoV-2 (COVID-19) virus RNA using colorimetric LAMP. *medRxiv* **2020**, *2*, doi:10.1101/2020.02.26.20028373.

[33] Broughton, J.P.; Deng, X.; Yu, G.; Fasching, C.L.; Servellita, V.; Singh, J.; Miao, X.; Streithorst, J.A.; Granados, A.; Sotomayor-Gonzalez, A.; et al. CRISPR–Cas12-based detection of SARS-CoV-2. Nat. Biotechnol. **2020**, *38*, 870-874, doi:10.1038/s41587-020-0513-4.

[34] Lau, Y.L.; Ismail, I. binti; Mustapa, N.I. binti; Lai, M.Y.; Soh, T.S.T.; Hassan, A.H.; Peariasamy, K.M.; Lee, Y.L.; Kahar, M.K.B.A.; Chong, J.; et al. Development of a reverse transcription recombinase polymerase amplification assay for rapid and direct visual detection of Severe Acute Respiratory Syndrome Coronavirus 2 (SARS-CoV-2). *PLoS One* **2021**, *16*, 2-9, doi:10.1371/journal.pone.0245164.

[35] Lassaunière, R.; Frische, A.; Harboe, Z.B.; Nielsen, A.C.Y.; Fomsgaard, A.; Krogfelt, K.A.; Jørgensen, C.S. Evaluation of nine commercial SARS-CoV-2 immunoassays. *medRxiv* **2020**, 1-15, doi:10.1101/2020.04.09.20056325.

[36] Mertens, P.; De Vos, N.; Martiny, D.; Jassoy, C.; Mirazimi, A.; Cuypers, L.; Van den Wijngaert, S.; Monteil, V.; Melin, P.; Stoffels, K.; et al. Development and Potential Usefulness of the COVID-19 Ag Respi-Strip Diagnostic Assay in a Pandemic Context. *Front. Med.* **2020**, *7*, doi:10.3389/fmed.2020.00225.

[37] Cai, X.F.; Chen, J.; Hu, J. li; Long, Q.X.; Deng, H.J.; Liu, P.; Fan, K.; Liao, P.; Liu, B.Z.; Wu, G.C.; et al. A peptide-based magnetic chemiluminescence enzyme immunoassay for serological diagnosis of coronavirus disease 2019. J. Infect. Dis. **2020**, *222*, 189-195, doi:10.1093/infdis/jiaa243.

[38] Giri, B.; Pandey, S.; Shrestha, R.; Pokharel, K.; Ligler, F.S.; Neupane, B.B. Review of analytical performance of COVID-19 detection methods. Anal. Bioanal. Chem. **2021**, *413*, 35-48, doi:10.1007/s00216-020-02889-x.

[39] Infantino, M.; Grossi, V.; Lari, B.; Bambi, R.; Perri, A.; Manneschi, M.; Terenzi, G.; Liotti, I.; Ciotta, G.; Taddei, C.; et al. Diagnostic accuracy of an automated chemiluminescent immunoassay for anti-SARS-CoV-2 IgM and IgG antibodies: an Italian experience. J. Med. Virol. **2020**, *92*, 1671-1675, doi:10.1002/jmv.25932.

[40] Russell, S.M.; Alba-Patiño, A.; Barón, E.; Borges, M.; Gonzalez-Freire, M.; De La Rica, R. Biosensors for Managing the COVID-19 Cytokine Storm: Challenges Ahead. ACS Sensors **2020**, *5*, 1506-1513, doi:10.1021/acssensors.0c00979.

[41] Fukumoto, T.; Iwasaki, S.; Fujisawa, S.; Hayasaka, K.; Sato, K.; Oguri, S.; Taki, K.; Nakakubo, S.; Kamada, K.; Yamashita, Y.; et al. Efficacy of a novel SARS-CoV-2 detection kit without RNA extraction and purification. Int. J. Infect. Dis. **2020**, *98*, 16-17, doi:10.1016/j.ijid.2020.06.074.

[42] Laghrib, F.; Saqrane, S.; El Bouabi, Y.; Farahi, A.; Bakasse, M.; Lahrich, S.; El Mhammedi, M.A. Current progress on COVID-19 related to biosensing technologies: New opportunity for detection and monitoring of viruses. Microchem. J. 2021, *160*, 105606.

[43] Xi, H.; Juhas, M.; Zhang, Y. G-quadruplex based biosensor: A potential tool for SARS-CoV-2 detection. Biosens. Bioelectron. **2020**, *167*, 112494, doi:10.1016/j.bios.2020.112494.

[44] Turner, A.P.F. Biosensors: Fundamentals and applications - Historic book now open access. Biosens. Bioelectron. 2015, *65*, A1.

[45] Ermolaeva, T.; Farafonova, O.; Karaseva, N. Possibilities and Prospects of Immunosensors for a Highly Sensitive Pesticide Detection in Vegetables and Fruits: a Review. Food Anal. Methods 2019, *12*, 2785-2801.

[46] Ramírez, N.B.; Salgado, A.M.; Valdman, B. The evolution and developments of immunosensors for health and environmental monitoring: Problems and perspectives. *Brazilian* J. Chem. Eng. **2009**, *26*, 227-249, doi:10.1590/s0104-66322009000200001.

[47] Goumi, Y. El Electrochemical Genosensors: Definition and Fields of Application. Int. J. Biosens. Bioelectron. **2017**, *3*, doi:10.15406/ijbsbe.2017.03.00080.

[48] Silva, A.C.A.; Silva, M.J.B.; Da Luz, F.A.C.; Silva, D.P.; De Deus, S.L.V.; Dantas, N.O. Controlling the cytotoxicity of CdSe magic-sized quantum dots as a function of surface defect density. Nano Lett. **2014**, *14*, 5452-5457, doi:10.1021/nl5028028.

[49] Silva, A.C.A.; Da Silva, S.W.; Morais, P.C.; Dantas, N.O. Shell thickness modulation in ultrasmall CdSe/CdSxSe 1-x/CdS core/shell quantum dots via 1-thioglycerol. ACS Nano **2014**, *8*, 1913-1922, doi:10.1021/nn406478f.

[50] Morais, P. V.; Gomes, V.F.; Silva, A.C.A.; Dantas, N.O.; Schöning, M.J.; Siqueira, J.R. Nanofilm of ZnO nanocrystals/carbon nanotubes as biocompatible layer for enzymatic

biosensors in capacitive field-effect devices. J. Mater. Sci. **2017**, *52*, 12314-12325, doi:10.1007/s10853-017-1369-y.

[51] Almeida Silva, A.C.; Gratens, X.; Chitta, V.A.; Franco, S.D.; Souza Da Silva, R.; Condeles, J.F.; Dantas, N.O. Effects of ultrasonic agitation on the structural and magnetic properties of CoFe2O4nanocrystals. *Eur. J. Inorg. Chem.* **2014**, doi:10.1002/ejic.201402563.

[52] Silva, A.C.A.; Freschi, A.P.P.; Rodrigues, C.M.; Matias, B.F.; Maia, L.P.; Goulart, L.R.; Dantas, N.O. Biological analysis and imaging applications of CdSe/CdSxSe1−x/CdS core–shell magic-sized quantum dot. *Nanomedicine Nanotechnology,* Biol. Med. **2016**, *12*, 1421-1430, doi:10.1016/j.nano.2016.01.001.

[53] Silva, A.C.A.; Azevedo, F.V.P.V.; Zóia, M.A.P.; Rodrigues, J.P.; Dantas, N.O.; Melo, V.R.Á.; Goulart, L.R. Magic Sized Quantum Dots as a Theranostic Tool for Breast Cancer. In *Recent Studies & Advances in Breast Cancer*; Open Access eBooks: Wilmington, 2017; pp. 1-10 ISBN 978-81-935757-2-7.

[54] Souza, G.L. de; Moura, C.C.G.; Silva, A.C.A.; Marinho, J.Z.; Silva, T.R.; Dantas, N.O.; Bonvicini, J.F.S.; Turrioni, A.P. Effects of zinc oxide and calcium–doped zinc oxide nanocrystals on cytotoxicity and reactive oxygen species production in different cell culture models. Restor. Dent. Endod. **2020**, *45*, 54, doi:10.5395/rde.2020.45.e54.

[55] Duarte, C.A.; Goulart, L.R.; Filice, L. de S.C.; Lima, I.L. de; Campos-Fernández, E.; Dantas, N.O.; Silva, A.C.A.; Soares, M.B.P.; Santos, R.R. dos; Cardoso, C.M.A.; et al. Characterization of Crystalline Phase of TiO2 Nanocrystals, Cytotoxicity and Cell Internalization Analysis on Human Adipose Tissue-Derived Mesenchymal Stem Cells. Materials (Basel). **2020**, *13*, 4071, doi:10.3390/ma13184071.

[56] Carvalho Naves, M.P.; de Morais, C.R.; Silva, A.C.A.; Dantas, N.O.; Spanó, M.A.; de Rezende, A.A.A. Assessment of mutagenic, recombinogenic and carcinogenic potential of titanium dioxide nanocristals in somatic cells of Drosophila melanogaster. Food Chem. Toxicol. **2018**, *112*, 273-228, doi:10.1016/j.fct.2017.12.040.

[57] Reis, É. de M.; de Rezende, A.A.A.; Santos, D.V.; de Oliveria, P.F.; Nicolella, H.D.; Tavares, D.C.; Silva, A.C.A.; Dantas, N.O.; Spanó, M.A. Assessment of the genotoxic potential of two zinc oxide sources (amorphous and nanoparticles) using the in vitro micronucleus test and the in vivo wing somatic mutation and recombination test. *Food Chem. Toxicol.* **2015**, *84*, 55-63, doi:10.1016/j.fct.2015.07.008.

[58] Reis, É. de M.; Rezende, A.A.A. de; Oliveira, P.F. de; Nicolella, H.D.; Tavares, D.C.; Silva, A.C.A.; Dantas, N.O.; Spanó, M.A. Evaluation of titanium dioxide nanocrystal-induced genotoxicity by the cytokinesis-block micronucleus assay and the Drosophila wing spot test. *Food Chem. Toxicol.* **2016**, *96*, 309-319, doi:10.1016/j.fct.2016.08.023.

[59] Silva, A.; Zóia, M.A.P.; Correia, L.I.V.; Azevedo, F.V.P.V.; Paula, A.T. de; Maia, L.P.; Carvalho, L.S. de; Carvalho, L.N.; Costa, M.P.C.; Giaretta, L.C.; et al. Biocompatibility of Doped Semiconductors Nanocrystals and Nanocomposites. In *Cytotoxicity*; InTech, 2018.

[60] Silva, A.C.A.; Dantas, N.O.; Silva, M.J.B.; Spanó, A.M.; Goulart, ; Luiz Ricardo Functional Nanocrystals : Towards Biocompatibility, Nontoxicity and. In *Advances in Biochemistry & Applications in Medicine*; 2017; pp. 1-27.

Rossiter, H.B.; Gao, W. SARS-CoV-2 RapidPlex: A Graphene-Based Multiplexed Telemedicine Platform for Rapid and Low-Cost COVID-19 Diagnosis and Monitoring. Matter **2020**, *3*, 1981-1998, doi:10.1016/j.matt.2020.09.027.

[86] Cui, F.; Zhou, H.S. Diagnostic methods and potential portable biosensors for coronavirus disease 2019. Biosens. Bioelectron. **2020**, *165*, 112349, doi:10.1016/j.bios.2020.112349.

Chapter 27

Role of Graphene and Graphene Derived Materials to Fight with COVID-19

Vamsi Krishna Kudapa, Ajay Mittal, Ishita Agrawal, Tejendra K. Gupta and Rajeev Gupta

Abstract

The COVID-19 pandemic is a genuine biosafety occasion that is causing an extreme effect on the worldwide society and economy. Various challenges associated with the outbreak of this pandemic include diagnosis, prevention, and proper medication. Engineered nanomaterials such as graphene and graphene derived materials could be the potential solution in preventing COVID-19. This study endeavors how the improvement of novel materials can assist researchers with handling the difficulties in biosafety. In recent years, 2D graphene had caught much consideration due to its efficient electrical properties and encouraging presentations, comprising methods to combat or identify drug-resistant bacterial contaminations. The bacteria lose its integrity when exposed to the graphene surface because of its efficient viral inhibition tendency.

Keywords: graphene, contact angle, superhydrophobic, mask, COVID-19

1. Introduction

Graphene belongs to the group of carbon comprising of a single layer of atoms organized in a 2D honeycomb structure [1]. Pristine graphene usage is limited due to its difficulty in bottom-up synthesis [2], lesser solubility [3], and the lower tendency of accumulation due to had proved challenging due to difficult van der Waals interactions [4]. To overcome the above limitations, alternative compounds may be derived from graphite or other carbon sources through top-down approaches, which can also incorporate functionalized oxygen groups on its surface. The protonated solvents has the tendency to form multi-layered graphene oxide by the process of graphene oxidation, which contains hexagraphene oxidenal based graphene structure. These derivatives are proven as efficient fillers in several polymer nanocomposite materials because of their uniform distribution across the polymer matrices [5]. This property has increased the functionality of graphene derivatives in paints, efficient and precise sensors, flexible displays, efficient solar panels, packing materials [6], sensitive electronic devices prevention [7], for resisting the corrosion on different materials [8] and in bio-imaging, biosensors, antibacterial agents, 3D bio printing, photo thermal therapy, drug delivery, gene therapy, and tissue engineering (**Figure 1**) [9].

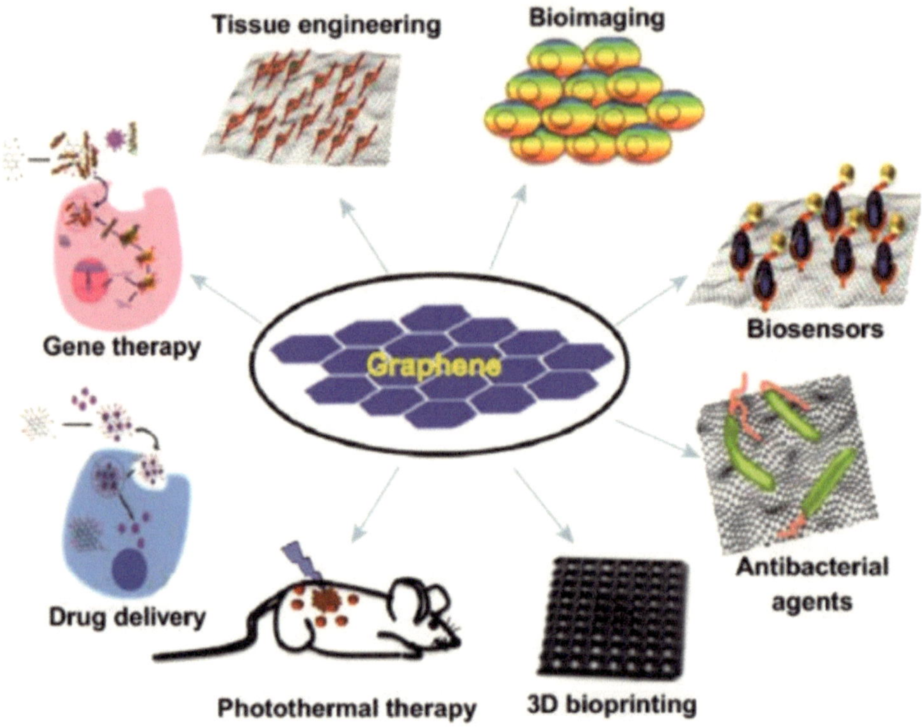

Figure 1.
Role of graphene in the area of bio-imaging, biosensors, antibacterial agents, 3D bio printing, photo thermal therapy, drug delivery, gene therapy and tissue engineering. Reprinted with the permission from [9].

Palmeri and Papi [10] studied different ways of interactions between various graphene-based materials and the viruses, which reveals that the graphene-based materials, can help in killing or blocking the viruses. Several recent studies have also revealed that graphene derivatives can be considered as a potential material for protecting from the COVID-19 virus [10, 11].

2. Mechanism of graphene based materials for prevention of COVID- 19

Earlier research suggests that graphene has a great viral hindrance limit. In 2012, the primary proof of graphene antiviral impacts was realized when fine layers of reduced graphene oxide -Tungsten oxide were misrepresented for photo inactivation of virus infecting bacteria under obvious light illumination [12]. Recent studies exhibited how the coronavirus spike S1 protein receptor-restricting area can cooperate with heparin and alternated compliance. It has suggestions for the advancement of initial remedial by adapting heparin and glycosamminoglycans-based antivirals [13], including treatment of graphene oxide based surface with sulfuric acid or sulfate. Sulfur reacted NPs functionalized with reduced graphene oxide had been effectively used to collect and photo thermally pulverize herpes simplex infection type 1 utilizing near-infrared (NIR) light [14]. This information brings up how graphene oxide detention could be combined with NIR medicines of lungs. As Gr and GrO absorbers fall under the NIR tissue transparency window, they allow the incident light deep into the body. The combination of carbon dots and natural antimicrobial polyphenol curcumin is proved to be an efficient model for preventing COVID-19 [15]. The respiratory syncytial infection is treated through the combination of Cyclodextrins-functionalized sulfonated graphene and curcumin-stacked cyclodextrins functionalized sulfonated graphene, GSCC. The sulfonate clusters on the GSCC can simulate the cell exterior and restrain RSV disease by an economical inhibition mechanism, recreating cell receptors utilized for infection connection. GSCC NPs impacts are because of a twofold component, by curcumin-intervened viral inactivation and by the self-consciousness of the infection connection to the host cell layers [16].

3. Fabrication of graphene based superhydrophobic coating

Revealed in December 2019, another lethal SAR-CoV-2 infection begins circling among the people [17] and spreads through the respiratory beds [18]. Additionally, an individual can likewise get in contact with this infection by interacting with the debased articles or exteriors and afterward getting in touch with mouth, nose, or eyes. A new report states that SAR-CoV-2 has a variable life span on different surfaces [19]. In comparison with Cu and cardboard, the adherence of coronavirus is estimated to be greater on the surfaces of plastic and tempered steel. Besides, the infection is affirmed to be steadier on smooth surfaces compared with uneven surfaces like printing/tissue papers, wood, and materials. Much more problematic is the discernible degree of the infection on the outside film of the surgical masks, which is 7 days [16]. These virus-infected touch surfaces, which can retain the virus for longer periods can spread the virus at a faster rate. In the current epidemic circumstance, where the coronavirus infections are dramatically expanding every day worldwide, improvement of the effective enemy of coronavirus protecting surfaces or coatings can be a potential solution for minimizing the spread of the virus through any source [20, 21]. Graphene or graphene derivatives are suitable for their antibacterial properties [22] and the study by Sametband [23] revealed the antiviral characteristics of graphene oxide and slightly reduced sulfuirnc acid treated graphene oxide against herpes simplex virus Type-1 by a specified unique mechanism. Comparable to receptor heparin sulfate cell surface, graphene oxide and its derivatives contain groups of negative charge elements and so the two moieties challenging each other in connection with HSV-1 as shown in **Figure 2**. Nanomaterials can be considered as main inhibitor in defending the Vero cell from the disease. The viral reduction effectiveness of graphene oxide, reduced graphene oxide, graphene oxide-polyvinylpyrrolidone (PVP) composite, graphene oxide poly (diallyl dimethyl ammonium chloride) composite with forerunners graphite

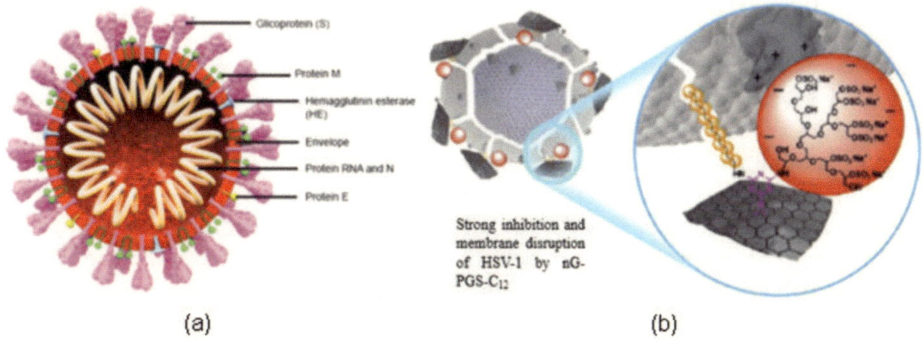

Figure 2.
(a) COVID-19 structure [2], (b) pictorial representation of the mechanism of breaking the long chain of virus envelope. Reprinted with the permission from [16].

and graphite oxide was analyzed by Ye et al. [24]. This research has opened a huge antiviral tendency of graphene oxide against Pseudorabies infection and porcine pestilence looseness of the bowels infection. He concludes that antiviral characteristics of graphene oxide are ascribed to its adversely charged, high-pitched structure. The graphene oxide formed with PVP, non-ionic polymer demonstrated intense antiviral movement, nonetheless, PDDA (cationic polymer) bound graphene oxide uncovered no infection hindrance, proposing negative charge as an essential for antiviral characteristics. Song and other authors [25] has revealed the graphene oxide based label-free technique to identify and sterilize natural infections, for example, Enterovirus 71 and endemic gastrointestinal avian flu an infection, which have incredible ecological strength and less affectability for carbon-based purifiers and detergents. Redox reactions between the graphene oxide layer and the viruses due to the physico-chemical process will act as an important parameter in destroying the viruses. Under higher temperature environment, the antiviral efficiency of the graphene oxide sheet will be improved. Chen and the co-authors [26] revealed that graphene oxide sheets are accounted for to display critical antiviral restraint possibilities towards covered feline COVID and connecting silver particles into graphene oxide structure widens its antiviral capability in the direction of non-enveloped infectious bursal disease virus. Yang et al. [27] synthesized curcumin stacked β-CD functionalized sulfonated graphene composite and researched its antiviral competence beside negative sense respiratory syncytial infection (RSV). The results demonstrated that GSCC could thwart RSV from tainting the host cells by deactivating the contamination clearly and blocking the association of the disease and have prophylactic and medicinal effects towards the contamination. Du et al. [28] researched the antiviral effect of graphene oxide - Silver nanoparticles composite as an afterthought impacts of porcine regenerative and respiratory problem disease. The outcomes propose that the presentation of infection with graphene oxide -Ag NPs composite block the infection to enter the host cell with a accuracy of 59.2% and advances the creation of IFN-invigorating qualities and interferon-α which hinders the infection expansion. Accordingly, Graphene-based surfaces have enormous probability in the improvement of antiviral surfaces and coatings for keeping fouling from harmful and infectious infections including corona virus, and could control the illness transmission [29]. Especially, for coronavirus infection, structures with higher carboxyl groups and less endurance of this infection on Cu surfaces, graphene oxide/reduced graphene oxide -SO_3 coatings enhanced with Cu nanoparticles/Cu particles could be a inspiring possibility for the advancement of hostile to coronavirus surfaces. These materials are important in successfully catching and destabilizing the infection structures and limiting their endurance time on different covered surfaces [30]. The schematic representation of the viral restriction process from the graphene or graphene derivative based coatings is understandable from **Figure 3**.

Zhong et al. [31] fabricated graphene layer-based superhydrophobic low-melting temperature nonwoven surgical masks through dual-mode laser-induced forward transfer method with excellent self-cleaning and photo thermal property. These functional masks are reusable after sunlight sterilization because the surface temperature can quickly increase to 80 °C under sunlight. In addition, these functional masks show the tendency of salt-rejection, which increases its usage lifetime. The superhydrophobic surgical masks, which are, produced through roll-to-roll production, give efficient protection against viruses. SEM image of pristine surgical mask reveals that the melt-blown fibers of 20 μm were smooth and exhibiting non-super hydrophobic properties. The wetting tendency of this mask is estimated through a static contact angle, which is observed to be 110°, representing a hydrophobic

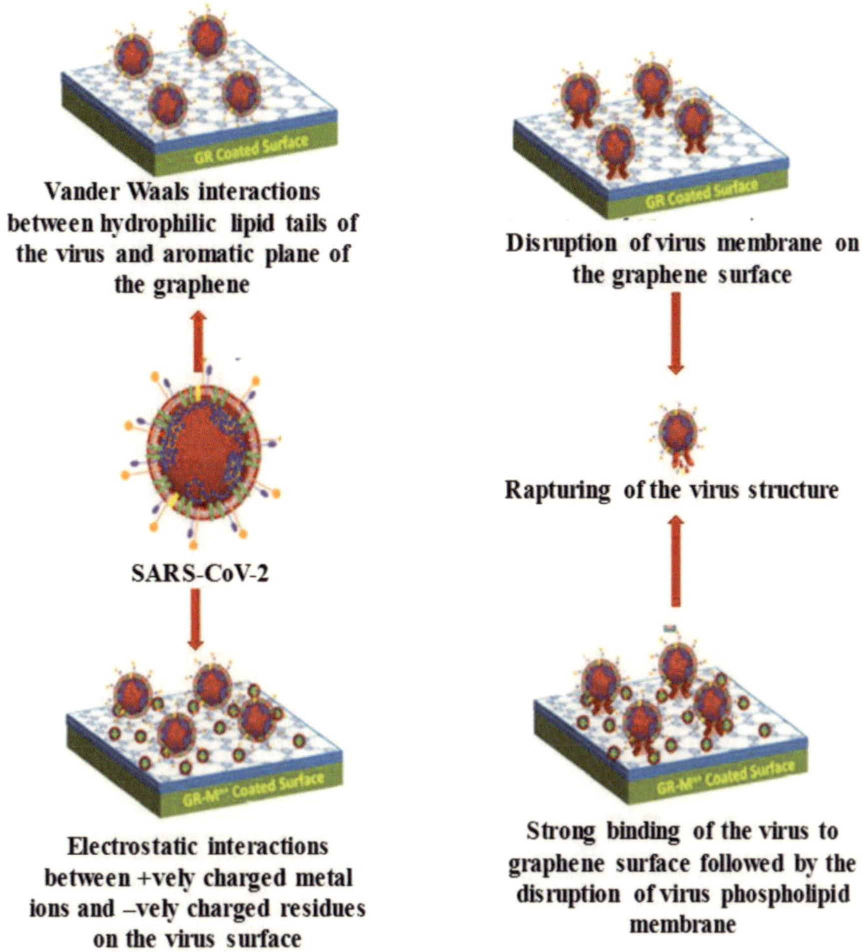

Figure 3.
Sequential representation of the graphene or graphene derivative based coatings in repelling various viruses including coronavirus. Adapted image [30].

surface. The disadvantage observed with this mask is that the droplets are attaching to the surface. After using dual-mode laser-induced forward transfer method, it was observed that nanostructured flakes were seen on the mask surface varying its size from 100 nm to few micrometers and the contact was observed to be 141°, which represents its superhydrophobicity (**Figure 4**).

The multi-layered masks for combatting COVID-19 need to be designed as per World Health Organization guidelines i.e. the innermost layer should behave like a hydrophilic surface and the rest two layers i.e. middle and outside layers are to be in hydrophobic nature. There are several combinations of different materials and fabrics, which have a greater tendency to increase the efficiency of filtration and breathability. As the porosity of the layer increases from the 3rd layer to the 1st layer, the extent of droplet filtration will also increase (**Figure 5**). He also reveals that tightly woven fabric in the third layer will attain 80% particle filtration efficiency and enhances breathability. The filtration effectiveness of any mas depends on the most penetrating particle size, which is in the range of 0.04–0.4 μm. The extent of MPPS filtration varies with the velocity at which filtration is done, fiber porosity & diameter, and particle size distribution [32].

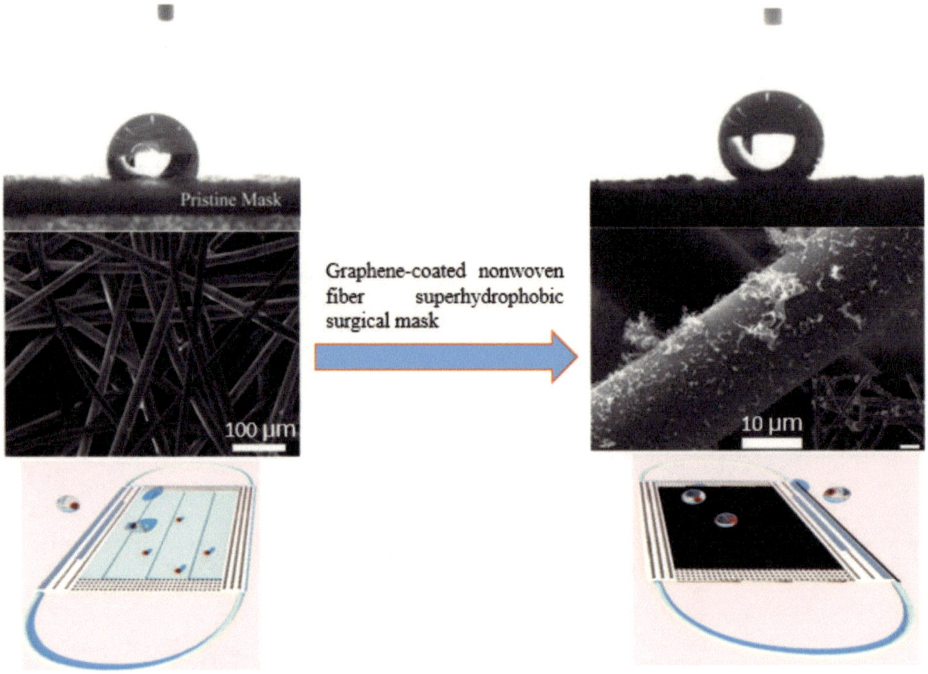

Figure 4.
Contact angle measurement and SEM images on uncoated and coated graphene nonwoven fiber surgical mask Reprinted with the permission from [31].

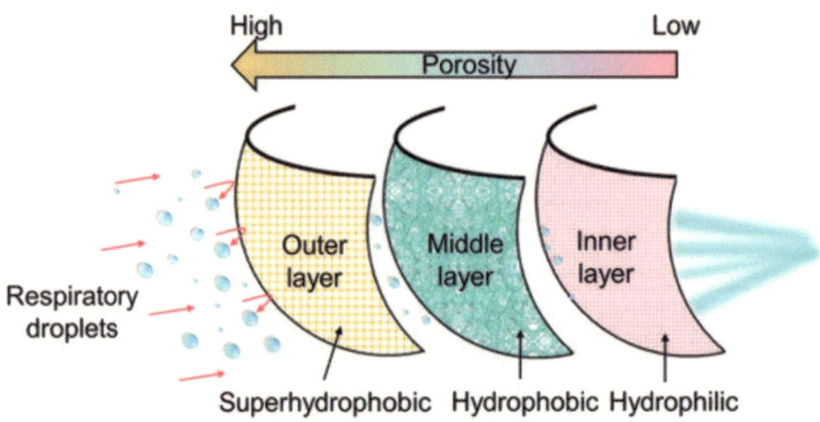

Figure 5.
Multi-layered masks with varying porosity from hydrophilicity to superhydrophobicity. Reprinted with the permission from [32].

4. Cytotoxicity of graphene

Cytotoxicity valuation of nanomaterials is important and beneficial for real understanding of their biological action. The *in-vitro* labeling of therapeutic cells with nanoparticles is becoming more and more common and the possible effects of the nanoparticles on the esthetic cells are increasing. In general, carbon based nanomaterials show specific antiviral activities and low cytotoxicity. It was found that the graphene based nanomedicines made for antiviral treatment have been tested for against a specific virus and these types of antiviral nanomedicines can also enhances the biocompatibility and reduces the cytotoxicity of the drug. The two-dimensional structure and negatively charged surfaces of graphene sheets can easily interact with bacteria and viruses and destroy them by disrupting their plasma membrane. Graphene sheets can also interact with living cells depending on its concentration [33]. Experimental evidences show that the graphene sheets inactivate the virus before it enters the cells and the sharp edges of graphene layers inactivate the infection by actual interruption of the construction through direct association. The antiviral movement of the graphene sheet can be powerful on both DNA and RNA infections, and reliant on fixation and incubation time. The *in-vitro* study shows that the carbon based materials disturb the membrane potential, membrane integrity, metabolic activity and cellular reproduction and they are blamed for DNA damage [34]. Ye et al. [24] reported the antimicrobial and antiviral activity of graphene and its derivatives and its cytotoxicity. In this study, he detailed the antiviral action of graphene oxide against pseudorabies infection and porcine pandemic the runs infection with non-cytotoxic concentration. In this experiment, antiviral activity along with the toxic effect of graphene was measured and it was found that at low concentration level, graphene show non-toxic effect with good antiviral behavior but at higher concentration level, graphene show low toxic effect. These results show that the graphene and its derivatives have low toxicity level compared to other carbon materials and it can be the promising candidate for the next generation antiviral materials.

5. Conclusion

Graphene and graphene derived materials have excellent antimicrobial, antiviral and self-cleaning properties and found application in various industries. Graphene and graphene-based material have recently received enormous attention due to their applicability in tacking lethal SAR-CoV-2 infection. The study suggests that the graphene-based coating on different surfaces tend to neutralize viruses and bacteria, to a varying degree, due to their antiviral and antimicrobial activity. The graphene coated surgical masks could control the transmission of virus and protection from the lethal covid-19 virus. It is to strengthen the research in this field to evaluate the effectiveness of graphene and graphene-based material for their applicability in fighting the Covid-19 virus.

Author details

Vamsi Krishna Kudapa[1], Ajay Mittal[1], Ishita Agrawal[2], Tejendra K. Gupta[3] and Rajeev Gupta[4*]

1 Department of Chemical Engineering, College of Engineering Studies, UPES, Dehradun, Uttarakhand, India

2 Department of Molecular and Human Genetics, Banaras Hindu University, Varanasi, U.P., India

3 Amity Institute of Applied Sciences, Amity University, Noida, India

4 Department of Physics, College of Engineering Studies, UPES, Dehradun, Uttarakhand, India

*Address all correspondence to: rajeev@ddn.upes.ac.in

'Biotechnology to Combat COVID-19' is a collaborative project with Biotechnology Kiosk

References

[1] P. Zhao *et al.*, "A new paradigm of ultrathin 2D nanomaterial adsorbents in aqueous media: Graphene and GO, MoS2, MXenes, and 2D MOFs," J. Mater. Chem. A, vol. 7, no. 28, pp. 16598-16621, 2019.

[2] Y. Zhu *et al.*, "Graphene and graphene oxide: Synthesis, properties, and applications," Adv. Mater., vol. 22, no. 35, pp. 3906-3924, 2010.

[3] S. Niyogi, E. Bekyarova, M. E. Itkis, J. L. McWilliams, M. A. Hamon, and R. C. Haddon, "Solution properties of graphite and graphene," J. Am. Chem. Soc., vol. 128, no. 24, pp. 7720-7721, 2006.

[4] T. Kuilla, S. Bhadra, D. Yao, N. H. Kim, S. Bose, and J. H. Lee, "Recent advances in graphene based polymer composites," Prog. Polym. Sci., vol. 35, no. 11, pp. 1350-1375, 2010.

[5] B. M. Yoo, H. J. Shin, H. W. Yoon, and H. B. Park, "Graphene and graphene oxide and their uses in barrier polymers," J. Appl. Polym. Sci., vol. 131, no. 1, pp. 1-23, 2014.

[6] C. Cheng, S. Li, A. Thomas, N. A. Kotov, and R. Haag, "Functional Graphene Nanomaterials Based Architectures: Biointeractions, Fabrications, and Emerging Biological Applications," Chem. Rev., vol. 117, no. 3, pp. 1826-1914, 2017.

[7] B. Tan and N. L. Thomas, "A review of the water barrier properties of polymer/clay and polymer/graphene nanocomposites," J. Memb. Sci., vol. 514, pp. 595-612, 2016.

[8] Y. N. Singhbabu, B. Sivakumar, S. K. Choudhary, S. Das, and R. K. Sahu, "Corrosion-protective reduced graphene oxide coated cold rolled steel prepared using industrial setup: A study of protocol feasibility for commercial production," Surf. Coatings Technol., vol. 349, no. 2017, pp. 119-132, 2018.

[9] S. Syama and P. V Mohanan, *Comprehensive Application of Graphene: Emphasis on Biomedical Concerns*, no. 0123456789. Springer Berlin Heidelberg, 2019.

[10] V. Palmieri and M. Papi, "Nano Today Can graphene take part in the fight against COVID-19 ?," Nano Today, vol. 33, p. 100883, 2020.

[11] B. Udugama *et al.*, "Diagnosing COVID-19 : The Disease and Tools for Detection," 2020.

[12] O. Akhavan, M. Choobtashani, and E. Ghaderi, "Protein degradation and RNA efflux of viruses photocatalyzed by graphene-tungsten oxide composite under visible light irradiation," J. Phys. Chem. C, vol. 116, no. 17, pp. 9653-9659, 2012.

[13] C. Mycroft-West *et al.*, "The 2019 coronavirus (SARS-CoV-2) surface protein (Spike) S1 Receptor Binding Domain undergoes conformational change upon heparin binding," pp. 1-9, 2020.

[14] A. P. S. Brogan, R. B. Sessions, A. W. Perriman, and S. Mann, "Molecular dynamics simulations reveal a dielectric-responsive coronal structure in protein-polymer surfactant hybrid nanoconstructs," J. Am. Chem. Soc., vol. 136, no. 48, pp. 16824-16831, 2014.

[15] D. Ting *et al.*, "Multisite inhibitors for enteric coronavirus: antiviral cationic carbon dots based on curcumin," ACS Appl. Nano Mater., vol. 1, no. 10, pp. 5451-5459, 2018.

[16] A. W. H. Chin *et al.*, "Stability of SARS-CoV-2 in different environmental conditions," *The Lancet Microbe*, vol. 1, no. 1, p. e10, 2020.

[17] F. Wu *et al.*, "A new coronavirus associated with human respiratory disease in China," Nature, vol. 579, no. 7798, pp. 265-269, 2020.

[18] V. Stadnytskyi, C. E. Bax, A. Bax, and P. Anfinrud, "The airborne lifetime of small speech droplets and their potential importance in SARS-CoV-2 transmission," Proc. Natl. Acad. Sci. U. S. A., vol. 117, no. 22, pp. 11875-11877, 2020.

[19] P. Neeltje van Doremalen, (National Institute of Allergy and Infectious, Diseases), B. S. N. I. of A. and Trenton Bushmaker, Diseases), and M. P. (Princeton U. Dylan H. Morris, "Aerosol and Surface Stability of SARS-CoV-2 as Compared with SARS-CoV-1," *N. Engl. J. Med.*, pp. 0-2, 2020.

[20] V. K. Kudapa, N. P. Nayak, R. Gupta, E. Studies, and E. Studies, "Mini Review MATERIALS FOR DIAGNOSIS, PREVENTION AND CONTROL OF COVID-19," vol. 2, no. 9, pp. 4-17, 2020.

[21] S. Arora, V. Yadav, P. Kumar, R. Gupta, and D. Kumar, "Polymer based antimicrobial coatings as potential biomaterial: A review," Int. J. Pharm. Sci. Rev. Res., vol. 23, no. 2, pp. 279-290, 2013.

[22] F. Perreault, A. F. De Faria, S. Nejati, and M. Elimelech, "Antimicrobial Properties of Graphene Oxide Nanosheets: Why Size Matters," ACS Nano, vol. 9, no. 7, pp. 7226-7236, 2015.

[23] M. Sametband, I. Kalt, A. Gedanken, and R. Sarid, "Herpes simplex virus type-1 attachment inhibition by functionalized graphene oxide," ACS Appl. Mater. Interfaces, vol. 6, no. 2, pp. 1228-1235, 2014.

[24] S. Ye *et al.*, "Antiviral Activity of Graphene Oxide: How Sharp Edged Structure and Charge Matter," ACS Appl. Mater. Interfaces, vol. 7, no. 38, pp. 21578-21579, 2015.

[25] Z. Song *et al.*, "Virus capture and destruction by label-free graphene oxide for detection and disinfection applications," Small, vol. 11, no. 9-10, pp. 1771-1776, 2015.

[26] Y. N. Chen, Y. H. Hsueh, C. Te Hsieh, D. Y. Tzou, and P. L. Chang, "Antiviral activity of graphene–silver nanocomposites against non-enveloped and enveloped viruses," Int. J. Environ. Res. Public Health, vol. 13, no. 4, pp. 4-6, 2016.

[27] X. X. Yang, C. M. Li, Y. F. Li, J. Wang, and C. Z. Huang, "Synergistic antiviral effect of curcumin functionalized graphene oxide against respiratory syncytial virus infection," Nanoscale, vol. 9, no. 41, pp. 16086-16092, 2017.

[28] T. Du *et al.*, "Antiviral Activity of Graphene Oxide-Silver Nanocomposites by Preventing Viral Entry and Activation of the Antiviral Innate Immune Response," ACS Appl. Bio Mater., vol. 1, no. 5, pp. 1286-1293, 2018.

[29] A. Hooda, M. S. Goyat, J. Kumar, A. Kumar, and R. Gupta, "Progress in Organic Coatings A review on fundamentals, constraints and fabrication techniques of superhydrophobic coatings," *Prog. Org. Coatings*, vol. 142, no. October 2019, p. 105557, 2020.

[30] A. K. Srivastava *et al.*, "Potential of graphene-based materials to combat COVID-19: properties, perspectives, and prospects," Mater. Today Chem., vol. 18, p. 100385, 2020.

[31] H. Zhong *et al.*, "Reusable and Recyclable Graphene Masks with Outstanding Superhydrophobic and Photothermal Performances," 2020.

[32] A. Aggarwal *et al.*, "Clinical & immunological erythematosus patients characteristics in systemic lupus Maryam," J. Dent. Educ., vol. 76, no. 11, pp. 1532-1539, 2012.

[33] P. Innocenzi and L. Stagi, "Carbon-based antiviral nanomaterials: Graphene, C-dots, and fullerenes. A perspective," Chem. Sci., vol. 11, no. 26, pp. 6606-6622, 2020.

[34] S. Gurunathan *et al.*, "Antiviral potential of nanoparticles—can nanoparticles fight against coronaviruses?," Nanomaterials, vol. 10, no. 9, pp. 1-29, 2020.

Section 8

Propagation and Electromagnetism in COVID

Chapter 28

Propagation Analysis of the Coronavirus Pandemic on the Light of the Percolation Theory

Moez Guettari and Ahmed El Aferni

Abstract

Efforts to combat the Covid-19 pandemic have not been limited to the processes of vaccine production, but they first began to analyze the dynamics of the epidemic's spread so that they could adopt barrier measures to bypass the spread. To do this, the works of modeling, predicting and analyzing the spread of the virus continue to increase day after day. In this context, the aim of this chapter is to analyze the propagation of the Coronavirus pandemic by using the percolation theory. In fact, an analogy was established between the electrical conductivity of reverse micelles under temperature variation and the spread of the Coronavirus pandemic. So, the percolation theory was used to describe the cumulate infected people versus time by using a modified Sigmoid Boltzman equation (MSBE) and several quantities are introduced such as: the pandemic percolation time, the maximum infected people, the time constant and the characteristic contamination frequency deduced from Arrhenius equation. Scaling laws and critical exponents are introduced to describe the spread nature near the percolation time. The speed of propagation is also proposed and expressed. The novel approach based on the percolation theory was used to study the Coronavirus (Covid-19) spread in five countries: France, Italy, Germany, China and Tunisia, during 6 months of the pandemic spread (the first wave). So, an explicit expression connecting the number of people infected versus time is proposed to analyze the pandemic percolation. The reported MSBE fit results for the studied countries showed high accuracy.

Keywords: Percolation theory, reverse micelles, electrical conductivity, sigmoid Boltzmann equation (SBE), Coronavirus, spread

1. Introduction

In late December 2019, the emerging epidemic of Coronavirus, Sars-Cov-2 (Covid-19) first appeared in China. Then, it spread on a very large scale to most of the world's countries. For this reason the World Health Organization (WHO) has declared it a global pandemic. The main distinguishing characteristic of this pandemic is its very high contagion power and subsequently, which gives it a spectacular speed of propagation. Recently [1], it was associated with the Spanish flu of 1918 in this regard. For this reason, efforts to forecast, predict, and model the spread of Coronavirus (Covid-19) global pandemic are accumulating to understand its contamination mode [2–6]. The objective of these efforts is to explore ways for predicting its evolution curve to be able to skirt the contamination, in the absence of an effective vaccine serving as an antidote against this disease.

In this context, in a recent study [7] on the spread of Covid-19 in 15 different countries, we have showed that the pandemic spread in a given population follows a sigmoidal law. Indeed, the curve of variation of the cumulative number of infected persons I is composed of 3 phases, a linear phase (slow growth) followed by second exponential phase (fast growth), then another stable phase (slow growth). Given that, in our laboratory, we are used to using the sigmoidal model to characterize the percolation phenomenon occurring in colloidal systems [8, 9].We suggest in the present work to apply the theory of percolation theory on the cumulative number of infected people in order to better understand the dynamics of the virus spread.

Percolation is a mathematical model which first introduced by S.R Braodblent and J. Hammersely in 1957 [10]. As a geometric phase transition, he described large-scale connectivity from other links that are randomly established on small scales. Such connectivity brought the studied system from one state of disorder to another more ordered state. This model has been widely applied to explain phase transitions in a very wide variety of physical systems such as alloys, complex fluids, semi-conductors, communication networks, etc. As examples of the application of the percolation model, we can cite the following transitions: Insulating conductive composite material (Insulator/conductor), Glass transition (Liquid/glass), Polymer gels (Liquid/gels), Quarks in nuclear matter (confinement/non confinement) [11].

Meanwhile, in our laboratory, we used to study several kinds of colloidal systems, in particular, the microemulsions water in oil, so-called reverse micelles. These are nano-droplets of water surrounded by monolayers of surfactant and dispersed in oily phases. In these systems, a percolation phenomenon has often been highlighted and widely studied. In fact, in reverse micelle systems, the percolation phenomenon was manifested by a spectacular increase in the transport properties (viscosity, dielectric constant electrical conductivity, etc.) of the micelles for a volume fraction, ϕ_d or a well-determined temperature T_p [8, 9]. The critical micellar volume fraction and the temperature signaling the appearance of percolation phenomenon are called the percolation thresholds ($\phi_{d,c}$,T_p). This increase has been explained by the fusion of neighboring micelles, a fusion which in turn leads to the formation of a percolating network and the exchange of charge carriers (or matter). In the bibliography, the studies were focused on the viscosity, the electrical conductivity [12] and, of the dielectric constant of the reverse micelles around the percolation threshold. Theoretically, two models have been proposed [13] to justify the percolation-related experimental observations: a static model and a dynamic model. In the static model, the sudden change in the conduction of the system is caused by the formation of a bicontinuous phase of the organic solvent and water at the percolation threshold. Otherwise, micellar fusions are established between the neighboring micelles giving rise to micellar exchanges of the charge and the material. Furthermore, concerning the dynamic model, it is a model that attributes this behavior to the Brownian movement of droplets. Such movement induces random mutual collisions between the different micelles accompanied by exchanges of charge and matter.

2. Electrical percolation versus Covid-19 pandemic percolation

2.1 Phenomenological description

It seems imperative to mention that we are dealing here with two systems with several similarities in dynamics. Regarding the reverse micellar systems, these are indeed spherical particles of nanometric sizes in Brownian (random) motion. This movement leads to permanent inter-micellar collisions giving rise to mutual exchanges of matter and electrical charges. Therefore, reverse micelles transport phenomena such as viscosity η and electrical conductivity σ increase exponentially. On the other side, they are infected people circulating randomly (carriers of the virus). This circulation leads to the virus spread in various ways (contamination of surfaces, the spread of droplets carrying the virus, handshaking with contaminated people...) which giving rise to cumulative number of infected people I_c. We report in **Figure 1** the schematic behavior of two systems. We also present in **Table 1** the detailed analogy between the two systems.

From a qualitative viewpoint, we find that the evolution of the number of people infected over time followed the same curve as the evolution of the micelles' electrical conductivity as a function of temperature. These are two trays separated by an exponential progression. We have measured the electrical conductivity of water/AOT/reverse micelles of composition $W_0 = \frac{[water]}{[AOT]} = 30, \phi_m = \frac{V_{AOT}}{V_{isooc\tan e}} = 0.1, 0.15, 0.2,$ with an increase in temperature. Results are reported in **Figure 2** and compared with the evolution of the cumulative number of detected cases of Covid-19 in china since the first case.

2.2 Theoretical background

2.2.1 Sigmoid Boltzmann equation

Authors [13, 14] are used to using the sigmoid Boltzmann equation (SBE) to model the percolation process in reverse micelles. It is important to elucidate some notions on the SBE equation so that both the relevance of this equation and the definitions of both of its terms are understood.

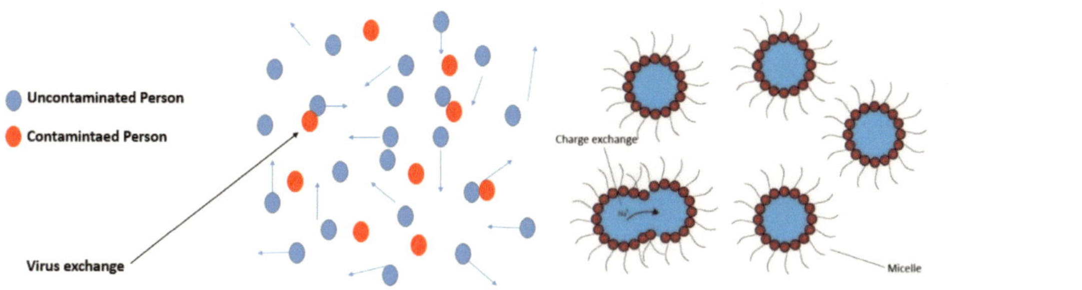

Figure 1.
Schematic representation of the analogy between reverse micelles and the virus spread.

Electrical percolation of reverse micelles	Spread of the virus (Covid-19)
σ : Electrical conductivity	N : Number of people infected
Reverse micelles: charge carriers	Infected people: carriers of the virus
Electrical charge (the Na^+ ion)	Virus
Nature of movement: Brownian (random)	Random
Micellar collision	Contamination of surfaces, spread of droplets carrying the virus, handshaking with contaminated people.

Table 1.
Detailed similarities between reverse micelles and the pandemic spread.

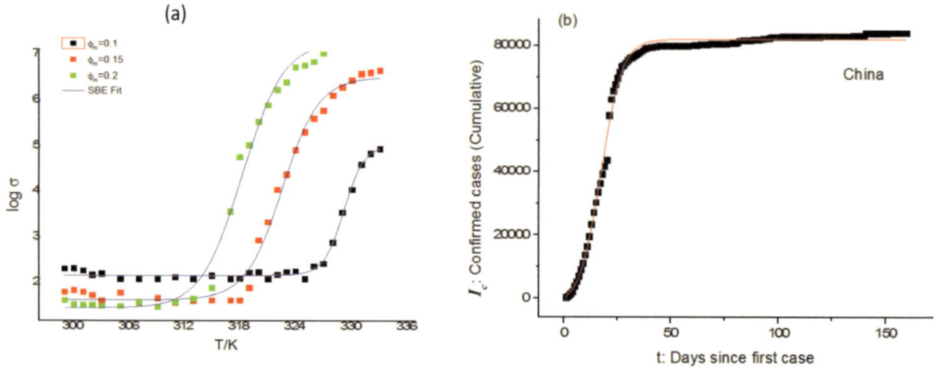

Figure 2.
(a) Electrical conductivity of water/AOT/isooctane reverse micelles ($W_o = 30, \phi_m = 0.1, 0.15, 0.2$ vs Temperature (b) Confirmed cases of infected persons with covid-19 since the first case in China.

To describe the evolution of a quantity evolving as a function of a variable, the Sigmoid-Boltzmann equation (SBE) has the following form:

$$y = \frac{y_i - y_r}{1 + \exp{(x - x_0)/\Delta x}} + y_r \tag{1}$$

Rearranging Eq. (1),

$$y = y_r \left[1 + \left(\frac{y_i - y_r}{y_r}\right) \times \{1 + \exp{(x - x_0)/\Delta x}\}^{-1}\right] \tag{2}$$

where y is the measured magnitude of the system which depends on x, y_i and y_r are the left and right asymptotes of y, x_0 is the center (where y returns the mean of y_i and y_r), and Δx is the constant interval of the independent variable that controls the rise profile or decrease from y_i to y_r(for a large Δx, the rise is gradual while for small Δx, the rise is rapid).

The equation therefore essentially deals with the switching of a variable from an initial state (state of y_i) to a final state (state of y_r) through a transition x_0.

2.2.2 Application for electrical percolation of reverse micelles

By applying this equation to the electrical conductivity of the inverse micelles, σ, evolving as a function of temperature, T, the equation, therefore, deals with the switching of the conductivity from an initial state, σ_i, to a final state, σ_f, passing through the transition, T_p, (percolation temperature).

$$\sigma = \sigma_f \left[1 + \left(\frac{\sigma_i - \sigma_f}{\sigma_f}\right) \times \{1 + \exp{(T - T_p)/\Delta T}\}^{-1}\right] \tag{3}$$

From an experimental point of view, it is often convenient to use the logarithmic scale to better highlight the variations. The equation therefore becomes:

$$\log \sigma = \log \sigma_f \left[1 + \left(\frac{\log \sigma_i - \log \sigma_f}{\log \sigma_f}\right) \times \{1 + \exp{(T - T_p)/\Delta T}\}^{-1}\right] \tag{4}$$

2.2.3 Application of SBE to the cumulative number of infected persons I_c with Covid-19

In a recent work, we modeled the evolution of the cumulative number of infected people I_c in 15 countries with the sigmoid Boltzmann equation (SBE), evolving as a function of time, t. The SBE equation deals with the switching of numbers, I_c, from an initial state, I_i, to a final state, $I_{\max}$, through the transition, t_p. At this point, we can consider that the transition, t_p, corresponds to what is called the pandemic peak.

$$I_c = I_{c,\max}\left[1 + \left(\frac{I_i - I_{c,\max}}{I_{\max}}\right) \times \left\{1 + \exp\left(t - t_p\right)/\Delta t\right\}^{-1}\right] \tag{5}$$

Knowing that at least one person is infected therefore $I_i = 1$ and taking into account that the maximum number of infected people, $I_{\max}$, takes huge values, so $I_{\max} >>> I_i$, the Eq. (5) becomes:

$$I_c = I_{c,\max}\left[1 - \left\{1 + \exp\left(t - t_p\right)/\Delta t\right\}^{-1}\right] \tag{6}$$

On a logarithmic scale, the sigmoid equation becomes:

$$\log I_c = \log I_{c,\max}\left[1 + \left(\frac{\log I_i - \log I_{c,\max}}{\log I_{c,\max}}\right) \times \left\{1 + \exp\left(t - t_p\right)/\Delta t\right\}^{-1}\right] \tag{7}$$

Considering that at least one person is infected, so $I_i = 1$, the Eq. (7) becomes:

$$\log I_c = \log I_{c,\max}\left[1 - \left\{1 + \exp\left(t - t_p\right)/\Delta t\right\}^{-1}\right] \tag{8}$$

For the spread of the pandemic in a given population, the Boltzmann equation (SBE) allows us to derive important parameters describing the spread of the virus. The most important parameters are the time interval, Δt, the percolation time, t_p, and the maximum number of infected persons, $I_{c,\max}$:

- The pandemic percolation time t_p

  This is the transition point corresponding to the pandemic percolation threshold. At this time, the number of infected people rises drastically until the day with the maximum propagation speed. After that time the speed of virus spread decreases and the number of infected cases per day begins to decrease. It represents the pandemic peak

- Maximum number of infected persons $I_{c,\max}$

  It is a cumulative number of infected people signaling the stabilization of the epidemic crisis in a population. The real maximum number of people infected is in the vicinity of this number.

- The time constant Δt

  It is called the time constant. It characterizes the rise of the exponential part (gradually or abrupt). Generally, the epidemic state stabilizes when the number of infected cases N reaches almost the maximum number of infected cases $I = 0.99 I_{c,\max}$ which corresponds to maximum time, $t_{\max}$ of pandemic spread:

Considering Eq. (6), the t_{max} value can be calculated from the following equation:

$$t_{max} = 2.19\Delta t + t_p \quad (9)$$

So, we can estimate the time necessary for the stabilization of the epidemic state of each country t_{max} from Eq. (9). From an epidemiological point of view, the Δt value must necessarily depend on the effectiveness of the precautionary and preventive measures taken by the authorities of each country.

2.2.4 The characteristic contamination frequency

For reverse micelles systems, the energy required to make two micelles appear and activate the exchange of charges between them is called the activation energy of percolation. This energy constitutes a barrier to be crossed for this energy constitutes a barrier to be crossed to put two micelles in contact and trigger the exchange of charges. It takes the form of the famous empirical law of Arrhenius [13]:

$$\sigma = A \exp\left(-E_p/RT\right) \quad (10)$$

Where σ is the electrical conductivity of the micelles. R is the universal constant of ideal gases. T is the temperature. A is a pre-exponential factor having the same unit as σ. Typically, the refinement of Arrhenius law was effected by the Eyring transition state theory [15, 16], where the pre-exponential factor A is shown as the entropic factor of the transition state. In this theory the transition kinetic constant k is correlated with temperature by law analogous to that of Arrhenius:

$$k = A \exp\left(-\Delta H/RT\right) \quad (11)$$

$$k = \frac{K_B T}{h} \exp\left(-\Delta S/R\right) \exp\left(-\Delta H/RT\right) \quad (12)$$

Where k is kinetic constant, ΔS and ΔH are the transition state entropy and enthalpy, K_B is the Boltzmann constant and h is the Planck constant. In another report [16], the pre-exponential factor A was also correlated to motion, rate, disorder, speed ... of particles. Tian Hao [6] considers that the movement of infected individuals and individuals exposed to contamination is analogous to that of the movement of particles in various systems such as granular systems, colloidal systems ... He suggests that the equations of conductivity and viscosity are also applicable in the description of the viruses spread. In his work, he asserts that Eyring Rate Process Theory and Free Volume Concept [6, 17] are applicable on the movement of individuals carrying viruses which means that the more the infected and exposed individuals have the more free volume to move, the higher the probability of transmission.

So, for the virus spread, Arrhenius law can be applied to the cumulative number of infected cases I as follows:

$$I = A_c \exp\left(-t_C/t\right) \quad (13)$$

Having the dimension of time, t_C is equivalent to the Arrhenius temperature $\frac{E_a}{R}$ [16], A_c is a pre-exponential factor considered as the contamination frequency factor and t is the number of days. The contamination frequency A_c can be determined from the slope of the linear portion of the curve:

$$\ln I = \ln A_C - \frac{t_C}{t} \quad (14)$$

2.2.5 Scaling laws and critical exponents

We have mentioned before that the rationalization of the experimental results resulted in two theoretical approaches discussing the state of a system during the percolation phenomenon. A static model which suggests that at the time of percolation, the charge carriers merge with their neighbors, thus establishing a network of connected particles exchanging charges. Besides, a dynamic model whose particles carrying the charges are in permanent collision, merge randomly at the percolation threshold, and exchange the charges. The scheme depicted in **Figure 3** simplifies the difference between the two percolation models.

Theoretically, scale laws have been established to identify the predominant model for a given system. These laws are explained by two equations, which are applied only around the percolation point. For electrical percolation in reverse micelles systems, induced by temperature variation, these equations take the following forms:

$$\sigma = \beta(T_p - T)^{-s}, T<T_p \tag{15}$$

$$\sigma = \gamma(\mathrm{T} - T_p)^{t_s}, T>T_p \tag{16}$$

Where β and γ are free parameters. S and t_s are called the critical exponents. These two laws are valid near to the temperature of the percolation, T_p. Critical exponent values exhibit the difference between static percolation and dynamic percolation [13]. In fact, in the case of static percolation, the predicted theoretical values of critical exponents were found to be $t_s = 1.6$ and $s = 0.7$. Divergence of these values was used to be the proof of dynamic percolation.

In the case of the propagation of Covid-19, these two equations apply to the vicinity of the peak pandemic as follows:

$$I = \beta(t_p - t)^{-s}, t<t_p \tag{17}$$

$$I = \gamma(t - t_p)^{t_s}, t>t_p \tag{18}$$

From an epidemiological point of view, the static percolation model corresponds to the formation of geolocated chains of transmission of the virus [17]. However, the dynamic model reflects randomly distributed chains of transmissions in space.

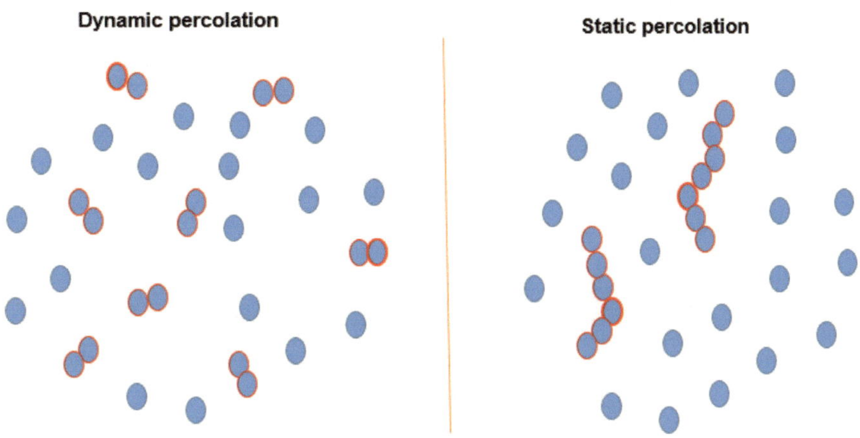

Figure 3.
Schematic representation of the two percolation models.

2.2.6 Speed of the pandemic spread

Typically, to detect the percolation threshold (temperature, volume fraction …), a differential method is used [9, 13]. The method consists of determining the maximum of the curve $\partial\sigma/\partial T$ versus the temperature (volume fraction...). This curve measures the speed of the variation of electrical conductivity as temperature varies.

Similarly, we can consider that the differential, $\partial I_c/\partial t$, measures the speed of propagation of the contamination V_p (and therefore of the virus) as a function of time. Thus, the maximum speed corresponds to the maximum curve $\partial I_c/\partial t$ versus time (Days).

$$V_p = \frac{\partial I_c}{\partial t} \tag{19}$$

3. Application to the cases of China, Tunisia, France, Italy and Germany

Using data provided by Johns Hopkins university resource center [19] on the number of infected cases in 5 countries (China, France, Germany, Italy and Tunisia) during 6 months of the virus spread since the day of the first case detection of until June 30.

3.1 The cumulative number of people infected I_c

We plotted in **Figure 4** the variation of the cumulative number of infected people in each country versus the number of days since the first detected case. The existence of 3 stages can be discerned: a first phase, where the number of cases varies gradually over time. A second phase in which the number of cases unexpectedly rises very quickly and a third phase in which the rate of increase in the number of cases is stabilized overtime. We have therefore adjusted all these curves with the

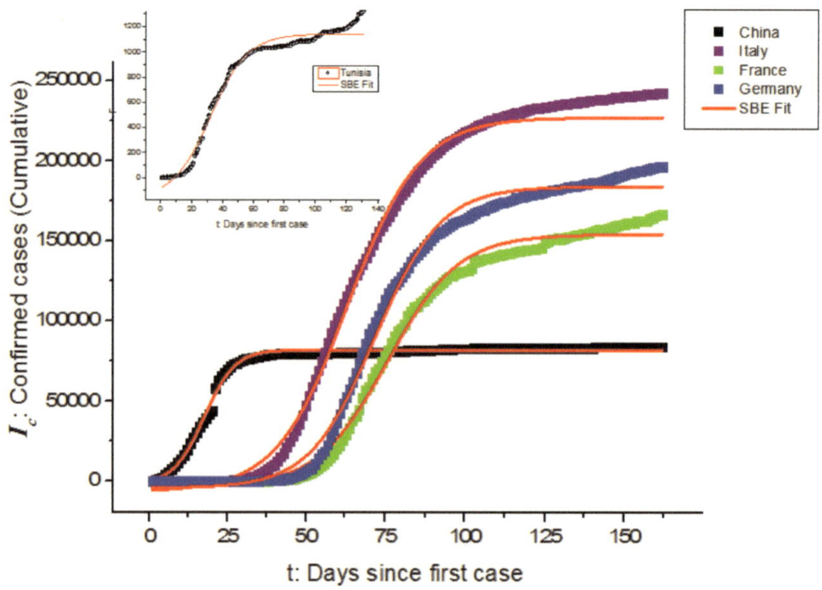

Figure 4.
Variation of the cumulative number of confirmed case I_c versus days since first case t. The red line (—) represents the sigmoid Boltzmann equation fit (SBE).

	N_{max}	t_p	Δt	t_{max}	R^2
China	82011.460	18	4 .944	28.827	0.993
Italy	227262.403	63	11.227	87.587	0.929
France	154264.941	75	10.901	98.873	0.993
Germany	184037.613	71	10.184	93.302	0.994
Tunisia	1142.577	32	12.184	58.682	0.994

Table 2.
Fit parameters of number of infected cases I_c (cumulative) with the SBE equation, for the different countries studied.

sigmoid Boltzmann equation (SBE) (Eq. (6)). The results are listed in **Table 2**. The fit results can therefore be interpreted with respect to the evolution of the epidemic situation as follows:

- **China**

  The number of infected cases reaches maximum of around 82011.46. The rise to this maximum lasts approximately 28 days. The transition point to a stable state is marked around day 18 (pandemic peak) since the first case detected.

- **Tunisia**

  The number of infected cases reaches maximum of around 1142.57. The rise to this maximum lasts for approximately 58 days. The transition point to a stable state is marked around day 32 (approximately 1 month) (pandemic peak) since the first case detected.

- **Italy**

  The number of infected cases reaches maximum of around 227262.40. The rise to this maximum lasts for approximately 87.58 days. The transition point to a stable state is marked around day 63 (approximately 2 months) (pandemic peak) since the first case detected.

- **Germany**

  The number of infected cases reaches maximum of around 227262.40. The rise to this maximum lasts approximately 93.302 days. The transition point to a stable state is marked at day 71 (approximately 2.5 months) (pandemic peak) since the first case detected.

- **France**

  The number of infected cases reaches maximum of around 154264.94. The rise to this maximum lasts approximately 98.873 days. The transition point to a stable state is marked around day 75 (pandemic peak) since the first case detected.

3.2 The contamination frequency A_c

By plotting the Arrhenius curve $Ln(I)$ versus $\frac{1}{t}$ (**Figure 5**), we have calculated the contamination frequency, A_c, from the intercept of its linear portion. The results for the 5 studied countries are listed in **Table 3**. The low values observed for China and

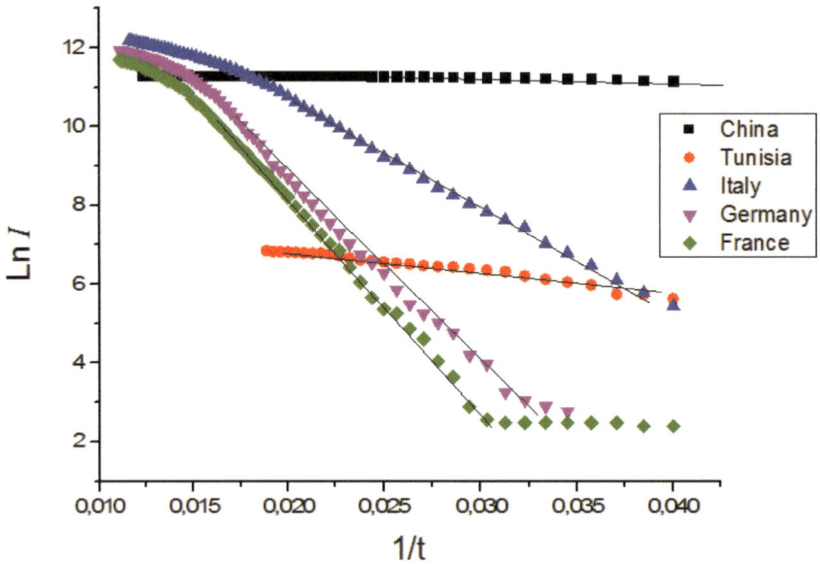

Figure 5.
Arrhenius plot of the number of cumulative infected persons Iversus days.

Tunisia reflect a reduction in the contamination frequency in these two countries. This can be attributed to the anticipation of the authorities of these two countries for reducing the mobility of people by imposing general confinement very early. However, the huge values observed for the 3 European countries reflect a very high contamination frequency. This can be explained by a delay in taking decisions relating to the restriction of people's movement.

3.3 The dynamic behavior of virus spread during the critical period

The determination of the critical exponents (Eqs. (17) and (18)) before (s) and after (t_s) the percolation point informed us about the percolation model which dominated the spread of the virus in each country. The results reported in **Table 3** show values have largely deviated from theoretical values. This represents a very strong tendency toward the dynamic model for all countries. This reveals that the chains of covid-19 virus transmission are randomly distributed in space and the contamination is dispersed in all regions. However, this general trend does not prevent us from observing deviations toward the static model, especially before the pandemic peak (s value), for Tunisia and China.

COUNTRY	S	$\Delta=\|(S-S_{th})\|$	t_s	$\Delta=\|(t_s-t_{th})\|$	A_c
TUNISIA	0.160	0.54	0.037	1.563	2416.317
CHINA	0.170	0.53	0.035	1.565	85819.368
GERMANY	0.123	0.577	0.053	1.547	$2.532.10^8$
FRANCE	0.121	0.579	0.051	1.549	$2.532.10^8$
ITALY	0.076	0.624	0.042	1.558	$1.436.10^7$

Table 3.
The critical exponents and contamination frequency for the 5 studied country.

3.4 Speed of the pandemic spread

In the first section of this article, we stated that the differential $\frac{\partial I}{\partial t}$ estimation of the variation rate in the number of people infected I as a function of the change in the number of days t since the first case is, therefore, the speed of the pandemic spread V_p (Eq. (19)). For the 5 studied countries, we measured this differential. The results were reported in **Figure 6**. As we can see, the speeds of the virus spread in the different countries gradually increase over time until they reach a maximum value $V_{p\,\max}$, then they start to decrease. It is crucial to note that the dates corresponding to the maximum speeds reached coincide with the dates recorded as pandemic peaks $t_p\left(\frac{t}{t_p}=1\right)$ that have been determined by the Boltzmann sigmoid equation (SBE).

Furthermore, we can also notice that the speeds achieved take on considerable values except for Tunisia ($V_{p\,\max} \approx 55$ cases per day), a country which Covid-19 did not greatly affect.

To assess the speed of propagation between the studied countries, we also have adjusted our findings by estimating the root mean square speed of propagation V_{PRMS} for each country:

$$V_{PRMS} = \sqrt{\frac{\sum_i V_{pi}^2}{n}} \tag{20}$$

Where V_{pi} the spread speed for day i and n is the number of days since the first case. In **Figure 7**, we have depicted the variation of the root mean square speed of Covid-19 in the studied 5 countries. As reported, the highest V_{PRMS} was recorded for Italy exceeding the speed of $V_{PRMS} = 2000$ cases/day. However, the lowest one was recorded for Tunisia with a value that does not exceed $V_{PRMS} = 19$ cases/day.

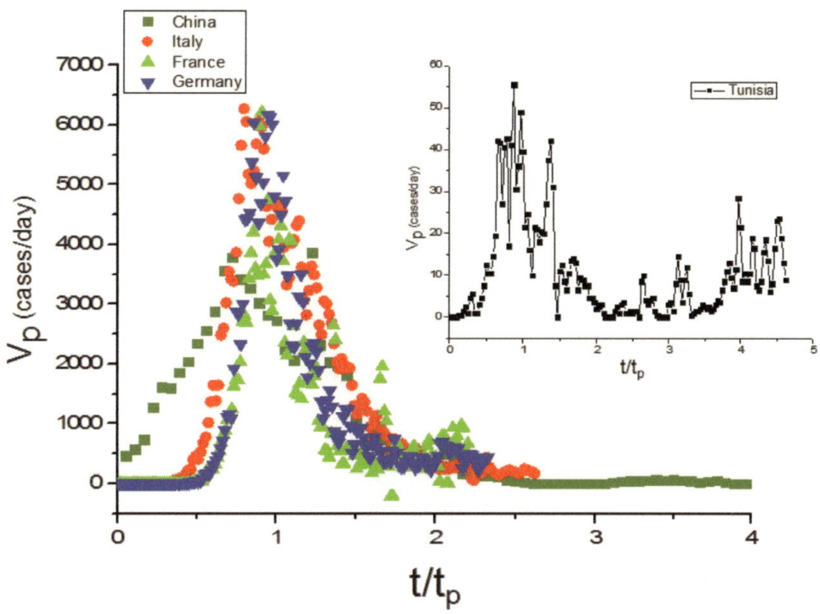

Figure 6.
Speed of the pandemic spread V_p versus $\frac{t}{t_p}$ for the 5 studied countries.

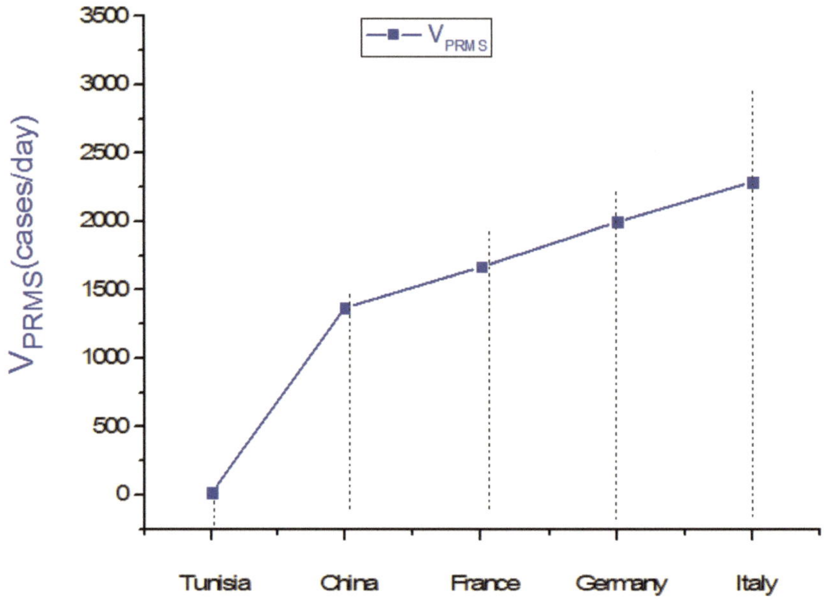

Figure 7.
The root mean square speed of propagation V_{PRMS} since the first case until 30 June, for the 5 studied country.

4. Conclusions

We analyzed epidemic data on the cumulative number of cases infected with covid-19 in 5 countries affected differently by the pandemic. The data describe the state of the virus spread during more than 6 months of its appearance (appeared at the beginning in China (December 2019)). This analysis was consisted of the application of the percolation theory on the evolution of the cumulative number of people infected I_c in each country. Based on an analogy between the spread of Covid-19 in a population and the electrical percolation of reverse micelles, we introduced the covid-19 pandemic percolation. First, adjusting the data using the Boltzmann sigmoid equation (SBE) made it possible to derive important parameters related to the spread of the pandemic: The first represents the cumulative number of people infected $I_{c,\,\max}$, from which the epidemic state in each country begins to stabilize. The second is the pandemic peak time t_p (threshold of pandemic percolation), this is a critical day corresponding to the transformation of the epidemic situation from serious to stable state. The third is a time interval Δt that we have called the time constant. This constant represents the momentum of exponential pandemic progression in each country. It allowed us to estimate the time necessary $t_{\max}$ for the stabilization of the epidemic state in each country. Comparing the value of this constant in each country makes it possible to assess the effectiveness of the preventive measures taken by the authorities.

By applying the Arrhenius law on the cumulative number of cases in each country, we introduced a characteristic contamination factor this rate measures the frequency of interpersonal contact in each country. This permits us to compare contamination frequency following the traffic restriction measures taken by each country (border closure, general confinement, geo-located confinement, etc.). The application of scale laws at the vicinity of the percolation threshold t_p has shown a total predominance of the dynamic percolation model of contamination. This predominance has been interpreted by the existence of transmission chains of the virus randomly distributed in each country (and not local chains).

Finally, the determination of the propagation speed V_p of covid-19 in each country showed that the maximum propagation speed was recorded during the pandemic peak t_p (previously determined by SBE equation). Moreover, the calculation of the quadratic mean root square speed of propagation V_{PRMS} allowed us to compare the evolution of the speed in each country.

Finally, all of the results show that Tunisia and China have implemented the most effective strategies to combat the first wave of Covid-19. Indeed, Tunisia's authorities have opted for general containment (lockdown) throughout the country since the second week after the first confirmed case of Covid-19 was discovered. According to our findings, this strategy significantly reduced the frequency of contact between individuals carrying the virus, as well as the speed of covid-19 propagation over the next three months. As a result, the total number of cases infected with covid-19 remained very low. This clearly demonstrates the effectiveness of this strategy in combating the pandemic. In addition, the second country which showed low propagation indicators (contact frequency, speed of propagation, total number of infected people) is China. This is due to China's adoption of a strategy known as targeted containment. That is, the confinement was limited to the city of Wuhan (the site of the virus's appearance). Such a strategy has clearly demonstrated its effectiveness by significantly slowing propagation. However, the three European countries (Italy, France, and Germany) experienced relatively high propagation rates as well as a high number of covid-19 cases. These outcomes are the result of the authorities' failure to implement general containment procedures on the right time.

This further proves that the most effective strategy to bypass the spread of covid-19 is either general containment or targeted containment.

Acknowledgements

The authors gratefully acknowledge financial support from the Tunisian Ministry of Education, Research, and Technology.

Conflict of interest

The authors declare that they have no competing interests.

Author details

Moez Guettari* and Ahmed El Aferni
Preparatory Institute for Engineering Studies of Tunis, Fluids and Materials Laboratory, University of Tunis, Tunis, Tunisia

*Address all correspondence to: gtarimoez@Yahoo.fr

References

[1] Fernandes N: Economic effects of coronavirus outbreak (COVID-19) on the world economy Nuno Fernandes Full Professor of Finance IESE Business School Spain. SSRN Electron. Journal, ISSN. 2020; 1556-5068, Elsevier BV, 0–29.

[2] Zhang X, Ma R, Wang L: Predicting turning point, duration and attack rate of COVID-19 outbreaks in major Western countries. Chaos, Solitons and Fractals. 2020; 135:. https://doi.org/10.1016/j.chaos.2020.109829

[3] Boudrioua MS, Boudrioua A: Predicting the COVID-19 epidemic in Algeria using the SIR model. 2020; 1–11. https://doi.org/10.1101/2020.04.25.20079467

[4] Fanelli D, Piazza F: Analysis and forecast of COVID-19 spreading in China, Italy and France. Chaos, Solitons and Fractals. 2020; 134:109761. https://doi.org/10.1016/j.chaos.2020.109761

[5] Chakraborty T, Ghosh I: Highlights ➢ Forecasting COVID-19 and assessing its risk are some real challenges. Chaos, Solitons Fractals Interdiscip J Nonlinear Sci Nonequilibrium Complex Phenom. 2020; 109850. https://doi.org/10.1016/j.chaos.2020.109850

[6] Hao T: Infection Dynamics of Coronavirus Disease 2019 (Covid-19) Modeled with the Integration of the Eyring Rate Process Theory and Free Volume Concept. medRxiv. 2020; https://doi.org/10.1101/2020.02.26.20028571

[7] El Aferni A, Guettari M, Tajouri T: Mathematical model of Boltzmann's sigmoidal equation applicable to the spreading of the coronavirus (Covid-19) waves. Environ Sci Pollut Res. 2020; https://doi.org/10.1007/s11356-020-11188-y

[8] Guettari M, Ben Naceur I, Kassab G, Tajouri T: Temperature effect on the inter-micellar collision and maximum packaging volume fraction in water/AOT/isooctane micro-emulsions. J Chem Thermodyn. 2016; 95:183–189. https://doi.org/10.1016/j.jct.2015.12.011

[9] Guettari M, Aferni AE, Tajouri T: Effect of micellar collisions and polyvinylpyrrolidone confinement on the electrical conductivity percolation parameters of water/AOT/isooctane reverse micelles. J Mol Struct. 2017; 1149:712–719. https://doi.org/10.1016/j.molstruc.2017.08.026

[10] Broadbent S.R., Hammersley J.M: Percolation processes: I. Crystals and mazes. Math. Proc. Cambridge Philos. Soc. 1957; 53, 629–641. https://doi.org/10.1017/S0305004100032680

[11] Stauffer D, Aharony A. Introduction to percolation theory. second edition (Taylor Francis), London ; 1992.

[12] Jada A, Lang J, Zana R: Relation between Electrical Percolation and Rate Constant for Exchange of Material between Droplets in Water in Oil Microemulsions. 1989; 10–12

[13] Mehta SK, Sharma S: Temperature-induced percolation behavior of AOT reverse micelles affected by poly (ethylene glycol)s. J Colloid Interface Sci. 2006; 296:690–699. https://doi.org/10.1016/j.jcis.2005.09.035

[14] Hait SK, Moulik SP, Palepu R: Refined method of assessment of parameters of micellization of surfactants and percolation of W/O microemulsions. Langmuir. 2002; 18: 2471–2476. https://doi.org/10.1021/la0110794

[15] Laidler, K.J., King M.C.: The development of transition-state theory. J. Phys. Chem. 1983; 87, 2657–2664. https://doi.org/10.1021/j100238a002

[16] Haj-Kacem RB, Ouerfelli N, Herráez J V: Contribution to modeling the viscosity Arrhenius-type equation for some solvents by statistical correlations analysis. Fluid Phase Equilib. 2014; 383: 11–20. https://doi.org/10.1016/j.fluid.2014.09.023

[17] Hao T: Analogous viscosity equations of granular powders based on Eyring's rate process theory and free volume concept. RSC Adv. 2015; 5: 95318–95333. https://doi.org/10.1039/c5ra16706j

[18] Davis S, Trapman P, Leirs H: The abundance threshold for plague as a critical percolation phenomenon. 2008; 454:2–5. https://doi.org/10.1038/nature07053

[19] COVID-19 Dashboard by the Center for Systems Science and Engineering (CSSE) at Johns Hopkins University (JHU). Available from: https://coronavirus.jhu.edu/map.html

Chapter 29

The Link between Electrical Properties of COVID-19 and Electromagnetic Radiation

Awaad K. Al Sarkhi

Abstract

The ability of a new vaccine design based on control the intracellular physiological consequences of both the electrical properties and the electromagnetic radiation interactions between a virus and a host cell, which is a method to strengthen immune system develop protection against COVID-19 and new strains. The capacity of COVID-19 to bind to angiotensin-converting enzyme 2 (ACE2) and immune evasion mechanisms are only one of the properties required to stimulate a preventative immune response. In this chapter, a multidimensional new strategy is used to exemplify the empowerment function intracellular and extracellular level information can play in the support of immunogen against COVID-19 pathogens. Besides during this chapter, the nature of electromagnetic radiation is described as a vibrating string based on a string-theory and unification of electromagnetic radiation and gravitational waves by supporting with multiple cites strong evidence. Overall, we demonstrate a new approach to understand the important role of the physiological consequences of the interplay between the immune system and COVID-19 and designing vaccine strategy immunogens that take advantage of that information against COVID-19 and new strains.

Keywords: COVID-19, Electrophysiology, Electrostatic Discharge (ESD), Electromagnetic Radiation (EMR), Voltage-Viral Channels, Zinc Homeostasis

1. Introduction

Vaccine design is either a method, or style, or programming to activate the immune system to help the immune system develop protection against infectious disease. Vaccination includes various strategies of immunogen designs [1–3]. In this chapter, we describe a new strategy based on events for the COVID-19 's journey to and interaction with the host cells, it seems to have the ability to induce a protective response against COVID-19 pathogens.

As known COVID-19 is adept at evasion host immune responses [4] and interfere with several receptor signaling pathways such as chemokine receptors to produce an active inflammatory response [5, 6]. Our previous work has shown the electrical properties of COVID-19 [7]. On another hand, many studies have shown a stronger electrotactic attraction over chemical gradients for human T cells led to migration [8]. This provides insight into the stronger electrotactic attraction for COVID-19 over chemical gradients for human T cell migration, and this reason virus interfered with several receptors signaling to prevent activation of the host innate immune system to allow for COVID-19 replication. This means the COVID-19 have electrical properties to evade interferon signaling and induction to avoid the antiviral agents of the host immune system. Evasion of the host antiviral immune response is critical for COVID-19 replication or spread. That is why some humans get very sick and may lead to death while some do not severely sick or even have no symptoms, and the reasons some humans have long-term impacts throughout their body, maybe get very sick and may lead to death.

In many types of the viral envelope, it has the viral ion channel in the small envelope membrane proteins like viroporins [9–12]. From a role and function in the viroporin life cycle standpoint, it has viral protein with viral ion channel proteins have been shown to play a significant role to help in multiple processes of the journey for viral to and interaction with the host cells, such as CoV (SARS-CoV), influenza A, Human immunodeficiency virus (HIV)-1 [13, 14].

2. COVID-19's journey to and interaction with the host cells

The electrical and electromagnetic radiation events are one of the first indications that virus is undergoing activation steps during infection to replicate the viral genome. There are four steps to and interaction with the host cells leads to having symptoms and long-term impacts throughout the body, maybe get very sick and may lead to death.

Step I. COVID-19 Migration: Virus is attracted by either chemical or electrical factors and which are released via the target cells. The behavioral response of a virus is the pattern of movement during an external stimulus such as electrotaxis and chemotaxis that leads the migration of the virus towards target cells. Several electrotaxis studies have shown that electrotaxis in the body in many cells plays an important role in physiological processes that can direct the migration of various cell types such as inflammation, cancer cells, and immune cells [15, 16]. Mutual electrotaxis and chemotaxis of the virus-host cell is a critical element of these events; electrical signals from the host cell investments induce spectacular changes in form and function of the virus, and the virus triggers the quiescent host cell into protease activation, cleavage and activation allow the virus to enter the host cell.

Step II. Binding and interaction of virus-host cell: After virus migration to the target cells to bind. Many studies have shown that a Spike protein on the virus can bind to angiotensin-converting enzyme 2 (ACE2) receptors on the host cells [5]. The angiotensin-converting enzyme 2 (ACE2) is a zinc-containing metalloenzyme [17]. An angiotensin-converting enzyme 2 (ACE2) does play an essential role in maintaining the physiological and homeostasis in the body [17]. The membrane proteins for COVID-19 sense electrical energy by electrotaxis according to the important role of zinc in angiotensin-converting enzyme 2 (ACE2) is converting chemical energy into electrical energy leads to binding to (ACE2) receptors that are found on the surface of many human cells. Angiotensin-converting enzyme 2 (ACE2) is located on the surface of cells such as (lung, arterial and venous endothelial, enterocytes of the small intestine, and other) cells [18, 19].

Step III Electrical events link with an emitted electromagnetic radiation: In the biological cell, contains ions (the potassium $K+$ and chloride anion $Cl–$) are inside the cell, and ions (sodium $Na+$, calcium $Ca2+$ cations, and chloride anion $Cl–$ (at higher concentration) are outside the cell [20]. After the virus enters a host cell leads it to changes the electrical steady state of the virus because the different distribution of electrical charges inside and outside the virus leads to an electrical gradient (voltage) across the membrane. This electrical gradient is a difference across the viral membrane that generates a store of potential energy in the form of an electrochemical gradient [21], which helps create the electric field or an electrical potential by the movement of ions across the two sides of the membrane [22, 23]. The viral membrane marks the border between the internal and external of the COVID-19 particle, which means, here the difference in electric potential between the inside and outside the COVID-19 particle. Thus, the viral membrane is responsible for the establishment of the electrical potential and serves as an insulator, all this indicates that there are lost or gained an electron, so there are lost or gained electrical charges. In another word, the viral membrane functions as an insulator and a diffusion channel to the movement of electrical charges, we will call it "Voltage-Viral Channels". The voltage-viral channels are formed by the movement of electrical charges that are activated by changes in the viral membrane potential close and open the viral channels. The viral membrane potential changes the modification of viral channels by complex mechanisms are regulating either closing or opening, and voltage-viral channels directionally diffuse the electrical signals. Virus enters host cells after binding via charges conductivity, the voltage-viral charges channels embedded in a COVID-19's envelope can actively collaborate in a COVID-19 entry through an endocytic process, whereas the customary view considered a spike protein is a part that appears to play a key role in entry to the host cell [4].

Moreover, the movement of ions generates an electric current by membrane depolarization (the influx of positive charge), in repeated motifs are regular by opening and closing of the channels because of a high potential difference. This electrical potential (high voltage) of the fluid surrounding a spike (S) protein is being electrically charged leads to generate corona discharge as results being a charged spike (S) protein have a sharp point, in adding to the protein–protein interactions (PPIs) leads to generate electrostatic force [24–26]. One of the side effects from an electrostatic discharge (ESD) is an induced to generate a corona discharge method, according to our previous work [7]. The corona discharge is a series reaction are creating a free electron that ionizes atoms surrounding it to create a positive ion and a free electron [24]. A corona discharge is classified into two general categories based on the type of attraction if all the electrons are attracted inward and the ions are repelled outwards, called a positive corona, else all the ions are attracted inward and all the electrons are repelled outwards, called a negative corona [24]. When the electrons from an inner orbit are released, the vacancy will be filled by the electrons from an outer orbit led to the excess energy from this shift is emitted as electromagnetic radiation, thus serve to ionize other atoms [27]. The emitted ionized radiation via the corona discharge method ionizes different cellular compartments inside the host cell. This emitted ionizing radiation can be damaged deoxyribonucleic acid (DNA) for host cell or many sorts of mutagens, thus cause host cell death via apoptosis [28].

Step IV. Fusion of virus-host cell: In the corona discharge method, occurs through a difference of electrical potential of the space surrounding a spike (S) protein, it in the COVID-19's envelope, that is electrically charged by voltage-viral channels. In adding to the protein–protein interactions (PPI) that occur between COVID-19 proteins (spike (S), envelope (E), membrane (M), and nucleocapsid (N), are disassembled under this high voltage condition, resulting in that form viral fusion, according to the phenomenon by Zimmermann [29, 30]. The fusion virus-host cell fusion finally triggers the fusion of the COVID-19 and endosomal membranes, leading to the release of virus RNA genome in the host cell cytoplasm, thus, the loss of ion homeostasis or fluctuation in the level of the ion triggered by COVID-19 activity excites the activation of the host defensive programmed cell death pathways, from stress responses to apoptosis [28]. Finally, COVID-19 is replication and secreted from the host cell through exocytosis [31].

Step V. Activation and the disorganized immune response: Besides modifying cellular processes to support COVID-19 propagation, the stress responses to apoptosis triggered by an electrical and an electromagnetic radiation events activity may have deleterious consequences for the host cell leads to inflammatory in response to virus such as the cytokines, chemokines in plasma, and chemokine-receptor, and interfere with several receptors signaling pathway [6]. Because the COVID-19 seems is an electrically excitable virus has a structure that permits virus to pass chemical signal or an electrical signal to another virus or to the host cell that actively responds to effects some change brings it about and a stimulus such as B cell, T cells, Cytokine, chemokine, chemokine receptor, cytokines, and mast cell that (involved in the development of asthma or allergic rhinitis). These cells and their receptors produce an incongruous signal cause by the disorganized immune responses. Sometimes the properties electrical for COVID-19 permit to pass an electrical signal without the need for angiotensin-converting enzyme 2 (ACE2) receptors to recognize chemical messengers, as known in neurons cells the electrical signal transmission is faster than that which occurs across the chemical signal. The COVID-19 factories will be able to direct the synthesis of viral proteins by they possess both fusion functions and encode their genetic information using an RNA genome by forcing them to rapidly-produce thousands of similar copies of COVID-19 in the human cell. In changes to membrane potential for host cell during the second step and third step, because the electric field is the gradient of the voltage distribution, in general, electrical signals within biological cells are driven by ions [29, 30]. This means that there is a change in membrane potential and property host cell excitability if it is considered to have an excitable membrane (e.g., taste receptors, beta cells, alpha cells, delta cells, enteroendocrine cells, and immune cells) [32]. Cell excitability. Such COVID-19 pump takes in virus from one side of the membrane (decreasing its concentration there) and releases them on the other side (increasing its concentration there) such as processes concentration gradients across the membrane [29, 30].

Finally, novel viruses are produced from infected cells by transport, thus that can infect other cells. While both a protease and a zinc metalloenzyme inside the (ACE2) uses electrical charges or electrical signal to push a non-spontaneous redox reaction such as process electrolysis. As known protease is often used to catalyzes the breakdown of proteins, with supplementary helping mechanisms from viruses [33]. Because the COVID-19 has an electric potential as discussed under Step III when COVID-19 migration to the (ACE2) this means occurs electrolysis.

3. Mechanisms of zinc metalloenzyme

In several studies have shown either the metal zinc, or ions zinc, or zinc transporters, or zinc signals, it has acted in different cellular functions and function of immune cells for both innate immune responses and adaptive immune responses [34–37]. This chapter explains the mechanisms of zinc metalloenzyme being necessary for regulating zinc homeostasis in the body. The angiotensin-converting enzyme 2 (ACE2), contains a zinc metalloenzyme [17], in addition to the angiotensin-converting enzyme 2 (ACE2) protein contains protease and amino acid [17], which means that both a protease and a zinc metalloenzyme in the angiotensin-converting enzyme 2 (ACE2) are often used to generate an electric current from spontaneous redox reactions like as electrical battery, has two different metalloenzymes connected by a salt bridge (amino acid) externally completing an angiotensin-converting enzyme 2 (ACE2). An angiotensin-converting enzyme 2 (ACE2) is using this electric current seemingly as signals.

To understand an (ACE2) is extensions of spontaneous redox reactions, in this redox reaction, zinc metalloenzyme or metal is oxidized to ions ($Zn2+$) and ions other electrode is reduced to metalloenzyme or metal such as two electrodes (a cathode and an anode). When electrons are transferred directly from Zn to ions another electrode, is allowing the chemical energy interconversion to electrical energy. In the zinc metalloenzyme such as (half-cell), which is inside the (ACE2), the zinc dissolves via oxidation into the oxidation ions ($Zn2+$), other words releasing electrons. Results the zinc ion concentration increased to recompense via amino acid, which is inside the (ACE2), the zinc ions leave, and anions enter the zinc. In the other electrode such as (another half-cell), the ions onto this electrode reduce, taking up electrons that are leaving the zinc.

4. Vaccine strategy

To optimize vaccine design, it seems relevant to investigate the relationship between the electrophysiology properties for COVID-19, which can include the COVID-19 's journey to and electrochemical interactions with the host cells, and the regulate zinc homeostasis on an intracellular level which includes (the mechanisms of zinc metalloenzyme inside the angiotensin-converting enzyme 2 (ACE2), zinc transporters, and zinc signals) through the physical processes. In several studies have shown the zinc is an essential supplement that serves to regulate different physiological mechanisms, it has antiviral properties [34–37]. It is well known that zinc homeostasis or the zinc metalloenzyme homeostasis is crucial for a single cell or even inside cell level, protects the cell against oxidative damages, and supports on functions of the immune system [34].

Consequently, by investigating from this relationship, the findings that are the regulated zinc homeostasis on the intracellular level is targeted to inhibit or prevent COVID-19 before infection or even infection has already occurred. Zinc-regulation plays a critical and essential role in maintaining immune cell numbers and activities. The surprising efficiency of the influence on influenza virus, HCV, SARS-CoV-2, treatment of COVID-19, suggest a novel strategy for the vaccine design of COVID-19. Continuous monitor every period of the zinc homeostasis in the body, and correct zinc homeostasis if there is a defect in zinc homeostasis. This strategy can enhance antiviral immunity and innate immunity functions, it holds promise as an effective vaccine design strategy that should be further explored.

5. The nature of electromagnetic radiation (EM radiation)

To exploitation of biophysics, electrochemical, and physical processes for combat infectious diseases by blocking or disrupting their electrostatic discharge (ESD) properties link with electromagnetic radiation (EM) interactions something in a skillful manner. Here, electromagnetic radiation is imagined as a flow of tones produce via the vibrating strings with free ends, whereas tones produce via the vibrating strings with fixed ends in the darkness. In nature the electromagnetic radiation, more studies have suggested that the electromagnetic radiation has behaved either a wave or a particle, and some of the studies have suggested, it behaves as a wave and a particle at the same time. In this chapter, we will raise the conjecture (the purport of which will hereafter be called the "Principle of Diplopia and String"), to the status of a postulate, and introduce another postulate, which is only apparently irreconcilable with the former, namely, that the introduction of a "gravitational wave" will prove to be necessary since the view here to be developed will require a unification of electromagnetic radiation and gravitational waves. Those two postulates suffice for the attainment of a simple and consistent theory of electromagnetic radiation. Thus, those two principles contribute as key to solve the mystery of the wave-particle duality for objects, the darkness, the dark energy.

5.1 Vibrating strings with free ends

To describe the electromagnetic radiation based on the principle of diplopia and string. We must imagine the electron, which that is a closed vibrating string loop or an opened vibrating string. To render our presentation more precise and to distinguish this electron verbally from others which will be introduced hereafter, we call it the "electronString" and the free electronString. Thus, that is an electronString, which is the quotient of a combination between energy, and its mass ($-$ 9.11 x 10^{-31} kg) [38].

If the electromagnetic radiation is imagined as a flow of tones, these tones we will call the "photonTone" with each photonTone carrying a separated packet of energy. To prove these tones means sound waves, and sound waves are part of the electromagnetic. First, according to several studies of electromagnetic radiation, which is a vibration of electric and magnetic fields at right angles. Accordingly, the tones or a sound wave are a disturbance that travels through a medium, this medium is a vibration of electric and magnetic fields, where here the tones, which is a vibration of electric and magnetic fields.

Let us apply the pair production [39, 40], based on the principle of diplopia and string when photonTone at extreme energy (gamma ray) can create two electronStrings. Here, the gamma ray or high photonTone, makes an electronString and its anti electronString, where the anti electronString is positively charged with the same mass as the electronString. By several studies have shown the sound waves carrying mass [41], and because the photonTone is a flow of tones carrying by a tones separated packet of energy, which means these photonTones carrying mass. Because we used a photonTone at extreme energy, this means the tones (sound wave) could carry much of mass to produces an electronString and its anti electronString. These two electronStrings can recombine with each other and create the photonTones. Thus, with the help of certain imaginary physical experiments we have settled what is to be understood by:

$$(\text{es}-) + \text{es} \rightarrow \text{pht} + \text{pht} \tag{1}$$

where,
(es−): an electronString = -9.11×10^{-31} kg + pht (its energy),
es: a positronString = 9.11×10^{-31} kg + pht (its energy), and
pht: an emitted photonString.

$$(-9.11 \text{ x } 10^{-31}\text{kg}) + \text{pht} + 9.11 \text{ x } 10^{-31}\text{kg} + \text{pht} \text{ -----> pht} + \text{pht} \tag{2}$$

Thus, when a number or amount (9.11 x 10^{-31} kg) is subtracted from itself, the results is zero.

$$\text{pht} + \text{pht} \rightarrow \text{pht} + \text{pht} \tag{3}$$

When applying the photoelectric effect as shown in **Figure 1** based on the principle of diplopia and string, when a photonTone incident on an atom transfers all its energy to this electronString, while the electronString containing the energy of the photonTone leaves the orbit of the atom.

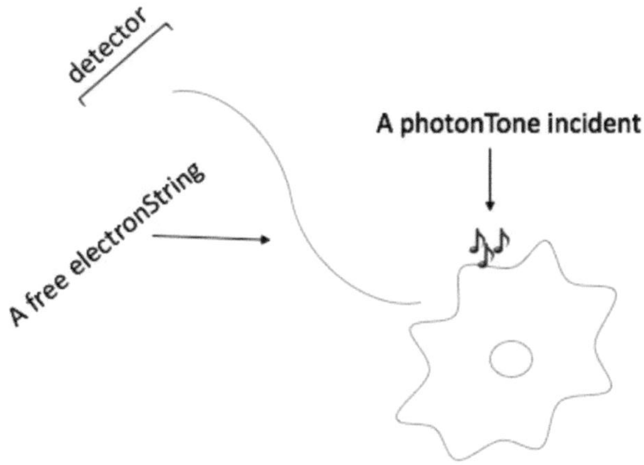

Figure 1.
Here, a photon incident on a hydrogen atom transfers its energy to an electronString, which leaves the orbit and is detected.

Each electronString has a certain amount of binding energy, which is the minimum energy that is required to remove an electronString from an atom, this electronString is held in place by the electrostatic pull of the positively charged nucleus. For example, when an electronString absorbs a photonTone incident, this electronString becomes the move to a higher energy shell or become a free electronString, when this electronString drops back down to a lower-energy shell. Thus, this electronString will release energy represent a photonTone. Now, the electromagnetic radiation can be pictured as a vibrating photonTone by oscillating electric and magnetic fields that move in a straight line at a constant velocity.

5.2 Vibrating strings with fixed ends

If darkness is imagined as a flow of tones, these tones are producing via the vibrating strings with fixed ends by the gravitational wave, thus can generate standing waves. Where the gravitational waves squeeze and stretch strings in their path as they pass by to vibrate the string produce their tones, these tones represent energy. The tones are standing wave modes that arise from the combination of reflection and interference such that the reflected waves interfere constructively with the incident waves.

In the musical instrument, the vibrating strings are squeeze and stretch the string in their path as they pass by to vibrate the string produce their tones [42], as in the darkness is created from two waves with equal frequency, amplitude, and wavelength traveling in opposite directions by applying superposition. Where occur the destructive or constructive interference of counter-propagating waves one form of energy decreases and the other increases such that the total energy remains constant, we will call this a pair of the superposition of standing waves "diplopia waves".

6. Conclusion

Effectiveness of vaccine against several types of viruses such as COVID-19 is mainly realized through investigating the relationship between the electrophysiology properties for a virus, and the regulate zinc homeostasis on intracellular level through the physical processes such as viral binding, membrane fusion, and infection. The regulated zinc homeostasis serves to stabilize the membrane potential which could play a role in preventing the virus of COVID-19 entry into the host cell. In additionally, the regulated zinc homeostasis serves to inhibit viral replication by protecting the deoxyribonucleic acid (DNA) from damage via an emitted ionizing radiation or mutagens as discussed under step III, protect the cells from exposure to oxidizing agents because the Zn2+ concentrations are directly belonging to the intracellular redox state. Interestingly, all this evidence used in this chapter supports the essential role for regulating zinc homeostasis to inhibit the physiological consequences as discussed under step III by this new vaccine strategy. This vaccine strategy is based on the properties of COVID-19, the voltage-viral charges channel activity required to inhibit the physiological consequences via dampening specific electrochemical functions associated with COVID-19's journey to and interaction with the host cells and to strengthen immune system develop protection against COVID-19 and new strains.

Conflict of interest

The author declares no conflict of interest.

Author details

Awaad K. Al Sarkhi
College of Science, Technology, Engineering, and Mathematics [CSTEM], University of Arkansas at Little Rock, USA

*Address all correspondence to: aalsarkhi@ualr.edu

'Biotechnology to Combat COVID-19' is a collaborative project with Biotechnology Kiosk

References

[1] Irvine DJ, Aung A, Silva M: Controlling timing and location in vaccines. Advanced Drug Delivery Reviews. 2020;158: 91-115. DOI: 10.1016/j.addr.2020.06.019

[2] Nabel GJ: Designing tomorrow's vaccines. New England Journal of Medicine. 2013;368:551-560. DOI: 10.1056/NEJMra1204186

[3] Haynes BF, Burton DR: Developing an HIV vaccine. Science. 2017;355:1129-1130. DOI: 10.1126/science.aan0662

[4] Taefehshokr N, Taefehshokr S, Hemmat N, Heit B: Covid-19: Perspectives on Innate Immune Evasion. Frontiers in immunology. 2020;11. DOI: 10.3389/fimmu.2020.580641

[5] Ni W, Yang X, Yang D, Bao J, Li R, Xiao Y, Hou C, Wang H, Liu J, Yang D, Xu Y: Role of angiotensin-converting enzyme 2 (ACE2) in COVID-19. Critical Care. 2020 Dec;24(1):1-0. DOI: 10.1186/s13054-020-03120-0

[6] Khalil BA, Elemam NM, Maghazachi AA: Chemokines and chemokine receptors during COVID-19 infection. Computational and Structural Biotechnology Journal. 2021;19: 976-988. DOI: 10.1016/j.csbj.2021.01.034

[7] Al Sarkhi AK: Hypothesis: The electrical properties of coronavirus. Electromagnetic biology and medicine. 2020 Oct 1;39(4):433-436. DOI: 10.1080/15368378.2020.1830794

[8] Wu J, Lin F: Recent developments in electrotaxis assays. Advances in wound care. 2014 Feb 1;3(2):149-155. DOI: 10.1089/wound.2013.0453

[9] Delcour A. H, editors. book of Electrophysiology of Unconventional Channels and Pores. Springer: Cham; 2015. DOI: 10.1007/978-3-319-20149-8

[10] Nieva JL, Madan V, Carrasco L: Viroporins: structure and biological functions. Nature Reviews Microbiology. 2012;10:563-574. DOI: 10.1038/nrmicro2820

[11] Giorda KM, Hebert DN: Viroporins customize host cells for efficient viral propagation. DNA and cell biology. 2013;32:557-564. DOI: 10.1089/dna.2013.2159

[12] Verdiá-Báguena C, Nieto-Torres JL, Alcaraz A, DeDiego ML, Torres J, Aguilella VM, Enjuanes L: Coronavirus E protein forms ion channels with functionally and structurally-involved membrane lipids. Virology. 2012 Oct 25;432(2):485-494. DOI: 10.1016/j.virol.2012.07.005

[13] Sze C, Tan YJ: Viral membrane channels: role and function in the virus life cycle. Viruses. 2015;7(6):3261-3284. DOI: 10.3390/v7062771

[14] Pinto LH, Holsinger LJ, Lamb RA: Influenza virus M2 protein has ion channel activity. Cell. 1992;69:517-528. DOI: 10.1016/0092-8674(92)90452-I.

[15] Wang SJ, Saadi W, Lin F, Nguyen CM, Jeon NL: Differential effects of EGF gradient profiles on MDA-MB-231 breast cancer cell chemotaxis. Experimental cell research. 2004 Oct 15;300(1):180-189. DOI: 10.1016/j.yexcr.2004.06.030

[16] Zigmond SH, Levitsky HI, Kreel BJ: Cell polarity: an examination of its behavioral expression and its consequences for polymorphonuclear leukocyte chemotaxis. The Journal of cell biology. 1981 Jun;89(3):585-592. DOI: 10.1083/jcb.89.3.585

[17] Turner AJ: ACE2 cell biology, regulation, and physiological functions. The Protective Arm of the Renin Angiotensin System

(RAS). 2015:185. DOI: 10.1016/B978-0-12-801364-9.00025-0

[18] Hamming I, Timens W, Bulthuis ML, Lely AT, Navis GV, van Goor H: Tissue distribution of ACE2 protein, the functional receptor for SARS coronavirus. A first step in understanding SARS pathogenesis. The Journal of Pathology: A Journal of the Pathological Society of Great Britain and Ireland. 2004 Jun;203(2):631-637. DOI: 10.1002/path.1570

[19] Kuba K, Imai Y, Penninger JM: Angiotensin-converting enzyme 2 in lung diseases. Current opinion in pharmacology. 2006 Jun 1;6(3):271-276. DOI: 10.1016/j.coph.2006.03.001

[20] Alberts B, Johnson A, Lewis J, Morgan D, Raff M, Roberts K, Walter P, Wilson J, Hunt T: Biologia molecular da célula. Artmed Editora; 2010; 1464. ISBN: 8582714238

[21] AZZONE GF, PIETROBON D, ZORATTI M: Determination of the proton electrochemical gradient across biological membranes. Current topics in bioenergetics. 1984 Jan 1;13:1-77. DOI: 10.1016/B978-0-12-152513-2.50008-8

[22] Mummert H, Gradmann D: Action potentials in Acetabularia: measurement and simulation of voltage-gated fluxes. The Journal of membrane biology. 1991 Dec;124(3):265-273. DOI: 10.1007/BF01994359

[23] Höhner R, Aboukila A, Kunz HH, Venema K: Proton gradients and proton-dependent transport processes in the chloroplast. Frontiers in plant science. 2016 Feb 29;7:218. DOI: 10.3389/fpls.2016.00218

[24] Kaiser KL: Electrostatic discharge. Technology & Engineering. 2005;344.

[25] Loeb LB: Electrical coronas, their basic physical mechanisms. University of California Press; 1965.

[26] Lüttgens G, Lüttgens S, Schubert W: Static Electricity: Understanding, Controlling, Applying. John Wiley & Sons; 2017 Aug 25.

[27] Curtiss LA, Raghavachari K, Redfern PC, Rassolov V, Pople JA: Gaussian-3 (G3) theory for molecules containing first and second-row atoms. The Journal of chemical physics. 1998 Nov 8;109(18):7764-7776. DOI: 10.1016/S0009-2614(01)01345-8

[28] Norbury CJ, Zhivotovsky B: DNA damage-induced apoptosis. Oncogene. 2004 Apr;23(16):2797-2808. DOI: 10.1038/sj.onc.1207532

[29] Scheurich, P. and Zimmermann, U: Giant human erythrocytes by electric-field-induced cell-to-cell fusion. Naturwissenschaften. 1981 Jan 1;68(1), pp.45-47. DOI: 10.1007%2FBF01047168

[30] Zimmermann U, Vienken J: Electric field-induced cell-to-cell fusion. The Journal of membrane biology. 1982 Dec;67(1):165-182.

[31] Nieto-Torres JL, Verdiá-Báguena C, Castaño-Rodriguez C, Aguilella VM, Enjuanes L: Relevance of viroporin ion channel activity on viral replication and pathogenesis. Viruses. 2015 Jul;7(7):3552-3573. DOI: 10.3390/v7072786

[32] Josephson RK, Schwab WE: Electrical properties of an excitable epithelium. The Journal of general physiology. 1979 Aug;74(2):213-236. DOI: 10.1085/jgp.74.2.213

[33] Dalabehera NR, Meher S, Bhusana Palai B, Sharma NK: Instability of Amide Bond with Trifluoroacetic Acid (20%): Synthesis, Conformational Analysis, and Mechanistic Insights into Cleavable Amide Bond Comprising β-Troponylhydrazino Acid. ACS omega. 2020 Oct 1;5(40):26141-26152. DOI: 10.1021/acsomega.0c03729

[34] Maywald M, Wessels I, Rink L: Zinc signals and immunity. International journal of molecular sciences. 2017;18(10):2222. DOI: 10.3390/ijms18102222

[35] Overbeck S, Rink L, Haase H: Modulating the immune response by oral zinc supplementation: a single approach for multiple diseases. Archivum immunological et therapiae experimentalis. 2008 Feb;56(1):15-30. DOI: 10.1007/s00005-008-0003-8

[36] Krężel A, Maret W: The biological inorganic chemistry of zinc ions. Archives of biochemistry and biophysics. 2016 Dec 1;611:3-19. DOI: 10.1016/j.abb.2016.04.010

[37] Kumar A, Kubota Y, Chernov M, Kasuya H: Potential role of zinc supplementation in prophylaxis and treatment of COVID-19. Medical hypotheses. 2020 Nov 1;144:109848. DOI:10.1016/j.mehy.2020.109848

[38] Muhammad S, Omama M: A New Approach to Duality of Electron. Energy. 2020;14(15):16. DOI: 10.5923/j.ijtmp.20201006.04

[39] Bomford K: Radiation protection. Walter and Miller's textbook of radiotherapy. New York: Churchill Livingstone. 2003;69-88.

[40] Bushberg JT: The AAPM/RSNA physics tutorial for residents. X-ray interactions. Radiographics. 1998;18 (2): 457-468. DOI: 10.1148/radiographics.18.2.9536489

[41] Esposito A, Krichevsky R, Nicolis A: Gravitational mass carried by sound waves. Physical review letters. 2019 Mar 1;122(8):084501. DOI: 10.1103/PhysRevLett.122.084501

[42] Perov P, Johnson W, Perova-Mello N. The physics of guitar string vibrations. American Journal of Physics. 2016 Jan;84(1):38-43. DOI: 10.1119/1.4935088

Section 9

Societal Effects Public Health Measures Meteorology Mortality Government and Media

Chapter 30

The Economic, Climate Change and Public Health Edges of the Geopolitics of COVID-19: An Exploratory Bibliometric Analysis

Jean Pierre Doussoulin and Benoît Mougenot

Abstract

We are in the middle of the storm and this does not allow us to see clearly what is coming. This often generates partial analyses of the issues of the situation. Therefore, this manuscript attempts to generate an integral perspective on the issues of the crisis. This chapter proposes a discussion of the Coronavirus crisis following analysis and comparison of the most important outstanding conversations of general public health, economics and environmental issues. The objective of this chapter is to travel on the far side of the discussion of the articles presently planned within the academic world and that were analyzed within the bibliometric review, that consist of these three issues. This analysis that integrates these dimensions allows to give an additional prospective answer to the queries exposed by the COVID crisis, conjointly taking into consideration geopolitics as a forgotten dimension within the public discussion. Our paper helps to indicate the positions of every one of those ideas and enrich the literature on the environmental sciences and public health by providing analysis of the consequences of international policies.

Keywords: COVID-19, health, growth, environment, geopolitics and bibliometric analysis

1. Introduction

Governments across the globe are putting into place unprecedented measures of lockdowns and social distancing measures and trillions of dollars in monetary and fiscal policies in the fight against COVID-19. These can only help slow down the spread while medical science works on a vaccine as a way to stop the disease. This is the ultimate solution. Everything else is temporary because of the prevalence of the contagious element and the seasonal peaks [1].

The objective of this chapter is to go beyond the discussion of the articles currently proposed in the academic world and which were analyzed in the bibliometric review, which deal with the issues of health, economics and the environment separately. This analysis that integrates these dimensions allows us to give a more prospective answer to the questions posed by the COVID crisis, also taking into account geopolitics as a forgotten dimension in the analysis.

Government has the vaccine but the question is who gets it first and why. It can be a sad reality in life that sometimes the people that desperately need the vaccine will not necessarily be the first to receive it. The other issue that arises is who can afford this vaccine because if it is only developed and rich countries that are able to reach this stage [2].

People genuinely believe that the only way to truly contain this, ultimately is the vaccine. That is why we have dozens of companies. Sampling is very important in the race to find an effective vaccine that involves researchers around the world at this point in time. There are over 50 companies looking into developing COVID-19 vaccine. It is quite unprecedented. This is a reflection, not only of the seriousness of the pandemic itself but, the state of science and biomedical science in particular. All around the world, China, Singapore, Europe and the US, there are a whole range of companies from the very traditional big multinational biopharmaceuticals to small biotech companies [3].

Governments and other groups have committed to hundreds of millions for vaccine research but aside from cost there are also questions over affordability and accessibility. It cannot be expensive because this is going to be something the governments will have to pay. This is something that is going to be very challenging which is why there are only a few companies that are pursuing this route [4].

Researchers think that in the case of COVID- 19 that governments are looking at a combined effort from both public and private sectors. The Singapore government has research for a vaccine to cover the country. The companies are working on a product which if successful, could vaccinate many people quickly and at a low cost. Right now the choice is half for manufacturing or vaccine for human trials. The industry is presently working with the Health Sciences Authority (HSA) in Singapore to identify a time for those for the first clinical trials. That is going to be relatively soon in the US and in China the first clinical trials on humans have already begun, this is just the initial stage in what is usually a long process [5–7].

2. Methodology

The methodology of this chapter considers two parts. We carry out a bibliometric analysis of the literature taking into account three dimensions: sustainability, health care, economic growth in order to provide an analysis related to COVID-19.

Figure 1 presents the examination of how these three measurements may be reconsidered utilizing the methodology used by Doussoulin [8, 9]. As demonstrated

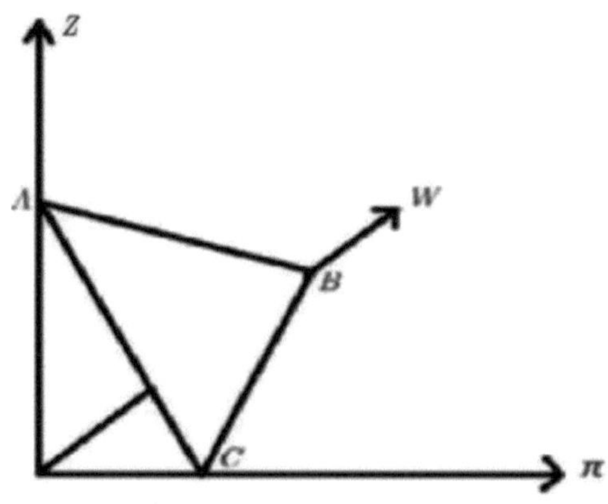

Figure 1.
Three dimensions: economic growth, health care and sustainability. Source: [8].

in **Figure 1**, when π = 100%, z = 0 and w = 0, all consideration devoted by the public authority are allocated to economic development. On the other hand, in the event that π = 0, z = 0 and w = 100%, at that point all consideration is given to medical services. It is additionally conceivable consideration regarding the earth as a characteristic asset which can be addressed where π =0, z = 100% and w = 0, which relates to a green future [1, 10].

In a second part and considering this bibliometric analysis, we will carry out an analysis of the three dimensions in search of characterizing the race for vaccines.

3. Conceptual evolution of COVID-19: a bibliometric analysis

3.1 Data sources and collection

This chapter selects the Scopus collection as the main data source (https://www.scopus.com/). The search terms are the followings: COVID-19 and economy or COVID-19 and environment or climate change or COVID-19 and public health. The period analyzed was from 2019 to 2021. All languages have been considered. Initially, the Scopus database considered various type of documents, but only original articles were included in the present analysis. 7806 documents were selected for the analysis but finally limited to the first 2000 due to the limitation of the Scopus importation in BibTex file and imported into Bibliometrix and Biblioshiny.

3.2 Research software

Bibliometrix and Biblioshiny open-source packages are used from the R language environment. Bibliometrix allows completing the full process of scientific literature analysis and data process. Biblioshiny captures the core Bibliometrix code and creates an online data analysis framework [3]. Biblioshiny enables users to perform pertinent bibliometric and visual analysis based on an interactive web interface.

Network analysis and mapping using the Bibliometrix and the Biblioshiny packages, the research allows showing bibliometric indicators on COVID-19 such as publication volume in number of articles, citation count, and keywords. Then, the article presents figures and maps such as a citation network diagram, thematic evolution map, and an international collaboration network map to identify research hotspots, research status and the dynamics of COVID.

3.3 Results of most relevant sources

The journal that published most articles about COVID-19 during the period were presented in **Figure 2**. International Journal of Environmental Research and Public Health was the journal that published the highest number of articles on COVID-19 during the period (72 articles). Frontiers in Public Health was the second leading journal with 63. The journal Frontiers in Public Health published 34 articles and the Journal of Medical Internet Research 23 articles. International Journal of Environmental Research and Public Health is the source with the higher impact, with an h index of 12.

3.4 Mapping the scientific collaboration

A map shown in **Figure 3** identifies the country collaboration of the main producing countries. Two countries hold a connection line indicating the status

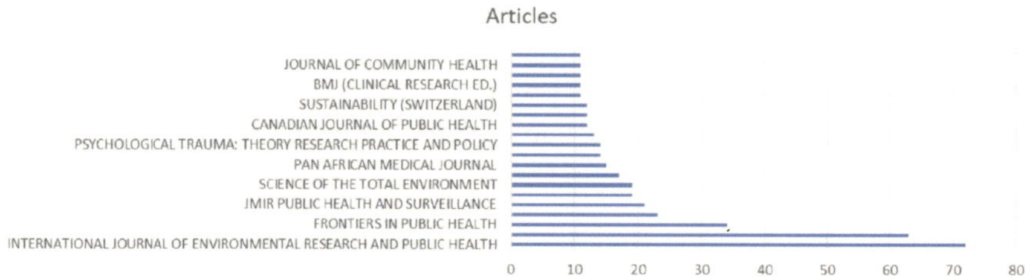

Figure 2.
Most relevant sources in the field of COVID-19.

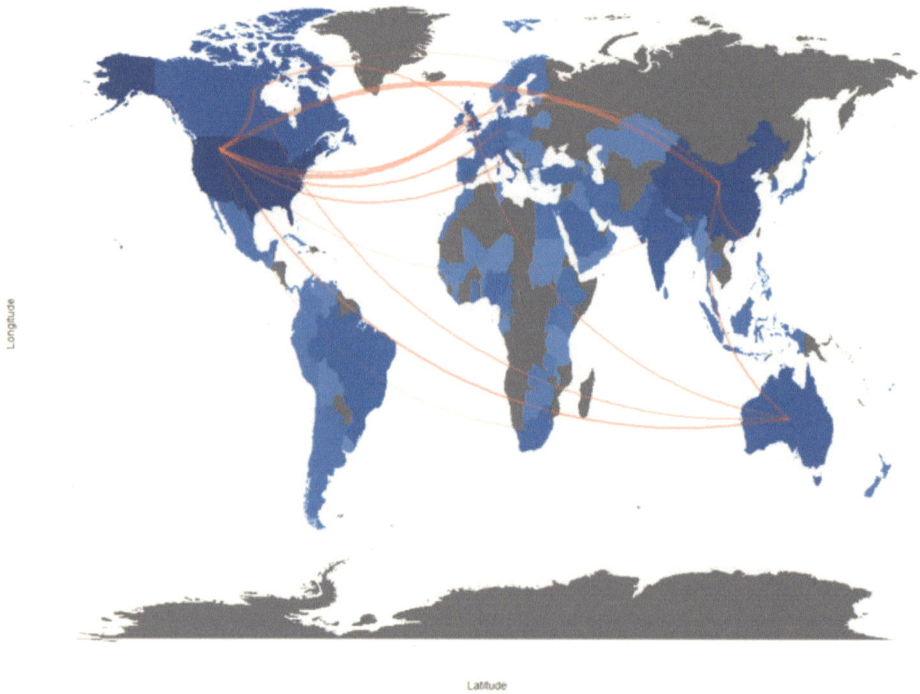

Figure 3.
Country collaboration map.

of collaboration among them. The scale of cooperation is represented through the thickness of the line. The United States, China, Australia, Western European countries showed deepened cooperation and exchange among scholars.

Figure 4 shows a co-citation analysis, with each box representing an article in the COVID literature. The size of the box indicates the volume of the citation (the larger the box, the more author's documents are cited) and the proximity of the boxes indicates a close relationship between the co-cited documents.

3.5 Analysis of keywords and co-keywords

Figure 5 illustrates the keyword co-occurrence network. The number of occurrences of the keywords is represented through the dimension of the box. When authors' keywords were more co-selected in the COVID-19 literature,

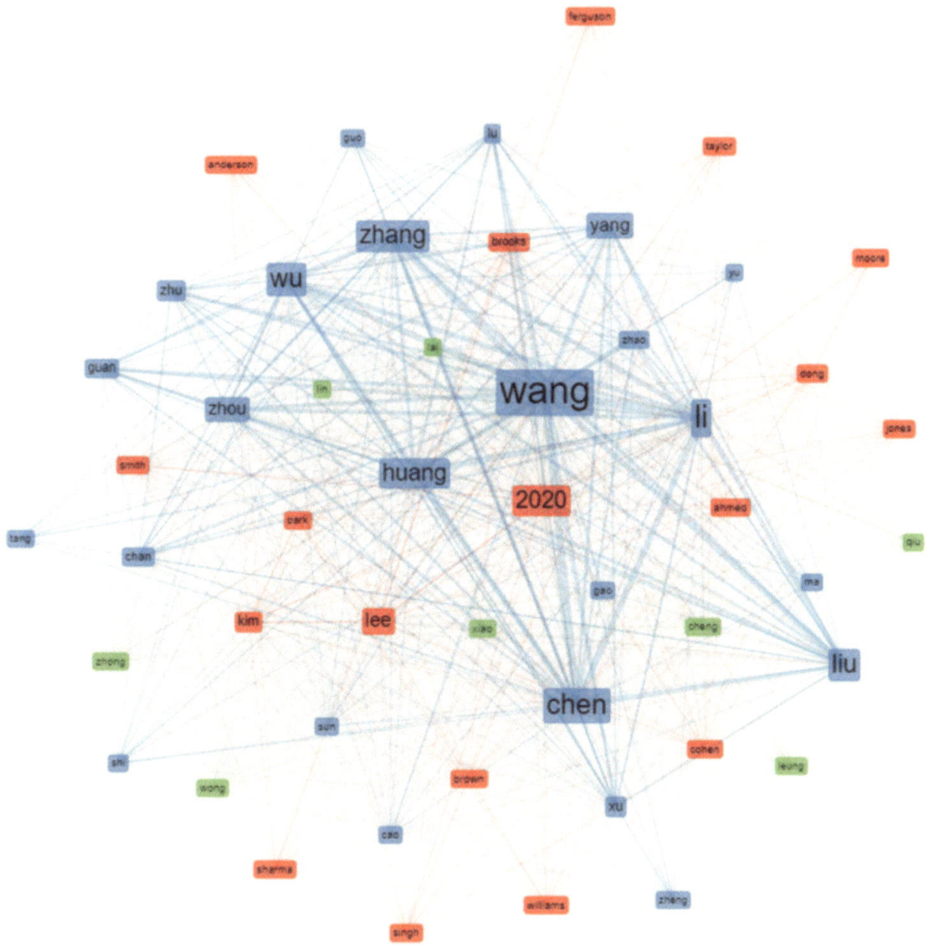

Figure 4.
Co-citation network.

the box is larger. The topic similarity and its relative strength is represented through the distance between the elements of individual pairs. Different box colors were assigned to individual clusters. A network of three distinct clusters are highlighted in **Figure 4**, representing individual subfields in COVID-19 research.

3.6 Keywords top authors and sources relations

In **Figure 6** a three fields graph represented the relationships between the keywords, the main authors' keywords and the sources. Therefore, the diagram of rectangles with distinct colors illustrated the main elements. The value of the sum of the relations appearing between the element represented by the rectangles and the diagram of the other elements designed the height of the rectangles. The size of the rectangles depends on more relations the element had.

The analysis showed in which research topics of the bioeconomy concept the authors of bioeconomy publications had explored and which sources they had most often published. The research topics were considered here as the keywords of the authors.

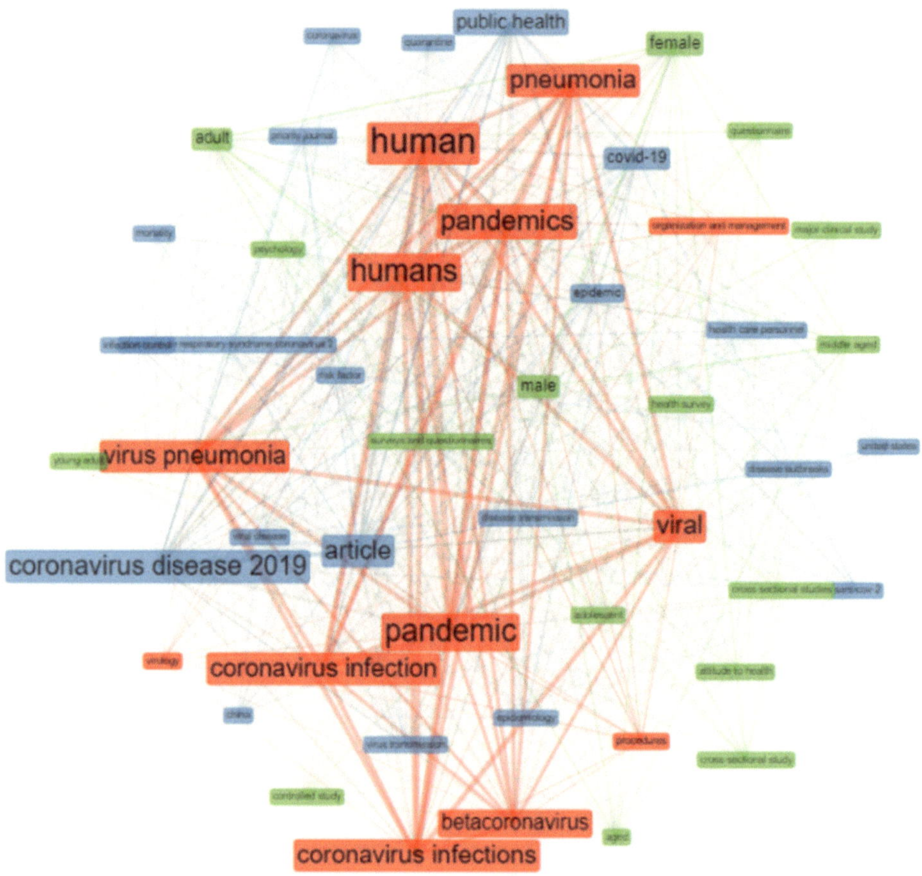

Figure 5.
Author keywords co-occurrence network in the COVID literature.

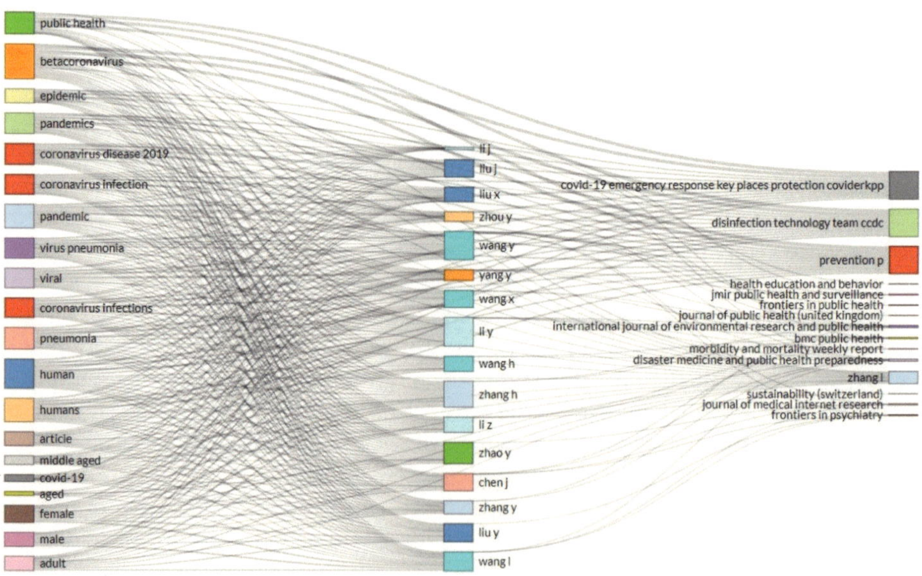

Figure 6.
Relationships between author keywords (left), authors (middle) and source (right).

4. Three dimensions of the Corona race

Ten COVID-19 vaccine candidates are now in late-stage trials. The world is celebrating what could be the breakthrough in fighting COVID-19. Pharmaceutical companies are also cheering the fact that the public sector has invested billions more in development. It is the private sector that will rake in the cash under existing agreements, they control the price and get profits. Pharmaceutical firms say that is fair as development is expensive and time-consuming and results are not announce. It is a gamble for governments too which are reserving millions of doses of a vaccine [11, 12].

Companies are taking billions of dollars in revenue, part of the funding for the vaccine researcher's public money but the profits stay in private hands. The companies can secure exclusive licenses to a vaccine and ultimately decide on a price because they have a monopoly [13–15]. For patents, the race to find the vaccine is in full swing and two German companies are among the leaders in the field, Cure Vac in Tübingen and BioNTech in Mainz which this weekend added promising early results from its phase 3 clinical trial. Both are working which added vaccines using messenger mRNA vaccines [16].

The vaccine takes a snippet of the coronavirus's genome to begin a defensive response without exposing it to the actual virus mRNA, essentially teaching the body to fight a dummy of the virus to help make it immune. Research into this technology has been going on for 20 years and has involved billions in public money and private investment but developing vaccines is highly risky and mixes of candidates active ingredient or vaccine candidate can fail at any stage in clinical trials because of a lack of efficacy or safety issues. Which is why pharmaceutical companies turn to public funding. This is then distributed by groups like the coalition for epidemic preparedness innovations (CEPI) which is co-funding development of some COVID-19 vaccine candidates. The main focus of this cooperation with CEPI is to produce a vaccine as quickly as possible and get it to the population. The commercial side is secondary for now although vaccine development is co-funded. The companies own licenses and distribution based on this the rules are relaxed [17–19]. That would have ensured that CEPI retains intellectual property rights to ensure a vaccine that is affordable for everyone and widely accessible. Pharmaceutical companies stand to make huge profits. If they succeed in coming up with a vaccine successfully which comes onto the market, that opens the door to a flood of similar vaccines and active ingredients that offers great opportunities so public funding could earn billions for private firms. The fear is biotech companies can name their price for access to this powerful pandemic fighting weapon according to professor of public economics Massimo Florio [20].

He argues that the problem with public funds being used to develop a vaccine for this coronavirus in the current emergency [15], that there is absolutely no alternative to disburse such funds. The government will be able to negotiate on prices and other conditions.

There are alternatives about the issue of what citizens are going to do the next time but the governments are in a bad negotiating position for what they are giving these big pharma companies. It is important in the future not to be stuck in this bad negotiating position and that governments or possibly a coalition of governments develop their own research and development capacity in this area [21, 22].

Private firms, of course, are about making a buck but that is that one of the reasons why individuals were not ready for this outbreak. The problem is that governments have entirely delegated to the private pharmaceutical industry the research and development of the weapons against pathogens and other diseases [23, 24].

There is a risk of disconnection or misalignment between the public health agenda and the private agenda if you are a pharmaceutical company. A manager of a pharmaceutical company has financial investors listed on the stock exchange [25, 26].

Some scholars, analyzed in **Figures 4** and **6**, will look into how people could solve the issue of a messenger RNA vaccine cold chain at a reasonable cost. People have heard it was minus 80 degrees Celsius if the interim results on efficacy from the candidate vaccine made by Biontech and Pfizer hold up to scrutiny [27]. By the end of November, if hurdles involving safety could be clear edit is hoped then some countries could approve it quickly maybe even by the end of the year. Companies will have already produced enough doses to vaccinate between 15 and 20 million people and should have production capacity for over a billion more in 2021. Manufacturing infrastructure has been set up in parallel with the trials to speed the whole process up [28, 29].

There is a big hurdle to overcome with this particular vaccine which is that it has to be kept at freezing temperatures minus 70 degrees Celsius to remain stable for any length of time and that the logistics will be expensive and problematic. Every step of the cold chain and the delivery process has to be as foolproof as you can make it, and you have to train people to work with products at such a low temperature [30].

Pfizer has even been building special containers for keeping its doses that could be good news and that they do not spoil instantly after thawing, but they also keep at normal refrigerator temperatures for around five days which makes the task maybe slightly less impossible [31]. There are many other vaccines going through late stage trials that might also prove safe and effective and some of them are based on other platforms with formulations that don not have to be kept at temperatures that low or anywhere close to it. With luck one or more of them will prove safe and effective too and can be used in places that don't have high-tech cold chain infrastructure [32].

This section outlines a set of matters involving the COVID-19 crisis through the exploration of three dimensions: sustainability, health care and economic growth.

4.1 Health care dimensions of COVID-19

It is common for vaccines to take 10 to 12 years to make it to the market but with a pandemic taking an unprecedented toll around the world, there are hopes that the timeline could be accelerated in this kind of situation. Things that generally might take several months to two years to go through are now being done in parallel. For example, the Coalition for epidemic preparedness innovation has set itself a very ambitious target of 16 weeks to try and do these kind of tests in parallel to find the same kind of information. This means that the regulatory authorities also have to change the approach in which they take the data on from the vaccine studies. They use what are called adaptive approaches or rolling submissions where small amounts of data based on the information found will come in sequence. They can sort of give provisional authorization along the way. It is a very different paradigm to assessing vaccines in this kind of pandemic situation compared to under normal circumstances [4–6].

Government agencies like the biomedical Advanced Research and Development Authority called Barda for short, are pushing to modernize the way the U.S. produces emergency vaccines like the flu shot. It is giving grants worth hundreds of millions of dollars to companies like Sanofi which uses recombinant DNA not chicken eggs to produce flu vaccines. One of its main jobs is to help create a market for drug companies to develop emergency vaccines through the use of its grants. In late January 2020, HSS secretary Alex declared an emergency and response to the coronavirus outbreak as part of that Barda announcement [7, 33].

The COVID-19 pandemic in the UK, may have subsided for now, but it is accelerating in many parts of the world. The search for treatments alongside a vaccine remains as urgent as ever. A landmark drug trial has revealed the steroid dexamethasone to be effective in reducing deaths by up to a third on many patients who come into the intensive care unit, who have a hyperimmune response. Their immune system goes into overdrive so it is the hyperimmune response which actually causes a lot of the damage to the lungs. Dexamethasone helped to just kind of dampen it all down for a 56-year-old. The patient believed that Dexamethasone saved his life because his body wasn't functioning, it was machines that were basically keeping him alive [34, 35].

It is backed by the Bill and Melinda Gates Foundation, as well as the governments of Germany, Japan and Norway. It is a relative newcomer to the global vaccine community. It was created in 2017 to help speed up the process of developing new vaccines. Furthermore, it invested about twenty-three point seven million dollars in the push to develop a COVID-19 vaccine and it plans to invest a total of 100 million dollars in order to get vaccine candidates to early-stage clinical trial [11, 36].

The Oslo based global coalition says it needs about two billion dollars more in additional funding to fully develop viable vaccines against COVID-19. Most of the Biotech companies working on vaccines or treatments already had a head start by previously working on SARS and Middle East respiratory syndrome which are part of the coronavirus family. Biotech firm Moderna has had one of the most promising starts [12].

Moderna is using a new technique had called messenger RNA or mRNA to develop its vaccine candidate. The drugmaker has already started to deliver its vaccine to national health officials. The vaccine was co-designed with the National Institute of Allergy and Infectious Diseases after Chinese scientists decoded the coronaviruses genetic sequence in January 2020 [13, 37]. Moderna set a record within the drug industry for the speed at which it developed its vaccine candidate using its mRNA method. It took Moderna about 42 days after the coronavirus's genome was sequenced, for comparison it took about 20 months to develop a vaccine to the human testing phase during the SARS outbreak in 2002 [14].

Moderna plans to start a small-scale human trial of the vaccine soon in Seattle Washington, an epicenter of the COVID-19 outbreak in the United States. It will take about three months or more to show that it is safe and then if persons show that it is safe, it has got to be put it into what is called a phase 2 trial to show that it works. The reason is that there are medical ethical and other considerations in giving this to normal people to prevent infection [15, 16].

Researchers must be sure of the medicial ethic first to do no harm. People need to make sure it is safe, citizens need to make sure it works. This entire process will take at least a year. In a year and a half Johnson & Johnson is also in the race, the company is working with Barda on a potential treatment [17].

It is also developing a vaccine using a deactivated version of the COVID-19 as mentioned earlier. Sanofi is also working with Barda on a COVID-19 vaccine, it plans to have a vaccine candidate to test in a lab within six months and on people within a year to eighteen months but approval could be as long as three years away. Inovio Pharmaceuticals has partnered with a Chinese company called Beijing to speed up the development of its DNA vaccine [18].

It received an initial grant of nine million dollars from the Coalition for epidemic preparedness. Innovations in Opium is using the same method for the COVID-19 vaccine as it did with its DNA vaccine against the Middle East respiratory syndrome. Currently there have not been any DNA vaccines approved for use on humans. Doctors and global health experts have tried to temper vaccine expectations saying that even though this stage has gone quickly, reviewing test results in getting a vaccine deployed to the public could take many more months or even a year to 18 months.

Likewise, it would still be the fastest people have ever seen a vaccine get developed and the way that breaks down right now for the lead program is that it is starting phase 1 clinical trials in people now, which will take about 3 to 4 months to determine the safety of the vaccine. Then they are going to move into phase 2 which will involve more people and remember these are healthy people.

4.2 Economics dimensions and chaos in global financial markets

The growing coronavirus outbreak is causing chaos in global financial markets. It is freezing supply chains, it is causing companies all over the world to create work from home plans and banned business travel. In late January 2020, Chinese scientists in Shanghai released the fully sequenced genome of the novel COVID-19 that was wreaking havoc in Hebei province which kicked off the race at drug companies and government labs to develop a cure for corona virus or at least its symptoms in terms of vaccines in the US [19].

The US has moved at a pace people have never seen before, still it is going to be at least a year to a year and a half until they have a vaccine broadly available to deploy. Among COVID-19 belongs to a larger family of corona viruses. That family of viruses includes the one that caused the SARS outbreak in 2002 and Middle East respiratory syndrome to spring up in 2012. The official name of the new COVID-19 is severe acute respiratory syndrome coronavirus - or SARS Cove - the one discovered in December 2019 in Wuhan China causes a disease that scientists decided to call COVID-19.

This naming convention works the same way with HIV and AIDS. HIV is the virus that causes AIDS. The disease symptoms of COVID-19 include fever fatigue and coughing. Some people become infected but don't develop any symptoms. Most people, around 80% recover without any special treatment, about 1 in 6 people with the disease end up developing a serious illness, older people and those with underlying medical conditions are most likely to come down with serious issues.

The disease travels through small droplets that spread when people cough or sneeze. Those droplets land on objects. People touch those objects and then touch their eyes, nose or mouth and that is how people catch the new COVID-19. There is no vaccine to prevent them from getting it, there is no vaccine for any of the corona viruses, for that matter. That is why vaccines have become a big market for drug companies' scientists and researchers no longer give them away. The Polio vaccine has become a thirty-five-billion-dollar market with strong and steady demand for vaccines against established diseases like polio measles and hepatitis. Creating vaccines for emergency pandemics becomes tricky.

Researchers are giving the vaccine to see if it can prevent disease, the risk tolerance is lower than if people were already sick. Companies are giving them a treatment, that is why people have to be so careful here, they say it could take perhaps eight months to get through phase two.

That is how it will take about a year before you even know if they have something that is safe and that works to protect people. Other drug companies are hurrying to develop various treatments for the coronavirus, and they could come much sooner.

The drug is already being tested at the epicenter of the outbreak in Wuhan China and Gilead is now expanding to other countries, including the United States. Researchers should know within a period of a few months whether this particular drug works. If it does the implementation of that would be almost immediate. The pressure to develop a corona virus vaccine grows each day as the number of infected people rises and the death toll climbs even higher but there is a real risk to pushing too hard and too fast. some drug companies plan to push testing schedules into human trials rather than spending months testing the vaccines on animals in labs.

That could lead to what is called immune enhancement where a person or animal who receives a vaccine ends up with a more serious disease than unvaccinated subjects according to Reuters. Leading health and drug company officials recently advocated for fast tracking human testing of coronavirus vaccines during a closed-door meeting convened by the World Health Organization.

The question facing health officials if accelerating testing schedules is worth these kinds of risks. That all depends on whether countries like the United States can contain the fast-spreading novel coronavirus.

4.3 Planet conservation and COVID

No war, no recession, no other pandemic, has had such an impact on CO_2 emissions during the last century as the one observed by COVID-19 in just a few months. For example: Germany might even reach its climate goals as the corona lockdown causes the economy to produce much less CO_2, the factories devoid of workers, thousands of flights cancelled, empty streets because people are working from home instead of driving to the office. Global economic activity has been put into an induced coma, bad for the world economy but from a climate perspective the corona virus pandemic is not entirely negative. Environmental activists might actually rejoice measures have been implemented immediately, thick smog has given way to blue skies [21, 22].

The current situation has seen people spending more time at home. They may have decided to have a spring-clean or get started on that bathroom renovation. Keep in mind you are responsible for the disposal of all the waste you produce [23]. Things like food scraps, demolition materials, hard rubbish and e-waste all have different requirements for correct disposal. Councils and the waste and recycling industry continue to provide waste services to the public. Like any business, some disruptions may occur from time-to-time due to physical distancing requirements, but they are not restricted activities and remain operating [24]. The regular curbside bin collections, such as recycling, household and garden waste continue as usual.

Hard rubbish collections are also available from your local council. Private waste collections, such as skip bin hire, are operating for waste such as construction and demolition materials [25]. For people working in the waste industry, the risk of transmission of coronavirus when handling waste is low. Waste handlers should continue using routine hygiene procedures such as wearing gloves and washing hands regularly for at least 20 seconds with soap. Keeping waste services operating helps reduce the potential for illegal dumping that costs millions of dollars to clean up [26].

Piling up disposable protective equipment and plastic packaging. Initially there had been a hope that the slowdown in the world economy would be good for the planet. Air traffic almost stopped completely, cruise ships were stranded in port and industrial pollution was reduced but the pandemic has had negative consequences for the environment, the world was already drowning under a sea of plastic waste but the pandemic has made the situation worse [38].

Face masks can stay in the environment for up to 450 years, it takes that long before they turn into invisible microplastic. This issue is quite serious as the human toll of the coronavirus mounts and the world economy struggles to adjust to the new normal. The wider impact on the environment is only now starting to become apparent. The global medical emergency has presented an opportunity to check on the health of the planet in the controversial new lockdown measures [39].

4.4 COVID's geopolitics: the dimension forgotten in the debate

Issues related to geopolitics and pandemics intersect through the sovereignty of the countries, to the logistics of vaccine distribution and power games. All of these issues are complex, urgent, and demand a solution through collective action based on their global and cross-border reach [22, 40].

As can be seen in **Figure 4**, the rich nations corner the market for COVID-19 vaccines and treatments. What does that mean for the world's poor? The world's largest trial of possible COVID-19 treatments has produced results that are already being used to save lives. The race to develop vaccines and treatments for the coronavirus pandemic is entering a crucial stage with large-scale trials underway [41].

The debate over opaque pricing has raised concerns that pharmaceutical companies could be charging way too much for COVID-19 treatments. The most recent disquiet was triggered by Gilead's Remdesivir at America's decision to monopolize supplies.

The U.S. government has cornered almost the entire global market of Remdesivir for the next several months. The drug has been found to shorten hospital stays for COVID-19 patients. This America first policy during the pandemic has led to expressions of outrage and dismay among some international leaders. U.S. coronavirus patients may not receive the drug if they do not have enough cash [27, 42].

The drug manufacturer Gilead says governments in the developed world will pay three hundred and ninety dollars for a treatment which will come to two thousand three hundred and forty dollars a patient. However each vial for the U.S. private health insurance system is five hundred and twenty dollars or an average cost of three thousand one hundred and twenty dollars a patient. It is not clear how much each patient will have to pay either out of pocket or in higher premiums as with many drugs that are eventually sold for profit by pharmaceutical companies. That was reported in the U.S. in January and many of those drugs are used to treat COVID-19 or used in intensive care units. Some economists wonder whether amid COVID-19 economic collapse, mass unemployment, the inability of millions to pay their rent and social unrest things may be changing. The perception of price gouging by pharmaceutical companies during a pandemic may become part of a wider reckoning for the U.S. [28–30].

Gilead says that because its drug reduces the time that COVID-19 patients spend in hospital, it priced Remdesivir fairly. Senator Bernie Sanders claimed that Remdesivir cost Gilead ten dollars a vial to manufacture and as you heard taxpayers have paid 70 million dollars towards the cost of development. That is crucial as many Americans do not have or have lost their health insurance and cannot afford to pay for the drug. The problem is Gilead has made the same claim before.

It bought the startup behind a ready to market hepatitis C drug for 11 billion dollars and began to market the drug for 84,000 allowing it to almost recoup the cost of acquisition in the first year according to Bloomberg [31, 32]. How much does big pharma spend on developing drugs? Well, on average 2.6 billion dollars according to Tufts university but advocacy group public citizen believes the cost is closer to 1.4 billion dollars as governments spend billions securing supplies of potential COVID-19 vaccines Pfizer is charging roughly 20 dollars for a dose which the company claims is 30 percent less.

Other drugmakers charge for seasonal flu jabs and because it is not receiving government money for research and development it can expect to make more than 15 billion dollars in revenue [43].

The opinion is, nothing else is working, nothing to lose. He had dexamethasone, his oxygen requirement came down and started to stay down and started to gradually decrease and for the first time there started to be talk of taking him off the ventilator which people couldn't even believe. The patient was given dexamethasone here at the hospital in Scotland, one of a large number taking part in a UK wide randomized drug trial being run by scientists at Oxford University. The aim to test a number of widely available off-the-shelf drugs with the hope of finding one or a combination that might work to ease some of the worst symptoms of COVID-19 [44].

The patient returning from the brink of death contributed to data that has seen dexamethasone approved as a breakthrough treatment for some of the worst cases of COVID-19. Dexamethasone has been a great result, and it now means that patients who are ventilated or an oxygen can be prescribed in a way they wouldn't been able to be before. The recovery trial has also been successful in ruling out the malaria drug hydroxychloroquine, once hailed as a game changer by president Donald Trump but found instead to be useless in treating COVID-19. As the world waits for a safe and effective vaccine that may yet be a long way off, recovery continues to look for treatments [45, 46]. Police officers in New Delhi are donating blood plasma, they are just some 2 500 police staff in the Indian capital who recovered from coronavirus but health minister Harsh Vardhan says few people have been willing to donate and has launched a campaign as the number of infections has increased [47].

This drive will encourage everyone, especially those who have recovered from coronavirus. to donate their plasma in large numbers. Plasma therapy is treating coronavirus patients around the world. Plasma from a former patient's blood is separated for a transfusion to an infected person. Plasma of recovered patients contains antibodies which can fight the virus. This person is the first person in Delhi to have donated his plasma after recovering from the coronavirus in April.

Trials to determine its effectiveness are continuing but researchers say the results so far are encouraging, it clearly reduces the need for increasing oxygen at the stage when the patient is deteriorating.

It does prevent a lot of patients from actually going onto a ventilator. Various centers across the world have shown mortality rates to be 50 to 80 percent when the patient goes on to a ventilator. By virtue of preventing a patient going onto a ventilator, it may be preventing excess deaths. Delhi state government is one of many around the country to set up plasma donation centers to make it easier for patients needing the therapy. People are struggling to find plasma from those who have recovered. Coronavirus is connected to the deaths of around 30,000 Indians with more than 1.2 million infections. As well as launching a donation campaign, the state government in Delhi is organizing transport for those willing to come to one of its centers. With far more recoveries than active infections health officials are urging Indians who were once sick to help patients who are suffering [48].

How can drug companies offset the cost of their research and offer cheaper drugs particularly to developing nations? That is a good and important question. A couple of things to note about research and development costs, first is the way that industry calculates research and development costs that include things that you and me would probably not consider research and development, for example the lost opportunity costs of foregoing investments with an annual return of over 10.

Some wealthier countries are being asked to pledge money to buy vaccines in advance which then will be distributed according to a global equitable allocation framework by the World Health Organization (WHO). Should all countries and companies adhere to this future framework? It is out there so that vaccine supply is truly allocated based on public health need, as said by the WHO and the Bill Gates foundation and not captured by narrow political or commercial interests. How that is going to work when the world has rich nations snapping up all the available supply? That is a big concern, these bilateral deals really help no one because it has been said before that no one is safe until everyone is safe.

For the world to have herd immunity, people are going to have to beat this thing, it will be crucial that this is successful and that countries commit a certain proportion of even the bilateral deals that they have struck to a facility that will share vaccines with the world. To be fair to the likes of companies like AstraZeneca and Johnson & Johnson, both have said that they are going to produce the vaccine on a not-for-profit basis.

What does that mean for poorer nations though even on a not-for-profit basis ? Can they afford them? That is a very good question, both companies should be applauded for their commitment to not profit from the pandemic. Unfortunately what companies say and what they do is not always the same. For instance, if you take Johnson & Johnson in the past, they have claimed that their lowest global price for an important drug called Bedaquiline was a not-for-profit price but which is disputed by independent academics.

It could be produced at profit for less than a quarter of that price. There have been calls for the price to be halved and just earlier this month they actually further dropped their supposedly not for profit price by over 30 percent following intensive campaigning. It is important to mention that these pledges only apply for the pandemic period and if SARS turns endemic [49].

What about the ethics of a vaccine treatment in a hurry? For strict ethical standards this should be the case too because vaccines and drugs act differently in different patient populations but what it definitely should also mean is that the very populations on which these vaccines and drugs are being tested should have equitable access to them in the future. It cannot be that they are just the guinea pigs for clinical trials but then will not be able to access the vaccines afterwards. In the midst of a global pandemic, should generically drugmakers be given licenses to produce much-needed treatment drugs? Generic drug reproduction will be crucial to meet the demands of this pandemic and national hoarding of physical supplies of drugs or vaccines is regrettable.

Should actively using intellectual property to prevent generic ground companies be avoided? There is a wealth of research into testing kits, there is one produced in Senegal for a dollar. Is there any way of commercializing that kind of expertise as a solution for developing nations?. People having accurate rapid diagnostic tests will be incredibly important to the global COVID-19 response given that they are simple to use, and while there are over 100 tests on the market the majority have limited to no evidence on diagnostic performance. An inaccurate test is worse than no test, quality assured rapid diagnostic tests are needed but once solid evidence for rapid diagnostic tests does emerge.

It will be crucial to scale up the production as quickly as possible. An example to cite is actually an excellent example of a private company in the UK collaborating with the Pasteur Institute to develop a rapid diagnostic test and then in the future locally producing it in Senegal for a price that is affordable for governments in the region. Some state actors have also been accused of attempting to hack laboratories and drug companies for COVID-19 research and vaccine secrets as more of us are lucky enough to work productively from home. Companies are stepping up cybersecurity for employees. One company that helps businesses replace usernames and passwords with biometrics is Silicon Valley based. The cost now is if a Silicon Valley social media platform like twitter can succumb to a hack.

5. Conclusions

We are in the middle of the storm, which does not allow us to see clearly what is coming and as can be seen in **Figure 4**, the keywords *pandemic* and *coronavirus infection* are positioned in the collective unconscious. People are told they may be ready by the end of the year probably more likely to be the middle of the next year.

What is going to be the fairest outcome for both drugmakers and developing nations. The fairest outcome for the public would be that no one dies from COVID-19 because they cannot access a drug or a vaccine and the fairest outcome for drug makers would be that of the experience with COVID-19. A new era of drug development which is collaborative, open and does not have profit as the sole motive for innovation manual.

From an economics viewpoint, they are used hopefully for a short period of time to address a problem that then individuals hope to be able to move past. It is not a big moneymaker for the industry, and it is very hard to predict flu vaccines for example grown in chicken eggs, this process takes a long time and it is not as reliable as newer methods such as incubating vaccines and cells as opposed to eggs. more than 100 national influenza centers in more than 100 countries monitor the flu throughout the year and make recommendations on how to create that seasons' flu vaccines.

Society needs something else. People need a mechanism not based on the priorities of financial investors. People need a mechanism based on the priorities of public health with a long term perspective. Just summing up really briefly SARS obviously didn't change anything. Will this outbreak change something because the alarm bells were there even 20 years ago but for some reasons they were in certain places and not such a global factor. Still more coronaviruses could come along. Vaccines could become big farmers new cash cow. One of the largest pharmaceutical companies only had four special vaccine units last year. Now everyone is getting in on the act, which is great, but they are using our money and can charge what they want. Some developers promise to only charge the cost price. It could even be cheaper than the flu vaccine, it is a race everyone wants to win whoever makes the first successful COVID-19 vaccine also stands to make a fortune.

The use of vaccines has a geopolitical dimension, there is no guarantee that prices will be affordable, especially for developing countries. In the Northern Hemisphere in winter, there is likely to be a second wave in the pandemic. Is a vaccine going to be in place by then to limit the effects of a second wave? What do you think the likely outcome will be? Well, individuals do not know. Citizens know that many groups are working very hard to still develop a vaccine but no vaccine candidate has passed phase three trials yet, people do not really know, how efficacious those vaccines are going to be and therefore also how likely they will be successful.

Finally, this text recognizes that there must be autonomous action priorities for each territory, which must consist of small victories in economic, health and environmental aspects within the territory. It is also relevant to incorporate into the discussion the geopolitical influence that recognizes and encourages unequal access to vaccines, generating a gap between rich, middle-income and poor countries.

Author details

Jean Pierre Doussoulin[1,2*] and Benoît Mougenot[3]

1 Universidad Austral de Chile, Economic Institute, Chile

2 Université Gustave Eiffel, Research Team on the Use of Panel Data in Economics, France

3 Universidad San Ignacio de Loyola, Lima, Peru

*Address all correspondence to: jean.doussoulin@uach.cl

'Biotechnology to Combat COVID-19' is a collaborative project with Biotechnology Kiosk

References

[1] Costanza R, Daly HE. Toward an ecological economics. Ecol Model. 1987;38(1-2):1-7.

[2] Walker PG, Whittaker C, Watson OJ, Baguelin M, Winskill P, Hamlet A, et al. The impact of COVID-19 and strategies for mitigation and suppression in low- and middle-income countries. Science. 2020;369(6502):413-422.

[3] Aria M, Cuccurullo C. bibliometrix: An R-tool for comprehensive science mapping analysis. J Informetr. 2017;11(4):959-975.

[4] Gary EN, Weiner DB. DNA vaccines: prime time is now. Curr Opin Immunol. 2020;65:21-27.

[5] Mahoney RT, Maynard JE. The introduction of new vaccines into developing countries. Vaccine. 1999;17(7-8):646-652.

[6] Robbins A, Freeman P. Obstacles to developing vaccines for the Third World. Sci Am. 1988;259(5):126-133.

[7] Hollingsworth R. Développement des vaccins candidats de Sanofi contre la COVID-19. Navigation. 2021;100.

[8] Doussoulin JP. A paradigm of the circular economy: the end of cheap nature? Energy Ecol Environ. 2020 Oct 1;5(5):359-368.

[9] Doussoulin JP. COVID-19: Turning a Threat into an Opportunity for the Circular Economy. In: Circular Economy-Recent Advances, New Perspectives and Applications. IntechOpen; 2020.

[10] Morlat C. Sustainable Production System: Eco-development versus Sustainable Development. John Wiley & Sons; 2020.

[11] Usher AD. COVID-19 vaccines for all? The Lancet. 2020;395(10240):1822-1823.

[12] Krause PR, Fleming TR, Ellenberg SS, Henao-Restrepo AM, Krause PR, Fleming T, et al. Maintaining confidentiality of emerging results in COVID-19 vaccine trials is essential. The Lancet. 2020;396(10263):1611-1613.

[13] Mozersky J, Mann DL, DuBois JM. The National Institute of Allergy and Infectious Diseases decision to stop the adaptive COVID-19 trial: on solid ethical and scientific grounds. American College of Cardiology Foundation Washington DC; 2020.

[14] Zhang N-N, Li X-F, Deng Y-Q, Zhao H, Huang Y-J, Yang G, et al. A thermostable mRNA vaccine against COVID-19. Cell. 2020;182(5):1271-1283. e16.

[15] Mahase E. Covid-19: Moderna vaccine is nearly 95% effective, trial involving high risk and elderly people shows. BMJ Br Med J Online. 2020;371.

[16] Corum J, Grady D, Wee S-L, Zimmer C. Coronavirus vaccine tracker. N Y Times. 2020;5.

[17] Cennimo DJ, Bergman SJ. Coronavirus disease 2019 (COVID-19) treatment & management. Medscape Updat. 2020;

[18] Wu S-C. Progress and concept for COVID-19 vaccine development. Biotechnol J. 2020;

[19] Xiong H, Wu Z, Hou F, Zhang J. Which firm-specific characteristics affect the market reaction of Chinese listed companies to the COVID-19 pandemic? Emerg Mark Finance Trade. 2020;56(10):2231-2242.

[20] Florio, M., 2020. Biomed Europa: after the coronavirus, a public infrastructure to overcome the pharmaceutical oligopoly.

[21] Hepburn C, O'Callaghan B, Stern N, Stiglitz J, Zenghelis D. Will COVID-19 fiscal recovery packages accelerate or retard progress on climate change? Oxf Rev Econ Policy. 2020;36.

[22] Cole J, Dodds K. Unhealthy geopolitics: can the response to COVID-19 reform climate change policy? Bull World Health Organ. 2021;99(2):148.

[23] Kalina M, Tilley E. "This is our next problem": cleaning up from the covid-19 response. Waste Manag. 2020;

[24] Vaverková MD, Paleologos EK, Dominijanni A, Koda E, Tang C-S, Małgorzata W, et al. Municipal Solid Waste Management under COVID-19: Challenges and Recommendations. Environ Geotech. 2020;1-15.

[25] Doussoulin JP, Bittencourt M. Analysing the circular economy opportunities in the French construction sector related to the sustainable supply chain: a waste input-output analysis. Int J Supply Chain Oper Resil. 2018;3(2):143-162.

[26] You S, Sonne C, Ok YS. COVID-19's unsustainable waste management. Science. 2020;368(6498):1438.

[27] Moynihan R, Macdonald H, Bero L, Godlee F. Commercial influence and covid-19. British Medical Journal Publishing Group; 2020.

[28] Brzezinski A, Kecht V, Van Dijcke D. The cost of staying open: voluntary social distancing and lockdowns in the US. Brzezinski Adam Kecht Val Van Dijcke David 2020 Cost Stay Open Volunt Soc Distancing Lockdowns US Econ Ser Work Pap. 2020;910.

[29] McCreary EK, Angus DC. Efficacy of Remdesivir in COVID-19. Jama. 2020;324(11):1041-1042.

[30] Diaz II, Mountz A. Intensifying fissures: Geopolitics, nationalism, militarism, and the US response to the novel coronavirus. Taylor & Francis; 2020.

[31] Beigel JH, Tomashek KM, Dodd LE, Mehta AK, Zingman BS, Kalil AC, et al. Remdesivir for the treatment of Covid-19. N Engl J Med. 2020;383(19):1813-1826.

[32] Al-Khatib IA, Arafat HA, Basheer T, Shawahneh H, Salahat A, Eid J, et al. Trends and problems of solid waste management in developing countries: A case study in seven Palestinian districts. Waste Manag. 2007;27(12):1910-1919.

[33] Le TT, Andreadakis Z, Kumar A, Román RG, Tollefsen S, Saville M, et al. The COVID-19 vaccine development landscape. Nat Rev Drug Discov. 2020;19(5):305-306.

[34] Mahase E. Covid-19: UK approves Oxford vaccine as cases of new variant surge. British Medical Journal Publishing Group; 2020.

[35] UK G. Coronavirus (COVID-19) in the UK. UK Gov. 2020;

[36] Gates B. Responding to Covid-19—a once-in-a-century pandemic? N Engl J Med. 2020;382(18):1677-1679.

[37] Mullard A. COVID-19 vaccine development pipeline gears up. The Lancet. 2020;395(10239):1751-1752.

[38] Klemeš JJ, Van Fan Y, Tan RR, Jiang P. Minimising the present and future plastic waste, energy and environmental footprints related to COVID-19. Renew Sustain Energy Rev. 2020;127:109883.

[39] Di Maria F, Beccaloni E, Bonadonna L, Cini C, Confalonieri E, La Rosa G, et al. Minimization of spreading of SARS-CoV-2 via household waste produced by subjects affected by COVID-19 or in quarantine. Sci Total Environ. 2020;743:140803.

[40] Cimmino J, Kroenig M, Pavel B. Taking Stock: Where Are Geopolitics Headed in the COVID-19 Era? 2020;

[41] Hale T, Petherick A, Phillips T, Webster S. Variation in government responses to COVID-19. Blavatnik Sch Gov Work Pap. 2020;31.

[42] Roussel Y, Raoult D. Influence of conflicts of interest on public positions in the COVID-19 era, the case of Gilead Sciences. New Microbes New Infect. 2020;38:100710.

[43] Kim DD, Neumann PJ. Analyzing the cost effectiveness of policy responses for COVID-19: the importance of capturing social consequences. Med Decis Making. 2020;40(3):251-253.

[44] Freeman D, Loe BS, Chadwick A, Vaccari C, Waite F, Rosebrock L, et al. COVID-19 vaccine hesitancy in the UK: the Oxford coronavirus explanations, attitudes, and narratives survey (Oceans) II. Psychol Med. 2020;1-15.

[45] Geleris J, Sun Y, Platt J, Zucker J, Baldwin M, Hripcsak G, et al. Observational study of hydroxychloroquine in hospitalized patients with Covid-19. N Engl J Med. 2020;382(25):2411-2418.

[46] Yamey G, Gonsalves G. Donald Trump: a political determinant of covid-19. British Medical Journal Publishing Group; 2020.

[47] Singh H, Sharma S. Concerns of frontline doctors in India during COVID-19: A cross-sectional survey. Indian J Public Health. 2020;64(6):237.

[48] Mahato S, Pal S, Ghosh KG. Effect of lockdown amid COVID-19 pandemic on air quality of the megacity Delhi, India. Sci Total Environ. 2020;730:139086.

[49] Pontali E, Sotgiu G, Tiberi S, Tadolini M, Visca D, D'Ambrosio L, et al. Combined treatment of drug-resistant tuberculosis with bedaquiline and delamanid: a systematic review. Eur Respir J. 2018;52(1).

Chapter 31

Consequence of Meteorological Parameters on the Transmission of Covid-19

Manish Sharma, Pargin Bangotra and Alok Sagar Gautam

Abstract

Coronavirus disease (COVID-19) was first detected in Wuhan, China in December 2019. The characteristics of the spread of COVID-19 infection from one person to another have led to an increasing number of infected cases and caused tremendous pressure around the world. The rapid spread of COVID-19 infection has made it a pandemic. In India, as of mid-May 2020, there were approximately 75,048 confirmed cases and 2,440 deaths due to COVID-19 alone. In order to break the COVID-19 chain, the Indian government decided to implement a lockdown, which was first implemented on March 23, 2020. The significant benefits of the lockdown have led to a reduction in air pollutants in cities around the world. The significant benefits of the lockdown have led to a reduction in air pollutants in cities around the world. The importance of particulate matter, temperature (°C) and relative humidity (%) to the spread of the COVID-19 virus and its correlation with the total number of cases (TC), active cases (AC), recovered cases (RC) and death cases (DC) Reference DEL will be discussed in detail in this chapter.

Keywords: COVID 19, Particulate matter, Meteorological parameters, Lockdown Impact

1. Introduction

Under the current circumstances, the entire world is at risk of widespread infection of COVID-19, a pandemic, affecting more than 208 countries [1]. According to recent research conducted by researcher [2], there were approximately 4,369,933 COVID-19 cases worldwide, of which 98% had mild infections, 2% have severe infections, and 15% of patients could not survived. On March 22, 2020, the Indian government decided to implement a complete lockdown to prevent the spread of COVID-19 infection.

COVID-19 showed a profound impact on human health as well as on the economies of most of the countries. According to the regulations of the World Health Organization (WHO), people over the age of 60 and children under 10 are severely affected by the coronavirus [3]. According to medical experts, this type of disease is somewhat similar to severe acute respiratory syndrome (SARS). In the earlier study [4] it was demonstrated the viral aerosol generation and airborne droplet transmission in case of SARS. As per some of the medical experts it was assumed the spread of the infection mainly through droplets, and sometimes through hand contact or indirect contact, but still the exact transmission route of this virus could not been recognized.

In India, as of May 13, 2020, there are approximately 75,048 confirmed cases and 2,440 deaths [5]. In view of the seriousness of the infection various activities and operations related to social gatherings, travel, and industry, including all modes of transportation, advertising, construction, and restaurants were restricted, but groceries, milk, fruits and vegetables, medicines, etc., were allowed in limited manner. However, during this lockdown period, the reduction of various air pollutants were observed over numerous countries [1, 6]. It was also reported the deterioration of pollutants PM2.5, PM10, SO2, CO and NO2 during the period of China's lockdown [7]. Prior to lockdown, most Indian cities had pollutant levels with a high proportion of the Indian urban population [8, 9].

The impact of the COVID-19 pandemic has led to a rapid increase in the number of COVID-19 cases in DEL (about 14 million people) in India. The importance of particulate matter, temperature (°C) and relative humidity (%) in the spread of COVID-19 virus and its correlation with the total number of cases (TC), active cases (AC), recovery cases (RC) and death cases (DC) are particularly discussed for the duration from January 1, 2020 to May 15, 2020 over Delhi (DEL) and one of the neighboring cities (Gurgaon (GW)).

Additionally the study conducted by a group of researchers [10], is in close understanding of relationship between air quality and COVID-19 cases in China. Air contamination estimated as particulate matter (PM) had additionally been demonstrated to be impeding to human wellbeing [11–14] and lead to expanded death rates [15, 16]. The prior examination exhibited the observable impact of meteorological parameters particularly surface air temperature and relative dampness on particulate issue [17]. Different pollutants were incorporated to characterize Air quality through the record of CO, Ozone, SO2, NO2, NH3, Pb, PM2.5 and PM10 (NAAQS). Anyway, the most responsible toxins answerable for helpless air quality list in India are presently PM2.5 and PM10.

In the investigation over DEL [18], the PM has been considered as one of the risky contaminations liable for persistent bronchitis and Asthma. Thusly, thinking about the criticality of PM and current lockdown circumstance, the investigation of fine (PM1.0 and PM2.5) and coarse (PM10) PM information for seven different places of Delhi (DEL) and Gurugram called Gurgaon (GW), India was done. During the previous (January 1, 2020 to March 22, 2020) and lock-in period (March

COVID-19	Coronavirus	Shantipath	SP
DEL	Delhi	Greater Kailash	GK
GW	Gurgaon	Lodhi Road	LR
PM	Particulate matter	WHO	World Health Organization
T	Temperature	TC	Total cases
RH	Relative Humidity	RC	Recovered cases
IIT-Delhi	IIT-DEL	AC	Active cases
US Embassy	USE	DC	Death cases
Mahant Gurmukh Singh	MGS	NAAQS	National Ambient Air Quality Standard

Table 1.
Abbreviations.

23, 2020 to May 15, 2020), the daily analysis and comparison corresponding to the abbreviations mentioned (**Table 1**), was accompanied. Since the optimized T (°C) and RH (%) support droplet stability in the local environment, this may be beneficial to the widespread spread of the virus [19]. According to research conducted in different cities in Italy and China, the association between high frequency of corona cases/fatalities and persistently high levels of air pollutants for more than four years were also noticed (www.downtoearth.org.in).

In this chapter, we strive to understand the relationship between PM, T (°C) and RH (%) and their synergy on COVID-19 cases through DEL, corresponding to the total number of cases (TC), active cases (AC), by considering the data available between April 1, 2020 and May 15, 2020, recover cases (RC) and death cases (DC).

2. Data and analysis techniques

This chapter covers the examined results of the study conducted over Delhi (DEL) and Gurgaon (GW), India (**Figure 1**). In the study the major pollutants i.e. PM of size ≤ 2.5 μm (PM2.5), ≤ 10 μm (PM10) and ≤ 1.0 (PM1.0) along with meteorological parameters, i.e., T (°C), RH (%) were downloaded through Purple Air sensors website (https://www.purpleair.com).The average PM and related T (°C) and RH (%) for consecutive 24 hours from January 1, 2020 to May 15, 2020 were used to covers seven different sites in Delhi, namely IIT-DEL, GK, LR, MGS, RJ, SP and USE, as well as two locations on GW.

The information comparing to TC just as RC were gathered from the source of New Delhi Television Limited (NDTV), an Indian TV media organization. (https://www.ndtv.com/coronavirus). The 2-tailed Bivariate Pearson correlations using Statistical Package for the Social Sciences (SPSS) was applied to verify the correlation among PM, T (°C),RH (%), TC, AC, RC and DC.

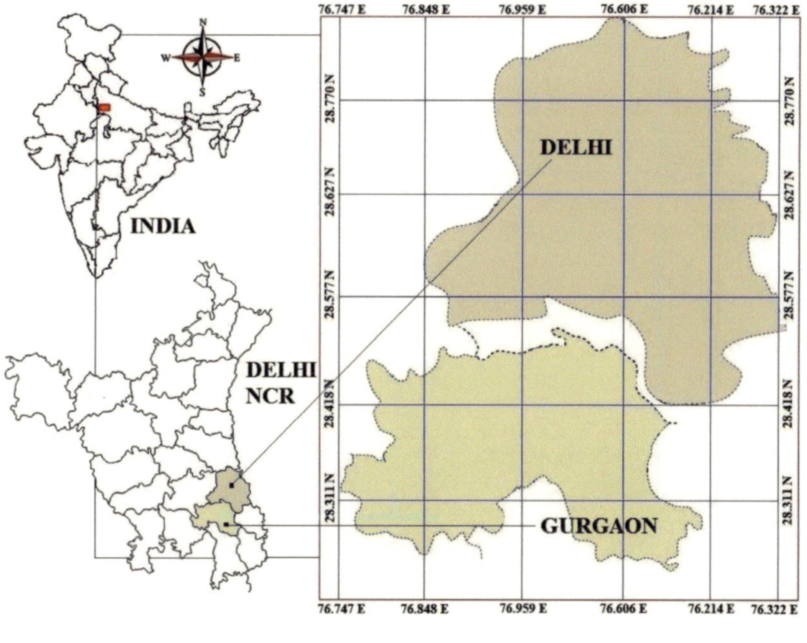

Figure 1.
Study location of Delhi (DEL) and Gurgaon (GW), India.

3. Results and discussion

This part of the chapter scrutinize the diversity in mean centralization of PM of size 1 micron, 2.5 micron and 10 micron generally perceived as PM 1.0, PM2.5 and PM10, over DEL and GW. The provocation of meteorology on PM and its relationship to TC and RC related to COVID-19 also covered here.

3.1 Dissemination of PM

The noteworthy distinction is clearly appearing for fine (PM1.0, PM 2.5) and coarse (PM10) over DEL and GW in box and whiskers charts view.

The dissimilar dispersal is clearly visible from the distribution pattern of PM concentration (PM1.0, PM2.5 and PM10) in above two sites during the period 1st January 2020 to 15th May 2020 (**Figure 2**). The concentrations are expressed in $\mu g.m^{-3}$ for PM1.0, PM2.5 and PM10.

The low mean convergence of PM (PM1.0, PM2.5 and PM10) over the site GW pronounce the better air quality as contrast with DEL. The entirety of the spans of PM were displayed divergent focus that shows the different wellsprings of contaminations over both of areas for example DEL and GW. The higher mean fixation and conspicuous trait of PM2.5 and PM10 showed in Box plot (**Figure 3**), propose street traffic [20] just as ventures, power plants and homegrown discharge.

In pattern investigation (**Figure 3a** and **b**) during first January 2020 to fifteenth May 2020, PM10 display a higher mean convergence of 127.61 $\mu g\text{-}m^{-3}$ (DEL) and 57.53 $\mu g\text{-}m^{-3}$ (GW) though PM1.0 and PM2.5, delineate the mean grouping of 69.22 $\mu g\text{-}m^{-3}$ (DEL), 34.20 $\mu g\text{-}m^{-3}$ (GW) and 111.75 $\mu g\text{-}m^{-3}$(DEL) and 53.10 $\mu g\text{-}m^{-3}$ (GW), separately.

The higher PM concentration during this period, obviously recommends the effect of vehicular emanation, modern outflow, and different types of burning cycle as the significant wellsprings of toxins. After execution of comprehensive lockdown through restricting various activities and operations related to social assembly, travel, industries operations and transport, started from 23rd March 2020, PM mass concentration in DEL (**Figure 3a**) and GW (**Figure 3b**) were significantly

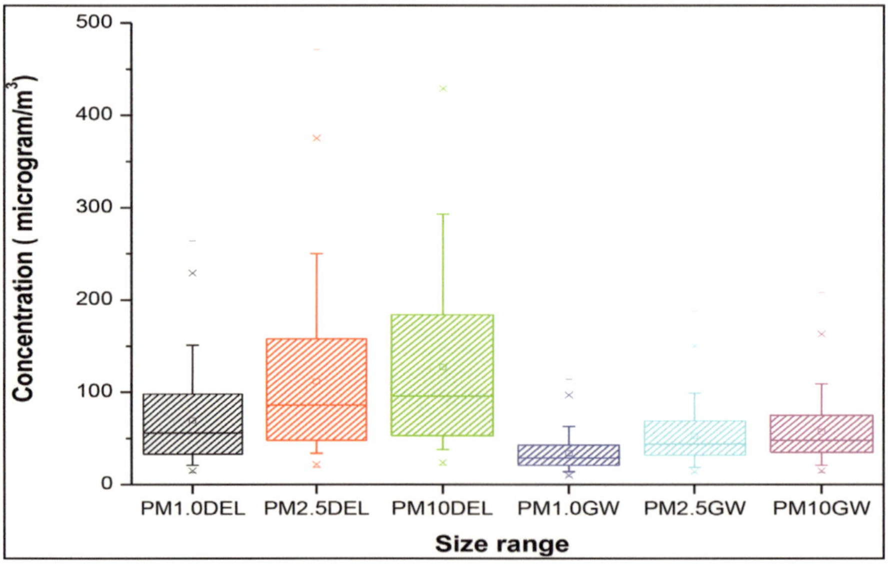

Figure 2.
Boxplots of daily concentrations of analyzed pollutants over Delhi and Gurgaon; the median is shown by the middle line of the box.

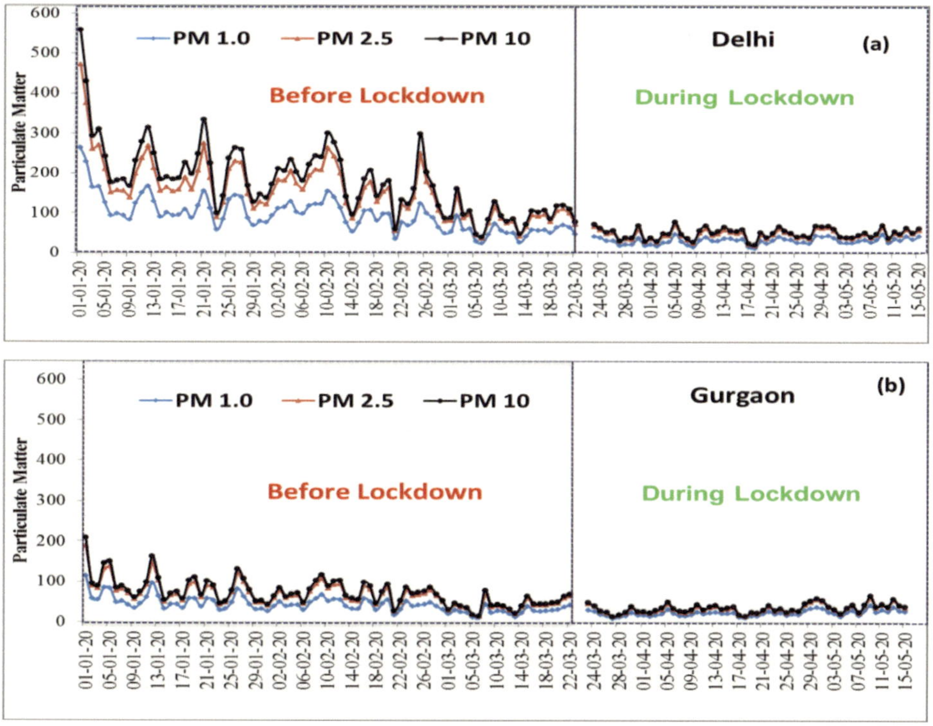

Figure 3.
(a, b). Trend analysis showing the effect of lockdown period on particulate matter in Delhi (a) and Gurgaon (b).

declined. The significant decline in the concentration of PM, clearly confirms the influence of the transport and traffic movement in the air quality of DEL. The tremendous decline of 48.21%, 51.82% and 52.45% in PM1.0 (21.90 $\mu g\text{-}m^{-3}$), PM2.5 (32.19 $\mu g\text{-}m^{-3}$) and (34.52 $\mu g\text{-}m^{-3}$) were witnessed the impact of lockdown over GW.

Because of discontinue of all kind of developments, mechanical emanation and transportation out and about, the fine (PM1.0 and PM2.5) and coarse (PM 10) particulate were essentially diminished over both of the areas (DEL and GW) and drew closer inside the restriction of NAAQS (PM2.5 = 60 $\mu g\text{-}m^{-3}$, PM10 = 100 $\mu g\text{-}m^{-3}$, in view of 24-hours normal [2] exhibiting the perceptible improvement in air quality. The huge abatement in climatic contamination credited to transportation and mechanical outflows over Beijing, Shanghai, Guangzhou, and Wuhan urban communities were likewise seen during the crown pandemic.

3.2 Effect of meteorology on PM

The past examinations exhibited the impact of meteorological factors, which influence the air quality [21, 22]. The complete example of the improvement of discretionary pollutions has the phenomenal relationship with the toxic substance release rate into the air all along, wind speed, unevenness level, air temperature, and precipitation [23]. Generally, T (°C) has a substantial involvement in air quality of the province therefore correlation analysis by considering the period of 1st March 2020 - 15th May 2020 between PM concentrations and T (°C) for the site DEL (**Figure 4**) and GW (**Figure 5**) were studied to understand the role of T (°C).

The results shows a significant negative correlation between T (°C) and PM1.0 (0.72), PM2. (0.73) and PM10 (0.73) in DEL while over GW, it is as 0.54 (PM1.0), 0.58 (PM2.5) and 0.25 (PM10). In the related **Figures 4** and **5**, the red, green and black dots indicate the data corresponding to PM1.0, PM2.5 and PM10, respectively.

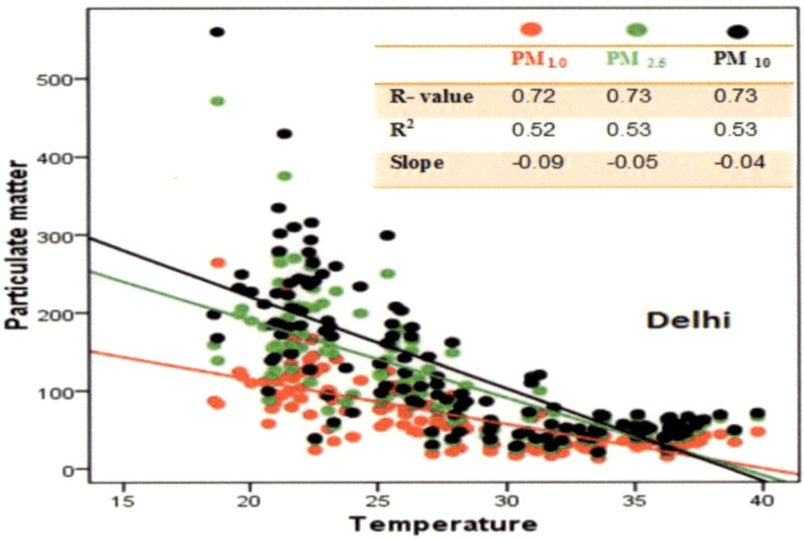

Figure 4.
Scatter plot among $PM_{1.0}$, $PM_{2.5}$ and PM_{10} and T (°C) over DEL.

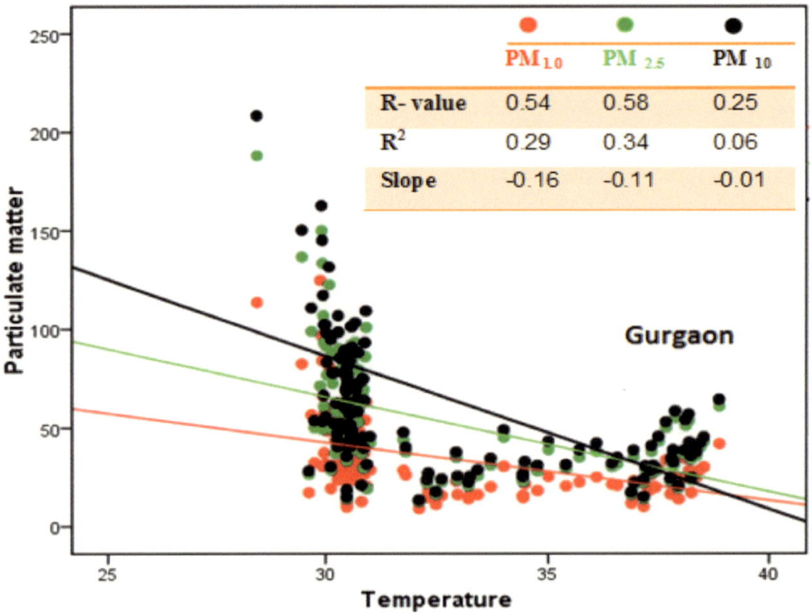

Figure 5.
Scatter plot among $PM_{1.0}$, $PM_{2.5}$ and PM_{10} and T (°C) over GW.

Here the regression analysis reveals significant negative correlation (r) of T (°C) with PM in DEL whereas GW has the low negative correlation of 0.25 with PM10. The total time of insight demonstrates the declining qualities of PM fixations on the increment of the T (°C).

3.3 PM over different locations of DEL and GW

As the long-range transport and buildup furthermore has a gigantic responsibility in the social event or dispersing of contaminations at metropolitan districts [24].

Further, the centralization of PM1.0, PM2.5 and PM10 for seven particular spaces of DEL and GW were bankrupt down and amazed for the situation and Box and whisker plot to perceive the possible impact of lockdown (**Figure 6a–c**).

Before lockdown and during lockdown season of the assessment are perceived by the letter B and A, independently. Preceding lockdown, the mean assembly of PM1.0 and PM2.5 over IIT-DEL, GK, LR, MGS, RJ, SP, and USE were noticed as 89.29 ± 45.51 µg-m^{-3}, 57.07 ± 32.70 µg-m^{-3}, 90.01 ± 40.72 µg-m^{-3}, 70.35 ± 28.33 µg-m^{-3}, 133.18 ± 68.15 µg-m^{-3}, 97.53 ± 49.39 µgm^{-3}, 121.31 ± 54.03 µgm^{-3} and 146.67 ± 78.63 µg-m^{-3}, 85.04 ± 51.02 µg-m^{-3}, 162.04 ± 91.42 µg-m^{-3}, 124.75 ± 57.26 µg-m^{-3}, 218.38 ± 144.20 µg-m^{-3}, 163 ± 88.94 µg-m^{-3},

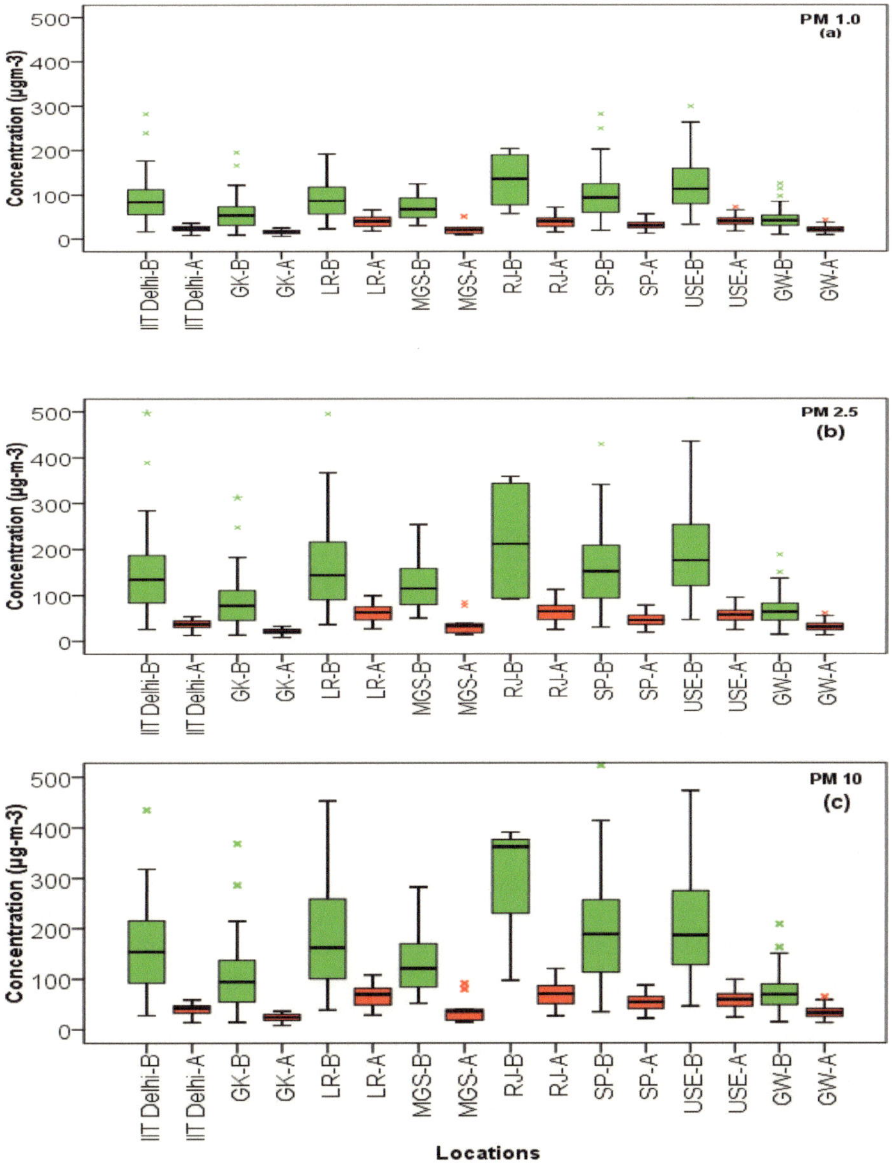

Figure 6.
Boxplots of daily concentrations of analyzed pollutants over different locations of Delhi and Gurgaon; median is shown by the middle line of the box. Concentrations are expressed in µg- m^{-3} for $PM_{1.0}$ (a), $PM_{2.5}$ (b) and PM_{10} (c). (letter "B" and "A" represents the boxes related to before lock down and during lockdown respectively).

191.09 ± 94.03 μg-m^{-3}, separately (**Figure 5a** and **b**). In any case, the mean assembly of PM1.0 in the above said regions was 166 ± 89.47 μg-m^{-3}, 103.33 ± 60.19 μg-m^{-3}, 187.32 ± 116.52 μg-m^{-3}, 134.78 ± 63.75 μg-m^{-3}, 283.46 ± 161.89 μg-m^{-3}, 200.83 ± 112.21 μg-m^{-3}, 205 ± 105.07 μg-m^{-3}, separately as portrayed in **Figure 6c**.

The GW area shows the lower PM fixation i.e. 43.31 ± 20.25 μg-m^{-3} (PM1.0), 66.55 ± 29.94 μg-m^{-3} (PM2.5) and 72.63 ± 33.10 μg-m^{-3} (PM 10) as contrast with DEL during the range of before lockdown. The normal PM2.5 and PM10 focuses over the distinctive examination site of DEL and GW districts are at higher side than the given furthest reaches of NAAQS (PM2.5 = 40 μg-m^{-3}) and PM10 = 60 μg-m^{-3}) [2]. Prior to lockdown circumstance, the most noteworthy PM1.0 esteems were found over the RJ showing mean of 133.18 μg-m^{-3} and is trailed by USE, SP, LR, IIT, MGS and GW, separately. The high interquartile range (RJ, USE, SP and LR) recommends that PM1.0 hold very extraordinary fixation exhibiting the enormous spread (56.95-203.85 μg-m^{-3}). The enormous upper stubble over the area IIT-DEL, SP and USE shows that the PM1.0 focus fluctuates among the best quartile bunch. The upper portions of the scale i.e. positive quartile bunch comparing to practically all areas with the exception of RJ shows the articulated inconstancy in the centralization of PM1.0, however, in case of least positive quartile group, the concentration spread is relatively less. However, the box plots related to before lockdown, show enormous focus disseminations of PM1.0 while the box plot associated to during lockdown shows the slight scattering that delineate the limit decrease in the grouping of PM1.0.

According to the past examinations, PM2.5 involves with various dangerous constituents, which may go into the lungs through the respiratory track and unsafe to the human wellbeing, chiefly to youngsters and the older individuals [25]. The recently directed investigation, uncover the particulate matter as one of prime explanation for damaging outcome on the human respiratory framework by stressing to take repetitive clinical remedy [11]. The spread and inconstancy of PM2.5 focus has been summed up in box plots as portrayed **Figure 6b**. The most noteworthy mean grouping of fine particulate matter PM2.5 (218.37 μg-m^{-3}), was seen over RJ during before lockdown period and 63.41 μg-m^{-3} during the lockdown period. The incredibly upper and lower stubbles (before lockdown) show the instance of least quartile that compares to less articulated conduct of PM2.5 focus because of the less number of information (4 days) over RJ locale. Notwithstanding that, the territories LR, SP and USE divulges the huge upper bristle shows the observable irregularity in the convergence of PM2.5.

As contrast with DEL district, GW locale (**Figure 6b**) clarify the low mean PM2.5 focus checking information as 73.51 μg-m^{-3} (13.98 μg-m^{-3}-188.04 μg-m^{-3}) related to earlier lockdown (GW-B) that decreased to 31.97 μg-m^{-3} (12 μg-m^{-3}-60.83 μg-m^{-3}) because of the lockdown (GW-A). The lockdown sway was liable for the unexpected fall in PM2.5 focuses because of cross country limitation on transport development and modern units that related to the emanation of essential toxins into the area. Prior to lockdown period, the relating areas of DEL and GW were high PM2.5 focus which upholds the finding of surrounding PM2.5 fixations higher more noteworthy than 60 μg-m^{-3} over New Delhi [6, 26]. This may be because of the area of the site that is near traffic and private contamination sources [20, 27]. According to above discoveries, an extremely different source of PM concentration has been seen in the examined area. **Figure 6c** divulges the mean convergence of PM10 by showing the most noteworthy worth over RJ (283.46 μg-m^{-3}) followed by USE (205.82 μg-m^{-3}) and SP (200.83 μg-m^{-3}) related to before lockdown period that further began to disintegrate to 69.36 μg-m^{-3}(RJ), 58.64 μg-m^{-3}(USE) and 53.59 μg-m^{-3} (SP) because of the lockdown impact. The area GW shows the mean convergence of 72.63 μg-m^{-3} (preceding lock down) and 34.28 μg-m^{-3}(during lockdown) which and both are extremely close endorsed breaking point of 60 μg-m^{-3} given by NAAQS.

3.4 COVID-19 and associated factor

DEL had been viewed as one of the focal points for Covid in India (https://indianexpress.com/article/india) and to comprehend the quick expansion in COVID-19 cases, it was important to comprehend the marvel and capable elements for its spreading. The aftereffects of 2-tailed Bivariate Pearson Correlation over DEL for the period 1 April 2020 to 15 May 2020 has been talked about here.

In light of 45 days information for period first April 2020 to fifteenth April 2020, it very well may be seen the normal TC, AC, RC, DC as 3003 ± 2393, 2137 ± 1514, 821 ± 877, 44 ± 28 individually. During this period the mean centralization of PM 1.0, PM 2.5 and PM10 has been seen as 31.42 μg-m^{-3}, 46.36 μg-m^{-3} and 50.78 μg-m^{-3}, separately. Be that as it may, normal T (°C) and RH (%) were 34.720C and 27.86% individually. The Pearson connection results (**Table 2**) over DEL uncovered the impressive relationship of T (°C) with TC (0.57, p = 0), AC (0.59, p = 0), RC (0.51, p = 0) and DC (0.58, p = 0) identified with COVID-19 and unmistakably demonstrates the expansion altogether and dynamic COVID-19 cases because of height of T (°C).

Because of inaccessibility of the information identified with different highlights that add to influence the pace of spread of COVID-19 disease inside a DEL area, the investigation does not bring up towards temperature as a solitary one factor answerable for the transmission of COVID-19. As the increment in the T (°C) over DEL during the period of April and May is likewise related to the occasional climate wonder, so it is hard to proclaim the precise relationship of T (°C) with the TC.

2-tailed Bivariate Pearson correlation										
		TC	AC	RC	DC	PM 1.0	PM 2.5	PM 10	Temp	RH
TC	Pearson Correlation	1.00	0.99**	0.98**	0.93**	0.34*	0.21	0.16	0.56**	0.28
	p value		0.00	0.00	0.00	0.02	0.16	0.29	0.00	0.06
AC	Pearson Correlation	0.99**	1.00	0.95**	0.92**	0.33*	0.20	0.15	0.58**	0.25
	p value	0.00		0.00	0.00	0.03	0.19	0.34	0.00	0.10
RC	Pearson Correlation	0.98**	0.95**	1.00	0.92**	0.36*	0.23	0.18	0.52**	0.33*
	p value	0.00	0.00		0.00	0.01	0.12	0.24	0.00	0.03
DC	Pearson Correlation	0.93**	0.92**	0.92**	1.00	0.32*	0.20	0.14	0.58**	0.26
	p value	0.00	0.00	0.00		0.03	0.20	0.37	0.00	0.08
RH	Pearson Correlation	0.28	0.25	0.33*	0.26	0.09	0.06	0.03	−0.07	1.00
	p value	0.06	0.10	0.03	0.08	0.55	0.70	0.85	0.65	

***shows here that correlation is significant at the 0.01 level (2-tailed).*
**showing that correlation is significant at the 0.05 level (2-tailed).*

Table 2.
Two-tailed bivariate Pearson correlation among Total cases (TC), active case (AC), recovered case (RC), PM1.0, PM2.5, PM10, temp, and RH over DEL.

The significant finding identified with the commendable certain connection (0.51, p = 0) of T (°C) and RC has been noticed yet likelihood of a critical expansion in RC with temperature alone is not sensible to come at some resolution.

There is a connection between RH (%) and the COVID-19 infection perseverance. Most infections endure best at low RH (<40%) and amazingly high RH (>90%). However, the connection between the endurance of COVID-19 infection and relative dampness should be elucidated. Here, the RH (%) shows minimal relationship with TC (0.28, p = 0.06), AC (0.25, p = 0.10), and DC (0.26, p = 0.08) and moderate connection with RC (0.33, p = 0.03). Such great connection of RH (%) with RC recommends the slight positive impact of RH on RC. The lower dampness upholds the mist concentrates molecule to decrease its size to remain suspended in air for longer time. As in the current month (April to May 2020) the mean RH (%) is lower (27.86%) and the disease spread might be because of the suspended mist concentrates molecule. In the event of COVID-19 infection scattering, these suspended vaporizers particles may assume a significant part in the transmission of infection starting with one then onto the next yet dependent upon some insufficient distance. To keep away from this disease, Government of India, pronounced the rules to keep up the social removing too least of 1 meter distance with someone else which was useful to stay away from the conceivable outcomes of contamination and enormous expansion in the quantity of TC (0.28, p = 0.06). The expansion of RH (%) with the presence of beads in the air supports to the substantial pressurized canned products particles to settle down on the ground surface. Thus, for this situation, when the contaminated individual, hack or sniffle around there, the mist concentrates drops because of its substantialness begins to settle down on a superficial level and further add to send the COVID-19 infection through the surface contact.

Some of prior examinations tracked down the critical job of T (°C) and RH (%) liable for the spread of numerous respiratory irresistible infections like flu [28, 29]. As claimed in the study [19], the urban areas with the common transmission of COVID-19 infection were high RH of 60% ~ 90% and low T (°C). To analyze the impact of the grouping of particulate poisons on all out number of COVID-19 cases, the spatio-transient investigation (**Figure 7**) was finished. It was tracked down the 154 number of affirmed instances of COVID-19 on dated 1 April 2020 which compares to the particulate mass centralization of 21.96 μg-m^{-3} (PM1.0), 34.69 μg-m^{-3} (PM2.5) and 39.04 μg-m^{-3} (PM10). Following 43 days (15th May 2020), the instances of COVID-19 in DEL came to up to a greatest number of 8470 with the increment of 98.02% and in the comparable example the PM fixation additionally quickly expanded by 48% (PM1.0), 40.47% (PM2.5) and 38.02% (PM10).

The increment in the quantity of COVID-19 cases with the expansion of particulate matter mass fixation over DEL recommend the impact of fine and coarse mode particulate matter on TC. The impact of variable sizes of PM on TC, AC, RC and DC were shown utilizing the Pearson connection (r) and Sig. 2-i.e. p-value.

The PM of different size i.e. PM1.0, PM2.5 and PM10 demonstrated the correlation (r) with TC, AC, RC and DC (**Table 2**). The PM1.0 has the moderate correlation with TC (0.34, p value = 0.02), AC (0.33, p value = 0.02), RC (0.36, p value = 0.01) and DC (0.32, p value = 0.02) whereas PM2.5 and PM10 were least correlation value (r) with TC, AC, RC and DC as 0.21 (p value = 0.15), 0.19 (p value = 0.19), 0.23 (p value = 0.12), 0.19 (p value = 0.19) and 0.16 (p value = 0.29), 0.14 (p value = 0.23), 0.18 (p value = 0.23) and 0.13 (p value = 0.36), respectively. Our studies indicate that PM1.0is relatively more associated with the various stages of COVID-19 patients i.e. TC, AC, RC and DC as compare to 2.5 and PM10. These observations propose that, while direct COVID-19 contamination is fundamental track of transmission, the part of PM1.0 in infection transmission may play a critical character. The RH (%) was related with the PM by meaning the relationship (r) as follows for

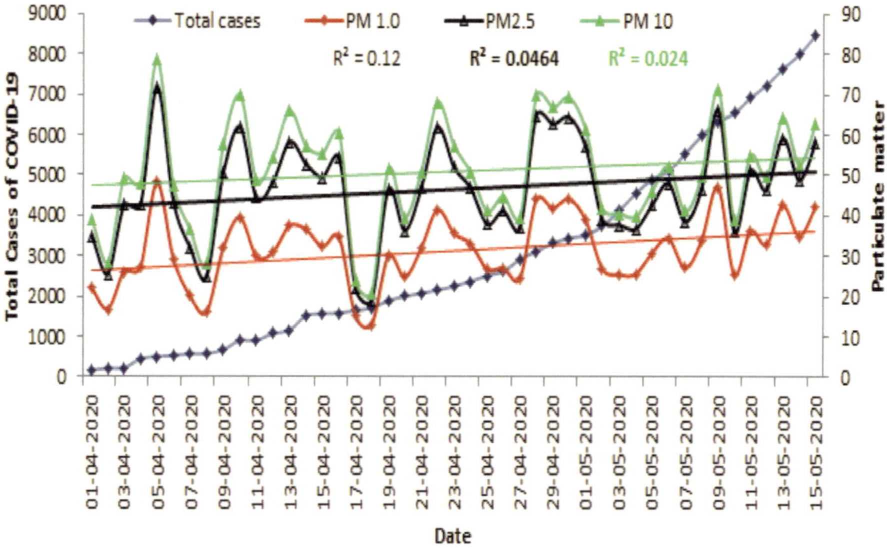

Figure 7.
Spatio-temporal observation between fine (PM1.0, PM2.5) and coarse (PM10) particulate pollutants and TC of COVID-19.

example 0.09 (PM1.0), 0.05 (PM2.5) and 0.03 (PM10). Likewise the Sig. (2-followed) for example p upsides of 0.54, 0.69 and 0.84 identified with PM1.0, PM2.5 and PM10 individually, exhibit the incredibly less impact of RH (%) on PM over DEL during the investigation time frame.

4. Conclusion

From last decade, numerous steps were taken by Delhi administration to tackle the pollution problem in distinct vicinities with main focus on air contamination over Delhi – NCR region. However, a pandemic (COVID - 19) forced to shut down all impurity sources in the form of transportation and industrial practices over this region.

The section supports the impact of lockdown over Delhi and Gurgaon on the particulate issue. It was the endeavors to exhibit the impacts of meteorological factors in COVID-19 in DEL. It was noticed the unmistakable impact of lockdown which show the decay of 67.31%, 70.29% and 71.66% more than Delhi and 48.21%, 51.82% and 52.45% over Gurgaon, in PM1.0, PM2.5 and PM10, separately. It was noticed that the Particulate Matter, Temperature and Relative Humidity (RH %) legitimize exceptional consideration. Relative humidity (RH %) was found as a considerable boundary that showed the huge connection with COVID 19 recuperated cases. For the investigation time frame chosen, the COVID-19 recuperated case in Delhi was seen to be supported by lower mean relative moistness (27.86°C) that was approved through the moderate relationship of 0.33 (p value = 0.03) with Recovered case. Such connection validate the impact of relative humidity (RH %) on COVID-19 recuperated cases. In light of double character of RH (%) on the scattering of COVID-19 infection, it was anticipated the expansion in the number COVID-19 cases in July and August through the surface transmission. However, it is essential to conduct an extensive study with long-term data, which might enhance the understanding between meteorological conditions and the COVID-19 transmissibility.

Acknowledgements

The authors are thankful to Purple Air for Particulate pollutants data. We also thank to New Delhi Television Limited (NDTV) for providing the updated information related to the COVID-19.

Conflict of interest

"The authors declare no conflict of interest."

Author details

Manish Sharma[1*], Pargin Bangotra[1] and Alok Sagar Gautam[2]

1 Atmospheric Research Laboratory, Department of Physics, School of Basic Sciences and Research, Sharda University, Greater Noida, India

2 Department of Physics, Hemvati Nandan Bahuguna Garhwal University, Uttarakhand, India

*Address all correspondence to: manish.sharma@sharda.ac.in

References

[1] Akshansha Chauhan, Ramesh P. Singh., Decline in PM2.5 concentrations over major cities around the world associated with COVID-19, Environmental Research 2020. 187109634

[2] Jain, S., Sharma, T. Social and Travel Lockdown Impact Considering Coronavirus Disease (COVID-19) on Air Quality in Megacities of India: Present Benefits, Future Challenges and Way Forward. Aerosol Air Qual Res. 2020. 20: 1222-1236.

[3] Donnelly, CA., Ghani, AC., Leung, GM., Hedley, AJ., Fraser, C., Riley, S., Radded, LAJ., Ho, LM., Thach, TQ., Chau, P., Chan, KP., Lam, TH., Tse, LY., Tsang, T., Liu, SH., Kong, JHB., Lau, mC., Ferguson, NM., Anderson, RM. Epidemiological determinants of spread of causal agent of severe acute respiratory syndrome in Hong Kong. *Lancet 2003.* 361 (9371): 1761-1766.

[4] Booth, TF., Kournikakis, B., Bastien, N., Ho, j., Kobasa, D., Stadnyk, L., Li, Y., Spence, M., Paton, S., Henry, B., Mederski, B., White, D., Low, DE., McGeer, A., Simor, A., Vearncombe, M., Downey, J., Jamieson, FB., Tang, P., Plummer, F. Detection of airborne severe acute respiratory syndrome (SARS) coronavirus and environmental contamination in SARS outbreak units. *J Infect Dis*. 2010. 91 (9): 1472-1477.

[5] MoHFW. 2020 https://www.mohfw.gov.in/

[6] Singh, DP., Gadi, R., Mandal, TK. Characterization of particulate-bound polycyclic aromatic hydrocarbons and trace metals composition of urban air in Delhi, India. *Atmos Environ*. 2011. 45: 7653-7663.

[7] Xu, K., Cui, K., Young, L.H., Hsieh, Y.K., Wang, Y.F., Zhang, J. and Wan, S. Impact of the COVID-19 event on air quality in central China. Aerosol Air Qual. Res., 2020. 20: 915-929. https://doi.org/10.4209/aaqr.2020.04.0150.

[8] Aggarwal, P. and Jain, S. Impact of air pollutants from surface transport sources on human health: A modeling and epidemiological approach. Environ. Int., 2015. 83: 146-157.

[9] Kumar, P., Jain, S., Gurjar, B.R., Sharma, P., Khare, M., Morawska, L. and Britter, R. New Directions: Can a "blue sky" return to Indian megacities? Atmos. Environ., 2013. 71: 198-201.

[10] Wu, X., Nethery, R.C., Sabath, B.M., Braun, D. and Dominici, F. Exposure to air pollution and COVID-19 mortality in the United States. medRxiv 2020.04.05.20054502. https://doi.org/10.1101/2020

[11] Anderson, J O., Thundiyil, JG., Stolbach, A., Clearing the air: a review of the effects of particulate matter air pollution on human health. J Med Toxicol 2012. 8(2): 166-175.

[12] Donaldson, K., Stone, V., Seaton, A., MacNee, W. Ambient particle inhalation and the cardiovascular system: potential mechanisms. Environ Health Persp. 2001. 109: 523-527.

[13] Pope, C., Bates, D., Raizenne, M. Health effects of particulate air pollution: time for reassessment. *Environ Health Persp* 1995. 103: 472-480.

[14] Puett, R., Hart, J., Yanosky, J., Spiegelman, D., Wang, M., Fisher, J., Hong, B., Laden, F. Particulate Matter Air Pollution Exposure, Distance to Road, and Incident Lung Cancer in the Nurses' Health Study Cohort. *Environ Health Persp* 2014. 122: 926-932.

[15] Dockery, D., Pope, C., Xu, X., Spengler, J., Ware, J., Fay, M., Ferris, B., Speizer, F. An association between air

pollution and mortality in six U.S. cities. *N Engl J Med*. 1993. 329: 1753-1759.

[16] Hales, S., Blakely, T., Woodward, A. Air Pollution and mortality in New Zealand: cohort study. *J Epidemiol Community Health*. 2010. 66: 468-473.

[17] Wang, P., Chen, K., et al., Severe air pollution events not avoided by reduced anthropogenic activities during COVID-19 outbreak. Resour. Conserv. Recycl. 2020. 158. https://doi.org/10.1016/j.resconrec.2020.104814.

[18] Saksena, S. and Dayal, V. Total exposure as a basis for the economic valuation of air pollution in India. Energy Environment Monitor, 2000. 13(2): 93-102.

[19] Chen, C. and Zhao, B. Makeshift hospitals for COVID-19 patients: Where health-care workers and patients need sufficient ventilation for more protection. J. Hosp. Infect. 2020. https://doi.org/10.1016/j.jhin.2020.03.008.

[20] Kumar, P., Gulia, S., Harrison, RM., Khare, M. The influence of odd-even car trial on fine and coarse particles in Delhi. *Environ Pollut*. 2017. 225: 20-30.

[21] Espinosa, AJF., Rodriguez, MT., Alvarez, FF. Source Characterisation of Fine Urban Particles by Multivariate Analysis of Trace Metal Speciation. *Atmos Environ*. 2004. 38: 873-886.

[22] Karar, K., Gupta, AK. Seasonal variations and chemical characterization of ambient PM_{10} at residential and industrial sites of an urban region of Kolkata (Calcutta), *India. Atmos Res.* 2006. 81: 36-53.

[23] Bhaskar, B V., Mehta, VM. Atmospheric Particulate Pollutants and their Relationship with Meteorology in Ahmedabad. *Aerosol and Air Quality Research* 2010. 10: 301-315.

[24] Arif, M., Kumar, R., Kumar, R., Eric, Z., Gourav, P. Ambient black carbon, PM2.5 and PM10 at Patna: Influence of anthropogenic emissions and brick kilns. The Science of the Total Environment ; 2018624:1387-1400.

[25] Daoru, L., Deng, Q., Zhou, Z., Lin, Y., Tao, J. Variation Trends of Fine Particulate Matter Concentration in Wuhan City from 2013 to 2017. Int J Environ Res Public Health. 2018. 15 (7): 1487.

[26] Tiwari, S., Bisht, DS., Srivastava, AK., Pipal, AS., Taneja, A., Srivastava, MK., Attri, SD. Variability in atmospheric particulates and meteorological effects on their mass concentrations over Delhi, India. *Atmos Res*. 2014. 45 – 46: 145 -146.

[27] Gulia, S., Mittal, A., Khare, M. Quantitative evaluation of source interventions for urban air quality improvement—A case study of Delhi city. Atmos Pollut Res. 2018. 9: 577-583.

[28] Barreca AI, Shimshack JP. Absolute humidity, temperature, and influenza mortality: 30 years of county-level evidence from the United States. *American journal of epidemiology*. 2012, 176(7): 114 - 122.

[29] Lowen, AC., Mubareka, S., Steel, J., Palese, P. Influenza Virus Transmission is Dependent on Relative Humidity and Temperature. *PLoSPathog*. 2007. 3 (10): 1470 - 1406.

Chapter 32

COVID-19 Lockdown and the Aerosphere in India: Lessons Learned on How to Reduce Air Pollution

Subhasmita Panda, Priyadatta Satpathy, Trutpi Das and Boopathy Ramasamy

Abstract

The giant increase in COVID-19 infection across India forced the government to impose strict lockdown in order to curb the pandemic. Although the stringent restrictions crippled India's economy and poor people's livelihood, it significantly improved the air quality of most of the polluted cities of India and rejuvenated the atmosphere. Thus, the major objective of this study is to provide a comprehensive overview of lockdown on pollutants prevailing in the atmosphere. A prominent decline in primary pollutants such as Particulate matter (PM), Black carbon (BC), Oxides of nitrogen (NOx), Carbon monoxide (CO) is observed across the country. However, lockdown had a trifling impact on Sulphur dioxide (SO2) concentration over some parts of India due to the constant operation of coal-fired thermal plants as a part of essential service. Furthermore, the sudden decline in NOx concentration disturbed the complex atmospheric chemistry and lead to an enhancement of surface ozone (O3) (secondary pollutant) in many cities of India. Thus, lockdown emerged as a unique opportunity for the atmospheric researchers, policymakers as well as stakeholders to collect baseline data of pollutants and their major sources. This will help to set new targets of air quality standards and to develop various mitigation processes to combat air pollution.

Keywords: COVID-19, lockdown, aerosols, trace gas, air quality index

1. Introduction

Air pollution has created wreaking havoc in many parts of the world. Over the decades, a rapid increase in population, especially in developing countries like India and China, has led to rapid urbanization, industrialization, energy consumption, and exponential growth in vehicles. Consequently, anthropogenic emissions have increased 2–6 folds, thus deteriorating the regional air quality and turning most of the Indian cities into non-attainment cities by the National Green Tribunal of India. Moreover, as per the latest IQAr 2020 report, India is the third most polluted country and is a home for 22 of the world's 30 worst polluted cities in 2020 [1]. Besides, they also stated Delhi as the most polluted capital that resides 10 most polluted cities of the world. Apart from this, there have been several reports in recent times on ambient air criteria pollutants, like, particulate matter, O3, CO and NOx that are at the helm of triggering several environmental health threats leading to comorbidity and premature deaths [2, 3]. According to the 2019 Global Burden disease report, ~1.67 million deaths were attributed to air pollution, which ascribed ~18% of the country's total death [4]. Short-term air pollution exposure is often associated with COPD (Chronic Obstructive Pulmonary Disease), shortness of breath, dizziness, nausea, asthma, cough, and an increase in rates of co-morbid symptoms [5]. However, long-term exposure leads to cardiovascular diseases, lung cancer, and respiratory diseases such as emphysema and is often also accountable for impairment of the nervous system, kidney, liver, and other organisms. Exposure of women to severe ambient pollution during pregnancy is related to a high risk of congenital disabilities, miscarriage and adverse long-term postnatal health [6, 7]. Air pollutants also affect plant growth by inducing changes in soil pH, decrease in photosynthesis rate (trace metals block the stomata opening) and retartded growths [8].

Over the last five decades, an increase in greenhouse gas emissions, especially CO2, has tremendously increased earth temperature globally by preventing solar radiation from getting reflected on the outer surface. Besides, short-lived climate pollutants (SLCPs) such as black carbon (BC), tropospheric/surface ozone (O3), methane (CH4) also significantly contribute to global warming, which in turn lead to prolonged heat waves, temperature variability, forest fires, droughts, flood, melting of ice, icebergs, and glaciers along with depletion of the stratospheric ozone layer [5, 9]. Also, a rampant rise in pollutants such as oxides of sulfur and nitrogen has led to acid rain ($pH<5$) which in turn affects surface water, soil, and lowers biodiversity. Acid rain damages limestone and marble buildings.

This havoc scenario has raised concern among researchers and environmentalists to focus on minor constituents of the atmosphere such as particulate matter and trace gases (mainly SO2, NOx, O3). These species vary enormously with space, time, meteorology, and climate. In this context, the Ministry of Environment, Forest and Climate Change initiated a National Air Quality Monitoring Program (NAMP) all over India. The network comprised of 543 operating stations in 240 cities/towns in 26 states and 5 Union Territories where monitoring is carried out collectively by the Central Pollution Control Board (CPCB); State Pollution Control Board (SPCB); Pollution Control Committees (PCC); National Environmental Engineering Research Institute (NEERI), Nagpur. Apart from these, the Space Physics Laboratory (SPL) of VSSC has set up more than 42 monitoring stations all over India under the project ISRO-GBP -ARFINET to study regional aerosol characterization, heterogeneous features, and radiative forcing. Robust monitoring helps assess the quality of air along with significant sources of pollutants and its negative impact on the ecosystem and humankind. It also aids in guarding against extreme events by alerting people through designing and implementing new air quality management programs into urban city planning platforms.

The main sources contributing to air pollution in India are transportation, industrial emission, commercial and residential biomass burning, coal-burning for energy production, agricultural stubble burning, brick kilns, municipal waste burning, etc. [10, 11]. Besides, the use of solid fuel such as wood, cow dung cakes, agricultural residue, coal, charcoal for cooking purposes in rural India is adding an extra burden of pollutants to the air [12]. In this challenging scenario, the Central government has recently launched *National Clean Air Programme (NCAP)* to develop a city-based clean air plan. In the first phase, 122 non-attainment cities were selected from Indo -Gangetic Plain (IGP) based on ambient air quality monitoring data of 2011–2015 [13]. The major objective is to reduce 20–30% of particulate pollution by 2024 compared to 2017. As a primary initiative of NCAP, the government has restricted older vehicles (10-year-old petrol vehicle, 15-year-old diesel vehicle), prioritized public transport, increased infrastructure for CNG and electric mobility, ordered to close older power plants in the vicinity (~300 km) of non-attainment cities and promoted conversion of brickkilns into induced draft zig-zag technology. In addition to the foregoing plan, the Central Government launched Pradhan Mantri Ujjawala Yojana in 2016 to distribute LPG connection to below poverty line women in order to reduce household pollution due to solid fuels. Another significant step taken by the Delhi government was the odd-even scheme for four-wheeler vehicles to reduce the city's vehicular fleet volume. However, a recent study at Delhi and Kolkata revealed that these policies could facilitate a maximum ~20% reduction of the primary emission, which in turn may not facilitate in achieving the desired goal of good air quality in these cities [14]. In such a situation, the national-level lockdown during 2020 to combat the spread of the novel coronavirus came up as a natural experiment to simulate the sensitivity of air pollutants. Several reports showed a significant plummet in primary emission sources or SLCPs (>30%) leading to the emergence of the blue sky after several decades in India [11, 15, 16]. Furthermore, a recent model-based study by our group predicted the drastic decline in fine particulate pollutant level during the lockdown had potentially avoided 73,853–92,116 mortalities during April–June 2020 that might have surpassed the fatality due to the pandemic [17]. Thus, lockdown provides a unique opportunity for environment researchers to collect baseline data of various pollutants, which could help develop new mitigation strategies in the future. In this context, we have provided a comprehensive overview of the impact of lockdown on different air pollutants in India.

1.1 Lockdown in India in brief

The government of India ensued lockdown in five phases from 25th March-31st May 2019. The lockdown phases are briefed below:

Lockdown 1: 1st March-23rd March 2020.

Lockdown 2: 24th March-14th April 2020.

Lockdown 3: 15th April-3rd May 2020.

Lockdown 4: 4th May-17th May 2020.

Lockdown 5: 18th May-31st May 2020.

Lockdown 1 marked the total suspension of all industrial activities, transportation, agricultural activities, educational institutions, government, and non-government offices. In addition to these, spiritual gatherings, parties, functions, and other non-essential gatherings were banned. This lead to a considerable reduction in anthropogenic emissions for a short period. During the 2nd lockdown, some relaxations were made in the movement of essential items like goods, medical equipment, private vehicles in the local area, and agricultural activities. However, public transportation such as bus, train, airways remained suspended along with inter-district and inter-state movement. Restrictions were further relaxed during lockdown-3 to 5 by allowing movement of vehicles (to a limited extent), re-opening of government offices and IT companies, small and medium-based industries, etc. However, educational institutions, cinema halls, public gathering places were closed during the entire lockdown. A more detailed description can be found in our recent publication [18, 19]. Whenever "lockdown" is mentioned in the running text it refers to all phases i.e. from 24th March to 31st May 2020. However, different researchers have taken different pre-lockdown periods for their reference. So, we have mentioned the pre-lockdown periods in the bracket.

2. Literature selection

This study includes relevant papers indexed in Google Scholar, a prominent online database for accessing scientific articles. The search string was intentionally designed to provide appropriate coverage of the diverse research. The search strategy used the following keywords: COVID-19 lockdown, the impact of lockdown on air quality, India. An initial search in Google Scholar returned 7500 articles. A brief screening revealed that many articles were not related to air quality but included only the term COVID-19 and its impact on water, health, etc. Therefore those articles were excluded. At the end of this stage, 457 articles remained in the database.

3. Impact of lockdown on different ambient air pollutants

3.1 Aerosols

3.1.1 Particulate matter (PM)

PM refers to the mixture of solid particles and liquid droplets suspended in the air. It is made up of a large variety of components like dust, smoke, soot (or BC), acids (such as nitrates and sulfate), metals, organic compounds. Some of the big particles or dark particles like soot/BC can be seen through the naked eye, while others can be detected under the microscope. The particles are introduced in the atmosphere from a wide variety of natural (sea-salt, mineral dust, volcanic eruptions, forest fires, etc) and anthropogenic sources (construction sites, unpaved roads, vehicles, industries, biomass burning, coal and oil combustion, solid waste burning) either directly (known as, primary sources) or through complex chemical reactions with gaseous precursors (known as, secondary sources), or both. Furthermore, based on aerodynamic diameter, PM can be classified as coarse (PM10; diameter ≤ 10 μm), fine (PM2.5; diameter ≤ 2.5 μm), and ultrafine (PM <1 μm). The different modes of PM originate separately, are transferred separately, and are removed by different mechanisms from the atmosphere [20]. Furthermore, the particles are known to influence climate and weather patterns by acting as cloud condensation nuclei (CCN), thus altering the microphysical properties of clouds and the hydrological cycle as well. In addition to this, aerosols disturb the earth's radiation budget, biogeochemistry of oceans and lakes, impair visibility, etc. The daily and annual threshold limit recommended by National ambient air quality (NAAQ) for PM10 is 60 and 100 $\mu g.m^{-3}$ while for PM2.5 is 40 and 60 $\mu g.m^{-3}$, respectively. In many recent studies, it is also hypothesized that chronic exposure to PM induces oxidative stress in the respiratory tract, triggering several health conditions starting from coughing and wheezing to severe asthma attacks, bronchitis to high blood pressure, heart attack, stroke, and premature deaths.

A remarkable reduction is observed in PM concentration across all cities during the lockdown. **Table 1** depicts the mean percentage change in PM loading over different Indian cities. A study over India with data from 200 air monitoring stations revealed PM10 and PM2.5 concentration decreased by 33% and 34% respectively, during lockdown (25th Mar-30th Apr 2020) as compared to the normal days (25th Feb-24th Mar 2020) [11]. New Delhi, the capital of India with the most hazardous air pollution level showed a drastic decline in PM10 and PM2.5 concentration (>50%) during the confinement period [21]. A recent study over Kolkata, the largest megacity in eastern India revealed that the average

City Studied	Period		Percentage change in PM		References
	Pre-Lockdown	Lockdown	PM 10	PM 2.5	
Delhi(34)	03-23 Mar 2020	24 Mar-14 April 2020	51.84 ↓	53.11↓	[21]
Delhi	01-24 Mar 2020	25 Mar-31 May 2020	-	37.1↓	[22]
Delhi	01-31 Mar 2019, 01-21 Mar 2020	22-31 Mar 2020	-	25.57↓	[23]
Delhi(63)	01st-24th Mar 2020	25 Mar-17 May 2020	46-58↓	49-55↓	[24]
Delhi(12)	01 Jan-14 Mar 2020	15 Mar-31 May 2020	89↓	95↓	[25]
Delhi	01 Jan-23 Mar 2020	24 Mar-31 May 2020	33↓	49↓	[26]
Delhi	25 Mar-03 May 2019	25 Mar-03 May 2020	57↓	47↓	[16]
Delhi	20 Mar-15 April (past 3-7 yrs)	20 Mar-15 April 2020	50↓	50↓	[27]
Hyderabad	01-31 Mar 2019, 01-21 Mar 2020	22 Mar-31 Mar 2020	-	3.99↓	[23]
Kolkata	01 Mar-31 Mar 2019, 01-21 Mar 2020	22 Mar-31 Mar 2020	-	34.52↓	[23]
Chennai			-	5.40↓	
Mumbai			-	19.25↓	
Pune	20 Mar-15 April (past 3-7 yrs)	20 Mar-15 April 2020	39↓	25↓	[27]
Mumbai			36↓	36↓	
Ahmedabad			47↓	50↓	
Kolkata(10)	22 Feb-23 Mar 2020	24 Mar-03 May 2020	57.92↓	58.71↓	[28]
Chennai	01-24 Mar 2020	25 Mar-31 May 2020	-	11.1↓	[22]
Kolkata			-	36.9↓	
Mumbai			-	24.4↓	
Hyderabad			-	2.9↑	
Mumbai	25 Mar-03 May 2019	25 Mar-03 May 2020	27↓	1↑	[16]
Mumbai			27↓	1↑	
Kolkata			47↓	38↓	
Chennai			-	48↓	
Bengaluru			54↓	52↓	
Hyderabad			41↓	23↓	
Jaipur			52↓	47↓	
Lucknow			-	49↓	
Chennai(5)	01 Mar-23 Mar	24 Mar-31 May	-	5.4-97↓	[29]

City Studied	Period		Percentage change in PM		References
	Pre-Lockdown	Lockdown	PM 10	PM 2.5	
Bengaluru	01 Mar-22 Apr 2019	01 Mar-22Apr 2020	-	15-22↓	[30]
Maharashtra	01 Jan-24 Mar 2020	25 Mar-01 Jul 2020	51↓	46↓	[31]
Kolkata	15 Mar-25 May 2017-2019	15 Mar-25 May 2020	20.91↓	20.04↓	[32]
Kolkata	24 Feb-23 Mar 2020	24 Mar-20 May	51.01↓		[33]
Kolkata	Jan-May 2019	Jan-May 2020	33↓	42↓	[34]
Ankleshwar	25 Mar-15 Jun 2019	25 Mar-15 Jun 2020	19↓		[35]
Vapi			51↓	40.73↓	
Andhra Pradesh (Gadanki)	15 Feb-31 May 2019	15 Feb-31 May 2020	50.4↓	46.7↓	[36]
Kolkata	01 Jan-23 Mar 2020	24 Mar-31 May 2020	63↓	73↓	[26]
Mumbai			47↓	73↓	
Chennai			17↓	54↓	
Bhubaneswar	24 Mar-31 May 2019	24 Mar-31 May 2020	1.92↑	40.26↑	[37]
Bhubaneswar	25 Mar-31 May 2017-2018	25 Mar-31 May 2020	33↓	38↓	[19]
Gujarat(9)	01 Jan-23 Mar	24 Mar-20 Apr	32-80↓	32-78↓	[38]
Kerala	Jan-May 2018-2019	Jan-May 2020	17-20↓	24-47↓	[39]
Kerala	01-24 Mar 2020, 10-17 May 2020	25 Mar-9 May 2020	61↓	53↓	[40]

The number of monitoring stations is mentioned within the bracket.

Table 1.
Percentage change in particulate matter concentration during the lockdown.

concentration of PM10 shows a significant plummet of 51% from pre-lockdown (17th Feb – 23rd Mar 2020) to lockdown (24th Mar-20th May 2020) with a decrement of 1 $\mu g.m^{-3}$ daily during the lockdown [33]. Other studies reported the impact of lockdown on Kolkata taking data from seven air quality monitoring stations [34]. A reduction in 33% and 42% for PM10 and PM2.5 respectively were observed over Kolkata during Jan-May 2020 as compared to the same time frame of 2019. Also, the average PM2.5 concentration was 20 $\mu g.m^{-3}$ during lockdown (1st Jan-23rd Mar 2020) while it was 80 $\mu g.m^{-3}$ in pre-lockdown days (1st Jan-23rd Mar 2020) representing a reduction of 75%. Similarly, a significant plummet in PM2.5 concentration in the peak hour (07:00–11:00 hour) during lockdown over Kolkata (63.4%), Mumbai (56.4%), Chennai (48.5%), New Delhi (21.3%) and Hyderabad (23.8%) compared to the pre-lockdown period (1st-24th Mar 2020) [22]. More studies over metro cities during the pandemic revealed that reduction in PM2.5 concentration shows large variability varying from 3–50% over Hyderabad, Delhi, Chennai, Ahmedabad, Pune compared to the previous year of the same time [23, 26, 27]. As per some studies, PM2.5 decreased from 102.17 $\mu g.m^{-3}$ to 51.66 $\mu g.m^{-3}$ (>50%) over Lucknow during lockdown compared to the previous year [16].

Furthermore, a prominent diminution in PM10 concentration is observed just after 4 days of nationwide lockdown at Dwarka river basin harboring 239 stone mining and 982 stone crushing areas [41]. PM10 loading was 100 $\mu g.m^{-3}$ on 12th Mar 2020 (before lockdown) which dropped to 60 $\mu g.m^{-3}$ (~40%) on 28th Mar 2020 (lockdown) with the temporary halt of industries. Similarly, studies over the industrial cities viz. Ankleshwar and Vapi of western India reported a drop in PM10 concentration by 19% and 51% respectively during the first phase of lockdown in comparison to the same period of 2019. Whereas, PM2.5 concentration shows a sharp decline from 72.23 to 43.60 $\mu g.m^{-3}$ at Vapi during the first phase of lockdown over the same time of the previous year [35]. A continuous drop in the concentration of PM2.5 and PM10 is also observed in eastern India i.e. Kolkata from 25th Mar -15th May 2020 in comparison to the previous 3 years (2017–2019) [32]. PM2.5 and PM10 loading curbed down to 38% and 33% respectively during lockdown (Mar-May 2020) over the former two years of the same time over Bhubaneswar, an urban coastal site in eastern India [19]. A significant reduction of PM2.5 in the range of 24–65% is observed at five different monitoring sites in Chennai, a tropical coastal site in South India [29]. However, the weekly analysis revealed that the decrement is not constant throughout the lockdown. There are some weeks with a higher value of PM2.5 due to the operation of coal-fired thermal power plants as a part of emergency services [29]. Nevertheless, in Chandigarh, the PM2.5 concentration was 20 $\mu g.m^{-3}$ just 21 days before lockdown which reduced to 14.3 $\mu g.m^{-3}$ (~28.5%) during the first phase of lockdown and then increased to 15.4 $\mu g.m^{-3}$ during the second phase because of some relaxations [42]. Maharastra, the worst-hit state by COVID-19 showed that during 1st-24th Mar 2020 the PM10 concentration was above the NAAQS threshold limit (> 100 $\mu g.m^{-3}$) which reduced sharply up to 51% during lockdown while PM2.5 dropped down by 46% over normalcy [31]. PM measurements over Gadanki, a rural site in south India revealed that PM2.5 and PM10 dropped down by ~47% and 50% respectively from pre-lockdown (15th Feb -21st Mar 2020) to lockdown [36]. Similarly, studies over south India reported that PM2.5 reduced by 53%, 15–22%, and 24–47% over Kunnur, Bengaluru and Kerala respectively during lockdown over pre-lockdown (1st Jan-22nd Mar 2020) [30, 39, 40]. Thus, a decrease in traffic density, human mobility, shutting of industries drastically reduced PM pollution over India leading to the emergence of blue sky after a decade [25, 43].

3.1.2 Black carbon (BC)

In recent years, with rapid modernization, India has become the second-largest emitter of BC in the world [44]. BC or soot (as discussed above) is an important anthropogenic component of atmospheric aerosol with residence time varying from several days to a week in the lower troposphere [45]. It is released into the atmosphere due to incomplete combustion of fossil fuel, biomass burning, and biogenic sources by the multiphase reaction [46, 47]. Furthermore, BC strongly absorbs solar radiation, affecting the Earth's radiation budget [48, 49], thermodynamics of the atmosphere [50], lifetime and optical properties of clouds [51], resulting in global warming. Moreover, inhalation of BC particles causes serious respiratory problems in humans [52] and aquatic animals [53] and is also responsible for crop damage. The real-time mass concentration of BC is measured using a seven-channel (370, 470, 520, 590, 660, 880, and 950 nm) instrument called *Aethelometer*. The instrument is based on spot technology and it measures the attenuation of light at seven different wavelengths passing through a quartz fiber filter tape, on which aerosols get deposited. The total mass concentration of BC is estimated from 880 nm wavelength. Being chemically inert under atmospheric conditions, BC is removed mostly by wet deposition from the atmosphere [52]. A recent study on primary BC measurement from ARFINET (Aerosol Radiative Forcing over India Network) reported 10–40% diminution in BC concentration during lockdown (24th Mar-31st May 2020) compared to pre-lockdown (4th -23rd Mar 2020) [54]. **Table 2** shows the reduction percentage of BC over different cities during confinement periods over normal days. Along with this, a significant reduction in the range of 16–60% over central and peninsular India and Himalayan and sub-Himalayan regions was observed during lockdown-2 compared to 2015–2020 at the same time [54]. However, Indo Gangetic Plain (IGP) showed a maximum reduction of >60% followed by north-eastern India (>30%) during lockdown-2 with respect to the preceding 5 years of the same period. Similarly, a study over Bhubaneswar depicted a 33% reduction in BC concentration during March–May 2020 compared to 2017–2018 of the same time frame [19]. BC concentration also showed a decline of 34% during lockdown over the same period of 2019 over Gadanki [36]. A notable dwindling in BC concentration (> 60%) during lockdown-1 over pre-lockdown (1st Jan-14th Mar 2020) is observed at Bengaluru, a megacity in southern India [55]. Nevertheless, a

City Studied	Period		Percentage change in BC	References
	Pre-Lockdown	Lockdown		
Andhra Pradesh (Gadanki)	15 Feb-31 May 2019	15 Feb-31 May 2020	34↓	[36]
Bhubaneswar	01 Mar-21 Mar 2020, 01 Jun-30 Jun 2020	22 Mar-31 May 2020	47↓	[18]
Bhubaneswar	25 Mar-31 May 2017-2018	25 Mar-31 May 2020	33↓	[19]
Bengaluru	24 Mar-01 Jul 2015-2019	24 Mar-01 Jul 2020	60↓	[55]
Hanle	04-24 Mar 2020	25 Mar-14 Apr 2020	31.4↓	[54]
Nainital			8.3↓	
Dehradun			45.5↓	
Kullu			67.5↓	
Lachung			47.7↓	
Agra			40.3↓	
Gorakhpur			68.3↓	
Agartala			44.6↓	
Bhubaneswar			8.7↓	
Nagpur			1.4↓	
Hyderabad			9.8↓	
Bengaluru			51.8↓	
Anantapur			26.0↓	
Goa			19.6↓	
Ooty			27.1↓	
Thiruvananthapuram			18.5↓	

Table 2.
Declining percentage of total BC during lockdown.

marginal reduction in BC concentration over Challakare (a remote rural location situated ~230 km away from Bengaluru) divulged that lockdown had a minimum impact on aerosol concentration over the rural location. Moreover, they re-emphasized that emissions from industries and the transport sector are the major sources of aerosols of urban and semi-urban locations whereas rural sites are mostly dominated by meteorological conditions and synoptic wind [55]. The study from ARFINET also disclosed that the most remarkable plummet is observed at the urban locations than remote and rural places [54]. Additionally, it was revealed that the sharp decline in BC concentration is due to strict restrictions in vehicular movement and other anthropogenic activities which resulted in a decrement of fossil fuel contribution to the overall BC load [19, 55]. However, no precipitable change is observed in BC from biomass burning because of domestic cooking activities as well as mass cooking by different Non-Governmental Organisations to feed the needy and homeless people.

3.1.3 Aerosol optical depth (AOD)

AOD is a comprehensive variable to measure the aerosol burden (such as dust, sea salt, smoke, urban haze, etc) distributed within the earth's surface to the top of the atmosphere. In other words, AOD gives information about how much direct sunlight is prevented from reaching the ground by aerosols. Furthermore, it gives an estimation of PM2.5 surface concentration [56]. Measurements using satellite-borne observation and aerosol reanalysis products revealed that during lockdown (24th Mar -22nd Apr 2020) maximum decrement in AOD value is observed in eastern IGP (~40% of pre-lockdown; 20th Feb-20th Mar 2020) followed by north-west (27%) and south-India (13%) [4]. In disparity, an increment of 20% is observed in central India, the most polluted part of India. It might be due to an increase in secondary aerosol formation, aerosol water content, and other meteorological conditions. Likely researchers observed a maximum reduction in AOD in the IGP region followed by western, southern and eastern parts of India [15]. Satellite visual maps over IGP showed a reduction in AOD during March 2020 compared to Jan-Feb 2020 and a much more reduction is observed in April 2020 (**Figure 1**). However, ground-based measurement revealed that the highest reduction in AOD is observed at Lahore (60%) followed by Kanpur (52%), Gandhi college (33%), Bhola near the Bay of Bengal (BoB) (12%). But Karachi, a coastal site near the Arabian sea showed an enhancement of 4% from pre-lockdown to lockdown. In addition, both ground-based and satellite measurements over Gadanki revealed a decrement of ~17% of AOD during lockdown over 2019 [36].

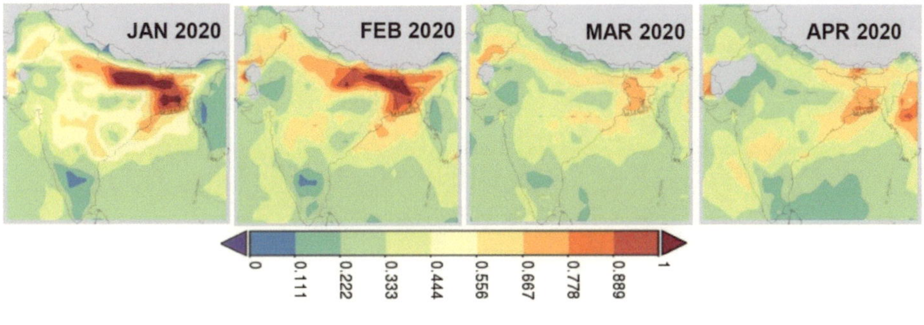

Figure 1.
AOD at 550 nm from January-April 2020 (source: [11]).

3.2 Trace gases

3.2.1 Carbon monoxide (CO)

CO is a very stable, odorless, colorless, and poisonous atmospheric pollutant with a lifetime of two to four months in the atmosphere [57]. However, CO is not considered as a direct greenhouse gas due to its low absorption in the infrared region but it increases the concentration of greenhouse gases (such as methane and ozone) by reacting with the hydroxyl radical of the atmosphere. The indirect radiative forcing by CO is 0.23 Wm^{-2} due to the formation of ozone, carbon dioxide, and methane (IPCC,2013). The major emission sources of CO include vehicular exhaust, waste incinerators, wildlife fires, power stations, biomass burning, furnaces, grills, stoves, and incomplete combustion of coal, wood, gasoline, plastics, fuel oils [58, 59]. The photooxidation of methane and other hydrocarbons also leads to the formation of CO as a by-product [18]. However, studies revealed biofuel burning in residential sites to be the major contributor of CO (~86%) followed by the transport section (~13%) in India. According to Occupational Safety and Health Association (OSHA), the personal exposure limit for CO is 50 ppm for 8 hours. However, chronic exposure to CO leads to a neurological disorder, cardiac dysfunction [60] in addition to fatigue, dizziness, food poisoning, stomach pain, etc. [61] Satellite images showed a significant reduction in surface CO concentration during the lockdown (**Figure 2**). Nationwide average CO concentration was observed to drop upto~21% during lockdown (25th Mar-30th Apr 2020) over pre-lockdown (25th Feb-24th Mar 2020) [11]. As per studies, CO concentration dropped by 15% during Jan-May 2020 over 2019 at Kolkata [34]. The lowest monthly average concentration of CO was reported during April and May 2020 compared to the preceding 3 years of the same month [32]. Studies over western India during the lockdown revealed a plummet of ~21% and 25% over Pune and Gujrat respectively, during 2020 in comparison to the same period during 2019, while no significant change is observed at Mumbai [38, 62]. Over Bhubaneswar, the eastern coastal city showed a reduction of ~14% in CO concentration during complete lockdown period compared to the earlier lockdown period (1st Mar-23rd Mar 2020) whereas it showed a diminution of 11.1% during March–May 2020 compared to the previous year of the same time [18, 37]. A lower reduction of CO compared to the early phase of lockdown might be attributed to its long residence time in the atmosphere. Similarly, a lower reduction in CO (~10%) compared to other primary pollutants is observed at Gadanki during lockdown over the previous year [36]. However, CO measurement at five different sites of Chennai showed a prominent plummet in the range of 5.60–90.72% during lockdown (**Table 3**) [29]. Similarly, a remarkable plummet of 4–44% is observed over Delhi, Uttar Pradesh and Haryana

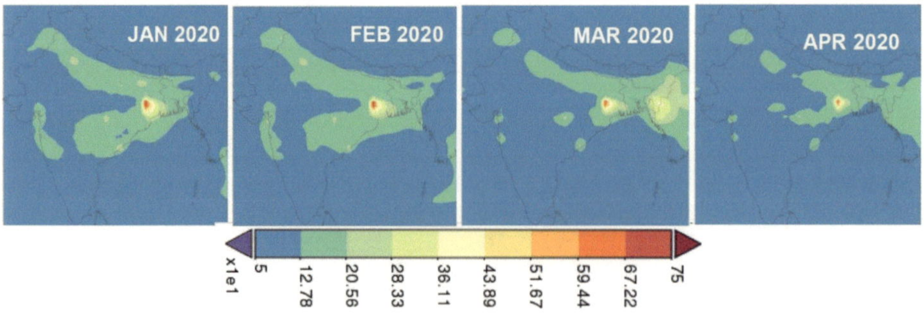

Figure 2.
Change in surface CO concentration during January-April 2020 (source: [11]).

City Studied	Period		Percentage change in CO	References
	Pre-Lockdown	Lockdown		
Delhi(34)	03 -23 Mar 2020	24 Mar-14 April 2020	30.35↓	[21]
Delhi(63)	01st-24th Mar 2020	25 Mar- 17 May 2020	4-44↓	[24]
Delhi(12)	01 Jan- 14 Mar 2020	15 Mar- 31 May 2020	82↓	[25]
Delhi	01 Jan- 23 Mar 2020	24 Mar- 31 May 2020	31↑	[26]
Delhi	25 Mar- 03 May 2019	25 Mar- 03 May 2020	43↓	[16]
Mumbai			75↓	
Kolkata			22↓	
Chennai			32↓	
Bengaluru			28↓	
Hyderabad			23↓	
Jaipur			46↓	
Lucknow			28↓	
Hyderabad	01 Feb–23 Mar 2020	24 Mar - 30 Apr 2020	27.25↓	[63]
Chennai	01 Jan- 23 Mar	24 Mar- 31 May	9↑	[26]
Kolkata	01 Jan- 23 Mar 2020	24 Mar- 31 May 2020	11↓	[26]
Mumbai	01 Jan- 23 Mar 2020	24 Mar- 31 May 2020	15↓	[26]
Chennai (5)	01 - 23 Mar 2020	24 Mar- 31 May 2020	18-25↓	[29]
Kolkata	Jan-May 2019	Jan-May 2020	15↓	[34]
Pune	17 Mar- 14 Apr 2019	17 Mar- 14 Apr 2020	21↓	[62]
Andhra Pradesh (Gadanki)	15 Feb- 31 May 2019	15 Feb- 31 May 2020	10↓	[36]
Bhubaneswar	01- 21 Mar 2020, 01 Jun- 30 Jun 2020	22 Mar-31 May 2020	14↓	[18]
	24 Mar- 31 May 2019	24 Mar- 31 May 2020	19-69↓	[37]
Kerala	Jan- May 2018-2019	Jan- May 2020	24-67↓	[39]
Kerala	01 Mar-24 Mar 2020, 10 May-17 May 2020	25 Mar-19 Apr 2020, 20 Apr-9 May 2020	67↓	[40]

Table 3.
Reduction in CO concentration during lockdown compared to pre-lockdown days.

during the lockdown. Chandigarh showed a decrement of 16.3% from 21-days before lockdown to the first phase of lockdown and then showed an enhancement of 5.4% in the second phase of lockdown compared to the first phase. A sharp reduction in the range of 24–67% is also reported over Kerala amid lockdown and meteorological changes [39].

3.2.2 Nitrogen oxides (NOx)

Nitrogen oxides (NOx = NO + NO2) are primary criteria air pollutants that play a vital role in tropospheric chemistry as the precursor of surface ozone and secondary aerosols apart from being responsible for acid rain and reddish-brown haze [64]. Besides, NOx affects human health causing several heart and lung diseases as well as unseasonable death worldwide. The NOx measurement over different parts of the country revealed that the major anthropogenic emitters of NOx are from vehicles followed by power plants [65, 66]. Apart from these, soil, lightning, and wildfire are some of the natural sources of NOx [67]. Owing to a very short lifetime (~2 days) NOx showed maximum reduction in concentration across all parts of India as compared to other primary pollutants (**Table 4**). Satellite data revealed major NO2 hotspots of India are Delhi, Haryana, Punjab, and in the eastern part of Bihar, Jharkhand, West-Bengal, and Odisha which disappeared completely during April 2020 [11] (**Figure 3**). Similarly, a 60–66% reduction in NO2 concentration was found over Delhi, Ahmedabad, Mumbai, and Pune [27]. Analysis of NO2 concentration at 63 locations of Delhi, Uttar Pradesh, Harayana revealed a plummet of 27–58% during lockdown [24]. In Lucknow, NO2 concentration reduced from 43.06 $\mu g.m^{-3}$ to 14.57 $\mu g.m^{-3}$ (66%) during lockdown 2020 compared to 2019. According to a recent study over Kolkata NOx showed a decline of 68% during lockdown (24th Mar-20 May 2020) in comparison to pre-lockdown (17th Feb – 23rd Mar 2020) with a daily decline of 0.373 $\mu g.m^{-3}$ during the lockdown [33]. Moreover, NO2 reduced up to 45% during Jan-May 2020 with respect to Jan-May 2019 over Kolkata [34]. On the same note, it was stated a sharp reduction in the average concentration of NO2 from 41.58 $\mu g.m^{-3}$ in Mar 2019 to 18.01 $\mu g.m^{-3}$ (~57%) in Mar 2020 [32]. A significant plummet in average NOx concentration is also observed on the eastern coast of India. Studies over Bhubaneswar revealed that average NOx concentration decreased by ~67% during quarantine days (24th Mar-31st May 2020) compared to pre-lockdown (1st -23rd Mar 2020) whereas 12.3% during Mar-May 2020 in comparison to 2019 of the same period [18, 37]. Similarly, NO and NO2 reduced by ~55 and 59% respectively, over Gadanki during lockdown with respect to 2019 [36]. Significant reduction in the range of 41–55% in NOx concentration is also observed at Chennai, the southern coastal site of India. Studies over Hyderabad and Kerala specified NO2 concentration dropped down by 33% and 48% respectively during lockdown over pre-lockdown [39, 63] . NO2 concentration curbed down by ~60% and 30–84% from pre-lockdown to lockdown over Maharashtra and Gujrat respectively [31, 38].

3.2.3 Sulphur dioxide (SO2)

SO2 is one of the potent anthropogenic sulphur-containing air pollutants responsible for smog and acid rain [20]. According to a 2019 report by Greenpeace, India has become the largest emitter of SO2 in the world with more than 15% of hotspots as detected by NASA OMI (Ozone Monitoring Instrument) satellite [68]. It is also revealed that coal-fired thermal power plants and industries are the major emitters of SO2 in India. In addition, emissions from vehicles, ships, locomotives, ore smelting are also contributing substantially to atmospheric SO2 concentration.

City Studied	Period		Percentage change in NOx	References
	Pre-Lockdown	Lockdown		
Delhi(34)	03 -23 Mar 2020	24 Mar-14 April 2020	52.68↓	[21]
Delhi(63)	01 -24 Mar 2020	25 Mar- 17 May 2020	27-58↓	[24]
Delhi(12)	01 Jan- 14 Mar 2020	15 Mar- 31 May 2020	92↓	[25]
Delhi(NO2)	25 Mar- 03 May 2019	25 Mar- 03 May 2020	59↓	[16]
Delhi(NO2)	20 Mar- 15 Apr (past 3-7 yrs)	20 Mar- 15 Apr 2020	66↓	[27]
Pune(NO2)			63↓	
Mumbai(NO2)			60↓	
Ahmedabad(NO2)			60↓	
Mumbai(NO2)	25 Mar- 03 May 2019	25 Mar- 03 May 2020	59↓	[16]
Kolkata (NO2)			68↓	
Chennai(NO2)			32↓	
Bengaluru(NO2)			64↓	
Hyderabad(NO2)			37↓	
Jaipur(NO2)			62↓	
Lucknow(NO2)			66↓	
Chennai(5) (NO2)	01 Mar- 23 Mar 2020	24 Mar- 31 May 2020	18-42↓	[29]
Ankleshwar	25 Mar- 15 Jun 2019	25 Mar- 15 Jun 2020	80↓	[35]
Vapi			91↓	
Chennai	01 Jan- 23 Mar 2020	24 Mar- 31 May 2020	7↑	[26]
Kolkata			79↓	
Mumbai			86↓	
Delhi (NO2)			29↓	
Kolkata	24 Feb- 23 Mar 2020	24 Mar-20 May 2020	68.38↓	[33]
Kolkata	Jan-May 2019	Jan-May 2020	45↓	[34]
Kolkata(10)	22 Feb- 23 Mar 2020	24 Mar- 03 May 2020	55.23	[28]
Mumbai	17 Mar- 14 Apr 2019	17 Mar- 14 Apr 2020	63↓	[62]
Pune			62↓	
Andhra Pradesh (Gadanki)	15 Feb- 31 May 2019	15 Feb- 31 May 2020	55-59↓	[36]
Hyderabad	01 Feb–23 Mar 2020	24 Mar - 30 Apr 2020	43.5↓	[63]

City Studied	Period		Percentage change in NOx	References
	Pre-Lockdown	Lockdown		
Bhubaneswar	01 - 21 Mar 2020	22 Mar-31 May 2020	67↓	[18]
Bhubaneswar	24 Mar- 31 May 2019	24 Mar- 31 May 2020	50↓	[37]
Maharashtra	01 Jan- 24 Mar 2020	25 Mar- 01Jul 2020	60↓	[31]
Gujarat(NO2)(9)	01 Jan- 23 Mar 2020	24 Mar- 20 Apr 2020	30-84↓	[38]
Kerala	Jan- May 2018-2019	Jan- May 2020	53-90↓	[39]
	01 -24 Mar 2020, 10-17 May 2020	25 Mar-19 Apr 2020, 20 Apr-9 May 2020	66↓	[40]

Table 4.
Percentage change in NOx over India during lockdown.

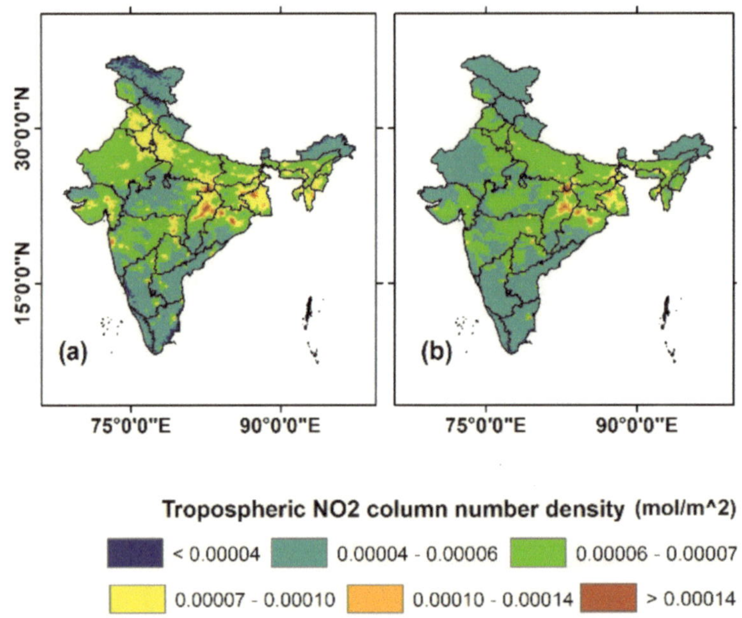

Figure 3.
Columunar distribution of NO2 during (a) 1st-24th March 2020 (b) 25th March-20th April 2020 (source: [15]).

Once released to the atmosphere, SO2 undergoes several reactions with the oxidants (O3 or H2O2) to form particulate of sulphate either as H2SO4 or ammonium sulphate. The particulate sulphate causes visibility degradation and poses a great threat to human health and plants. Nonetheless, short-term exposure to a higher level of SO2 (>5 ppm) leads to lung damage, inflammation of the eyes, nose, and throats. Also, it disturbs the plant photosynthesis process leading to foliar injury.

The average concentration of SO2 over Kolkata was 15.35 $\mu g.m^{-3}$ before lockdown (17th Feb – 23rd Mar 2020) which reduced drastically to 9.15 $\mu g.m^{-3}$

lockdown (24th Mar-20 May 2020) with an average reduction of 40%. However, the daily decrement of SO2 was found to be 0.153 μg.m^{-3} [33]. A reduction of 3% in SO2 Jan-May 2020 compared to the previous year of the same time [34]. Similarly, the monthly average concentration of SO2 during April 2017, 2018, and 2019 was found to be 7.59, 9.47 and 8.27 μg.m^{-3} respectively which dwindled up to 5.36 μg. m^{-3} during complete lockdown (i.e. Apr 2020), depicting a plummet of ~37% compared to the past three years [32]. A sharp decline in SO2 ~63% and ~16% is also observed over Gadanki and Lucknow respectively during lockdown than in 2019 [16, 36]. Kannur (the hotspot of corona) in Kerala showed a decrement of ~62% in SO2 concentration during the quarantine days (25th Mar-9th May 2020) over normal days (1st -24th Mar 2020 & 10th -17th May 2020) [40]. A reduction of ~40% is also observed over the industrial state of western India during Jan-Apr

City Studied	Period		Percentage change in SO2	References
	Pre-Lockdown	Lockdown		
Delhi(34)	03 Mar-23 Mar 2020	24 Mar-14 Apr 2020	17.97↓	[21]
Delhi	01 Jan- 23 Mar 2020	24 Mar- 31 May 2020	24↓	[26]
Ankleshwar	25 Mar- 15 Jun 2019	25 Mar- 15 Jun 2020	67↓	[35]
Vapi			80↓	
Chennai	01 Jan- 23 Mar 2020	24 Mar- 31 May 2020	39↓	[26]
Kolkata			15↓	
Mumbai			58↓	
Delhi	25 Mar- 03 May 2019	25 Mar- 03 May 2020	32↓	[16]
Mumbai			48↓	
Kolkata			25↑	
Chennai			22↓	
Bengaluru			9↑	
Hyderabad			9↓	
Jaipur			9↓	
Lucknow			16↓	
Kolkata	24 Feb- 23 Mar 2020	24 Mar-20 May 2020	40.38↓	[33]
Kolkata	Jan-May 2019	Jan-May 2020	3↓	[34]
Chennai(5)	01 Mar- 23 Mar 2020	24 Mar- 31 May 2020	25-69↓	[29]
Kerala	01 -24 Mar 2020, 10-17 May 2020	25 Mar-19 Apr, 20 Apr-9 May	62↓	[40]
Andhra Pradesh (Gadanki)	15 Feb- 31 May 2019	15 Feb- 31 May 2020	63↓	[36]

Table 5.
Mean percentage change in the mean percentage change in SO2 concentration over India during lockdown.

2020 over the previous year [38]. Likely, SO2 concentration reduced from 28.99 to 9.43 μg.m^{-3} (~67%) and 19.14 to 9.43 μg.m^{-3} (~51%) over Ankleshwar and Vapi respectively located in Gujrat during the first phase of lockdown than the previous year [35]. However, amid lockdown, an increase in SO2 concentration is observed at the commercial cum residential sites of Chennai namely Teynampet (40%) and Velacherry (70%) due to the use of fossil fuels (coal, wood) for cooking purposes and constant operation of thermal power plants [29]. Chandigarh also showed an increment in SO2 concentration from 9.9 μg.m^{-3} (before lockdown) to 10.0 (~1%) and 11.4 μg.m^{-3} (15%) during the first and second phases of lockdown respectively. Similarly, no significant change in SO2 intensity is observed from satellite data over eastern Odisha, West-Bengal, and South-west industrial regions of Maharashtra and Gujrat [11]. This is due to the presence of excessive coal mining and the constant operation of power plants as part of emergency service. Likewise, SO2 measurement over Singrauli, which is home to several coal-fired thermal power plants showed an increment of 12% during lockdown over normalcy (1st-24th Mar 2020). **Table 5** describes the mean percentage change in SO2 concentration over India during lockdown.

3.2.4 Ozone (O3)

Surface O3 is a secondary pollutant formed majorly by photooxidation of CO, methane (CH4), or volatile organic carbons (VOCs) in presence of a sufficient amount of NOx. The major formation pathways are shown below

$$CO + OH \rightarrow CO_2 + H \tag{1}$$

$$H + O_2 + M \rightarrow HO_2 + M \tag{2}$$

$$HO_2 + NO \rightarrow NO_2 + OH \tag{3}$$

$$NO_2 + hv \rightarrow O(3P) + NO \tag{4}$$

$$O(3P) + O_2 + M \rightarrow O_3 + M \tag{5}$$

Net: $CO + 2O_2 + hv \rightarrow CO_2 + O_3$

During this process, NOx acts as a catalyst until it is removed by surface deposition or converted to other NOy compounds. Also, we can say NO2 helps in O3 formation while NO destroys O3. Being a powerful oxidizing agent, O3 controls the lifetime of many primary pollutants in the atmosphere. Nonetheless, O3 is a potent greenhouse gas that substantially contributes to global warming and affects human health, crop yield, natural ecosystem, and climate.

Table 6 summarises the mean percentage change in O3 concentration over different parts of India. During lockdown (24th Mar-20th May 2020), O3 concentration shows a sizeable daily reduction of 0.571 μg.m^{-3} with an average of 42% compared to pre-lockdown (17th Feb– 23rd Mar 2020) over Kolkata [33]. A reduction of ~7% is also observed during lockdown over 2019 at Gadanki [36]. Similarly, an 18% decrement in O3 concentration is observed over Maharashtra during lockdown with respect to pre-lockdown (1st -24th Mar 2020) [31]. In contrast, an enhancement of 4–6% of O3 concentration is observed at 63 different stations of Delhi, Uttar Pradesh, and Haryana during lockdown [24]. Some studies revealed concentration of O3 increased by 32% and 6% over Kolkata and Gujarat during the lockdown year as compared to the previous year [34, 38]. Likely, an increment of 3% and 2% was observed over Mumbai and Pune respectively during lockdown over the previous year [62]. Similarly, O3 concentration gets amplified by 5.59%, 9.73%, 3.56% during March, April, and May 2020 compared to the same month of

City Studied	Period		Percentage change in O3	Author
	Pre-Lockdown	Lockdown		
Delhi(34)	03 -23 Mar 2020	24 Mar-14 April 2020	>10 ↑	[21]
Delhi(63)	01-24 Mar 2020	25 Mar- 17 May 2020	6↑	[24]
Delhi	01 Jan- 23 Mar 2020	24 Mar- 31 May 2020	109↑	[26]
Chennai			80↑	
Kolkata			77↑	
Mumbai			60↓	
Delhi	25 Mar- 03 May 2019	25 Mar- 03 May 2020	6↓	[16]
Mumbai			2↓	
Kolkata			63↑	
Chennai			51↑	
Bengaluru			25↓	
Hyderabad			29↓	
Jaipur			17↓	
Lucknow			28↓	
Gujarat(9)	01 Jan- 23 Mar 2020	24 Mar- 20 Apr 2020	16-48↑	[38]
Bhubaneswar	24 Mar- 31 May 2019	24 Mar- 31 May 2020	13-93↑	[37]
Bhubaneswar	01- 21 Mar 2020	22 Mar-15 Apr 2020	3↑	[18]
Chennai(5)	01- 23 Mar 2020	24 Mar- 31 May 2020	3-47↑	[29]
Maharashtra	01 Jan- 24 Mar 2020	25 Mar- 01Jul 2020	18↓	[31]
Hyderabad	01 Feb–23 Mar 2020	24 Mar - 30 Apr 2020	41.73↑	[63]
Kerala	01 -24 Mar 2020, 10 -17 May 2020	25 Mar-19 Apr 2020, 20 Apr-9 May 2020	22↑	[40]
Kolkata	24 Feb- 23 Mar 2020	24 Mar-20 May 2020	42.58↓	[33]
Kolkata	Jan-May 2019	Jan-May 2020	32↑	[34]
Mumbai	17 Mar- 14 Apr 2019	17 Mar- 14 Apr 2020	3↑	[62]
Pune			2↑	
Andhra Pradesh (Gadanki)	15 Feb- 31 May 2019	15 Feb- 31 May 2020	7↓	[36]

Table 6.
Percentage change in O3 concentration over India amid lockdown.

2019. Two times enhancement in O3 concentration is also observed at Hyderabad during COVID-19 lockdown over normal days [63]. An increment of 3% in O3 concentration was also found during the 22nd March-14th April 2020 over the past weeks (1st - 21st Mar 2020) at Bhubaneswar [18]. Similarly, an 12% increment in O3 concentration was reported during Mar-May 2020 over 2019 [37]. O3 concentration enhancement is also observed at the commercial (Teynampat) and residential (Velachery) sites of Chennai by 48 and 5% respectively [29]. O3 concentration over Chandigarh sharply increases from 38.7 μgm^{-3} (21 days before lockdown) to 91.4 $\mu g.m^{-3}$ (136%) and 128.9 $\mu g.m^{-3}$ (233%) during first and second phase lockdown respectively. The enhancement in O3 is due to insufficient NO concentration as discussed in the previous section which resulted in the accumulation of O3 in the troposphere.

AQI	Possible health implications
Good (0-50)	Nominal impact
Satisfactory (51-100)	Slight discomfort in breathing for sensitive people
Moderately (101-200)	Discomfort in breathing for older people having a co-morbid system such as asthma, lung disease, heart disease.
Poor (201-300)	Long-term exposure gives rise to breathing problems, especially for heart patients.
Very poor (301-400)	Chronic exposure lead to breathing issue and respiratory inflammation.
Severe (401-500)	Serious respiratory problem for healthy people too

Table 7.
Air quality index and possible health impact.

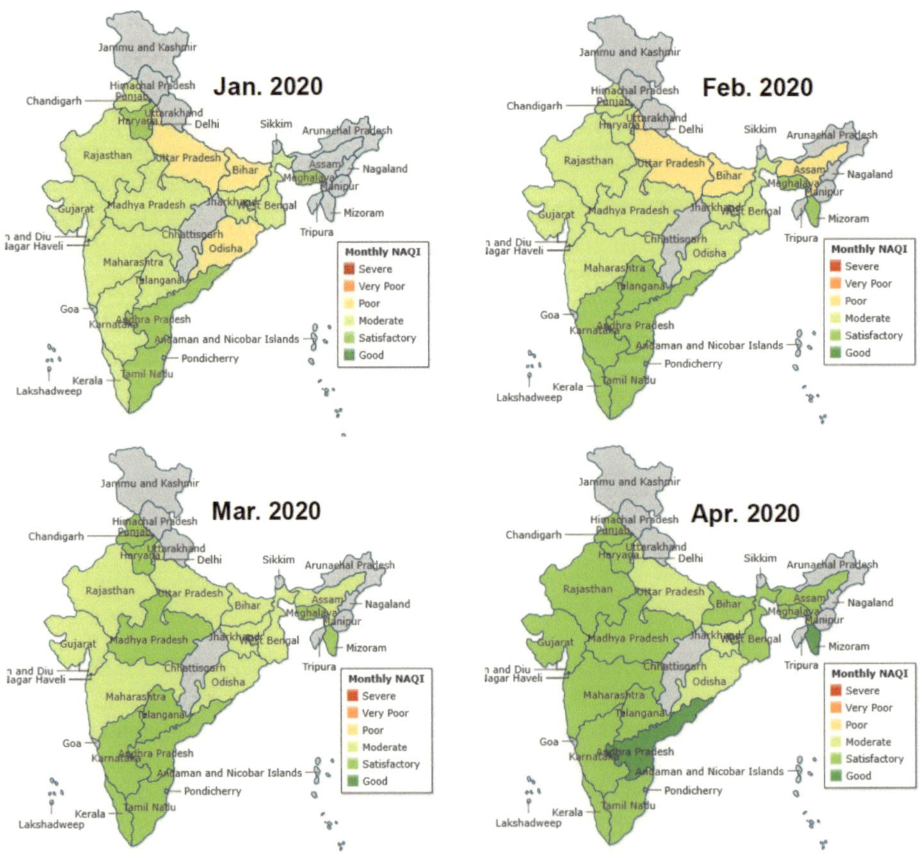

Figure 4.
Change in Air quality index from January-April 2020 (source: [11]).

3.3 Air Quality Index (AQI)

AQI gives information about daily air quality and related public health risks. In general, there are six AQI categories as shown in **Table 7**. The Indian national predicted the daily air quality data taking 24 hour average of eight criteria pollutants such as (PM10, PM2.5, NO2, SO2, CO, O3, NH3 and Pb), however, for CO and O3 8-hour average. Exposure to an enhanced AQI leads to acute and chronic health issues, especially for older age people and children.

Studies in this context stated AQI decreased drastically over Delhi (51%), Mumbai (30%), Kolkata (19%), Chennai (32%), Bangalore (52%), Hyderabad (35%), Jaipur (42%) and Lucknow (52%) during 2020 over 2019 [16]. Further, the order of AQI in lockdown 2020 satisfied > moderate > good > poor while for 2019 the order was moderate > satisfied > poor > good > very poor. It was also stated a deduction of anthropogenic activities because of strict lockdown in and around Kolkata has improved AQI from 'poor' to 'good' or 'satisfactory' [28, 69]. In addition, AQI analysis amid April 2020 over 115 Indian cities revealed AQI in all states were good or satisfactory except Odisha and Jharkhand where AQI was moderate (**Figure 4**) [11]. A decrement of 60–75% in AQI is observed over the industrial cities of western India such as Ahmedabad, Gandhinagar, Jamnagar, Rajkot while 34–39% reduction is observed at Surat, Ankleshwar, Vadodra, Bhuj and Panipat [38]. However, despite the significant reduction of pollutants during lockdown over Gadanki no change in the AQI category is observed [36].

4. Summary and recommendation

This review clearly illustrates that the strict imposition of lockdown by the Indian Government not only helped to curb the pandemic spread but also significantly improved the air quality during quarantine days across numerous cities nested within different states of India. Thus, this unique scenario emerged as a natural experiment to get the baseline data of pollutants which will be useful for policymakers and stakeholders to develop new targets to tweak air quality standards and various mitigation processes to combat air pollution. However, it is important to keep in mind the atmospheric chemistry while developing mitigation strategies for the abatement of primary pollutants. As it is observed, a sudden reduction in NOx concentration during lockdown leads to an enhancement of O3 concentration over many parts of India. So, time demands a better understanding of pollutant sources and the development of extenuation policies.

We are suggesting a few science-driven measures which can lead to the co-existence of a sustainable economy and environment hand to hand

a. Decentralization of metro cities and some urban sites.

b. Fossil fuel consumption should be replaced with solar/wind/hydro/CNG/battery/nuclear energy.

c. A focal shift from fossil fuel-based economy to bio-energy-based economy.

d. Development of clean coal technology to generate electricity.

e. Reducing vehicle density by encouraging the use of public transport, carpooling, and bicycle

f. Development in geoengineering technique to improve road conditions and substitute metallic brakes with ceramic.

g. Development of indigenous processes to arrest the PM polluted generated through biomass and stable burning at various locations in the country.

h. Always encouraging and choosing sustainable ways of existence.

Acknowledgements

The authors are thankful to the Director, CSIR-IMMT, and the Head,Environment and Sustainability Department, CSIR-IMMT for their encouragement. TD and BR are grateful to ISRO-GBP (ATCTM and ARFI) for the financial support.

Conflict of interest

The authors declare that they have no know competing interests.

Nomenclature

PM	Particulate matter
BC	Black carbon
AOD	Aerosol optical depth
CO	Carbon Monoxide
NOx	Nitrogen oxides
SO2	Sulphur dioxide
O3	Ozone
AQI	Air quality index
SLCPs	short lived climatic pollutants

Author details

Subhasmita Panda, Priyadatta Satpathy, Trutpi Das and Boopathy Ramasamy*
CSIR-Institute of Minerals and Materials Technology, Bhubaneswar, Odisha, India

*Address all correspondence to: boopathy@immt.res.in

References

[1] The World Air Quality Report 2020. https://www.insightsonindia.com/2021/03/17/the-world-air-quality-report-2020/

[2] Cohen AJ, Brauer M, Burnett R, Anderson HR, Frostad J, Estep K, Balakrishnan K, Brunekreef B, Dandona L, Dandona R, Feigin V, Freedman G, Hubbell B, Jobling A, Kan H, Knibbs L, Liu Y, Martin R, Morawska L, Pope CA 3rd, Shin H, Straif K, Shaddick G, Thomas M, van Dingenen R, van Donkelaar A, Vos T, Murray CJL, Forouzanfar MH, Estimates and 25-year trends of the global burden of disease attributable to ambient air pollution: an analysis of data from the Global Burden of Diseases Study 2015. Lancet2017 May 13;389 (10082):1907-1918.DOI: 10.1016/S0140-6736(17)30505-6

[3] Genc S, Zadeoglulari Z, Fuss SH, Genc K. The Adverse Effects of Air Pollution on the Nervous System. J Toxicol 2012;782462. DOI: 10.1155/2012/782462.

[4] Pandey SK, Vinoj, V. Surprising Changes in Aerosol Loading over India amid COVID-19 Lockdown. Aerosol Air Qual. Res. 2021; 200466. DOI: 10.4209/aaqr.2020.07.0466

[5] Manisalidis, I, Stavropoulou E, Stavropoulos A, Bezirtzoglou E,. Environmental and Health Impacts of Air Pollution: A Review. Front Public Health 8, 2020;14-14. DOI: 10.3389/fpubh.2020.00014

[6] Wu G, Brown J, Zamora M.L , Miller A, Satterfield M.C, Meininger C J, Steinhauser C B, Johnson G A, Burghardt R C, Bazer F W, Li Y, Johnson N M, Molina M J, Zhang R. Adverse organogenesis and predisposed long-term metabolic syndrome from prenatal exposure to fine particulate matter. PNAS 2019 ; 116, 11590-11595. DOI: 10.1073/pnas.1902925116

[7] Xiong L, Xu Z, Wang H, Liu Z, Xie D, Wang A, Kong F. The association between ambient air pollution and birth defects in four cities in Hunan province, China, from 2014 to 2016. Medicine (Baltimore) 2019; 98, e14253-e14253. DOI: 10.1097/MD.0000000000014253

[8] Iuliana F, Barbu I. The effects of air pollutants on vegetation and the role of vegetation in reducing atmospheric pollution, The impact of air pollution on health, economy, environment and agriculture sources, Mohamed Khallaf (Ed). 2011; ISBN:978 953 307 528 0, Intech

[9] D'Amato G, Pawankar R, Vitale C, Lanza M, Molino A, Stanziola A, Sanduzzi A, Vatrella A, D'Amato M. Climate Change and Air Pollution: Effects on Respiratory Allergy. Allergy Asthma Immunol Res 2016;8, 391-395. DOI: 10.4168/aair.2016.8.5.391

[10] Guttikunda S K, Goel R, Pant P. Nature of air pollution, emission sources, and management in the Indian cities. Atmospheric Environment 2014; 95, 501-510. DOI: 10.1016/j.atmosenv.2014.07.006

[11] Verma R L, Kamyotra J S. Impacts of COVID-19 on Air Quality in India. Aerosol and Air Quality Research 2021; 21, 200482. DOI: 10.4209/aaqr.200482

[12] Arku R E, Birch A., Shupler M, Yusuf S, Hystad P, Brauer M. Characterizing exposure to household air pollution within the Prospective Urban Rural Epidemiology (PURE) study. Environ Int 2018; 114, 307-317. DOI: 10.1016/j.envint.2018.02.033.

[13] https://www.nrdc.org/sites/default/files/10-city-plans-fight-air-pollution-india-202001.pdf.

[14] Majumdar D. How are the Two Most Polluted Metro-cities of India

Combating Air Pollution? Way Forward after Lifting of COVID-19 Lockdown. Aerosol and Air Quality Research 2021; 21, 200463. DOI: 10.4209/aaqr. 2020.07.0463

[15] Lal, P., Kumar, A., Bharti, S., Saikia, P., Adhikari, D., Khan, M.L., Lockdown to Contain the COVID-19 Pandemic: An Opportunity to Create a Less Polluted Environment in India. Aerosol and Air Quality Research 2021;21, 200229. DOI: 10.4209/aaqr.2020.05.0229

[16] Rathore D S, Nagda C, Shaktawat B S, Kain T, Chouhan C S, Purohit R, Harish, Khangarot R K, Nagda G, Jhala LS. COVID-19 lockdown: a boon in boosting the air quality of major Indian Metropolitan Cities. Aerobiologia 2021; 37, 79-103. DOI: 10.1007/s10453-020-09673-5

[17] Patra S S, Das T, Ramasamy B. Estimating the Inadvertent Decrement in Mortality due to Reduction in Ambient Fine Particulate Concentrations During COVID-19 Lockdown in India. Aerosol Sci Eng. 2021; Mar 12: 1–6. DOI: 10.1007/s41810-021-00097-3

[18] Panda S, Mallik C, Nath J, Das T, Ramasamy B 2021. A study on variation of atmospheric pollutants over Bhubaneswar during imposition of nationwide lockdown in India for the COVID-19 pandemic. Air Qual Atmos Health 2021; 14, 97–108 . DOI: 10.1007/s11869-020-00916-5

[19] Nath J, Panda S, Patra S S, Ramasamy B, 2021.Variation of black carbon and particulate matter in Bhubaneswar during the pre-monsoon : possible impact of meteorology and COVID-19 lockdown. CURRENT SCIENCE 2021; 120, 2.DOI:10.18520/cs/v120/i2/313-321

[20] Seinfeld J H, Pandis S N. From air pollution to climate change. Atmospheric Chemistry and Physics. Wiley, New York 1998p; 1326pp. DOI: 10.1063/1.882420

[21] Mahato S, Pal S, Ghosh K G. Effect of lockdown amid COVID-19 pandemic on air quality of the megacity Delhi, India.. Sci. Total Environ 2020;730, 139086. DOI: 10.1016/j.scitotenv. 2020.139086.

[22] Ravindra K, Singh T, Biswal A, Singh V, Mor S, 2021. Impact of COVID-19 lockdown on ambient air quality in megacities of India and implication for air pollution control strategies. Environ Sci Pollut Res Int. 2021;1-12.DOI: 10.1007/s11356-020-11808-7

[23] Singh R P, Chauhan A. Impact of lockdown on air quality in India during COVID-19 pandemic. Air Qual Atmos Health 2020; 13, 921-928. DOI: 10.1007/s11869-020-00863-1

[24] Dumka U C , Kaskaoutis DG , Verma S , Ningombam S S, Kumar S, Ghosh S. Silver linings in the dark clouds of COVID-19: Improvement of air quality over India and Delhi metropolitan area from measurements and WRF-CHIMERE model simulations. Atmos. Pollut. Res 2021;12, 225-242. DOI: 10.1016/j.apr.2020.11.005

[25] Kotnala G, Mandal T K, Sharma S K, Kotnala R K. Emergence of Blue Sky Over Delhi Due to Coronavirus Disease (COVID-19) Lockdown Implications. Aerosol Sci Eng. 2020; 1-11. DOI: 10.1007/s41810-020-00062-6.

[26] Pant G, Alka, Garlapati D, Gaur A, Hossain K, Singh S V, Gupta A K, 2020. Air quality assessment among populous sites of major metropolitan cities in India during COVID-19 pandemic confinement. Environ Sci Pollut Res Int. 2020;27, 44629-44636. DOI: 10.1007/s11356-020-11061-y

[27] Yadav R, Korhale N, Anand V, Rathod A, Bano S, Shinde R, Latha R,

Sahu S K, Murthy B S, Beig G. COVID-19 lockdown and air quality of SAFAR-India metro cities. Urban Clim 2020; 34, 100729. DOI: 10.1016/j.envres.2020.110121

[28] Sarkar M, Das A, Mukhopadhyay S. Assessing the immediate impact of COVID-19 lockdown on the air quality of Kolkata and Howrah, West Bengal, India. Environ Dev Sustain. 2020 ;Sep 22 : 1–30. DOI: 10.1007/s10668-020-00985-7

[29] Singh J, Tyagi B. Transformation of Air Quality over a Coastal Tropical Station Chennai during COVID-19 Lockdown in India. AEROSOL AIR QUAL RES 2021;21, 200490-200490. DOI: 10.4209/aaqr.200490

[30] Sreekanth V, Kushwaha M, Kulkarni P, Upadhya A R, Spandana B, Prabhu V. Impact of COVID-19 lockdown on the fine particulate matter concentration levels: Results from Bengaluru megacity, India. ADV SPACE RES 2021 67, 2140-2150. DOI: 10.1016/j.asr.2021.01.017

[31] Sahoo P K , Mangla S, Pathak A K, Salãmao G N, Sarkar D. Pre-to-post lockdown impact on air quality and the role of environmental factors in spreading the COVID-19 cases - a study from a worst-hit state of India. Int. J. Biometeorol. 2021; 65, 205-222. DOI: 10.1007/s00484-020-02019-3

[32] Bera B, Bhattacharjee S, Shit P K, Sengupta N, Saha S. Significant impacts of COVID-19 lockdown on urban air pollution in Kolkata (India) and amelioration of environmental health. Environ Dev Sustain 2020; Jul 28 : 1–28. DOI: 10.1007/s10668-020-00898-5

[33] Chowdhuri I, Pal S C, Saha A, Chakrabortty R, Ghosh M, Roy P. Significant decrease of lightning activities during COVID-19 lockdown period over Kolkata megacity in India. Sci. Total Environ 2020; 747, 141321. DOI: 10.1016/j.scitotenv.2020.141321

[34] Kabiraj S, Gavli N V. Impact of SARS-CoV-2 Pandemic Lockdown on Air Quality Using Satellite Imagery with Ground Station Monitoring Data in Most Polluted City Kolkata, India. Ae rosol Sci Eng. 2020;4, 320-330. DOI: 10.1007/s41810-020-00077-z

[35] Nigam R, Pandya K, Luis A J, Sengupta R, Kotha M. Positive effects of COVID-19 lockdown on air quality of industrial cities (Ankleshwar and Vapi) of Western India. Scientific Reports 2021; 11, 4285. DOI: 10.1038/s41598-021-83393-9

[36] Jain C D, Madhavan, B L, Singh V, Prasad P, Sai Krishnaveni A, Ravi Kiran V, Venkat Ratnam M. Phase-wise analysis of the COVID-19 lockdown impact on aerosol, radiation and trace gases and associated chemistry in a tropical rural environment. Environ. Res 2021;194, 110665. DOI: 10.1016/j.envres.2020.110665

[37] Sahu S K, Tyagi B, Beig G, Mangaraj P, Pradhan C, Khuntia S, Singh V. Significant change in air quality parameters during the year 2020 over 1st smart city of India: Bhubaneswar. SN Applied Sciences 2020;2, 1990. DOI: 10.1007/s42452-020-03831-7

[38] Selvam S, Muthukumar P , Venkatramanan S , Roy P D, Manikanda Bharath K, Jesuraja K. SARS-CoV-2 pandemic lockdown: Effects on air quality in the industrialized Gujarat state of India. Sci. Total Environ, 2020; 737, 140391. DOI: 10.1016/j.scitotenv.2020.140391

[39] Thomas J, Jainet P J, Sudheer K P. Ambient air quality of a less industrialized region of India (Kerala) during the COVID-19 lockdown. Anthropocene 2020; 32, 100270. DOI: 10.1016/j.ancene.2020.100270

[40] Resmi C T, Nishanth T, Kumar M K S, Manoj M G. Air quality improvement during triple-lockdown in the coastal city of Kannur, Kerala to combat Covid-19 transmission. PeerJ. 2020; 8: e9642 1–20. DOI: 10.7717/peerj.9642

[41] Mandal I, Pal S. COVID-19 pandemic persuaded lockdown effects on environment over stone quarrying and crushing areas. Sci. Total Environ 2020; 732, 139281. DOI: 10.1016/j.scitotenv.2020.139281

[42] Mor S, Kumar S, Singh T, Dogra S, Pandey V, Ravindra K. Impact of COVID-19 lockdown on air quality in Chandigarh, India: Understanding the emission sources during controlled anthropogenic activities. Chemosphere 2021; 263, 127978. DOI: 10.1016/j.chemosphere.2020.127978

[43] Patra S S, Chilukuri B R, Vanajakshi L. Analysis of road traffic pattern changes due to activity restrictions during COVID-19 pandemic in Chennai. TRANSP LETT 2021a;1-9. DOI: 10.1080/19427867.2021.1899580

[44] Rana A, Jia S, Sarkar S. Black carbon aerosol in India: A comprehensive review of current status and future prospects. Atmos. Res. 2019;218, 207-230. DOI: 10.1016/j.atmosres.2018.12.002

[45] Mahapatra P S, Panda S, Das N, Rath S, Das T. Variation in black carbon mass concentration over an urban site in the eastern coastal plains of the Indian sub-continent. Theor. Appl. Climatol 2014;117, 133-147. DOI: 10.1007/s00704-013-0984-z

[46] Kumar R, Barth MC, Pfister G G, Nair V S, Ghude S D, Ojha N. What controls the seasonal cycle of black carbon aerosols in India? J. Geophys. Res. Atmos,2015;120, 7788-7812. DOI: 10.1002/2015JD023298

[47] Verma S, Pani S K, Bhanja S N. Sources and radiative effects of wintertime black carbon aerosols in an urban atmosphere in east India. Chemosphere 2013;90, 260-269. DOI: 10.1016/j.chemosphere.2012.06.063

[48] Adhikary B, Carmichael G R, Tang Y, Leung L R, Qian Y, Schauer J J, Stone E A, Ramanathan V, Ramana M V. Characterization of the seasonal cycle of south Asian aerosols: A regional-scale modeling analysis. J. Geophys. Res. Atmos 2007;112. DOI: 10.1029/2006JD008143, 2007

[49] Babu S S, Moorthy K K. Aerosol black carbon over a tropical coastal station in India. Geophys. Res. Lett. 2002;29, 13-11-13-14. DOI: 10.1029/2002GL015662

[50] Satheesh S K, Ramanathan V. Large differences in tropical aerosol forcing at the top of the atmosphere and Earth's surface. Nature 2000;405, 60-63. DOI: 10.1038/35011039

[51] Koch D, Del Genio A D. Black carbon semi-direct effects on cloud cover: review and synthesis. Atmos. Chem. Phys. 2010;10, 7685-7696. DOI: https://doi.org/10.5194/acp-10-7685-2010

[52] Beegum S N, Moorthy K K, Babu S S, Satheesh S K, Vinoj V, Badarinath K V S, Safai P D, Devara P C S, Singh S, Vinod, Dumka U C, Pant P. Spatial distribution of aerosol black carbon over India during pre-monsoon season. Atmos. Environ. 2009;43, 1071-1078. DOI: 10.1016/j.atmosenv.2008.11.042

[53] Forbes M S, Raison R J, Skjemstad J O. Formation, transformation and transport of black carbon (charcoal) in terrestrial and aquatic ecosystems. Sci. Total Environ. 2006;370, 190-206. DOI: 10.1016/j.scitotenv.2006.06.007

[54] Gogoi M M, Babu S S, Arun B S, Moorthy K K, Shaikh A, Pathak B, Gharai B , Ramasamy B. Response of ambient BC concentration across the Indian region to the nation-wide lockdown : results from the ARFINET

measurements of ISRO-GBP. Current Science 2021; 120, 2 DOI: 10.18520/cs/v120/i2/341-351

[55] Ajay A, Moorthy KK, Satheesh S K, Ilavazhagan G. Impact of lockdown-related reduction in anthropogenic emissions on aerosol characteristics in the megacity, Bengaluru Current Science 2021b;120,2. DOI: 10.18520/cs/v120/i2/287-295

[56] Wang Q, Zeng Q , Tao J, Sun L, Zhang L, Gu T , Wang Z , Chen L. Estimating PM2.5 Concentrations Based on MODIS AOD and NAQPMS Data over Beijing–Tianjin–Hebei. Sensors 2019;19. DOI: 10.3390/s19051207

[57] Miller BG. The Effect of Coal Usage on Human Health and the Environment, in: Miller, B.G. (Ed.), Clean Coal Engineering Technology. Butterworth-Heinemann 2011, Boston, pp. 85-132.

[58] Kubba S. Chapter Seven - Indoor Environmental Quality, in: Kubba, S. (Ed.), Handbook of Green Building Design and Construction (Second Edition). Butterworth-Heinemann, pp. 353-412. Elsevier Science,2017. DOI: 10.1016/C2009-0-64483-4

[59] Vakkilainen EK. Solid Biofuels and Combustion, in: Vakkilainen, E.K. (Ed.), Steam Generation from Biomass. Butterworth-Heinemann2017, pp. 18-56.

[60] Rose J J , Wang L , Xu Q , McTiernan C F, Shiva S, Tejero J, Gladwin M T. Carbon Monoxide Poisoning: Pathogenesis, Management, and Future Directions of Therapy. Am J Respir Crit Care Med 2017;195, 596-606. DOI: 10.1164/rccm.201606-1275CI

[61] Stork C M, 2014. Carbon Monoxide, in: Wexler, P. (Ed.), Encyclopedia of Toxicology (Third Edition). Academic Press, Oxford, pp. 682-684.

[62] Korhale N, Anand V, Beig G. Disparity in ozone trends under COVID-19 lockdown in a closely located coastal and hillocky metropolis of India. Air Qual Atmos Health 2020; Oct 31 : 1–10. DOI: 10.1007/s11869-020-00958-9

[63] Allu S K, Reddy A, Srinivasan S, Maddala R K, Anupoju G R. Surface Ozone and its Precursor Gases Concentrations during COVID-19 Lockdown and Pre-Lockdown Periods in Hyderabad City, India. Environ Proce ss. 2021; Feb 16: 1–14. DOI: 10.1007/s40710-020-00490-z

[64] Brusseau M L , Matthias A D, Comrie A C, Musil S A. Chapter 17 - Atmospheric Pollution, in: Brusseau, M. L., Pepper, I.L., Gerba, C.P. (Eds.), Environmental and Pollution Science (Third Edition). Academic Press 2019; pp. 293-309.

[65] Garg A, Shukla P R, Kapshe M. The sectoral trends of multigas emissions inventory of India. Atmos. Environ 2006; 40, 4608-4620. DOI:.1016/j.atmosenv.2006.03.045

[66] Mallik C, Lal S , Venkataramani S. Trace gases at a semi-arid urban site in western India: variability and inter-correlations. J. Atmos. Chem. 2015; 72, 143-164. DOI: 10.1007/s10874-015-9311-7

[67] Zhang R, Zhang Y, Lin H , Feng X, Fu T-M , Wang Y, NOx Emission Reduction and Recovery during COVID-19 in East China. Atmosphere 2020;11,433. DOI: 10.3390/atmos11040433

[68] https://www.greenpeace.org/india/en/press/4015/india-largest-so2-emitter-in-the-world-says-greenpeaces-new-analysis/

[69] Das N, Sutradhar S, Ghosh R, Mondal P. Asymmetric nexus between air quality index and nationwide lockdown for COVID-19 pandemic in a part of Kolkata metropolitan, India. Urban Clim 2021; 36, 100789. DOI: 10.1016/j.uclim.2021.100789

Chapter 33

A Qualitative Study of Pre-Vaccine Decrease of Mortality from COVID-19

Vugar Mammadov and Lala Jafarova

Abstract

More than a year has passed since the appearance of disease called COVID-19 in the world. This disease became the reason for unprecedented measures taken so far, having received the classification of pandemic. The world has faced with pandemics before, but society has not yet taken such unprecedented restrictive measures. The restrictions of not only local but even of global nature, such as the suspension of international flights, various scientific and political events were adopted around the world. Media resources have played a key role in the formation and development of the attitude towards the disease in people. Despite all the depressing news, the facts showed a low mortality rate, which is often ignored by the media. As a result, medical staff around the world have faced psychological health issues among the different groups of the population, especially vulnerable ones such as people with chronic disease and with weak immunity. At present, it is early to talk about the results and outcomes of the pandemic. However, previous year has taught us many lessons and can become a key factor in understanding the role of the media in pandemic times, developing strategies for combating diseases and protecting public health.

Keywords: coronavirus, coronavirus pandemics, COVID-19, media and coronavirus, infodemic, fake-news, coronavirus and social media, coronavirus and internet, coronavirus and healthcare, quarantine, lockdown, coronavirus pandemics and politics, coronavirus pandemics and economics, telemedicine

1. Introduction

COVID-19 pandemic has changed the world. More than half of the planet's population, namely, more than five billion people have been isolated during the last year, changing regular life, habits and thoughts. Most international flights, travels, events and gatherings, sports and cultural programs including World Expo, World Sport Cups, and the Olympic Games have been cancelled, political and scientific events moved to the online format. The global economy has collapsed and prognosis for the next year includes the increase in hunger and poverty. International organisations, national and international leaders could not shade their own weaknesses and disorientation. Wrong decisions, non-justified actions and declarations were made... Being medico-legal expert who used to look into facts rather than rumoured and unproven information, the mortality rate is the first thing that is taken into consideration. According to our analysis of mortality rates in different continents and countries that have been made from the beginning of pandemic we have seen that panic in the countries, frightening messages from TV screens, media speculations in newspapers have been developing in a similar scenario to aggravate dangers of the pandemic, which is probably more beneficial for certain political reasons rather than economic, scientific, medical or public. Our definite conclusion is that this pandemic is not only medical and biological problem. From other side, our observations shown it may have great value for the world if to take right lessons from its global effects on our future lives.

Thus, the article provides a qualitative analysis of the factors associated with the pandemic in the field of biotechnology and other spheres of life through their reflection in the media.

2. The development of biotechnology as one of the factors of the positive impact of the pandemic

Despite its negative impact, the pandemic primarily gave impetus to the development of biotechnology that ensured creation of effective tools to combat the coronavirus. Biotechnology, in addition to traditional fields such as genetics or molecular biology, is also based on information technology. Computer modelling tools provide wide opportunities for modern biotechnologies. Those tools ensure faster study of viruses, identification of their genome and, as a consequence, development of new testing methods and disease prevention. The innovative biotechnology tools accelerated study of sequence of the new coronavirus genome. As a result of their application in just a few weeks after discovery of the disease [1, 2], its virus genome has been analysed.

Prompt decoding and computer modelling of the virus created conditions for development of express coronavirus tests [3]. Moreover, biotechnologies ensured the development of various types of vaccines against the virus [4] based on different methods. In that context, biotech companies have become a kind of founders in the hope of fighting against the pandemic as they are at the forefront of research to develop vaccines and treatments.

It is the development of modern biotechnology that has led to such a rapid development of various vaccines in such a short time. Considering urgency of the situation U.S. Food and Drug Administration (FDA) has authorised several vaccines for emergency use. Thus, based on clinical research results as of March 2, 2021 CDC information confirms [5–7] the efficacy of the approved vaccines as shown in **Figure 1**.

Although vaccines are the most important tool developed because of the application of biotechnology in the fight against coronavirus, their effectiveness at the initial stage caused a heated discussion in the media. Moreover, their use and side effects have become the subject of massive misinformation and rumours among population. In order to avoid similar phenomena in the future and to help

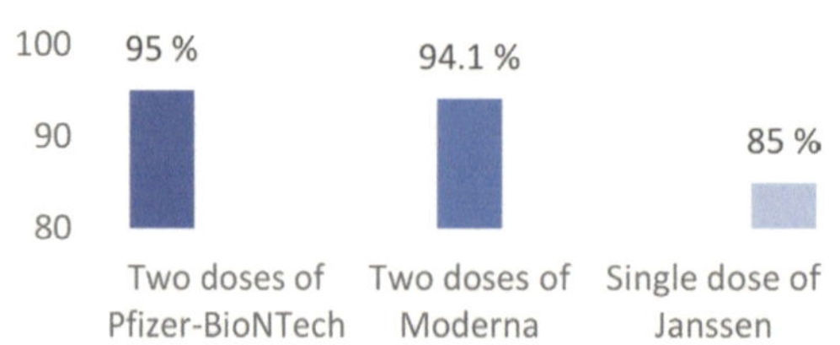

Figure 1.
Efficacy of the CDC approved vaccines. Data of 2 March 2021.

biotechnological companies and states to correctly develop their strategy for working with the media, we consider it necessary to analyse information and most common media cases related to the pandemic in this context.

3. Coronavirus and the role of the media

Today, computer technology has become an integral part or even a fundamental tool for scientific research, especially in high-tech research such as biotechnology. However, development of information technology is inherently associated with the Internet and media in general. Scientists and biotechnology companies analyse media resources in order to study the social aspects of people's lives and conduct relevant research. Moreover, media resources such as social networks create opportunities not only for the communication of scientists, but also for identifying trends in public discussions and sharing their research or developments. Thus, the Biotech-careers web-resource conducted an analysis in their database and found 109 companies in 364 localities working on COVID-19 as of April 06, 2020 [8]. We presume that those numbers are increasing. During the pandemic, reports on biotechnology found wide media coverage but what did the pandemic represent for society?

The COVID-19 pandemic has become one of the largest threats facing humanity. However, can we say that it was the disease, fight against which was worth such unprecedented measures as complete lockdowns, the cancellation of all public events, depriving people of such a basic right as freedom of movement? What became the hallmark of the disease besides the fact that it was a new strain of the coronavirus infection?

The humanity has already faced epidemics and pandemics earlier. The diseases such as tuberculosis, smallpox, the virus called "Spanish flu" killed thousands of people. In our opinion, in addition to purely medical and epidemiological factors, the key factor that distinguishes COVID-19 is the role of the media. In contrast with the 19th or early 20th centuries when there was no Internet, social media, so many TV and radio companies, today the number of such sources of information is innumerable. The era when people had to wait for a new issue of the newspaper to get information is outdated. Today, thanks to media resources and the Internet, information is updated every second. The presence of social networks contributes to the prompt dissemination of the information. However, it is often distorted or even "overgrown with rumours" on the Internet.

Various viruses coexist with humanity. For example, although the influenza virus is activated every year, lockdowns and other global restrictions are not enforced. Successful fight against seasonal flu is a prime example of biotech progress. Experts have learned how to cope with the influenza virus [9], which infects thousands of people every year. However, modern biotechnologies allow not only to cure people from influenza, but also to prevent its spread.

Because of enforcement of the measures to combat COVID-19, all areas of life were paralysed. Even biotech companies faced difficulties in their research due to lockdowns and morbidity risk among staff.

Closing the borders of states, stopping civil interstate flights and other measures led to many social and economic problems. Thus, the Azerbaijan citizens who used to travel abroad for the medical tourism purposes had to postpone planned procedures because of the closure of borders and the suspension of air traffic for some time. Although restrictions on air traffic had a positive effect on the environment, it is difficult to assess the balance of harm and benefit when comparing the social activities, economy and the environment. Restrictions and associated social, economic problems, depression and increased anxiety in society, the violation of all social contacts, when people were afraid or prohibited from meeting with relatives and friends, were weighed against the risk of spread of the disease. Therefore, it is difficult to assess the benefit of restrictive measures as both economic and medical areas play the key role in life of the world community. However, there were also exceptions. The Republic of Belarus has not implemented the restrictive measures and, nevertheless, the mortality rate in the state was "one of the lowest in the world" [10]. If in Azerbaijan throughout all the investigated period of the last 11 months mortality rate was not above 1,5%, in Belarus this was less than 0,7%. If today in Azerbaijan we have about quarter of million contaminated during last year COVID patients, Belarus had slightly more for a few dozen thousands people, but mortality was twice less. Moreover, this is in a situation, when they did not close schools, universities, stadiums, public transport, nothing. They made a military parade of Victory Day 9 May 2020, presidential elections, had millions on the meetings and demonstrations after but COVID did not appear as frightening as in the rest of the world. Belarus and Azerbaijan both have similar geography and population about 10 million but management of pandemics were very different, and they succeeded even more than Azerbaijan and the rest of the world. In one of our past articles, we mentioned that the main reason was that the genotype of neither Azerbaijani nor Belarus was a target for COVID-19.

Talking about social and other factors, we return to the role of the media. What was their role and remains today? At first glance, the media simply broadcast the latest summaries of information about the disease and its mortality. The provision of statistical information, which often did not represent any value for the average reader, caused panic and fear. Therefore, it often had more negative than positive significance. Obviously, in pursuit of the rating, the media often published data on the most rare consequences and symptoms of the coronavirus infection [11, 12]. Although the experts later explained the reason for the incident, rumours continued to spread, especially on social networks and telephone voice messengers. The example of such misleading information is the change in skin colour from the coronavirus. Publication and replication of such incomplete information to attract visitors is an example of the so-called "hype" [13]. People reading such headings and sometimes without even opening the whole article begin to panic and spread this information.

3.1 "Infodemic" – new realities

Information resources on various platforms both at the beginning of the emergence of a new virus and today are full of headlines that "the world will no longer be the same" [14]. Many new terms have appeared during the pandemic. They either did not exist before or were not widely used. Terms such as "fake news", "lockdown", "covidiot", "doom scrolling", etc. entered our daily life. Another example of such terms is "infodemic" [15]. In our opinion, this word most clearly shows how large-scale the flow of information associated with the new virus has become. This term, highlighted by the WHO, described the unfounded information, which does not reflect the truth. It includes panic news and in some cases concealment of the essence of the information, rumours, and conspiracy theories aimed only at misleading the society. Human beings tend to believe and share alarm warnings. Such information in addition attracts more readers, which is of higher importance for the media resources. That became a key factor of the development of infodemic.

Often, the official media unintentionally sowed panic among the population, reporting on the upcoming lockdown, disinfection, etc. Thus, such panic gripped the society in Baku, as in other cities of the world, during the announcement of the complete lockdown [16]. People rushed to the markets buying almost everything after hearing such news [17]. Although full lockdowns in Baku lasted no more than two days, people bought several times more bread than usual. Society affected by the impact of the panic experienced as a result of the unexpected announcement of the news about the restriction exaggerated by rumours that flooded social networks and voice messengers have only fuelled peoples' fears. On the contrary, along with panic and socio-economic tensions, so-called memes or funny pictures about the coronavirus [18] were also spreading on the Internet. Of course, this does not mean that we should not take the virus seriously. All medical advice must be followed, but one must not be afraid. In addition, even if in social isolation, we should do it without fear. We should strictly follow personal hygiene and distancing but not fear.

A lot of information, which was often fake, had a detrimental effect on both the psychological health of people and hindered an effective fight against the pandemic. People, left in complete isolation, were forced to search for information on the Internet in order to understand what was happening, how to protect themselves from the virus. Given the high interest in the subject matter, the unscrupulous media, accordingly, published and updated information, which did not always reflect reliable data, at lightning speed. Regular users who did not have in-depth knowledge of the topic and were unable to distinguish scientific data from rumours started to panic at such fake information. People prone to depression, who are in chronic stress, suspecting they have a coronavirus, lost their ability to adequately assess the situation. A large number of news, often-fake ones, about the coronavirus, and their even greater spread on social networks, indicate that the criticality of information perception in times of turmoil decreases sharply. This is what the mass distribution of infodemic is based on.

Cybercriminals on the Internet have also contributed to the increase in the scale of the infodemic. Thus, they created hundreds of so-called bad bots [19]. These programs, imitating the behaviour of a real person, spread deliberately false and misleading information. However, during the pandemic, positive bots created by official structures served to provide help. Thus, a bot launched in Azerbaijan [20] allowed people to check themselves for the signs of the coronavirus infection.

However, is it right to say that the pandemic was accompanied only by false news? It is not only the information itself that is very important, but the context in which it is presented and its emotional colouring. Thus, national media in all countries of the world, as well as global media, began to publish "shocking" data on death toll from the coronavirus. Media headlines were mostly representing data on negative facts about the coronavirus. In this context, wasn't it a manipulation of readers aimed only at increasing the "clickability" of the title? It is obvious that the worse the news about the disease, the more readers it will attract. Haven't people before that die of AIDS, cardiovascular diseases and other diseases? How important is the context of presenting information? Infodemic, when information or misinformation spreads virally, like the spread of the viral infection itself, has become the result of the work of the media and social networks. Pure statistics, even if it concerns mortality, can be frightening or neutral depending on different contexts [21]. 3000+ deaths from COVID-19 in Azerbaijan during 12 months repeated everyday from TV channels impact deleteriously to the mental health of the people and make them panic. This is natural for public to be afraid. However, as forensic experts in Azerbaijan we know that the average mortality of the country about 60 thousands deaths in the past year makes three thousands less than even 10% of mortality. Is this a justified reason for things we observed in last year? We do not think so. Majority of people continue to die from traditional diseases and most of dying COVID patients are also dying from own main diseases aggravated by concomitant coronavirus infections, which was always happened in past when influenza made complications for such categories of diabetic, cardiac, oncology, hepatic and renal patients.

Literally recently, from a historical point of view, humanity has been fighting epidemics such as "SARS (2002, 10% of deaths from those infected), avian flu (2003, 50% of deaths from those infected), MERS (2012, 35% of deaths from those infected), Ebola (2014, 40% of deaths from those infected)" [22]. At those times, the media was also filled with information of a frightening nature. However, humanity coped and literally until 2020, people lived a normal life, and only virologists and epidemiologists spoke about viruses in everyday life, to a lesser extent - representatives of other medical specialties.

Aimed at creation of sensation impressions and mass distribution, and in the case of social networks to get more shares, likes, views, journalists and bloggers, ordinary users, knowing nothing about medicine, or knowing at the level of the non-professional, write about the pandemic, the virus and even give treatment advices. How ethical in that context is writing of news by a person who does not have professional education in this area? What shall be the criteria? What medical, epidemiology and other information can and cannot be published by a non-professional? We usually do not look into the education of the author of news but is it important in the era of pandemics? There are no definite answers, since everyone is entitled to the right to have personal point of view. From a legal standpoint, freedom of thought and expression of will is an inalienable human right. However, if a person disseminates knowingly false information, gives advice of medical nature without a licence, then personal opinion becomes an example of violation of the law. If the advice caused harm to health, then this action entails criminal liability. At the same time, we know many examples of medical errors done by professionals [23]. Therefore, it is impossible to mark the availability of medical education as the standard for authors writing or speaking about the pandemic. We can conclude that the coronavirus pandemic has led not only to medical but also to many ethical and legal issues in society as well.

3.2 Information about the virus: myths and facts in the media

If earlier the society experienced a lack of information, now there is a surplus of it. A person is simply not able to assess the scale of the incoming information. Thus, the query "coronavirus" in the popular search engine Google as of mid-February 2021 gives out about 2.220 million [24] search results. Publication of such a large amount of information is often accompanied by a decrease in its quality. Unfortunately, in this case we have to rely on the search engine and hope that it will show the most truthful, complete and interesting information in response to our request. Most people in a fast-paced world have neither the time nor the energy to browse through a large amount of resources. In the old days, people went to libraries, where there was a large, but limited number of sources. Today, their number on the Internet is simply physically incalculable.

In times when only government agencies were the sources of information, it was possible to trace its author and purpose for which the publication was made. It is clear that at all times the media are always engaged to some degree. It is difficult to say, in our opinion that the media is independent when they have sponsors thanks to which they actually exist. However, there are state and large private media holdings committed to publishing clear information in order to maintain their status as a reliable source. In addition, even in the event of an error, they tend to publish an immediate rebuttal. Nevertheless, even they can hardly be called completely independent. Rating and audience coverage are also important for them.

In the context of the coronavirus, many types of media, both private and public, have sought to convey information as quickly as possible. However, if the "prestigious" resources that treasure their name gave out only official information, then the rest of the media, guided only by attracting the audience, often published an outright fake. Often, the media, referring to famous doctors on their behalf, published information that did not belong to the author at all. What the author indicated either as possible or researched was published as accurate information.

Spreading of false information (or so-called "fake news") has also become a serious problem. Such news are distinguished by their manipulative nature [25]. Often the authors of publications publish them not by mistake but purposefully. To attract the attention of the population media especially online publications for which traffic is especially important, often referred to the unconfirmed or even false information contributing to its spread. Misleading information can be related to both the disease itself and the methods of its treatment. Thus, information about folk remedies and methods of disease treatment, with the protocols for the use of alternative medicine, which often only worsened the patient's condition, has filled the Internet.

Lack of medical knowledge and panic among politicians contributed to the dissemination of such information by the media at the initial stage of the emergence of a new virus.

Often, even before the confirmation of the effectiveness of the drug or treatment method and protocol, the media began to spread information about it. Thus, at the initial stage of the pandemic, there were reports of the possible efficacy of certain drugs such as antimalarial one. Media resources began to replicate information about this medicine; even some famous personalities claimed its effectiveness [26], which further increased the public interest. Based on unproven information, some people began to use this drug without a prescription, which led to serious side effects, and in some cases even death [27]. Only after clinical trials, scientists and medical professionals concluded that the drug is not only ineffective but can be even dangerous for use by certain parts of the population [28]. Nevertheless, unfortunately, despite further denial in the media, there was already data on mortality caused by the use of the unverified information. However, at the initial stage, in early 2020, COVID-19 was a new type of disease for the medical and scientific community. This significantly complicated the work of doctors and less of the media. In the beginning, when there were no approved and proven effective treatment protocols, doctors had to verify any information empirically, that is, to use all available treatment options to save lives. However, the media, in pursuit of the rating, immediately publishing these data, albeit even if unintentionally, misled people.

Since the appearance of a new type of virus, many theories about its origin began to appear on the Internet. At an early stage, various rumours that have spread on the Internet, in the absence of scientifically proven facts caused distrust among people [29]. This fact largely contributed to the emergence of conspiracy theories. The so-called conspiracy theories put forward different ideas massively replicated in the media. In addition, even when experts denied the causes stated as the reason for the emergence of the virus in theory or the resources themselves published a refutation, people continued to spread information through social media networks. The most popular was the theory of the spread of the virus by the communication stations, which led to dozens of cases of the destruction of stations by the population [30]. Spreading of such misleading information forced internet resources such as popular social media [31] to mark the information about the coronavirus as unverified and in some cases to even delete or block it.

In response to mass disinformation the WHO as well as UNESCO, European Commission and other organisations have created special web platform such as "mythbusters" to in an understandable form with the help of specialists to debunk each of the myths and provide scientifically based information [32–34].

We think reality we have now and experience we gained in last year could make us taking very positive lessons as well: decrease of mortality started in the second half of the last year and continued to present levels even in pre-vaccine era, 80% of contaminated population had mild course of disease, more than 90% of population has recovered, young people and children were ill much rare than the older age groups, panic took more people to the death rather the disease itself.

3.3 Vaccination and role of the media

Since the very appearance of vaccines in the media, unverified and often false information about vaccines began to spread. As well as it was with the coronavirus itself. The most widespread conspiracy theory, of course, was the "chipping". This fake appeared at the beginning of the pandemic and explained its appearance as the desire of certain forces to microchip all of humanity by means of vaccination.

The efficacy and safety of vaccines has been the subject of debates. Although vaccines appeared just a couple of months ago, the media were already filled with information about mortality after their introduction [35]. Unfortunately, mortality from the vaccine as a reaction of the body (anaphylactic shock) is quite possible, even in the case of the administration of long-used, well-studied vaccines.

COVID-19 vaccine has recently appeared. Due to its urgency, it has not passed long-term clinical trials, which usually take 2–3 years. However, preliminary data made it possible to speak about their effectiveness and safety, which gave the WHO reason to approve the first yet vaccine.

The media circulating conspiracy theories and other fakes earlier are now publishing news about the need for vaccination. An interesting fact is that even now the Internet is filled with information about vaccines' side effects, which alternates with a call for vaccination. The media, with their fast-changing and sometimes diametrically opposed news, is often misleading their viewers and readers. Many people, reading about mortality from coronavirus, want to be vaccinated immediately, while others, reading about its side effects, start to panic.

Publishing only information on side effects and mortality from vaccinations, the media rarely covers how many people were successfully vaccinated. How many and at what level developed antibodies after? That is, one gets the impression that the media are not engaged in providing information, but in only attracting an audience or so-called hype.

It is also necessary to note the inadmissibility of discrimination against people who refuse vaccination. Coercion violates a constitutional human right and right for autonomy and dignity. Moreover, for some people, vaccination is contraindicated due to the medical reasons, such as allergies to its components. However, media are actively broadcasting information about "covid passports", manipulating peoples' fears.

Azerbaijan is the first country in the South Caucasus region and is one of the first in the world that ensured vaccines' delivery and has launched vaccination on 18th of January 2021. Vaccination is implemented free of charge for the citizens and on voluntary basis thus protecting the autonomy of decision-making.

The Cabinet of Ministers approved the "Strategy of vaccination against COVID-19 in the Republic of Azerbaijan for 2021-2022" on 16 January 2021 by the Order No. 48 s. The phased vaccination strategy implemented in the country prioritises the elderly and medical workers.

The vaccines approved so far by the CDC are not yet available in Azerbaijan due to the lack of sufficient amount of them at the manufactures and high demand.

However, the country has contributed $21 million [36] to the COVAX [37] initiative and supports all international activities in the fight against the coronavirus [38]. Moreover, as the delivery of vaccines within the COVAX is still expected [39], Azerbaijan has already purchased 4 million vaccines of Coronavac from China [40] to start the vaccination early. The procedure takes time because it includes an examination of those wishing to be vaccinated. For check-up and vaccination purpose, the State Agency for Compulsory Medical Insurance has launched a new electronic service called "COVID-19 vaccine appointment" [41]. Vaccinated citizens will be issued an electronic certificate in case of need a vaccination document when travelling abroad.

3.4 Social networks and phone messengers as a source of disinformation

Today, in addition to official state and private information companies, social networks have become a great source of information. Conceived to create a means of convenient communication and exchange of information between people, social networks have become independent sources of information. Although most of the official media, government officials and various international and other structures have official pages in the networks, in addition to them, there are millions of other pages. Some pretend to be original, creating fake profiles on behalf of the official or structure. Others share information at the rumour level, creating a false impression of credible awareness.

Smartphone messengers posed a special threat in this sense specifically when messages were sent from person to person, and the author could only be identified by involving law enforcement agencies. Thus, one of the most "egregious" fakes, widespread in Azerbaijan, was a voice message about the alleged disinfection of the entire country from a helicopter [42]. Unfortunately, doctors themselves often participated in the spread of such fakes, as they later explained "under the influence of panic" [43] or, more horribly, for the sake of joke [44].

During the pandemic, Azerbaijan had to introduce fines, administrative or criminal liability for spreading rumours about the coronavirus [45]. Of course, doctors, like the rest of the population were in fear and stress during the peak period of the pandemic in the country and in even more risk of being in constant contact with patients. However, the role of the media, especially unofficial ones that disseminated such information should not be underestimated. In the case of instant messengers, the situation is even more complicated for a number of reasons. First, they guarantee the confidentiality of the information sent through their platform. Secondly, personal correspondence is not an official source of information and only expresses the opinion of the author, to which everyone is entitled by law. Moreover, since the information is private it does not imply distribution. However, unfortunately, the pandemic has shown that information can be disseminated through instant messengers even faster and on a larger scale than through publications on the Internet. For example, some messengers had to mark frequently sent messages as a possible fake or even prohibit their forwarding [46]. However, these restrictions are sometimes ineffective. The user can not only simply forward the message to others, but also write a new one, referring to initial information as "heard" one, "it was said that...". As a result, the original message is further distorted and overgrown with rumours. There is no responsibility of messengers in this context. It is impossible, since they do not break the law by their work. They only do what they were created for, namely they represent the means of communication.

People who use social media or phone messengers should understand their responsibility by sending comic messages on such a serious topic as the coronavirus. In addition, it is the personal responsibility to trust rumours or not. The only possibility to protect our safety in this regard is to verify all the incoming information with the official sources, such as the state ministries' websites and think critically about the news we get.

3.5 COVID-19: role of media in the positive effects of the pandemic

Along with high uncertainty and anxiety, the pandemic has created conditions for development in some areas. As a result of total lockdown the digitalization of society has accelerated. People were forced to spend more time on the Internet. Many workers were transferred to the so-called remote job. Online shopping began to develop in those countries where it was not popular before. Even areas that previously seemed impossible online have begun to adapt to the new environment. Thus, online pharmacies began to appear in Azerbaijan, school and university studies also switched to online training, and special training platforms were launched. Telemedicine has started to be developing.

Online commerce and marketing are the areas that have benefited most from the coronavirus-related restrictions. Clothing manufacturers often used the coronavirus theme. Advertisements for T-shirts with various inscriptions and images on the topic of coronavirus appeared on the Internet. Some companies have supported healthcare [47] by producing medical equipment, which was also a good marketing strategy.

Although internet commerce has grown rapidly due to the pandemic, it is difficult to say that it will permanently eliminate shopping malls, at least not in the next decades. Hiking to the malls often has nothing to do with shopping. People, especially the youth, went to shopping malls, which usually have restaurants, cinemas, and a lot of entertainment such as bowling, to spend their leisure time and meet with friends.

The field of telemedicine is perhaps one of the few that has evolved during the pandemic. Today it is still too early to talk about general surgical interventions that can be performed remotely via the Internet (although such experiments have been implemented already [48]). However, telemedicine in today's conditions has become a real salvation for both patients and doctors. First, patients could save the time they usually spend travelling to the hospital. Secondly, the doctor and the patient were both protected from possible infection, since often people themselves did not even suspect that they were infected (the so-called "asymptomatic patients"). In addition, in some cases, the patient does not need a real examination, but a consultation, an adjustment of the treatment course. The psychological effect is also important when the patient turns to the doctor "to calm down his fears". In the case of the field of psychology, telemedicine was easily possible, and it did not lose its meaning either. Since in psychological practice the factor of communication prevails and does not require physical contact such as, for example, in the case of traumatology.

4. General information about the impact of the disease in Azerbaijan and around the world

The coronavirus pandemic is a unique phenomenon. Right after the emergence of the virus and information from China, people around the world were locked-up in their homes. Cities and streets became empty. The world community divided into groups of those who feared the new virus and those who did not believe in it. Fear changed the world. Politicians had to enforce restrictive measures to create a sense of security among citizens. Moreover, the population blamed politicians who did not act. However, there was also another part of the population that was left without income because of restrictive measures, whose business went bankrupt. On the contrary, they wanted the restrictions to be lifted as soon as possible. Many people came out to mass demonstrations against the mask regime and other restrictions in such big cities such as London, Berlin, Madrid, Amsterdam [49–52].

Comparative statistics analysis for 9 months (March 2020 – February 2021) shows more than two fold growth in morbidity and mortality in the world. Coronavirus cases at the end of February 2021 almost doubled compared to May 2020 (about 112 million compared to more than 5 million) [53]. The coronavirus death toll also increased significantly. Thus, for the mentioned period it has increased from 351,886 in May 2020 to more than 2 million 400 thousand deaths to date. However, recovery rate also has increased indicating that more than 87 million or about 80 percent of patients have already recovered [54]. The above data give us reason to believe that most of the people currently undergoing treatment will fully recover. 99,6% of those who are active cases now have a high chance to be recovered. So, our observations of global mortality rate being 6–7% in early months of March – April, went down to 5–5,5% in May – June, then to 4% in August and to 2,2% from the fall of the year till start of the vaccination. This says a lot. So present mortality rate at 2,2% is not a result of vaccination but this is result of natural processes, which can be scientifically explained or not, but this is a fact which all of us should accept.

The disease, which was classified as the pandemic by the WHO, which affected more than 100 million people in one year has been also registered in Azerbaijan. At the beginning of January 2020, when there were no cases of infection among the population, epidemiological and overall situation in Azerbaijan was not so tense. Even before the first officially documented coronavirus case, the authorities have started the development of the antiviral measures. These measures included the adoption of the Action Plan to prevent the spread of the new coronavirus disease in the Azerbaijan Republic, and then the creation of the Task Force under the Cabinet of Ministers (Task Force or Operative Headquarter under Prime-Minister) to combat coronavirus [55]. However, the escalation of the situation in the media made the situation worse. Global and local media resources covered information of a purely medical or biological nature. This information was not familiar for the average reader, but aggravated fear in society.

The first case of the coronavirus infection was registered at the end of February 2020 in Azerbaijan [56]. The shocking news from other countries by that time have already scared people. Subsequently, after the first death case that followed in March [57] social situation deteriorated. The massive information flow, which was accompanied by frightening statistics about the rapid spread of the virus and lack of treatment of the unknown disease filled local media. The further introduction of quarantine measures led not only to the deterioration in the emotional state of people, but also disrupted the work of almost all areas.

Throughout the year, easing and tightening of the quarantine regime have changed alternately several times, that had a negative impact on the psyche of the people and the economy of Azerbaijan. Thus, according to the latest data, the state spent 2 billion manats (local currency, 1 USD = 1,7 AZN manat) to fight the coronavirus in the country in 2020 [58]. The imminent recession in the economy, business activity, tourism and other spheres negatively affected the economic condition of people. As a result, the income of the population has significantly decreased or stopped altogether. Although the state has provided financial support [59] to the citizens and entrepreneurs [60], people accustomed to the certain level of incomes, who took out a flat or a bank loan on a mortgage, found themselves in very difficult circumstances. The most difficult situation was observed in the tourism, restaurant, and entertainment sectors. Under the conditions of quarantine measures, their work was either prohibited or significantly restricted. Consequently, the economic factor has become an additional reason for the deterioration of the psychological health of the population. Moreover, under the conditions of the strict quarantine, restrictions and even ban to leave home were applied in the country [61].

Implemented during the quarantine time limit for leaving home [62] negatively affected people's everyday life. In fact, people were limited to outdoor walks. The time restrictions on leaving the house forced people to make a choice between visiting, for example, a bank and taking a walk in the park or even doctor visit.

The ban on the work of gyms and admission to parks has become an additional fact of the aggravation of not only the physical but also the psychological health of the people. Accustomed to a sports lifestyle were limited even to visiting parks and the sea. Morning jogging along the embankment was allowed only in compliance with epidemiological measures, such as wearing a medical mask, which questioned the benefits of such a run. In our opinion, in Azerbaijan, where the summer season is very hot wearing a medical mask during that times was more harmful than beneficial especially while morning jogging. Wearing a mask limited calm breathing, caused shortness of breath and additional sweating. In general, from a medical point of view, the value of wearing a mask in the hot summer season, weighed down by the high levels of humidity that is observed in the most parts of the country, from our point of view, are not just controversial, but rather negative. Thus, sweaty masks, in conditions of poor air exchange during summer season, often absent or very weak wind attracts bacteria more than protects health. Such measures had an extremely negative impact on both the physical and emotional state of people. Moreover, unfortunately, masks were not distributed free of charge on a massive scale to the country's whole population. Therefore, some people ignored the need to change the mask every 2 hours, and there was no point in it due to the high air temperature, which some days was above 40 degrees Celsius, and high humidity.

Even during the hot summer months, within the framework of quarantine measures people were deprived of the opportunity to visit the beaches. Access to the beaches was opened only at the beginning of August when the beach season in Baku was already ending [63]. Moreover, the opening also took place subject to the necessary epidemiological measures [64] such as social distance between beach loungers and limiting the number of people on the beach. To this end, a website was created where people could book their place in advance on the beach and estimate how many people are there.

Places of religious worship were also closed in Azerbaijan during the tough quarantine as well as in many countries. However, people who were already in the stressful state and used to find peace only in such places through prayer were deprived of this opportunity. The pilgrims were deprived of the opportunity to perform the Hajj [65], the devout deprived of carrying out religious rites in relation to those who died from the coronavirus. The closure of churches [66], temples, mosques and other places of worship at certain times has been implemented around the world. Unfortunately, it is difficult to maintain social distance in places of worship. There were also recorded cases of mass infection in such places [67, 68] that ensured the restrictive measures. Nevertheless, such restrictive measures have created an additional burden on the psychological health of people and have disrupted the usual way of life. The mosques remain closed even at present. Moreover, the closure of the religious sites while restaurants are open is also causing debates in the society.

We believe that one of the unjustified measures taken in the fight against coronavirus in Azerbaijan as well as in many other countries was the disinfection of the streets. The chemicals used for the disinfection were further absorbed into the soil, disrupting the ecology and harming biodiversity. Moreover, these substances posed a particular threat on people's health, especially of those suffering from allergies and lung diseases. Therefore, both from an environmental and a medical point of view, this measure caused more damage than benefit. Large financial resources were allocated for its implementation, which in the conditions of the economic downturn was spending that could be directed to health care needs. An additional, albeit not so important, negative factor of disinfection is the inconvenience of the population. Often people were advised not to leave the house during disinfection.

From the epidemiological point of view, mentioned restrictive measures might be justified if they made sense in terms of reducing the rate of increase in the incidence. However, the statistics, unfortunately, show the opposite. Moreover, the negative influence of the lack of sports activity and walking in the fresh air, the importance of vitamin D produced by the body under the influence of sunlight is widely known. That is, the restriction on walking in the fresh air led to stress and an even greater weakening of natural immunity, which is so important in the fight against the virus.

Restrictive measures in connection with the coronavirus in Azerbaijan have been further tightened as a result of the introduction of martial law at the end of 2020. Coronavirus disease during the war has become an additional burden on the healthcare system. The outbreak of the Patriotic War or the Second Karabakh 44-day war [69] at the end of September created tension in society. News reports from the front line were combined with statistics on the spread of coronavirus infection. Moreover, the restrictive measures have been further tightened in connection with the introduction of martial law in the country. The country's health care had to solve a difficult task of allocation of resources between the needs of the front and coronavirus hospitals. In this respect, this period was especially difficult for doctors. Consequently, the health care system was overloaded during this period.

The Task Force significantly weakened the quarantine regime, however, has not completely lifted it as of February 2021. Thus, a number of restrictions such as the necessity to wear medical masks, large shopping centres and metro remain closed, public transport does not work on the weekends, will remain valid until April 2021 [70].

The coronavirus emergence also gave impetus to the development of domestic healthcare in Azerbaijan. Thus, foreign experts from China, Russia, Italy and Cuba were repeatedly invited to the country to exchange experience and help to fight coronavirus [71–74]. For the first time in the country, modular hospitals were opened [75]. Factories for the production of medical masks and even disinfection tunnels [76] for domestic use and export have been launched.

As of February 2021, statistics on coronavirus in Azerbaijan show about 80 percent recovery [77]. At present, some patients are still in hospitals, some are being treated at home, so it is difficult to give a final figure yet. However, based on one-year observation we can assume that the final death rate from the disease in the country will be low and not more than 2 percent.

Not only Azerbaijan experienced coronavirus-related restrictions. Worldwide unprecedented control measures have been taken. Thus, all international sporting, cultural and scientific events have been cancelled. Many events such as international chess tournaments and even political meetings with the participation of state officials were held in the online format.

Restrictive measures of unprecedented scale and often-conflicting media coverage may have resulted from the lack of timely action by the WHO [78], which declared pandemic and gave appropriate medical advice to the member-states quite late. Were these measures justified? Experts have yet to figure it out. At the initial stage, when the world was gripped by panic due to the unknown type of virus, such measures may have been necessary. However, by the middle of 2020, their destructive side in relation to the economy and the psychological health of people became clear. A similar situation and restrictive measures were observed in many countries of the world and for now, people still do not have the opportunity to return to their usual way of life. For now, continuation of quarantines around the world, restrictive measures when the coronavirus infection has already been studied and vaccines have been developed and made available, is questionable and causes controversial ideas among the world community.

5. Conclusion

Despite all the restrictive measures taken in the world, the pandemic did not stop, and only a year after its emergence the European Commissioner admitted that "the borders do not prevent the coronavirus" [79]. Unfortunately, society has gone through practically a halt in all social life. It has been deprived of the opportunity to visit other states for more than a year. However, today there is no decision to completely lift restrictions by all states. Some countries announce quarantines even in 2021 [80]. The Internet today is filled with "predictions" about how the world has changed, that it will no longer be the same again after COVID-19. Positive ideas are replaced by negative ones and vice versa. All this information affects the psychological state of readers. For some, coronavirus is depressing, for the others it has opened up new opportunities and ideas. "What will the world be like after...?" Journalists and representatives of other spheres argue. A little over a year has passed since the emergence of the new virus. What can we conclude for today? First, the impulse that the virus gave to the development of biotechnologies and medicine. In just a year, several effective vaccines for coronavirus appeared at once in particular thanks to the development of biotechnology. Have we encountered such lightning-fast vaccine development before? Perhaps, the developments scientists have launched today will give positive results for medicine in the future. Despite all the seeming global changes, if we remove the noise created in the media, then nothing has essentially changed. At each stage of human development, one can note the events that "changed" life. Thus, "Spanish flu" has led to the death of millions of people. At that time, it seemed that society would not return to normal life. Nevertheless, humanity coped with the disease and continued its development.

However, we consider the role of the media to be the most important aspect of the pandemic. Media resources are the most important source of information. We have witnessed how misrepresentation of information or its deliberate distortion can harm society, how it affects psychological health. Nor should the role of the state be underestimated in this regard. Politicians, heads of states are interested in the development of society, elimination of threats and maintenance of public health. However, inappropriate or unnecessarily strict measures can sometimes only exacerbate the situation. In this context, a well-coordinated and close cooperation between representatives of the health system, scientists and the media is necessary. State should not allow the spread of fakes, or vice versa, withhold information. The average citizen cannot and does not have to be a scientist to understand a situation. Moreover, the main task of the media is to convey reliable information not through scary headlines, but through proven science-based information. Oftentimes, politicians or lawyers with no medical knowledge make decisions that are medically unfounded. However, there are also opposite situations, when the opinion of a specialist is expressed in the media, but it is so full of terminology that it is not clear to readers or viewers.

From a historical point of view, the significance of the pandemic in our opinion should be assessed as a unique experience, thanks to which people got the opportunity to re-evaluate approaches to the digital transformation of society, rethink its economic, socio-political, ecological fields and outline the main conclusions about the priorities for the further development of humanity.

For Azerbaijan as well as other countries, it is necessary to develop popular science journalism. Such journalism should research on how to balance the information flow during such a hard times as a pandemic. It is necessary to conduct an objective assessment of media work, effectiveness of healthcare management, identify its weak sides and develop new strategies. The organisation of the healthcare system should ensure its preparedness for extreme situations such as pandemic.

We hope people will not face such pandemics in the future but we – the world community must be prepared for that and do not let panic destroy our lives.

Author details

Vugar Mammadov[1*] and Lala Jafarova[2]

1 Azerbaijan Medical University, Law Faculty, Baku State University, Baku, Azerbaijan

2 ANAS, Institute on Law and Human Rights, European Association of Health Law, Baku, Azerbaijan

*Address all correspondence to: vumammadov@yahoo.com

References

[1] Asian Scientist Magazine. Chinese Scientists Sequence Genome Of COVID-19. [Internet]. Feb. 25 2020. Available from: https://www.asianscientist.com/2020/02/topnews/china-coronavirus-covid-19-study/ [Accessed: 2021 Mar 01].

[2] Institut Pasteur. Whole genome of novel coronavirus, 2019-nCoV, sequenced. [Internet] ScienceDaily. 2020. Available from: www.sciencedaily.com/releases/2020/01/200131114748.htm [Accessed: 2021 Mar 01].

[3] Guglielmi G. Rapid coronavirus tests: a guide for the perplexed [Internet]. Nature. 2021. Available from: doi: https://doi.org/10.1038/d41586-021-00332-4 [Accessed: 2021 Mar 01].

[4] The different types of COVID-19 vaccines. [Internet] WHO. 2021. Available from: https://www.who.int/news-room/feature-stories/detail/the-race-for-a-covid-19-vaccine-explained [Accessed: 2021 Mar 01].

[5] Pfizer-BioNTech COVID-19 Vaccine Questions [Internet] CDC. Available from: https://www.cdc.gov/vaccines/covid-19/info-by-product/pfizer/pfizer-bioNTech-faqs.html [Accessed: 2021 Mar 02].

[6] Moderna COVID-19 Vaccine Questions [Internet] CDC. Available from: https://www.cdc.gov/vaccines/covid-19/info-by-product/moderna/moderna-faqs.html [Accessed: 2021 Mar 02].

[7] FDA Issues Emergency Use Authorization for Third COVID-19 Vaccine [Internet] FDA. Available from: https://www.fda.gov/news-events/press-announcements/fda-issues-emergency-use-authorization-third-covid-19-vaccine [Accessed: 2021 Mar 02].

[8] Smith T. Companies working on COVID-19 also work on ... [Internet] Biotech-careers.org. 06 Apr 2020. Available from: https://biotech-careers.org/articles/companies-working-covid-19-also-work [Accessed: 2021 Mar 01].

[9] WHO. Influenza (Seasonal). [Online]. Available from: https://www.who.int/news-room/fact-sheets/detail/influenza-(seasonal) [Accessed: 2021 Feb 13].

[10] Karáth K. Covid-19: How does Belarus have one of the lowest death rates in Europe? BMJ. 2020;370:m3543.

[11] Pavlova V. The man turns yellow completely due to a rare reaction to the coronavirus. [Internet]. Lenta.ru. 2021 Available from: https://lenta.ru/news/2021/02/07/yellow/ [Accessed: 2021 Feb 13]. In Russian.

[12] Ershad A. Did these Chinese doctors' skin turn black after getting Covid-19? There's more to this story... [Internet]. The Observers - France 24. 2020. Available from: https://observers.france24.com/en/20200424-chinese-doctors-skin-black-covid-19 [Accessed: 2021 Feb 13].

[13] hype [Internet]. Cambridge.org. Available from: https://dictionary.cambridge.org/dictionary/english/hype [Accessed: 2021 Feb 13].

[14] Otorbaev D. Valdai Club [Internet]. Valdaiclub.com. Available from: https://valdaiclub.com/a/highlights/after-the-pandemic-the-world-will-never-be/ [Accessed: 2021 Feb 14].

[15] De Caro W. Infodemia and COVID-19: a text mining analysis. Eur J Public Health [Internet]. 2020;30(Supplement_5). Available from: https://academic.oup.com/

eurpub/article/30/Supplement_5/ckaa165.065/5914289 [Accessed: 2021 Feb 14].

[16] TASS. People in Baku and other cities of Azerbaijan will spend the weekend in complete isolation. [Internet]. TASS. 2020. Available from: https://tass.ru/obschestvo/8663927 [Accessed: 2021 Feb 14].

[17] BBC News. Coronavirus: Supermarkets ask shoppers to be "considerate" and stop stockpiling. BBC [Internet]. 2020. Available from: https://www.bbc.com/news/business-51883440 [Accessed: 2021 Feb 14].

[18] Gazeta.ru. Laughter versus Panic: Coronavirus memes. Internet. 2020. Accessed from: https://www.gazeta.ru/tech/2020/03/22/13014397/coronamemes.shtml. [Accessed: 2021 Feb 14]. In Russian.

[19] Cloudflare.com. What Is a Bot? | Bot Definition. [Internet]. Available from: https://www.cloudflare.com/learning/bots/what-is-a-bot/ [Accessed: 2021 Feb 16].

[20] Ministry of health and UNDP launch Coronavirus self-checker bot in Azerbaijan [Internet]. UNDP. 2020. Available from: https://www.az.undp.org/content/azerbaijan/en/home/presscenter/pressreleases/2018/UNDP-AZE-Self-Checker-Bot-launched.html [Accessed: 2021 Feb 16].

[21] Novoprudskiy S. Infodemia: how it works? Gazeta.ru. 2020. Internet]. Available from: https://www.gazeta.ru/comments/column/novoprudsky/13404962.shtml. [Accessed: 2021 Feb 14].

[22] Pestova M.E., Safonov E.A. Pandemic of a new decade: coverage of coronavirus in the media [Internet]. Media environment; 2020. Available from: http://dx.doi.org/10.24411/2070-0717-2020-10136. [Accessed: 2021 Feb 14]. In Russian.

[23] Mammadov V. Doctor's responsibility [Internet]. Anl.az. Available from: http://anl.az/down/meqale/azerbaycan/2010/may/121298.htm [Accessed: 2021 Feb 14]. In Azerbaijani.

[24] Google.com. coronavirus - Google Search [Internet]. Available from: https://www.google.com/search?q=coronavirus&oq=coronavirus&aqs=chrome..69i57j69i59l4j69i60l3.5187j0j7&sourceid=chrome&ie=UTF-8 [Accessed: 2021 Feb 15].

[25] Muratova N., Toshpulatova N., Alimova G. Fake News Disinformation in the media. [Internet] Uzbekistan, Tashkent: UNESCO, Great Britain Embassy to Tashkent, University of Journalism and Mass Communications of Uzbekistan; 2020. Available from: https://ru.unesco.org/sites/default/files/fake_news_rus_0.pdf [Accessed: 2021 Feb 13].

[26] Deutsche Welle. Hydroxychloroquine: Using anti-malaria drug is a risky business [Internet]. Available from: https://www.dw.com/en/chloroquine-is-ineffective-and-dangerous/a-53188219 [Accessed: 2021 Feb 10].

[27] FDA reports of deaths and injuries from use of antimalarial hydroxychloroquine in COVID-19 patients [Internet]. Dicardiology.com. 2020. Available from: https://www.dicardiology.com/article/fda-reports-deaths-and-injuries-use-antimalarial-hydroxychloroquine-covid-19-patients [Accessed: 2021 Feb 10].

[28] Reuters. Malaria drug touted by Trump fails to prevent COVID-19 in high profile study. [Internet]. 2020 Jun 4. Available from: https://www.reuters.com/article/health-coronavirus-hydroxychloroquine-idINKBN23B069 [Accessed: 2021 Feb 10].

[29] BBC. [Anatomy of "covid dissidence". Why is it so easy to believe in a conspiracy amid a pandemic?] [Internet]. 2020. Available from: https://www.bbc.com/russian/features-55438177 [Accessed: 2021 Feb 11] in Russian.

[30] Satariano A, Alba D. Burning cell towers, out of baseless fear they spread the virus. The New York times [Internet]. 2020. Available from: https://www.nytimes.com/2020/04/10/technology/coronavirus-5g-uk.html [Accessed: 2021 Feb 10].

[31] Twitter Help Center. COVID-19 misleading information policy [Internet]. 2021. Available from: https://help.twitter.com/en/rules-and-policies/medical-misinformation-policy [Accessed: 2021 Feb 10].

[32] Coronavirus disease (COVID-19) advice for the public: Mythbusters [Internet] WHO. Available from: https://www.who.int/emergencies/diseases/novel-coronavirus-2019/advice-for-public/myth-busters [Accessed: 2021 Mar 01].

[33] Fighting disinformation [Internet]. European Commission. Available from: https://ec.europa.eu/info/live-work-travel-eu/coronavirus-response/fighting-disinformation_en#separating-facts-from-fiction-on-vaccines [Accessed: 2021 Mar 02].

[34] #ThinkBeforeSharing - Stop the spread of conspiracy theories [Internet]. UNESCO. Available from: https://en.unesco.org/themes/gced/thinkbeforesharing [Accessed: 2021 Mar 02].

[35] Deutsche Welle. Fact check: Are COVID-19 vaccines causing deaths? [Internet]. 2021. Available from: https://www.dw.com/en/fact-check-are-covid-19-vaccines-causing-deaths/a-56458746 [Accessed: 2021 Feb 15].

[36] Trend News Agency. Azerbaijan joins COVAX with $ 21 million contribution. 2020. Available from: https://az.trend.az/azerbaijan/politics/3356794.html [Accessed: 2021 Feb 16].

[37] WHO. COVAX [Internet]. Available from: https://www.who.int/initiatives/act-accelerator/covax [Accessed: 2021 Feb 16].

[38] Official web-site of President of Azerbaijan Republic - NEWS » Events. President of the Republic of Azerbaijan, chairman of the Non-Aligned Movement Ilham Aliyev addressed the Special Session of the United Nations General Assembly in Response to the Coronavirus Disease (COVID-19) Pandemic in a video format. 2020. [Internet]. Available from: https://en.president.az/articles/48460 [Accessed: 2021 Feb 16].

[39] APA. Delivery of vaccines to Azerbaijan under COVAX program expected in April. 2021. [Internet]. Available from: https://apa.az/az/sosial_xeberler/COVAX-proqrami-crcivsind-Azrbaycana-peyvndin-aprel-ayinda-gtirilmsi-gozlnilir-626068 [Accessed: 2021 Feb 16].

[40] AZERNEWS. Azerbaijan to start vaccination against COVID-19 on January 18 [Internet]. 2021. Available from: https://www.azernews.az/healthcare/175097.html [Accessed: 2021 Feb 16].

[41] The State Agency on Mandatory Health Insurance, "COVID-19 vaccination appointment". [Internet]. 2021. Available from: https://randevu.its.gov.az/ [Accessed: 2021 Feb 16]. In Azerbaijani.

[42] 1News.az. "Helicopters will spray Baku": Operational headquarters denied yet another fake - AUDIO [Internet].2020.

Available from: https://1news.az/news/20200312050634765-Vertolety-budut-opryskivat-Baku-Operativnyi-shtab-oproverg-ocherednoi-feik-AUDIO [Accessed: 2021 Feb 16]. In Russian.

[43] Azerbaijan24. The person who spread rumours about the mass infection among children on Whatsapp was a doctor - VIDEO. [Internet]. 2021. Available from: https://www.azerbaycan24.com/votsapda-usaqlarin-kutlevi-yoluxmasi-ile-bagli-sesi-yayan-hekim-imis-video/ [Accessed: 2021 Feb 16]. In Azerbaijani.

[44] Qafqazinfo. Person who distributed the audio about the coronavirus was the doctor... [Internet]. 2020. Available from: https://qafqazinfo.az/news/detail/koronavirusla-bagli-sesyazisini-yayan-hekim-imis-278657 [Accessed: 2021 Feb 16]. In Azerbaijani.

[45] 1News.az. In Azerbaijan, the spread of false rumors in connection with the coronavirus will be prosecuted [Internet]. 2020. Available from: https://1news.az/news/20200312083706713-V-Azerbaidzhane-rasprostranitelei-lozhnykh-slukhov-v-svyazi-s-koronavirusom-budut-privlekat-k-otvetstvennosti [Accessed: 2021 Feb 16]. In Russian.

[46] Deutsche Welle. WhatsApp restricts spread of coronavirus misinformation [Internet]. Available from: https://www.dw.com/en/whatsapp-restricts-spread-of-coronavirus-misinformation/a-53046901 [Accessed: 2021 Feb 16].

[47] Ria.ru. A subsidiary of Roskosmos started production of ventilators. [Internet]. 2020. Available from: https://ria.ru/20200416/1570133831.html [Accessed: 2021 Feb 15]. In Russian.

[48] Frost C. 5G is being used to perform remote surgery from thousands of miles away, and it could transform the healthcare industry. Business Insider [Internet]. 2019. Available from: https://www.businessinsider.com/5g-surgery-could-transform-healthcare-industry-2019-8 [Accessed: 2021 Feb 16].

[49] Gayle D. Thousands march in London in fourth anti-lockdown protest. The Guardian [Internet]. 2020. Available from: http://www.theguardian.com/world/2020/oct/24/london-braces-for-fourth-protest-against-covid-19-restrictions [Accessed: 2021 Feb 13].

[50] AFP. Berlin police stop mass 'anti-corona' protest. Arab news [Internet]. 2020 Aug 29; Available from: https://www.arabnews.com/node/1726486/world [Accessed: 2021 Feb 13].

[51] Coronavirus: Hundreds gather in Madrid for anti-mask protest. BBC [Internet]. 2020. Available from: https://www.bbc.com/news/av/world-europe-53802226 [Accessed: 2021 Feb 13].

[52] Didili Z. Mass anti-lockdown protest in Amsterdam [Internet]. Neweurope.eu. 2021. Available from: https://www.neweurope.eu/article/mass-anti-lockdown-protest-in-amsterdam/ [Accessed: 2021 Feb 13].

[53] Mammadov, V. Political, scientific and management aspects of coronavirus pandemics: considerations from Azerbaijan perspective. Medicine and Law. 2020;39(2): 115-128.

[54] Worldometers.info. Coronavirus update (live): 110,070,257 cases and 2,430,794 deaths from COVID-19 virus pandemic - worldometer [Internet]. 2021. Available from: https://www.worldometers.info/coronavirus/ [Accessed: 2021 Feb 17].

[55] APA news. Azərbaycanda koronavirus təhlükəsi ilə əlaqədar

qərargah yaradılıb [Internet]. 2020. Available from: https://apa.az/az/sosial_xeberler/Azrbaycanda-koronavirus-thluksi-il-laqdar-qrargah-yaradilib-574026 [Accessed: 2021 Feb 10].

[56] AzTv. First coronavirus case registered in Azerbaijan [Internet]. 2020. Available from: http://www.aztv.az/az/news/5509/azerbaycanda-koronavirusa-ilk-yoluxma-fakti-qeyde-alindi [Accessed: 2021 Feb 10].

[57] Azerbaijan State News Agency. Azerbaijan reports first coronavirus death [Internet] 2020. Available from: https://azertag.az/en/xeber/Azerbaijan_reports_first_coronavirus_death-1439123 [Accessed: 2021 Feb 10].

[58] APA news. Last year, the state budget spent about 2 billion manat on the fight against coronavirus in Azerbaijan. [Internet] 2020. Available from: https://apa.az/az/sosial_xeberler/Azrbaycanda-otn-il-dovlt-budcsindn-koronavirusla-mubarizy-2-milyard-manata-yaxin-vsait-srf-olunub-628680 [Accessed: 2021 Feb 12].

[59] AZERTAC. Aslanov A., Great challenge and leader's rescue mission. [Internet]. Available from: https://azertag.az/en/xeber/Great_challenge_and_leaders_rescue_mission-1478567 [Accessed: 2021 Feb 12].

[60] Banker. STS: due to pandemic 115 million manats were discounted to the entrepreneurs. [Internet]. 2021. Available from: https://banker.az/dvx-pandemiyaya-gor%c9%99-115-mln-manat-guz%c9%99st-olunub/ [Accessed: 2021 Feb 13]. In Azerbaijani.

[61] Anadoly Agency. Rahimov R., Aydin, H.K. Azerbaijan to impose curfew amid coronavirus outbreak. Stay-home order to enter into force across country as of March 31. [Internet]. 2020. Available from: https://www.aa.com.tr/en/latest-on-coronavirus-outbreak/azerbaijan-to-impose-curfew-amid-coronavirus-outbreak/1785680# [Accessed: 2021 Feb 12].

[62] Eurasianet.org. Kucera J, Kumenov A. Azerbaijanis to need police permission to leave home [Internet].2020. Available from: https://eurasianet.org/azerbaijanis-to-need-police-permission-to-leave-home [Accessed: 12 Feb 2021]

[63] Azernews.az. Eight beaches fit for use in Baku amid COVID-19 [VIDEO] [Internet]. 2020. Available from: https://www.azernews.az/nation/167680.html [Accessed: 12 Feb 2021]

[64] APA news. Mehdiyev U.: "From August 5, website 'cimerlik.az' to start to operate" [Internet]. 2020. Available from: https://apa.az/en/social-news/Ulvi-Mehdiyev:-%22From-August-5-website-%22cimerlik.az%22-to-start-to-operate%22-327144 [Accessed: 2021 Feb 12].

[65] Gehrke L. Saudi Arabia imposes ban on international pilgrims for hajj [Internet]. POLITICO. 2020. Available from: https://www.politico.eu/article/saudi-arabia-imposes-ban-on-international-pilgrims-for-hajj/ [Accessed: 2021 Feb 12]

[66] Conger K, Healy J, Tompkins L. Churches were eager to reopen. Now they are confronting Coronavirus cases. The New York Times [Internet]. 2020. Available from: https://www.nytimes.com/2020/07/08/us/coronavirus-churches-outbreaks.html [Accessed: 2021 Feb 12].

[67] Deutsche Welle (www. dw.com). German church at the center of over 100 coronavirus cases [Internet]. 2020. Available from: https://www.dw.com/en/german-church-at-the-center-of-over-100-coronavirus-cases/a-53804687 [Accessed: 2021 Feb 12].

[68] James A, Eagle L, Phillips C, et al. High COVID-19 Attack Rate Among Attendees at Events at a Church — Arkansas, March 2020. MMWR Morb Mortal Wkly Rep 2020;69:632-635. DOI: http://dx.doi.org/10.15585/mmwr.mm6920e2external icon

[69] The Second Karabakh War [Internet]. Virtualkarabakh.az. Available from: https://www.virtualkarabakh.az/en/post-item/52/2871/ikinci-qarabag-muharibesi.html [Accessed: 2021 Feb 14].

[70] APA news. Azerbaijan extends special quarantine regime until 1 April. [Internet]. 2020. Available from: https://apa.az/en/social-news/Azerbaijan-extends-special-quarantine-regime-until-1-April-340340 [Accessed: 2021 Feb 11].

[71] APA news. A group of Turkish and Russian experts on COVID-19 arrived in Azerbaijan - VIDEO. [Internet]. 2020. Available from: https://apa.az/en/social-news/A-group-of-Turkish-and-Russian-experts-on-COVID-19-arrived-in-Azerbaijan-colorredVIDEOcolor-325283 [Accessed: 2021 Feb 12].

[72] Global times. Chinese expert team helps Azerbaijan fight COVID-19: FM. [Internet]. 2020. Available from: https://www.globaltimes.cn/content/1197430.shtml [Accessed: 2021 Feb 12].

[73] Caspian news. Italian Specialists Join Azerbaijani Experts On Covid-19 Frontline. [Internet]. 2020. Available from: https://caspiannews.com/news-detail/italian-specialists-join-azerbaijani-experts-on-covid-19-frontline-2020-8-4-37/ [Accessed: 2021 Feb 12].

[74] AZERTAC. Another team of Cuban doctors on COVID-19 arrive in Azerbaijan. [Internet]. 2020. Available from: https://azertag.az/en/xeber/Another_team_of_Cuban_doctors_on_COVID_19_arrive_in_Azerbaijan-1635853 [Accessed: 2021 Feb 12].

[75] Mehriban Aliyeva First Lady of Azerbaijan official website. First modular hospital complex is inaugurated in Baku. [Internet]. Available from: https://mehriban-aliyeva.az/en/news/node/848336 [Accessed: 2021 Feb 12].

[76] APA news. Azerbaijan starts production of disinfection tunnels - PHOTOSESSION. [Internet]. Available from: https://apa.az/en/social-news/Azerbaijan-starts-production-of-disinfection-tunnels-colorredPHOTOSESSIONcolor-323602 [Accessed: 2021Feb 12]

[77] The State Agency on mandatory Health Insurance [Internet]. Available from: https://its.gov.az/ [Accessed: 2021 Feb 11].

[78] WHO. WHO Director-General's opening remarks at the media briefing on COVID-19 - 11 March 2020 [Internet]. Available from: https://www.who.int/director-general/speeches/detail/who-director-general-s-opening-remarks-at-the-media-briefing-on-covid-19---11-march-2020 [Accessed: 2021 Feb 10].

[79] "Closing borders does not prevent the virus" — European Commissioner [Internet]. Qafqazinfo.az. 2021. Available from: https://qafqazinfo.az/news/detail/serhedlerin-baglanmasi-virusun-qarsisini-almir-avropa-komissari-314773 [Accessed: 2021 Feb 15]. In Azerbaijani.

[80] Bloomberg. Covid Lockdowns Are Spreading a Year After China Shocked World [Internet]. Available from: https://www.bloomberg.com/news/articles/2021-01-17/from-the-bubonic-plague-to-2021-why-lockdowns-look-set-to-stay [Accessed: 2021 Feb 15].